Paul L. Marino, MD, PhD, FCCM

Clinical Associate Professor
Weill Cornell Medical College
New York, New York

With contributions from:
Samuel M. Galvagno Jr., DO, PhD, MS, FCCM

Associate Professor
Division Chief, Critical Care Medicine
Associate Medical Director, Surgical Intensive Care Unit
Shock Trauma Center
Program in Trauma and Division of Critical Care Medicine
Department of Anesthesiology
The University of Maryland School of Medicine
Baltimore, Maryland

Lt. Col, USAFR, MC, SFS
Director of Critical Care Air Transport Team (CCATT) Operations
943rd Aerospace Medicine Squadron
943rd Rescue Group Davis-Monthan Air Force Base, Arizona

Illustrations by Patricia Gast

MARINO'S

The *Little*

ICU

Book

Second Edition

Wolters Kluwer

Philadelphia • Baltimore • New York • London
Buenos Aires • Hong Kong • Sydney • Tokyo

Acquisitions Editor: Keith Donnellan
Product Development Editor: Kate Heaney
Production Project Manager: Bridgett Dougherty
Manufacturing Coordinator: Beth Welsh
Marketing Manager: Dan Dressler
Design Coordinator: Teresa Mallon
Production Service: Aptara, Inc.

9 8 7 6 5 4 3 2 1

Printed in China

Library of Congress Cataloging-in-Publication Data

Names: Marino, Paul L., author. | Galvagno, Samuel M., Jr., author. |
  Supplement to (work): Marino, Paul L. Marino's the ICU book. 4e.
Title: Marino's the little ICU book / Paul L. Marino ; with contributions
  from Samuel M. Galvagno, Jr. ; illustrations by Patricia Gast.
Other titles: Little ICU book of facts and formulas | Marino's the little
  intensive care unit book | Little ICU book
Description: 2nd edition. | Philadelphia : Wolters Kluwer, [2017] | Preceded
  by The little ICU book of facts and formulas / Paul L. Marino ; with
  contributions from Kenneth M. Sutin. c2008. | Includes bibliographical
  references and index.
Identifiers: LCCN 2016047340 | ISBN 9781451194586 (alk. paper)
Subjects: | MESH: Critical Care | Intensive Care Units | Handbooks
Classification: LCC RC86.7 | NLM WX 39 | DDC 616/.028–dc23
LC record available at https://lccn.loc.gov/2016047340

To Daniel Joseph Marino,
my 29 year-old son,
who is well into manhood,
but didn't forget
to bring the boy along.

Seek simplicity, and distrust it.

ALFRED NORTH WHITEHEAD
The Concept of Nature, 1919

Acknowledgements

This book owes its look and texture to the considerable skills of Patricia Gast, who is responsible for all the illustrations, tables, and page layouts in the book. This is our fourth book together, and I continue to marvel at her talent and work ethic.

Also to Keith Donnellan, my editor at Wolters Kluwer, who has that rare capacity to understand the exigencies of an author and his work. He is a true professional, and it shows. And finally, to Kate Heaney, project development editor, for her firm footing in guiding the gestation of this book.

The second edition of *The Little ICU Book* retains the intent of the first edition; i.e., to create a distilled version of the parent textbook, *The ICU Book,* that presents the essentials of critical care practice in a succinct and easily retrievable format. The organization and chapter titles in the "little book" mirror those in the "big book", but all the chapters have been rewritten and updated, with heavy emphasis on the recommendations in evidence-based clinical practice guidelines. This edition also bears the fruits of a collaboration with Sam Galvagno, DO, PhD, who lent his wisdom and encyclopedic knowledge to several chapters in the text.

The Little ICU Book may be short in stature, but it is a densely packed, generic resource for the care of critically ill adults in any ICU.

Table of Contents

Chapter 1

Central Venous Access

Vascular access in critically ill patients often involves the insertion of long, flexible catheters into large veins entering the thorax or abdomen. This type of *central venous access* is the focus of the current chapter.

I. INFECTION CONTROL

The infection control measures recommended for central venous cannulation are shown in Table 1.1 (1,2). When used together (as a "bundle"), these five measures have been effective in reducing the incidence of catheter-related bloodstream infections (3). The following is a brief description of these preventive measures.

A. Skin Antisepsis

1. Handwashing is recommended before and after palpating catheter insertion sites, and before and after glove use (1). Alcohol-based hand rubs are preferred if available (1,4); otherwise, handwashing with soap (plain or antimicrobial soap) and water is acceptable (4).

2. The skin around the catheter insertion site should be decontaminated just prior to cannulation, and the preferred antiseptic agent is chlorhexidine (1).

   a. The advantage of chlorhexidine is its prolonged antimicrobial activity, which lasts for at least 6 hours after a single application.

   b. Antimicrobial activity is maximized if chlorhexidine

1

it is allowed to air-dry on the skin for at least two minutes (1).

Table 1.1	The Central Line Bundle
Components	**Recommendations**
Hand Hygiene	Use an alcohol-based handrub or a soap and water handwash before and after inserting or manipulating catheters.
Barrier Precautions	Use maximal barrier precautions, including cap, mask, sterile gloves, sterile gown, and sterile full body drape, for catheter insertion or guidewire exchange.
Skin Antisepsis	Apply a chlorhexidine-based solution to the catheter insertion site and allow 2 minutes to air-dry.
Cannulation Site	When possible, avoid femoral vein cannulation.
Catheter Removal	Remove catheter promptly when it is no longer needed.

From the Institute for Healthcare Improvement (2).

B. Sterile Barriers

All central venous (and arterial) cannulation procedures should be performed using full sterile barrier precautions, which includes caps, masks, sterile gloves, sterile gowns, and a sterile drape from head to foot (1).

C. Site Selection

According to published guidelines (1) femoral vein cannulation should be avoided to reduce the risk of catheter-associated septicemia. However, clinical studies indicate that the incidence of septicemia from femoral vein catheters (2–3 infections per 1000 catheter days) is no different than the incidence of septicemia from subclavian or internal jugular vein catheters (5,6).

II. CATHETERS

A. Catheter Size

1. The size of vascular catheters is expressed in terms of their outside diameter. Size can be expressed in a metric-based *French* size or a wire-based *gauge* size.

   a. The French size is a series of whole numbers that increases in increments of 0.33 millimeters (e.g., 1 French = 0.33 mm, 2 French = 0.66 mm).

   b. The gauge size (originally developed for solid wires) has no definable relationship to other units of measurement, and requires a table of reference values (like the one in Appendix 3).

B. Central Venous Catheters

1. The term *central venous catheter* (CVC) refers to catheters inserted into the internal jugular, subclavian, or femoral veins and advanced into one of the vena cavae.

2. Modern CVCs have multiple infusion channels, like the popular triple-lumen catheter shown in Figure 1.1. This catheter has an outside diameter of 2.3 mm (French size 7), and is available in lengths of 16 cm (6 in), 20 cm (8 in), and 30 cm (12 in). (Dimensions may vary by manufacturer.)

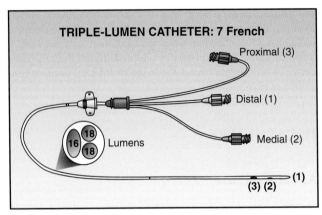

FIGURE 1.1 Triple-lumen central venous catheter, showing the gauge size of each lumen and the position of the outflow ports at the distal end of the catheter.

C. Antimicrobial Coating

1. CVCs are available with two types of antimicrobial coating: (*a*) chlorhexidine and silver sulfadiazine (available from Arrow International), and (*b*) minocylcine and rifampin (available from Cook Critical Care). Each of these coatings can reduce the risk of catheter-related bloodstream infections (7).

2. According to published guidelines (1), antimicrobial-coated catheters should be considered if the expected duration of catheterization is >5 days *and* if the incidence of catheter-related infections in an ICU is unacceptably high.

D. Peripherally-Inserted Central Catheters

1. The term *peripherally-inserted central catheter* (PICC) refers to long catheters that are inserted into the basilic or cephalic vein in the arm (just above the antecubital fossa) and advanced into the superior vena cava.

2. PICCs are available with multiple infusion channels, like CVCs, but they are narrower than CVCs (typically 5 French or 1.65 mm in diameter), and are considerably longer than CVCs. PICCS are available in lengths of 50 cm (19.5 in) and 70 cm (27.5 in).

3. As a result of the smaller diameter and longer length of PICCs, flow through PICCs is considerably slower than flow through CVCs. (See Appendix 3 for charts showing the flow rates through PICCs and CVCs.)

III. CANNULATION SITES

The following is a brief description of central venous cannulation at four different access sites: i.e., the internal jugular vein, the subclavian vein, the femoral vein, and the veins emerging from the antecubital fossa.

A. Internal Jugular Vein

1. Anatomy

   a. The internal jugular vein (IJV) is located under the sternocleidomastoid muscle (see Figure 1.2), and runs obliquely down the neck along a line drawn from the pinna of the ear to the sternoclavicular joint. In the lower neck region, the vein is often located just anterior and lateral to the carotid artery, but anatomic relationships can vary (16).

   b. At the base of the neck, the IJV joins the subclavian vein to form the innominate vein, and the convergence of the right and left innominate veins forms the superior vena cava.

   c. The right side of the neck is preferred for cannulation of the IJV because the vessels run a straight course to the right atrium. The distance from cannulation site

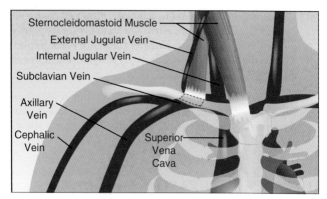

FIGURE 1.2 The large veins entering the thorax.

to the right atrium is about 15 cm, so the shortest CVCs (~15 cm) should be used for right-sided cannulations (to avoid advancing the catheter tip into the right atrium).

2. **Positioning**

   a. A head-down body tilt to 15° below horizontal (Trendelenburg position) results in a 20–25% increase in the diameter of the IJV (8). Further increases in the degree of body tilt has no incremental effect (8).

   b. A head-down body tilt of 15° can be used to facilitate IJV cannulation, particularly in hypovolemic patients, but is not necessary in patients with venous congestion, and is not advised in patients with increased intracranial pressure.

   c. The head should be turned slightly in the opposite direction to straighten the course of the vein, but turning the head beyond 30° from midline is counterproductive because it stretches the vein and reduces its diameter (16).

3. Locating the Vein

a. Ultrasound imaging has been recommended as a standard practice for locating and cannulating the IJV (9). Ultrasound guidance is associated with a higher success rate, fewer cannulation attempts, a shorter time to cannulation, and a reduced risk of carotid artery puncture (9-11).

b. To obtain a cross-sectional image of the IJV and carotid artery, place the ultrasound probe across the triangle created by the two heads of the sternocleidomastoid muscle (see Figure 1.2). This produces images like the ones shown in Figure 1.3. The image on the left shows the IJV situated anterior and lateral to the carotid artery. The image on the right shows the IJV collapsing when downward pressure is applied to the overlying skin (a simple maneuver for distinguishing between arteries and veins).

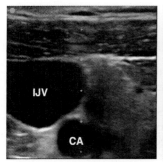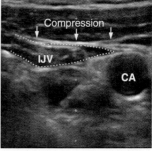

FIGURE 1.3 Ultrasound images of the internal jugular vein (IJV) and carotid artery (CA) on the right side of the neck. The image on the right shows collapse of the vein when pressure is applied to the overlying skin. The green dots mark the lateral side of each image. (Images courtesy of Cynthia Sullivan, RN and Shaun Newvine, RN)

4. Complications

a. Carotid artery puncture is the most feared complication of IJV cannulation. The reported incidence is 0.5–11% when surface landmarks are used (10-12), and 1% when ultrasound imaging is employed (10).

b. Pneumothorax is not expected at the IJV cannulation site (because it is located in the neck), however this complication is reported in 1.3% of IJV cannulations when surface landmarks are used to guide cannulation (10).

B. The Subclavian Vein

1. Anatomy

a. The subclavian vein (SCV) is a continuation of the axillary vein as it passes over the first rib (see Figure 1.2). It runs most of its course along the underside of the clavicle and continues to the thoracic inlet, where it joins the internal jugular vein to form the innominate vein.

b. The underside of the SCV sits on the anterior scalene muscle along with the phrenic nerve, which comes in contact with the vein along its posteroinferior side. On the underside of the anterior scalene muscle is the subclavian artery and brachial plexus.

c. The diameter of the SCV (7–12 mm in the supine position) does not vary with respiration (unlike the IJV), which is attributed to strong fascial attachments that fix the vein to surrounding structures and hold it open (13). This is also the basis for the claim that volume depletion does not collapse the SCV (14), which is unproven.

2. Positioning

a. The head-down body tilt distends the SCV by 8–10% (13), and could facilitate cannulation.

b. Other maneuvers believed to facilitate cannulation, such as arching the shoulders or placing a rolled towel under the shoulder, actually cause a decrease in the cross-sectional area of the SCV (13,15).

3. Locating the Vessel

a. The SCV is difficult to visualize with ultrasound imaging because the overlying clavicle blocks transmission of ultrasound waves. As a result, the use of surface landmarks continues to be the standard method of cannulating the SCV.

b. The SCV can be located by identifying the clavicular head of the sterno-cleidomastoid muscle (see Figure 1.2): the vein lies just underneath the clavicle at this point, and can be cannulated from above or below the clavicle. This portion of the clavicle can be marked with a small rectangle, as shown in Figure 1.2, to guide insertion of the probe needle.

4. Complications

a. Complications of SCV cannulation (using the landmark method of location) include puncture of the subclavian artery (≤5%), pneumothorax (≤5%), brachial plexus injury (≤3%), and phrenic nerve injury (≤1.5%) (11,14).

b. Stenosis of the SCV can appear days or months after catheter removal, and has a reported incidence of 15–50% (16). This complication is the principal reason to avoid SCV cannulation in patients who might require hemodialysis access (via an arteriovenous fistula) in the ipsilateral arm (16).

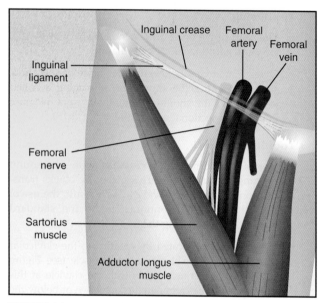

FIGURE 1.4 Anatomy of the femoral triangle.

C. Femoral Vein

1. Anatomy

The femoral vein (FV) is a continuation of the long saphenous vein in the groin, where it is located in the femoral triangle along with the femoral artery and nerve, as shown in Figure 1.4. At the level of the inguinal crease, the vein lies just medial to the artery, and is only a few centimeters from the skin. The FV is easier to cannulate when the leg is placed in abduction.

2. Locating the Vein

The FV is easier to cannulate when the leg is placed in abduction.

a. Locating the FV begins by palpating the femoral artery pulse, which is typically located just below and medial to the midpoint of the inguinal crease.

b. If available, an ultrasound probe should be placed at the point where the femoral artery pulse is palpable to obtain cross-sectional images of the underlying vessels. The vein is then identified by its compressibility, as demonstrated in Figure 1.3.

c. If ultrasound imaging is not available, first palpate the femoral artery pulse, and insert the probe needle (with the bevel at 12 o'clock) 1–2 cm medial to the pulse; the FV should be entered at a depth of 2–4 cm from the skin.

3. Complications

a. The principal complications of FV cannulation are femoral artery puncture, FV thrombosis, and catheter-related septicemia.

b. Catheter-related thrombosis is more common than suspected, but is clinically silent in most cases. In one study of indwelling FV catheters, thrombosis was detected by ultrasound in 10% of patients, but clinically apparent thrombosis occurred in <1% of patients (17).

c. As mentioned earlier (Section I, C), the risk of septicemia from FV cannulation is no different than the risk at other sites of central venous cannulation (5,6).

D. Peripherally-Inserted Central Catheters

1. Peripherally-inserted central catheters (PICCs) are long catheters (50–70 cm) inserted into the basilic or cephalic vein in the arm (see Figure 1.5) and advanced into the superior vena cava. The basilic vein, which runs up the medial aspect of the arm, is preferred for PICC place-

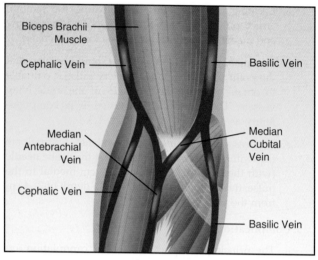

FIGURE 1.5 The major veins in the region of the antecubital fossa of the right arm.

ment because it has a larger diameter than the cephalic vein, and it runs a straighter course up the arm.

2. The benefits of PICCs over CVCs include enhanced patient comfort and mobility, and eliminating certain risks associated with CVC placement (e.g., pneumothorax).

3. The most common complication of PICCs is catheter-induced thrombosis of the axillary and subclavian veins. Occlusive thrombosis with swelling of the upper arm is reported in 2–11% of patients with indwelling PICCs (18,19); the highest incidence occurs in patients with a history of venous thrombosis (18) and in cancer patients (19).

4. Septicemia from PICCs occurs at a rate of one infection per 1000 catheter days (20), which is similar to the rate of infection from CVCs.

IV. IMMEDIATE CONCERNS

A. Venous Air Embolism

Air entry into the central veins is a potentially lethal complication of central venous cannulation (21,22).

1. Pathophysiology

a. When a vascular catheter is advanced into the thorax, the negative intrathoracic pressure generated during spontaneous breathing can draw air into the venous circulation if the catheter hub is open to the atmosphere.

b. Both the volume and rate of air entry determine the consequences of venous air embolism. The consequences can be fatal when air entry reaches 200–300 mL (3–5 mL/kg) over a few seconds (22).

c. The adverse consequences of venous air embolism include acute right heart failure (from an air lock in the right ventricle), leaky-capillary pulmonary edema, and acute embolic stroke (from air bubbles that pass through a patent foramen ovale) (22).

2. Preventive Measures

Positive-pressure ventilation is a deterrent to venous air embolism, and can eliminate the problem if the intrathoracic pressure remains positive throughout the respiratory cycle. In spontaneously breathing patients, head-down body tilt (Trendelenburg position) can reduce the risk of air entry during internal jugular and subclavian vein cannulation. Using appropriate precautions, the risk of symptomatic venous air embolism is <1% (21).

3. Clinical Presentation

a. Venous air embolism can be clinically silent (21).

b. In symptomatic cases, the earliest manifestation is sudden onset of dyspnea, which may be accompanied by a distressing cough.

c. In severe cases, there is rapid progression to hypotension, oliguria, and depressed consciousness (from cardiogenic shock). The mixing of air and blood in the right ventricle can produce a drum-like, *mill wheel murmur* just prior to cardiovascular collapse (22).

4. **Diagnosis**

a. Venous air embolism is usually a clinical diagnosis.

b. If time permits, transthoracic Doppler ultrasound is a sensitive method of detecting air in the heart (22). (Doppler ultrasound converts flow velocities into sounds, and air in the cardiac chambers produces a characteristic high-pitched sound.)

5. **Management**

The management of venous air embolism primarily involves cardiorespiratory support. The following maneuvers deserve mention, although each is without documented benefit (22).

a. If air entrainment is suspected through an indwelling catheter, you can attach a syringe to the hub of the catheter and attempt to aspirate air from the bloodstream.

b. Pure oxygen breathing can reduce the volume of air in the pulmonary circulation promoting the egress of nitrogen from the pulmonary capillaries.

c. Placing the patient in the left lateral decubitus position is a traditional maneuver aimed at relieving an air lock at the outflow of the right ventricle.

d. Chest compressions can help to force air out of the pulmonary outflow tract and into the pulmonary circulation.

B. Pneumothorax

1. Pneumothorax is primarily a concern with subclavian vein catheterization; the reported incidence is ≤5% (11,14).

2. Portable chest x-rays are insensitive for the detection of pleural air, particularly in the supine position, where air collects anterior to the lung (23).

3. Ultrasonography is a much more sensitive method of detecting pleural air when compared with portable chest radiography (24). If immediately available, bedside ultrasonography is the method of choice for the detection of pleural air in ICU patients.

C. Catheter Location

Because malposition of catheters occurs in 5–25% of CVC and PICC insertions (11,20), post-procedural chest x-rays are obtained routinely to evaluate catheter location.

1. Proper Placement

A properly placed CVC or PICC should be in the superior vena cava, with the catheter tip 1–2 cm above the right atrium. The tracheal carina (i.e., the bifurcation of the trachea to form the right and left mainstem bronchi) is located just above the junction between the superior vena cava and the right atrium, which makes it a useful landmark for evaluating catheter tip location (26). The appropriate position of a CVC is shown in Figure 1.6. Note that the tip of the catheter is just above the tracheal carina.

2. Catheter Tip in Right Atrium

A catheter tip that extends below the tracheal carina on a portable chest x-ray is likely to be in the right atrium. This creates a risk of right atrial perforation and cardiac tamponade (27), so retraction of catheters is generally advised when the tip is located below the carina.

However, right atrial placement of CVCs is a common occurrence, with an incidence of 25% in one study (28), while right atrial perforation is a rare complication of CVC placement (27), so the need to reposition catheters advanced into the right atrium is questionable.

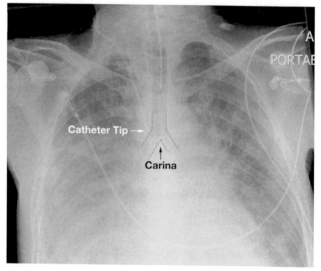

FIGURE 1.6 Portable chest x-ray showing the proper placement of a central venous catheter, with the tip just above the tracheal carina. (Catheter image digitally enhanced.)

REFERENCES

1. O'Grady NP, Alexander M, Burns LA, et al. and the Healthcare Infection Control Practices Advisory Committee (HICPAC). Guidelines for the Prevention of Intravascular Catheter-related Infections. Clin Infect Dis 2011; 52:e1–e32.

2. Institute for Healthcare Improvement. Implement the central line bundle. Available at www.ihi.org/resources/Pages/Changes/

ImplementtheCentralLineBundle.aspx (Accessed July 11, 2014).

3. Furuya EY, Dick A, Perencevich EN, et al. Central line bundle implementation in U.S. intensive care units and impact on bloodstream infection. PLoS ONE 2011; 6(1):e15452. (Open access journal available at www.plosone.org (Accessed November 5, 2011).)

4. Tschudin-Sutter S, Pargger H, and Widmer AF. Hand hygiene in the intensive care unit. Crit Care Med 2010; 38(Suppl):S299–S305.

5. Deshpande K, Hatem C, Ulrich H, et al. The incidence of infectious complications of central venous catheters at the subclavian, internal jugular, and femoral sites in an intensive care unit population. Crit Care Med 2005; 33:13–20.

6. Parienti J-J, Thirion M, Megarbane B, et al. Femoral vs jugular venous catheterization and risk of nosocomial events in adults requiring acute renal replacement therapy. JAMA 2008; 299:2413–2422.

7. Casey AL, Mermel LA, Nightingale P, Elliott TSJ. Antimicrobial central venous catheters in adults: a systematic review and meta-analysis. Lancet Infect Dis 2008; 8:763–776.

8. Clenaghan S, McLaughlin RE, Martyn C, et al. Relationship between Trendelenburg tilt and internal jugular vein diameter. Emerg Med J 2005; 22:867–868.

9. Feller-Kopman D. Ultrasound-guided internal jugular access. Chest 2007; 132:302–309.

10. Hayashi H, Amano M. Does ultrasound imaging before puncture facilitate internal jugular vein cannulation? Prospective, randomized comparison with landmark-guided puncture in ventilated patients. J Cardiothorac Vasc Anesth 2002; 16:572–575.

11. Ruesch S, Walder B, Tramer M. Complications of central venous catheters: internal jugular versus subclavian access – A systematic review. Crit Care Med 2002; 30:454–460.

12. Reuber M, Dunkley LA, Turton EP, et al. Stroke after internal jugular venous cannulation. Acta Neurol Scand 2002; 105:235–239.

13. Fortune JB, Feustel. Effect of patient position on size and location of the subclavian vein for percutaneous puncture. Arch Surg 2003; 138:996–1000.

14. Fragou M, Gravvanis A, Dimitriou V, et al. Real-time ultrasound-guided subclavian vein cannulation versus the landmark

method in critical care patients: A prospective randomized study. Crit Care Med 2011; 39:1607–1612.

15. Rodriguez CJ, Bolanowski A, Patel K, et al. Classic positioning decreases cross-sectional area of the subclavian vein. Am J Surg 2006; 192:135–137.

16. Hernandez D, Diaz F, Rufino M, et al. Subclavian vascular access stenosis in dialysis patients: Natural history and risk factors. J Am Soc Nephrol 1998; 9:1507–1510.

17. Parienti J-J, Thirion M, Megarbane B, et al. Femoral vs jugular venous catheterization and risk of nosocomial events in adults requiring acute renal replacement therapy. JAMA 2008; 299:2413–2422.

18. Evans RS, Sharp JH, Linford LH, et al. Risk of symptomatic DVT associated with peripherally inserted central catheters. Chest 2010; 138:803–810.

19. Hughes ME. PICC-related thrombosis: pathophysiology, incidence, morbidity, and the effect of ultrasound guided placement technique on occurrence in cancer patients. JAVA 2011; 16:8–18.

20. Ng P, Ault M, Ellrodt AG, Maldonado L. Peripherally inserted central catheters in general medicine. Mayo Clin Proc 1997; 72:225–233.

21. Vesely TM. Air embolism during insertion of central venous catheters. J Vasc Interv Radiol 2001; 12:1291–1295.

22. Mirski MA, Lele AV, Fitzsimmons L, Toung TJK. Diagnosis and treatment of vascular air embolism. Anesthesiology 2007; 106:164–177.

23. Tocino IM, Miller MH, Fairfax WR. Distribution of pneumothorax in the supine and semirecumbent critically ill adult. Am J Radiol 1985; 144:901–905.

24. Collin GR, Clarke LE. Delayed pneumothorax: a complication of central venous catheterization. Surg Rounds 1994; 17:589–594.

25. Xirouchaki N, Magkanas E, Vaporidi K, et al. Lung ultrasound in critically ill patients: comparison with bedside chest radiography. Intensive Care Med 2011; 37:1488–1493.

26. Stonelake PA, Bodenham AR. The carina as a radiological landmark for central venous catheter tip position. Br J Anesthesia 2006; 96:335–340.

27. Booth SA, Norton B, Mulvey DA. Central venous catheterization and fatal cardiac tamponade. Br J Anesth 2001; 87:298–302.

28. Vezzani A, Brusasco C, Palermo S, et al. Ultrasound localization of central vein catheter and detection of postprocedural pneumothorax: an alternative to chest radiography. Crit Care Med 2010; 38:533–538.

Chapter 2

The Indwelling Vascular Catheter

This chapter describes the routine care and adverse consequences of indwelling vascular catheters, with emphasis on central venous catheters.

I. ROUTINE CATHETER CARE

The recommendations for routine catheter care are summarized in Table 2.1.

A. Catheter Site Dressing

1. Catheter insertion sites should be covered with a sterile dressing for the life of the catheter. This can be a covering of sterile gauze pads, or an adhesive, transparent plastic membrane (called *occlusive dressings*).

2. The transparent membrane in occlusive dressings is semipermeable, and allows the loss of water vapor, but not liquid secretions, from the underlying skin. This prevents excessive drying of the underlying skin to promote wound healing.

3. Occlusive dressings are favored because the transparent membrane allows daily inspection of the catheter insertion site. Sterile gauze dressings are preferred when the catheter insertion site is difficult to keep dry (1).

4. Sterile gauze dressings and occlusive dressings are roughly equivalent in their ability to limit catheter colonization and infection (1,2). However, occlusive dressings can promote colonization when moisture accumulates under the sealed dressing (2), so occlusive dressings should be changed when fluid accumulates under the transparent membrane.

Table 2.1	Recommendations for Routine Catheter Care
	Recommendations
Sterile Dressings	Adhesive transparent dressings are favored because they allow inspection of the catheter insertion site.
	Sterile gauze dressings are used for skin areas that are difficult to keep dry.
	Adhesive transparent dressings and sterile gauze dressings provide equivalent protection against catheter colonization.
Antimicrobial Gels	Do not apply antimicrobial gels to catheter insertion sites, except for hemodialysis catheters.
Replacing Catheters	Regular replacement of central venous catheters is not recommended.
Flushing Catheters	Avoid using heparin in catheter flush solutions.

From the clinical practice guidelines in Reference 1.

B. Antimicrobial Gels

The application of antimicrobial gels to the catheter insertion site does not reduce the incidence of catheter-related infections (1), with the possible exception of hemodialysis catheters (3). As a result, topical antimicrobial gels are recommended only for hemodialysis catheters (1), and should be applied after each dialysis.

C. Flushing Catheters

1. Vascular catheters are flushed at regular intervals to prevent thrombotic occlusion.

2. The traditional flush solution is heparinized saline (10–1000 units/mL), but avoiding heparin flushes is advised because of the risk of heparin-induced thrombocytopenia (see Chapter 12).

3. Saline alone is as effective as heparinized saline for flushing venous catheters (4), but this is not the case for arterial catheters (5): in the latter case, 1.4% sodium citrate is a suitable alternative for maintaining catheter patency (6).

D. Replacing Catheters

1. Replacing central venous catheters at regular intervals (using either guidewire exchange or a new venipuncture site) does not reduce the incidence of catheter-related infections (7), and can actually promote complications (both mechanical and infectious) (8). As a result, *routine replacement of central venous catheters is not recommended* (1). This also applies to peripherally-inserted central catheters (PICCs), hemodialysis catheters, and pulmonary artery catheters (1).

2. Replacing central venous catheters is not necessary when there is erythema around the catheter insertion site, since erythema alone is not evidence of infection (9).

3. Purulent drainage from the catheter insertion site is an absolute indication for catheter replacement, using a new venipuncture site for the replacement catheter.

II. NONINFECTIOUS COMPLICATIONS

A. Occluded Catheters

Occlusion of central venous catheters can be the result of thrombosis or insoluble precipitates from the infusates. Advancing a guidewire to dislodge an obstructing mass is not advised because of the risk of embolization. Instead, chemical dissolution of the obstructing mass (described next) is the preferred intervention.

1. **Thrombotic Occlusion**

   Thrombosis (from backwash of blood into the catheter) is the most common cause of catheter obstruction (10), and instillation of the thrombolytic agent alteplase (recombinant tissue plasminogen activator) can restore patency in 80–90% of occluded catheters (11,12). Cathflo Activase™ (Genentech, Inc.) is a popular alteplase preparation for occluded catheters (12).

2. **Non-Thrombotic Occlusion**

   a. Occlusion from insoluble precipitates can be the result of water-insoluble drugs (e.g., diazepam, digoxin, phenytoin, trimethoprim-sulfa) or anion–cation complexes (e.g., calcium phosphate) (13). Instillation of a dilute acid (0.1N HCL) can promote dissolution of these precipitates (14).

   b. Obstruction can be the result of lipid residues (from propofol infusions or lipid emulsions used for parenteral nutrition). In this case, instillation of 70% ethanol can restore catheter patency (13).

B. Venous Thrombosis

Thrombosis around the catheter tip is demonstrated (by routine ultrasonography or contrast venography) in 40–65% of indwelling central venous catheters (15,16), and is most prevalent in patients with cancer (16). However, symptomatic (occlusive) thrombosis is uncommon (15-17), and occurs most frequently with femoral vein catheters (3.4%) and peripherally-inserted central catheters (3%) (17,18).

1. **Upper Extremity Thrombosis**

   a. Thrombotic occlusion of the axillary or subclavian vein produces swelling of the upper arm, which can be accompanied by paresthesias and arm weakness (19). Propagation of the thrombi into the superior vena cava, with subsequent *superior vena cava syndrome* (i.e., facial swelling, etc.) is rare (20).

   b. Symptomatic pulmonary embolism occurs in fewer than 10% of cases of occlusive upper extremity thrombosis (19).

   c. Compression ultrasonography is the diagnostic test of choice for upper extremity thrombosis (see Figure 1.3 for an example of this method), with a sensitivity and specificity that exceeds 95% (19).

   d. Anticoagulant therapy is recommended for upper extremity thrombosis (19), using the same regimens recommended for lower-extremity thrombosis (see Chapter 4). Removal of the offending catheter is not mandatory, but is advised when arm swelling is severe or painful, or when anticoagulant therapy is contraindicated (19).

C. Vascular Perforation

1. **Superior Vena Cava Perforation**

   a. Perforation of the superior vena cava is most often caused by left-sided central venous catheters that are aligned perpendicular to the lateral wall of the superior vena cava.

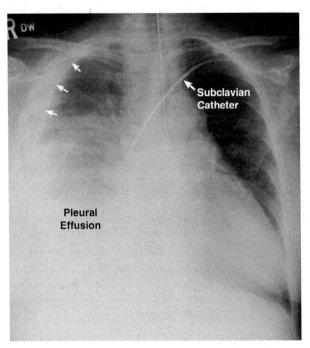

FIGURE 2.1 Chest x-ray showing a large right-sided pleural effusion, which is the result of a perforated superior vena cava caused by the tip of a left-sided central venous catheter. Image courtesy of John E. Heffner, MD (from Reference 21).

b. The clinical presentation is nonspecific, and suspicion of perforation is usually prompted by the sudden appearance of mediastinal widening or a pleural effusion on chest radiography (see Figure 2.1) (21).

c. If vena cava perforation is suspected, the infusion should be stopped immediately. The diagnosis is supported by thoracentesis showing pleural fluid with a similar composition of the infusate fluid. Diagnosis is confirmed by injecting radiocontrast dye through the catheter, and noting the presence of dye in the mediastinum.

d. If the diagnosis is confirmed, the catheter should be removed immediately (this does not provoke mediastinal bleeding) (21). Antibiotic therapy is not necessary unless there is evidence of infection in the pleural fluid (21).

2. **Right Atrial Perforation**

a. Perforation of the right atrium (with subsequent cardiac tamponade) is a rare complication of central venous cannulation, but is often overlooked, and has a mortality rate of 40–100% (22).

b. The first sign of tamponade is usually the abrupt onset of dyspnea, which can progress to cardiovascular collapse within an hour. The diagnosis requires ultrasound evidence of a pericardial effusion with diastolic collapse of the right atrium.

c. Immediate pericardiocentesis is necessary, and emergency thoracotomy may be required for recurrent hemopericardium.

d. The most effective approach to this condition is prevention, which requires proper positioning of catheters so the tip does not extend below the level of the tracheal carina (see Figure 1.6).

III. CATHETER–RELATED SEPTICEMIA

(*Note:* The information in this section does not pertain to peripheral venous catheters, which are not involved in catheter-related bloodstream infections.) Pathogenic organisms can colonize the intravascular portion of central venous catheters and then disseminate in the bloodstream. The incidence of these bloodstream infections in different types of

ICUs is shown in Table 2.2 (23). Note that the frequency of infections is expressed in terms of the number of catheter-days (because each day that a catheter remains in place carries a risk of infection).

Table 2.2	Incidence of Catheter-Associated Bloodstream Infections (CABI) in the United States in 2010	
Type of ICU	**Infections per 1000 catheter-days**	
	Pooled Mean	**Range (10–90%)**
Burn Units	3.5	0 – 8.0
Trauma Units	1.9	0 – 4.0
Medical ICUs	1.8	0 – 3.5
Surgical ICUs	1.4	0 – 3.2
Med/Surg ICUs	1.4	0 – 3.1
Coronary Care Units	1.3	0 – 2.7
Neurosurgical ICUs	1.3	0 – 2.7
Cardiothoracic ICUs	0.9	0 – 2.0

From the National Healthcare Safety Network (23). Includes only ICUs in major teaching hospitals.

A. Definitions

The following definitions are used to identify infections attributed to central venous catheters:

1. Catheter-*Associated* Bloodstream Infections (CABIs) are bloodstream infections that have no apparent source other than a vascular catheter. This is the definition used in clinical surveys (like the one in Table 2.2), and it requires no evidence of microbial growth on the suspected catheter.

2. Catheter-*Related* Bloodstream Infections (CRBIs) are bloodstream infections where the organism identified in peripheral blood is also present in significant quantities on the tip of the catheter or in a blood sample drawn through the catheter (the criteria for a significant quantity is presented later). This is the definition used in clinical practice, and it requires evidence of catheter involvement with the same organism present in peripheral blood.

3. Since the diagnostic criteria for CABIs (which are used in clinical surveys) are far less rigorous than the diagnostic criteria for CRBIs (which are used in clinical practice), clinical surveys overestimate the incidence of CRBIs in clinical practice (24).

Table 2.3	Culture Methods for the Diagnosis of Catheter-Related Bloodstream Infections (CRBI)
Culture Method	**Diagnosis Criteria for CRBI†**
Semiquantitative Culture of the Catheter Tip	Same organism on catheter tip and in peripheral blood, and growth from the catheter tip >15 colony-forming units (CFU) in 24 hrs.
Differential Quantitative Blood Cultures	Same organism in peripheral blood and catheter blood, and colony count from catheter blood ≥3 times greater than colony count from peripheral blood.

†From Reference 25.

B. Clinical Features

1. CRBIs do not appear in the first 48 hours after catheter insertion.

2. The clinical manifestations of CRBIs are non-specific (e.g., fever, leukocytosis).

3. Inflammation at the catheter insertion site has no predictive value for the presence of septicemia (12), and purulent drainage from the catheter insertion site can be a manifestation of an exit-site infection without bloodstream invasion (2).

4. The diagnosis of CRBI is not possible on clinical grounds, and one of the culture methods described next is required to confirm or exclude the diagnosis (see Table 2.3).

C. Catheter Tip Cultures

The traditional approach to suspected CRBI is to combine a culture of the catheter tip with a blood culture obtained from a peripheral vein. This method requires removal of the indwelling catheter.

1. The catheter is removed using sterile technique, and a 2-inch segment is severed from the distal end of the catheter and placed in a sterile culturette tube.

2. The catheter tip should be cultured using a semiquantitative "roll-plate" method, where the catheter tip is rolled directly over the surface of a blood agar plate, and growth is measured as the number of colony forming units (CFUs) on the plate in 24 hours.

3. The diagnosis of CRBI requires growth of at least 15 CFUs on the culture plate plus isolation of the same organism from the blood culture (25).

4. This is the "gold standard" method for the diagnosis of CRBI, but has the following drawbacks:

   a. It requires removal of an indwelling catheter, and more than $2/3$ of catheters removed for presumed CRBI are sterile when cultured (26).

   b. It will not detect infection confined to the luminal surface of the catheter (which is the surface involved if microbes are introduced via the hub of the catheter).

D. Differential Blood Cultures

This method does not require catheter removal, and is based on the expectation that, if a catheter is the source of septicemia, blood withdrawn through the catheter will have a higher microbial density than blood withdrawn through a peripheral vein. This method requires a quantitative assessment of microbial density in the blood, where culture results are expressed as colony forming units per mL (CFU/mL).

1. Blood samples must be collected in specialized tubes (Isolator Culture System, Dupont, Wilmington, DE), which contain a substance that lyses cells to release intracellular organisms.

2. Two blood samples are obtained for culture: one sample is withdrawn through the indwelling catheter (use the distal lumen in multilumen catheters) and the other sample is taken from a peripheral vein.

3. The diagnosis of CRBI is confirmed if the same organism is isolated from both blood samples and the microbial density (CFU/mL) in the catheter blood sample is at least 3 times greater than the microbial density in peripheral blood. An example of the comparative growth density in a case of CRBI is shown in Figure 2.2 (27).

4. This method does not detect infection on the outer surface of the catheter, but it has a diagnostic accuracy of 94% when compared with catheter tip cultures (the gold standard) (24).

E. The Microbial Spectrum

1. The organisms involved in CRBI are (in order of prevalence) coagulase-negative staphylococci, gram-negative aerobic bacilli (*Pseudomonas aeruginosa,* etc.), enterococci, *Staph aureus*, and *Candida* species (28).

2. Coagulase-negative staphylococci (mostly *Staph epider-*

midis) are responsible for about one-third of CRBIs, while enteric pathogens (i.e., enterococci and gram-negative aerobic bacilli) are involved in about half the infections.

3. *Candida* CRBIs are becoming more prevalent; e.g., a recent survey of North American ICUs revealed that *Candida* species were the third leading cause of CRBIs (29).

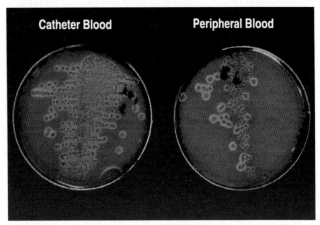

FIGURE 2.2 Culture plates showing colonies of bacterial growth from blood samples drawn from a central venous catheter and a peripheral vein. The denser growth in "catheter blood" is evidence of catheter-related septicemia. From Reference 27; image colorized digitally.

F. Empiric Antibiotic Coverage

Empiric antibiotic therapy is recommended for all patients with suspected CRBI, and should be started immediately after cultures are obtained. Recommendations for empiric antibiotic coverage (25) are shown in Table 2.4.

1. Vancomycin is a staple of empiric antibiotic coverage because it is the most active agent against staphylococci (including coagulase-negative and methicillin-resistant

strains), and enterococci, which together are responsible for about 50% of catheter-related infections (28). Daptomycin can substitute for vancomycin if there is a risk of infection with vancomycin-resistant enterococci.

Table 2.4	Empiric Antibiotics for Possible Isolates in Catheter-Related Infections
Organism	**Recommendations**
Staphylococci	*Antibiotic:* Vancomycin *Comment:* If MRSA isolstes with MIC >2 mg/mL are prevalent, use daptomycin.
Enterococci	*Antibiotic:* Vancomycin *Comment:* If vancomycin resistance is a concern, use daptomycin.
Gram-Negative Bacilli	*Antibiotic:* Either pipericillin-tazobactam, cefepime, or a carbapenem.[a] *Comment:* Add aminoglycoside for neutropenia or high risk of multidrug-resistant organisms.
Candida spp.	*Antibiotic:* An echinocandin[b] *Comment:* Risk factors for candidemia include recent abdominal surgery, recent transplant, immunosuppression, broad-spectrum antibiotic R_x, and *Candida* spp. at multiple sites.

From the guidelines in Reference 25. See Chapter 44 for antibiotic dosing.
[a]Carbapenems include imipenem, meropenem, and doripenem.
[b]Echinocandins include caspofungin, micafungin, and anidulafungin.

2. Empiric coverage for enteric gram-negative bacilli is advised because these organisms are the second most common isolates in ICU patients with CRBI (28). The antibiotics best-suited for empiric gram-negative cover-

age include the carbapenems (e.g., meropenem), the fourth-generation cephalosporins (e.g., cefepime), and the β-lactam/β-lactamase inhibitor combinations (e.g., pipericillin/tazobactam).

3. Empiric coverage for candidemia should be considered for patients with the high-risk conditions mentioned in Table 2.4, particularly when when there is no response to 72 hours of empiric antibacterial therapy. The echinocandins (e.g., caspofungin) are favored for empiric coverage because some *Candida* species (i.e., *Candida krusei* and *Candida glabrata*) are resistant to azoles (e.g., fluconazole).

4. Dosing recommendations for the antibiotics mentioned can be found in Chapter 44.

G. Culture-Confirmed Infections

1. If the culture results confirm the diagnosis of CRBI, further antibiotic therapy is dictated by the identified organisms and antibiotic susceptibilities.

2. When the diagnosis of CRBI is confirmed, catheters that were left in place or changed over a guidewire should be removed and reinserted at a new venipuncture site, unless the offending organism is a coagulase-negative staphylococcus or an enterococcus, and the patient shows a favorable response to empiric antimicrobial therapy (25).

3. Some experts recommend that all cases of *Staph aureus* bacteremia should include an evaluation for endocarditis (with transesophageal ultrasound) 5–7 days after the onset of bacteremia (25).

4. Duration of Therapy

   The duration of antibiotic therapy is determined by the offending pathogen, the status of the catheter (i.e., replaced or retained), and the clinical response. For patients who show a favorable response in the first 72 hours of systemic antibiotic therapy, the recommended duration of treatment is as follows (25):

a. For coagulase-negative staphylococci infections, antibiotic therapy is continued for 5–7 days if the catheter is removed, and for 10–14 days if the catheter is left in place.

b. If *S. aureus* is the culprit, antibiotic therapy can be limited to 14 days if the catheter is removed and the the patient is not immunosuppressed, and has no evidence of endocarditis (25). For these latter conditions, 4–6 weeks of antibiotic therapy is recommended.

c. For infections caused by enterococci or gram-negative bacilli, 7–14 days of antibiotic therapy is recommended, regardless of whether the catheter is replaced or retained (25).

d. For uncomplicated *Candida* infections, antifungal therapy should be continued for 14 days after the first negative blood culture (25).

H. Persistent Sepsis

Continued signs of sepsis or persistent septicemia after 72 hours of antimicrobial therapy should prompt an evaluation for the following conditions.

1. **Suppurative Thrombophlebitis**

   As mentioned earlier, thrombus formation on in-dwelling catheters is common, and if the thrombus becomes infected, it can transform into an intravascular abscess. The most common offending organism is *Staph aureus* (25).

   a. Clinical manifestations are often absent, but can include purulent drainage from the catheter insertion site, limb swelling from thrombotic venous occlusion, and cavitary lesions in the lungs from septic emboli.

b. The diagnosis of septic thrombophlebitis requires evidence of thrombosis in the cannulated blood vessel (e.g., by ultrasound) and persistent septicemia with no other apparent source. (Purulent drainage from the catheter insertion site can represent an exit-site infection rather than a suppurative phlebitis.)

c. Treatment includes catheter removal and systemic antibiotic therapy for 4–6 weeks (25). Surgical excision of the infected thrombus is usually not necessary, and is reserved for cases of refractory septicemia.

d. There is no consensus on the use of heparin anticoagulation in this condition; recent guidelines on CRBIs state that heparin therapy is a consideration (not a requirement) (25).

2. **Endocarditis**

a. CRBIs are responsible for 30–50% of cases of nosocomial endocarditis, and staphylococci (mostly *S. aureus*) are the offending organisms in up to 75% of cases (30,31). Methicillin-resistant strains of *S. aureus* (MRSA) predominate in some reports (32).

b. Typical manifestations of endocarditis (e.g., new or changing cardiac murmur) can be absent in as many as two-thirds of patients with nosocomial endocarditis involving *S. aureus* (31). As a result, endocarditis should be considered in all cases of *S. aureus* bacteremia, including patients who appear to respond to antimicrobial therapy (25).

c. The diagnostic procedure of choice for endocarditis is transesophageal (not transthoracic) ultrasound.

d. Antimicrobial therapy for 4–6 weeks is recommended for endocarditis, although about 30% of patients do not survive the illness (30-32).

3. **Disseminated Candidiasis**

a. Because *Candida* species can be difficult to grow on

blood cultures, disseminated candidiasis should be considered in any case of suspected CRBI where there is no response to empiric antibacterial therapy and blood cultures show no growth. Patients with risk factors for candidemia (see Table 2.4) are of particular concern.

b. The diagnosis of disseminated candidiasis can be elusive, and serum biomarkers such as $(1,3)$-β-D-glucan (a cell wall constituent in *Candida* species) are gaining popularity for the detection of invasive *Candida* infections (33).

c. Antifungal therapy with an echinocandin (e.g., caspofungin) is adequate for cases of candidemia without apparent end-organ involvement, while amphotericin B may be more appropriate for end-organ infections (e.g., endocarditis) (33).

REFERENCES

1. O'Grady NP, Alexander M, Burns LA, et al. and the Healthcare Infection Control Practices Advisory Committee (HICPAC). Guidelines for the Prevention of Intravascular Catheter-related Infections. Clin Infect Dis 2011; 52:e1–e32.

2. Maki DG, Stolz SS, Wheeler S, Mermi LA. A prospective, randomized trial of gauze and two polyurethane dressings for site care of pulmonary artery catheters: implications for catheter management. Crit Care Med 1994; 22:1729–1737.

3. Lok CE, Stanle KE, Hux JE, et al. Hemodialysis infection prevention with polysporin ointment. J Am Soc Nephrol 2003; 14:169–179.

4. Peterson FY, Kirchhoff KT. Analysis of research about heparinized versus non-heparinized intravascular lines. Heart Lung 1991; 20:631–642.

5. American Association of Critical Care Nurses. Evaluation of the effects of heparinized and nonheparinized flush solutions on the patency of arterial pressure monitoring lines: the AACN Thunder Project. Am J Crit Care 1993; 2:3–15.

6. Branson PK, McCoy RA, Phillips BA, Clifton GD. Efficacy of 1.4% sodium citrate in maintaining arterial catheter patency in patients in a medical ICU. Chest 1993; 103:882–885.

7. Cook D, Randolph A, Kernerman P, et al. Central venous replacement strategies: a systematic review of the literature. Crit Care Med 1997; 25:1417–1424.

8. Cobb DK, High KP, Sawyer RP, et al. A controlled trial of scheduled replacement of central venous and pulmonary artery catheters. N Engl J Med 1992; 327:1062–1068.

9. Safdar N, Maki D. Inflammation at the insertion site is not predictive of catheter-related bloodstream infection with short-term, non-cuffed central venous catheters. Crit Care Med 2002; 30:2632–2635.

10. Jacobs BR. Central venous catheter occlusion and thrombosis. Crit Care Clin 2003; 19:489–514.

11. Deitcher SR, Fesen MR, Kiproff PM, et al. Safety and efficacy of alteplase for restoring function in occluded central venous catheters: results of the cardiovascular thrombolytic to open occluded lines trial. J Clin Oncol 2002; 20:317–324.

12. Cathflo Activase (Alteplase) Drug Monograph. San Francisco, CA: Genentech, Inc, 2005.

13. Trissel LA. Drug stability and compatibility issues in drug delivery. Cancer Bull 1990; 42:393–398.

14. Shulman RJ, Reed T, Pitre D, Laine L. Use of hydrochloric acid to clear obstructed central venous catheters. J Parent Ent Nutr 1988; 12:509–510.

15. Timsit J-F, Farkas J-C, Boyer J-M, et al. Central vein catheter-related thrombosis in intensive care patients. Chest 1998; 114:207–213.

16. Verso M, Agnelli G. Venous thromboembolism associated with long-term use of central venous cathters in cancer patients. J Clin Oncol 2003; 21:3665–3675.

17. Evans RS, Sharp JH, Linford LH, et al. Risk of symptomatic DVT associated with peripherally inserted central catheters. Chest 2010; 138:803–810.

18. Joynt GM, Kew J, Gomersall CD, et al. Deep venous thrombosis caused by femoral venous catheters in critically ill adult patients. Chest 2000; 117:178–183.

19. Kucher N. Deep-vein thrombosis of the upper extremities. N Engl J Med 2011; 364:861–869.

20. Otten TR, Stein PD, Patel KC, et al. Thromboembolic disease involving the superior vena cava and brachiocephalic veins. Chest 2003; 123:809–812.

21. Heffner JE. A 49-year-old man with tachypnea and a rapidly enlarging pleural effusion. J Crit Illness 1994; 9:101–109.

22. Booth SA, Norton B, Mulvey DA. Central venous catheterization and fatal cardiac tamponade. Br J Anesth 2001; 87:298–302.

23. Dudeck MA, Horan TC, Peterson KD, et al. National Healthcare Safety Network (NHSN) Report, data summary for 2010, device-associated module. Am J Infect Control 2011; 39:798–816.

24. Bouza E, Alvaredo N, Alcela L, et al. A randomized and prospective study of 3 procedures for the diagnosis of catheter-related bloodstream infection without catheter withdrawal. Clin Infect Dis 2007; 44:820–826.

25. Mermel LA, Allon M, Bouza E, et al. Clinical practice guidelines for the diagnosis and management of intravascular catheter-related infection: 2009 update by the Infectious Diseases Society of America. Clin Infect Dis 2009; 49:1–45.

26. Mermel LA, Farr BM, Sherertz RJ, et al. Guidelines for the management of intravascular catheter-related infections. Clin Infect Dis 2001; 32:1249–1272.

27. Curtas S, Tramposch K. Culture methods to evaluate central venous catheter sepsis. Nutr Clin Pract 1991;6:43–51.

28. Richards M, Edwards J, Culver D, Gaynes R. Nosocomial infections in medical intensive care units in the United States. Crit Care Med 1999; 27:887–892.

29. Vincent JL, Rello J, Marshall J, et al. International study of the prevalence and outcomes of infection in intensive care units. JAMA 2009; 302:2323–2329.

30. Martin-Davila P, Fortun J, Navas E, et al. Nosocomial endocarditis in a tertiary hospital. Chest 2005; 128:772–779.

31. Gouello JP, Asfar P, Brenet O, et al. Nosocomial endocarditis in the intensive care unit: an analysis of 22 cases. Crit Care Med 2000; 28:377–382.

32. Fowler VG, Miro JM, Hoen B, et al. *Staphylococcus aureus* endocarditis: a consequence of medical progress. JAMA 2005; 293:3012–3021.

33. Leon C, Ostrosky-Zeichner L, Schuster M. What's new in the clinical and diagnostic management of invasive candidiasis in critically ill patients. Intensive Care Med 2014; 40:808–819.

Chapter 3

Alimentary Prophylaxis

This chapter describes the following preventive practices in the alimentary tract (which extends from the mouth to the rectum):

1. Gastric acid suppression to prevent bleeding from stress ulcers.

2. Decontamination of the oral cavity to prevent nosocomial pneumonia.

3. Decontamination of the gastrointestinal tract to prevent systemic spread of enteric pathogens.

I. STRESS-RELATED MUCOSAL INJURY

A. Introduction

1. Erosions on the surface of the gastric mucosa are visible in 75–100% of patients within 24 hours of ICU admission (1). These erosions (called *stress ulcers*) are usually confined to the gastric mucosa, and are clinically silent. However, erosions can extend into the submucosa and produce visible bleeding.

2. Clinically apparent bleeding from stress ulcers is reported in up to 15% of ICU patients (2), but clinically significant bleeding (i.e., requires a blood transfusion) occurs in only 3–4% of patients (3).

3. All of the preventive measures described next have been shown to reduce the incidence of stress ulcer bleeding

(2), but much of this effect is for clinically apparent bleeding, which usually has no adverse consequences.

B. Risk Factors

1. Surveys indicate that about 90% of ICU patients receive prophylaxis for stress ulcer bleeding (4), but this is excessive. Preventive measures are indicated only for patients with proven risk factors for stress ulcer bleeding.

2. The risk factors for stress ulcer bleeding are listed in Table 3.1 (5,6). Note that the only independent risk factors (i.e., require no other risk factors to promote bleeding) are mechanical ventilation for longer than 48 hours, significant coagulopathies, and extensive burn injury.

3. *Prophylaxis is indicated for any of the independent risk factors, and for patients with 2 or more of the other risk factors in Table 3.1.*

Table 3.1	Risk Factors for Stress Ulcer Bleeding
Independent Risk Factors	**Other Risk Factors**

1. Mechanical Ventilation (>48 h)
2. Coagulopathy
   a. platelets <50,000 or
   b. INR >1.5 or
   c. PTT >2x control
3. Burns involving >30% of the
   body surface
	1. Circulatory Shock
	2. Severe Sepsis
	3. Multisystem Trauma
	4. Traumatic Brain
	   & Spinal Cord Injury
	5. Renal Failure
	6. Steroid Therapy

C. Gastric Acid Suppression

The principal preventive measure for stress ulcer bleeding is inhibition of gastric acid secretion with histamine type-2 receptor antagonists or proton pump inhibitors. The goal is a pH >4 in gastric secretions, but this is rarely monitored.

1. **Histamine H$_2$-Receptor Antagonists**

   a. Histamine H$_2$-receptor antagonists (H$_2$RAs) are the most frequently used drugs for stress ulcer prophylaxis (4).

   b. Ranitidine and famotidine are the H$_2$RAs used most often for stress ulcer prophylaxis. Both can be given intravenously using the dosing regimens shown in Table 3.2 (7,8). Famotidine has a longer duration of action than ranitidine, and is given less frequently. Both drugs are considered equally effective in preventing stress ulcer bleeding.

   c. H$_2$RAs are less effective in reducing gastric acidity with continued use, but this does not reduce their effectiveness in preventing stress ulcer bleeding (9).

   d. H$_2$RAs can accumulate in renal insufficiency and produce a neurotoxic syndrome characterized by confusion, agitation and seizures (10). Dose reduction is therefore required in renal failure. This can be accomplished by increasing the dosing interval (to 24 hours for ranitidine, and 36–48 hours for famotidine) (10).

2. **Proton Pump Inhibitors**

   a. Proton pump inhibitors (PPIs) are replacing H$_2$RAs for stress ulcer prophylaxis because they produce a more complete inhibition of gastric acid secretion, and there is no response attenuation with continued use (11).

   b. Despite their pharmacological advantages, *PPIs are not more effective than H$_2$RAs for preventing stress ulcer bleeding* (2,12).

   c. The prophylactic dosing regimens for two PPIs are shown in Table 3.2. Both drugs are given intravenously, which is the recommended route for stress ulcer prophylaxis (11). One of the drugs (lansoprazole) requires an in-line filter to trap particulate matter, and must be given slowly (over 30 min) (11). The other drug (pantoprazole) does not have these restrictions, and thus is the favored PPI for stress ulcer prophylaxis.

d. Adverse effects of PPIs are primarily related to the reduced gastric acidity (see next section). One drug interaction deserves mention: PPIs impede the activation of clopidogrel (a popular antiplatelet agent) in the liver (13). Although the significance of this interaction is unclear, current opinion favors avoiding PPIs, if possible, during antiplatelet therapy with clopidogrel.

Table 3.2	Drug Regimens for Prophylaxis of Stress Ulcer Bleeding	
Drug	**Class**	**Usual Dose**
Famotidine	H₂RA	20 mg IV every 12 hrs[1]
Ranitidine	H₂RA	50 mg IV every 8 hrs[2]
Lansoprazole	PPI	30 mg IV once daily
Pantoprazole	PPI	40 mg IV once daily
Sucralfate	Cytoprotective Agent	1 gram PO/IG every 6 hrs

Abbreviations: H_2RA=H_2-receptor antagonist; PPI=proton pump inhibitor; IG=intragastric.

[1]Increase dosing interval to 36–48 hrs in renal failure.

[2]Increase dosing interval to 24 hrs in renal failure.

3. **Infectious Risks**

a. The stomach is a relatively sterile environment, thanks to the bactericidal actions of gastric acid, as demonstrated in Figure 3.1 (14). In this case, pathogenic salmonella organisms were completely eradi-

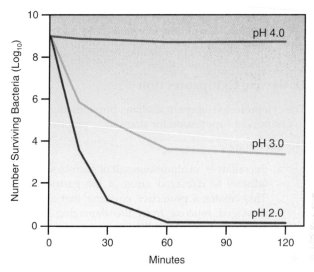

FIGURE 3.1 The influence of gastric pH on the growth of *Salmonella typhimurium*, a common cause of infectious enteritis. From Reference 14.

cated in one hour when the gastric pH was reduced from 4 to 2.

b. Observations like the one in Figure 3.1 have led to the notion that *gastric acid is an antimicrobial defense system* that eradicates pathogens swallowed in food or transmitted via the fecal-oral route.

c. Three infections have been linked to gastric acid suppression: pneumonia (from aspiration of microbe-laden gastric secretions into the airways) (8,15,16), spontaneous bacterial peritonitis (10), and *Clostridium difficile* enterocolitis (17-20). PPIs create a much higher risk of these infections than H₂RAs (16,18).

d. Because PPIs offer no advantage over H₂RAs for the prevention of stress ulcer bleeding (2,12), it seems wise to *avoid PPIs for the prophylaxis of stress ulcer bleeding*, to avoid the infectious risks associated with these agents.

D. Gastric Cytoprotection

The cytoprotective agent, sucralfate, provides an alternative to gastric acid suppression for stress ulcer prophylaxis.

1. Sucralfate

    a. Sucralfate is an aluminum salt of sucrose sulfate that adheres to damaged areas of the gastric mucosa. This creates a protective covering that shields the damaged mucosa from the damaging effects of pepsin and gastric acidity.

    b. *Sucralfate does not inhibit gastric acid secretion, and thus does not create a heightened risk of infection.*

    c. The preferred preparation for sucralfate is a suspension (1 g/10 mL) that can be instilled into the stomach through a feeding tube. A single dose (1 gram) of sucralfate remains adherent to the gastric mucosa for about 6 hours, so a 6-hour dosing interval is recommended (see Table 3.2).

    d. Sucralfate binds to several drugs in the bowel lumen, which can reduce their bioavailability (21). These drugs include ciprofloxacin, norfloxacin, digoxin, ketoconazole, phenytoin, ranitidine, thyroxin, and warfarin. When these drugs are given orally or via a feeding tube, sucralfate doses should be separated by at least 2 hours to minimize drug interactions.

    e. The aluminum in sucralfate can bind phosphate in the bowel, but hypophosphatemia is uncommon (22). Sucralfate does not elevate plasma aluminum levels, even with prolonged use (23).

2. **Sucralfate vs. Ranitidine**

   There are several clinical trials that have compared sucralfate and ranitidine for stress ulcer prophylaxis, and the combined observations in these studies can be summarized as follows (9):

   a. Clinically significant stress ulcer bleeding occurs less frequently with ranitidine, although the difference is small (2%).

   b. The advantage of ranitidine for stress ulcer bleeding is offset by a higher incidence of nosocomial pneumonia associated with ranitidine.

   c. Since nosocomial pneumonia has a higher mortality than stress ulcer bleeding (50% vs. 10%), sucralfate could be preferred to ranitidine because of fewer lives lost (from fewer pneumonias) despite the higher risk of stress ulcer bleeding.

   d. The above observations indicate that neither agent has a convincing advantage over the other, and surveys show that the choice of agent for stress ulcer prophylaxis is dictated by personal preference (4).

II. ORAL DECONTAMINATION

The aspiration of oral secretions into the upper airways is the inciting event in most cases of ventilator-associated pneumonia (24,25).

A. Colonization of Oral Mucosa

1. The microbes that populate the oropharynx in healthy subjects are harmless saprophytes, but the oropharynx in critically ill patients is colonized by pathogenic organisms, predominantly gram-negative bacilli like *Pseudomonas aeruginosa* (24,26).

2. The change in microbial spectrum in the mouth is not environmentally driven, but is a function of the presence and severity of illness. This is shown in Figure 3.2 (26).

3. A change in bacterial adherence to epithelial cells has been identified as the mechanism for the change in microflora. Epithelial cells have specialized surface receptors that bind specific bacteria, and serious illness in the host somehow triggers the expression of different surface receptors on epithelial cells, allowing different microorganisms to colonize the oral mucosa.

4. Since gram-negative bacilli are the most common cause of ventilator-associated pneumonia (see Chapter 16), colonization of the oral mucosa with gram-negative bacilli can be viewed as a red flag that signals a heightened risk for pneumonia. This is the rationale for oral decontamination in ventilator-dependent patients.

B. Chlorhexidine

Chlorhexidine is the most popular antiseptic agent for the skin, largely because of its prolonged activity (6 hours). It has also been adopted for oral decontamination, and has become the standard method of oral decontamination in ventilator-dependent patients.

1. **Regimen**

   Using a gloved hand, 15 mL of a 0.12% chlorhexidine solution is applied to the oral mucosa every 4 hours, and this is continued for the duration of mechanical ventilation.

2. **Efficacy**

   a. The success of chlorhexidine has been variable. To date, only 4 of 7 studies have shown a significant decline in ventilator-associated pneumonias associated with chlorhexidine oral care (27).

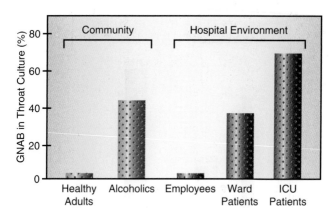

FIGURE 3.2 The prevalence of colonization of the oropharynx with gram-negative aerobic bacilli (GNAB) in subjects with varying degrees of illness. From Reference 26.

b. One explanation for this limited success is the limited spectrum of activity for chlorhexidine; i.e., *chlorhexidine is active against gram-positive organisms (28), but gram-negative organisms are the predominant inhabitants of the oral cavity in seriously ill patients* (see Figure 3.2) (26). This problem deserves attention.

B. Nonabsorbable Antibiotics

1. The traditional method of oral decontamination involves the topical application of nonabsorbable antibiotics. The use of multiple antibiotics provides an advantage over chlorhexidine because of a broader spectrum of antimicrobial activity.

2. Clinical studies show a consistent reduction in ventilator-associated pneumonias when multiple nonabsorbable antibiotics are used for oral decontamination (see later). An example of an effective antibiotic regimen is presented next (29).

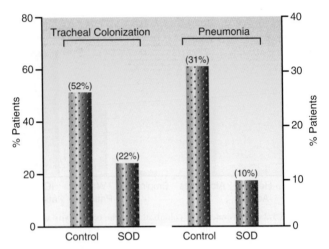

FIGURE 3.3 The effect of selective oral decontamination (SOD) on the incidence of tracheal colonization and pneumonia in ventilator-dependent patients. Data from Reference 29.

3. **Regimen**

   Have the hospital pharmacist prepare a mixture of 2% gentamicin, 2% colistin, and 2% vancomycin in an Orabase gel. Apply this gel to the oral mucosa every 6 hours until the patient is extubated.

   a. This antibiotic mixture is active against staphylococci, gram-negative aerobic bacilli, and *Candida* species. There is little activity against normal mouth flora, which will hasten restoration of the normal microbial population in the mouth.

   b. Because of the selective nature of the antibiotic coverage, this regimen is known as *selective oral decontamination* (SOD).

4. **Efficacy**

   The impact of SOD (same regimen just described) on

colonization and infection in the lungs is demonstrated in Figure 3.3. In this case, SOD was associated with a 57% (relative) decrease in the incidence of tracheal colonization, and a 67% (relative) decrease in the incidence of ventilator-associated pneumonia. Other studies have reported similar results (30).

III. SELECTIVE DIGESTIVE DECONTAMINATION

Selective digestive decontamination (SDD) is similar in principle to selective oral decontamination (SOD); i.e., the goal is to eradicate pathogens and leave the normal microflora intact. The target in SDD is the entire alimentary tract, from mouth to rectum. SDD is intended for all patients who will remain in the ICU for longer than 72 hours, and it is continued for the length of the ICU stay.

A. Regimen

1. A popular SDD regimen with proven efficacy is shown in Table 3.3. Like SOD regimens, SDD regimens employ multiple nonabsorbable antibiotics to eradicate staphylococci, gram-negative aerobic bacilli, and *Candida* species. Normal bowel inhabitants (e.g., anaerobes) are spared, to prevent colonization with opportunistic pathogens like *Clostridium difficile*.

2. A systemic antibiotic is employed for the first few days of SDD to prevent dissemination of bowel pathogens while the decontamination is incomplete.

3. Full decontamination of the bowel requires about 7 days.

B. Efficacy

1. Numerous studies have demonstrated the ability of SDD to reduce the frequency of ICU-acquired infections

(31-33), and the results of one of these studies is shown in Figure 3.4 (32). This study evaluated the influence of SDD on the incidence of ICU-acquired bacteremias involving gram-negative bacilli. Two expressions of incidence are included in the figure, and SDD was associated with a 70% decrease in both expressions of incidence. Although not indicated, the decline in bacteremias in this study was accompanied by a decrease in mortality rate.

2. Early studies of SDD showed no impact on survival, but a survival benefit is apparent in larger, more recent clinical trials (33,34).

Table 3.3	Selective Digestive Decontamination
Target	**Regimen**
Oral Cavity	Create a mixture of 2% tobramycin, 2% amphotericin, and 2% polymyxin in an Orabase gel, and apply this mixture to the oral mucosa every 4 hrs for the duration of the ICU stay.
GI Tract	Create a solution containing 80 mg tobramycin, 500 mg amphotericin, and 100 mg polymyxin in 10 mL of isotonic saline, and deliver this solution through a nasogastric tube every 6 hrs for the duration of the ICU stay.
Systemic Circulation	Intravenous cefuroxime, 1.5 grams every 8 hrs for the first 4 days.

From Reference 31.

C. Antibiotic Resistance

The prolonged exposure to antibiotics with SDD has raised concerns about the emergence of antibiotic resistant organisms. However, there is no evidence of developing antibiotic resistance in the numerous clinical studies of SDD (30-35).

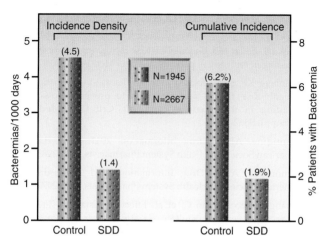

FIGURE 3.4 The effect of selective digestive decontamination (SDD) on the incidence of ICU-acquired, gram-negative bacteremias, expressed as the number of bacteremias per 1000 days (incidence density), and the percentage of patients with bacteremia (cumulative incidence). *N* is the number of patients in the intervention and control groups. Data from Reference 32.

One study that is particularly relevant showed no increase in antibiotic resistance with long-term use of SDD over a 5-year period (35).

REFERENCES

1. Fennerty MB. Pathophysiology of the upper gastrointestinal tract in the critically ill patient: rationale for the therapeutic benefits of acid suppression. Crit Care Med 2002; 30(Suppl):S351–S355.

2. Krag M, Perner A, Wetterslev J, et al. Stress ulcer prophylaxis versus placebo or no prophylaxis in critically ill patients. Intensive Care Med 2014; 40:11–22.

3. Mutlu GM, Mutlu EA, Factor P. GI complications in patients receiving mechanical ventilation. Chest 2001; 119:1222–1241.

4. Daley RJ, Rebuck JA, Welage LS, et al. Prevention of stress ulceration: current trends in critical care. Crit Care Med 2004; 32:2008–2013.

5. Cook DJ, Fuller MB, Guyatt GH. Risk factors for gastrointestinal bleeding in critically ill patients. N Engl J Med 1994; 330:377–381.

6. Steinberg KP. Stress-related mucosal disease in the critically ill patient: Risk factors and strategies to prevent stress-related bleeding in the intensive care unit. Crit Care Med 2002; 30(Suppl):S362–S364.

7. Ranitidine. AHFS Drug Information, 2011. Bethesda, MD: American Society of Health System Pharmacists, 2011:2983–2990.

8. Famotidine. AHFS Drug Information, 2011. Bethesda, MD: American Society of Health System Pharmacists, 2011:2977–2983.

9. Huang J, Cao Y, Liao C, et al. Effect of histamine-2-receptor antagonists versus sucralfate on stress ulcer prophylaxis in mechanically ventilated patients: A meta-analysis of 10 randomized controlled trials. Crit Care 2010; 14:R194–R204.

10. Self TH. Mental confusion induced by H2-receptor antagonists. How to avoid. J Crit Illness 2000; 15:47–48.

11. Pang SH, Graham DY. A clinical guide to using intravenous proton pump inhibitors in reflux and peptic ulcers. Ther Adv Gastroenterol 2010; 3:11–22.

12. Lin P-C, Chang C-H, Hsu P-I, et al. The efficacy and safety of proton pump inhibitors vs histamine-2 receptor antagonists for stress ulcer bleeding prophylaxis among critical care patients: A meta-analysis. Crit Care Med 2010; 38:1197–1205.

13. Egred M. Clopidogrel and proton-pump inhibitor interaction. Br J Cardiol 2011; 18:84–87.

14. Gianella RA, Broitman SA, Zamcheck N. Gastric acid barrier to ingested microorganisms in man: studies in vivo and in vitro. Gut 1972; 13:251–256.

15. Gulmez SE, Holm A, Frederiksen H, et al. Use of proton pump inhibitors and the risk of community-acquired pneumonia. Arch Intern Med 2007; 167:950–955.

16. Herzig SJ, Howell MD, Ngo LH, Marcantonio ER. Acid-suppressive medication use and the risk for hospital-acquired pneumonia. JAMA 2009; 301:2120–2128.

17. Dial S, Delaney JAC, Barkun AN, Suissa S. Use of gastric acid-suppressing agents and the risk of community-acquired *Clostridium difficile*-associated disease. JAMA 2005; 294:2989–2994.

18. Dial S, Alrasadi K, Manoukian C, et al. Risk of *Clostridium-difficile* diarrhea among hospitalized patients prescribed proton pump inhibitors: cohort and case-control studies. Canad Med Assoc J 2004; 171:33–38.

19. Lowe DO, Mamdani MM, Kopp A, et al. Proton pump inhibitors and hospitalization for *Clostridium difficile*-associated disease: a population-based study. Clin Infect Dis 2006; 43:1272–1276.

20. Aseri M, Schroeder T, Kramer J, Kackula R. Gastric acid suppression by proton pump inhibitors as a risk factor for *Clostridium difficile*-associated diarrhea in hospitalized patients. Am J Gastroenterol 2008; 103:2308–2313.

21. Sucralfate. AHFS Drug Information, 2011. Bethesda, MD: American Society of Health System Pharmacists, 2011:2996–2998.

22. Miller SJ, Simpson J. Medication–nutrient interactions: hypophosphatemia associated with sucralfate in the intensive care unit. Nutr Clin Pract 1991; 6:199–201.

23. Tryba M, Kurz-Muller K, Donner B. Plasma aluminum concentrations in long-term mechanically ventilated patients receiving stress ulcer prophylaxis with sucralfate. Crit Care Med 1994; 22:1769–1773.

24. Estes RJ, Meduri GU. The pathogenesis of ventilator-associated pneumonia: I. Mechanisms of bacterial transcolonization and airway inoculation. Intensive Care Med 1995; 21:365–383.

25. Higuchi JH, Johanson WG. Colonization and bronchopulmonary infection. Clin Chest Med 1982; 3:133–142.

26. Johanson WG, Pierce AK, Sanford JP. Changing pharyngeal bacterial flora of hospitalized patients. Emergence of gram-negative bacilli. N Engl J Med 1969; 281:1137–1140.

27. Chlebicki MP, Safdar N. Topical chlorhexidine for prevention of ventilator-associated pneumonia: a meta-analysis. Crit Care Med 2007; 35:595–602.

28. Emilson CG. Susceptibility of various microorganisms to chlorhexidine. Scand J Dent Res 1977; 85:255–265

29. Bergmans C, Bonten M, Gaillard C, et al. Prevention of ventilator-associated pneumonia by oral decontamination. Am J Respir Crit Care Med 2001; 164:382–388.

30. van Nieuwenhoven CA, Buskens E, Bergmans DC, et al. Oral decontamination is cost-saving in the prevention of ventilator associated pneumonia in intensive care units. Crit Care Med 2004; 32:126–130.

31. Stoutenbeek CP, van Saene HKF, Miranda DR, Zandstra DF. The effect of selective decontamination of the digestive tract on colonization and infection rate in multiple trauma patients. Intensive Care Med 1984; 10:185–192.

32. Oostdijk EA, de Smet AM, Kesecioglu J, et al. The role of intestinal colonization with Gram-negative bacteria as a source for intensive care unit-acquired bacteremia. Crit Care Med 2011; 39:961–966.

33. de Smet AMGA, Kluytmans JAJW, Cooper BS, et al. Decontamination of the digestive tract and oropharynx in ICU patients. N Engl J Med 2009; 360:20–31.

34. de Jonge E, Schultz MJ, Spanjaard L, et al. Effects of selective decontamination of digestive tract on mortality and acquisition of resistant bacteria in intensive care: a randomized controlled trial. Lancet 2003; 362:1011–1016.

35. Ochoa-Ardila ME, Garcia-Canas A, Gomez-Mediavilla K, et al. Long-term use of selective decontamination of the digestive tract does not increase antibiotic resistance: a 5-year prospective cohort study. Intensive Care Med 2011; 37:1458–1465.

Chapter 4

Venous Thromboembolism

This chapter presents the current practices for the prevention, diagnosis, and treatment of venous thrombosis and pulmonary embolism (*venous thromboembolism* or VTE). The major focus is on prevention, because VTE is considered the leading cause of preventable deaths in hospitalized patients (1).

I. RISK FACTORS

A. Major Surgery

1. Major surgery (i.e., performed under general or spinal anesthesia that lasts longer than 30 minutes) is the leading source of VTE in hospitalized patients (2-4). Contributing factors include vascular injury and thromboplastin release during the surgical procedure.

2. The highest incidence of postoperative VTE occurs after major procedures involving the hip and knee (3,4).

B. Major Trauma

1. Victims of major trauma have a greater than 50% chance of developing VTE, and pulmonary embolism is the third leading cause of death in those who survive the first day (3). Contributing factors in trauma-related VTE are vascular injury and thromboplastin release from damaged tissues (similar to surgery-related VTE).

57

2. Traumatic injuries with the highest risk of VTE include spinal cord injuries and fractures of the spine, hip and pelvis (3,4).

C. Acute Medical Illness

1. Hospitalization for acute medical illness is associated with an 8-fold increase in the risk of VTE (5).

2. Conditions with the highest risk of VTE include acute stroke, neuromuscular weakness syndromes, severe sepsis, cancer, and right-sided heart failure.

3. The risk of VTE is lower in acute medical illness than in major surgery or trauma (2-4), but the majority (70–80%) of deaths from VTE occur in medical patients (3).

D. ICU-Related Risks

1. ICU-related risk factors for VTE include prolonged mechanical ventilation (>48 hrs), central venous catheters, vasopressor infusions, drug-induced paralysis, and prolonged immobility.

2. ICU patients often have one of the high-risk conditions mentioned previously, in addition to the ICU-related risk factors for VTE; as a result, *all ICU patients are considered to have a high risk of VTE* (3), and are therefore candidates for thromboprophylaxis (see next).

II. THROMBOPROPHYLAXIS

Prophylaxis for VTE is a standard measure for all ICU patients (except those that are fully anticoagulated), and is started on the day of admission. Appropriate preventive measures can vary in different high-risk conditions, as indicated in Table 4.1.

Table 4.1	Thromboprophylaxis for Selected Conditions
Conditions	**Regimens**
Acute Medical Illness	LDUH or LMWH
Major Abdominal Surgery	(LDUH or LMWH) + (GCS or IPC)
Thoracic Surgery	(LDUH or LMWH) + (GCS or IPC)
Cardiac Surgery with Complications	(LDUH or LMWH) + IPC
Craniotomy	IPC
Hip or Knee Surgery	LMWH
Major Trauma	LDUH or LMWH or IPC
Head or Spinal Cord Injury	(LDUH or LMWH) + IPC
Any of the above + active bleeding or high risk of bleeding	IPC

From Reference 3. Abbreviations: LDUH = low-dose unfractionated heparin; LMWH = low-molecular weight heparin; GCS = graded compression stockings; IPC = intermittent pneumatic compression.

A. Unfractionated Heparin

Standard or *unfractionated* heparin is a heterogeneous mix of mucopolysaccharide molecules that vary in size and anticoagulant activity.

1. **Actions**

   a. Heparin is an indirect-acting drug that must bind to a cofactor (antithrombin III or AT) to produce an anticoagulant effect. The heparin-AT complex inactivates several coagulation factors, and inactivation of factor IIa (antithrombin effect) is 10 times more sensitive than the other anticoagulant reactions (6).

b. Heparin also binds to a specific protein on platelets to form an antigenic complex that induces the formation of IgG antibodies. These antibodies can cross-react with the platelet binding site and activate platelets, which promotes thrombosis and a consumptive thrombocytopenia. This is the mechanism for *heparin-induced thrombocytopenia*, which is described in more detail in Chapter 12.

2. **Prophylactic Dosing**

The potent antithrombin activity of the heparin-AT complex allows low doses of heparin to inhibit thrombogenesis without producing systemic anticoagulation.

a. The standard regimen of *low-dose unfractionated heparin* (LDUH) is 5000 units by subcutaneous injection every 12 hours. There is a more frequent dosing regimen (5000 units every 8 hours), but there is no evidence of superiority over twice daily dosing (2,7).

b. Studies in ICU patients (8) and postoperative patients (9) have shown a 50–60% reduction in the incidence of leg vein thrombosis with LDUH.

c. The standard LDUH regimen may be less effective in obese patients because of the increased volume of drug distribution in obesity. The recommended dosing for LDUH in obesity is included in Table 4.2 (10).

3. **Complications**

a. The risk of major bleeding with LDUH is <1% (7), and anticoagulation monitoring is not necessary.

b. Heparin-induced thrombocytopenia has been reported in 2.6% of patients receiving LDUH (11).

4. Indications

LDUH is suitable for thromboprophylaxis in all high-risk conditions except hip and knee surgery (see Table 4.1) (3).

Table 4.2	Anticoagulant Regimens for Thromboprophylaxis

Unfractionated Heparin

Usual Dose:	5000 Units SC every 12 hrs
High-Risk Dose:	5000 Units SC every 8 hrs
Obesity:	5000 Units SC every 8 hrs (BMI < 50)
	7500 Units SC every 8 hrs (BMI ≥ 50)

Enoxaparin (LMWH)

Usual Dose:	40 mg SC once daily
High-Risk Dose:	30 mg SC twice daily
Obesity:	0.5 mg/kg SC once daily (BMI > 40)
Renal Failure:	30 mg once daily (for CrCL < 30 mL/min)

Dalteparin (LMWH)

Usual Dose:	2500 Units SC once daily
High-Risk Dose:	5000 Units SC once daily
Renal Failure:	No recommended dose adjustment

From References 2, 10, 13–16. CrCL = creatinine clearance, SC = subcutaneous.

B. Low-Molecular-Weight Heparin

Low-molecular-weight heparin (LMWH) is produced by enzymatic cleavage of heparin molecules, which produces smaller molecules of more uniform size. This results in more potent and predictable anticoagulation than occurs with unfractionated heparin. LMWH must still bind to anti-thrombin III, and the major anticoagulant reaction is inactivation of Factor Xa.

1. **Advantages**

   LMWH has the following advantages over unfractionated heparin:

   a. A more predictable dose-response relationship, and no routine monitoring of anticoagulant activity (5).

   b. Less frequent dosing due to a longer duration of action.

   c. A much lower risk of heparin-induced thrombocytopenia (0.2% for LMWH vs. 2.6% for LDUH) (11).

2. **Disadvantages**

   The major disadvantage of LMWH is its clearance by the kidneys, which creates the need for dosage adjustments in patients with renal failure. However, the tendency to accumulate in renal failure varies with individual LMWH preparations (see later).

3. **Relative Efficacy**

   LMWH is equivalent to LDUH for all high-risk conditions encountered in the ICU (11), and is superior to LDUH for prophylaxis of VTE in hip and knee surgery (3,4).

4. **Prophylactic Dosing**

   The LMWH preparations studied most extensively for thromboprophylaxis are enoxaparin (Lovenox) and dalteparin (Fragmin). Prophylactic dosing regimens for these agents are summarized in Table 4.2.

   a. ENOXAPARIN: The standard enoxaparin dose for thromboprophylaxis is 40 mg by subcutaneous injection once daily (13). In conditions with a very high risk of VTE (e.g., major trauma, hip and knee surgery), the dose is 30 mg twice daily (13). Dosing adjustments for renal failure (13) and morbid obesity (14) are shown in Table 4.2.

b. DALTEPARIN: Dalteparin has two advantages over enoxaparin: (*a*) It is given only once daily (15), and (*b*) it has been used safely without dose reduction in renal failure (16). The appropriate dose of dalteparin in morbid obesity is not known.

C. Neuraxial Analgesia

Anticoagulant prophylaxis can promote hematoma formation during the insertion and removal of intrathecal and epidural catheters. To limit this risk, the insertion and removal of intrathecal and epidural catheters should be performed at a time when anticoagulant effects are minimal, and at least 2 hours should elapse after these procedures before an anticoagulant dose is administered (2).

D. Mechanical Aids

External compression of the lower extremities can promote venous outflow from the legs and reduce the risk of VTE. This approach is typically used as a replacement for anticoagulant drugs in patients who are bleeding or have a high risk of bleeding, but it can also be used as an adjunct to anticoagulant prophylaxis in selected patients (see Table 4.2). There are two methods of external leg compression, as described next.

1. Graded Compression Stockings

   Graded compression stockings (GCS) are designed to create 18 mm Hg external pressure at the ankles and 8 mm Hg external pressure in the thigh (17). The resulting 10 mm Hg pressure gradient acts as a driving force for venous outflow from the legs.

   a. These stocking have been shown to reduce the incidence of VTE when used alone after major surgery (18), but they are not recommended as the sole method of thromboprophylaxis in ICU patients (3).

2. **Intermittent Pneumatic Compression**

Intermittent pneumatic compression (IPC) is achieved with inflatable bladders that are wrapped around the lower extremities and connected to a pneumatic pump. Bladder inflation creates 35 mm Hg external compression at the ankle and 20 mm Hg external compression at the thigh, and repeated inflation and deflation of the bladders creates a pumping action that augments venous outflow from the legs (17).

a. IPC is more effective than graded compression stockings (3,4), and can be used alone for thromboprophylaxis after craniotomy (3).

III. DIAGNOSTIC EVALUATION

Deep vein thrombosis in the legs is often clinically silent, and VTE is suspected only when a symptomatic pulmonary embolus appears. Therefore, the diagnostic evaluation described here is for suspected pulmonary embolism.

A. Initial Evaluation

The diagnosis of pulmonary embolism (PE) is confirmed in only 10% of suspected cases (19), which reflects the nonspecific clinical presentation of PE.

1. The predictive value of clinical and laboratory findings in suspected PE is shown in Table 4.3 (20). Note that none of the findings is reliable for confirming or excluding the presence of PE.

2. Plasma D-dimer levels (a reflection of fibrinolysis) are frequently elevated in patients with VTE. However, several other conditions can elevate plasma D-dimer levels

(e.g., sepsis, heart failure, and renal failure), and a majority (up to 80%) of ICU patients have elevated plasma D-dimer levels in the absence of VTE (21). Therefore, the D-dimer assay is not reliable in the ICU setting.

Table 4.3	Predictive Value of Clinical and Laboratory Findings in Suspected Pulmonary Embolism	
Findings	**Positive Predictive Value†**	**Negative Predictive Value§**
Dyspnea	37%	75%
Tachycardia	47%	86%
Tachypnea	48%	75%
Pleuritic Chest Pain	39%	71%
Hemoptysis	32%	67%
Pulmonary Infiltrate	33%	71%
Pleural Effusion	40%	69%
Hypoxemia	34%	70%

†Positive predictive value is the percentage of patients with the finding who have a pulmonary embolus.

§Negative predictive value is the percentage of patients without the finding who do not have a pulmonary embolus.

From Reference 20.

3. Since the diagnosis of PE is not possible with clinical or laboratory findings, one or more of the diagnostic tests described next is required. The use of these tests can proceed as shown in the flow diagram in Figure 4.1.

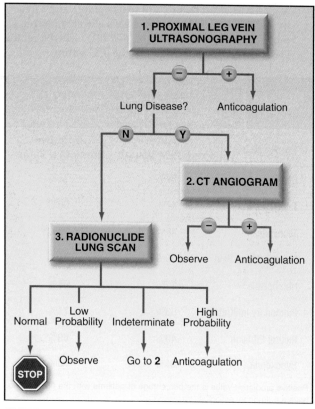

FIGURE 4.1 Flow diagram for the evaluation of suspected pulmonary embolism.

B. Vascular Ultrasound

Pulmonary emboli originate primarily from thrombi in proximal leg veins (22), so the evaluation of suspected PE can begin with a search for thrombosis in the proximal leg veins using this approach. Vascular ultrasound has 2 advantages: it can be done at the bedside, and it does not require radiocontrast dye.

1. For the detection of proximal deep vein thrombosis (proximal DVT) in the legs, vascular ultrasound has a sensitivity ≥95% and a specificity ≥97% (23). This confirms the reliability of vascular ultrasound as a diagnostic test.

2. In patients with documented PE, vascular ultrasound shows evidence of proximal DVT in the legs in 45% of patients (24). In these patients, no further evaluation for PE is necessary (since the treatment of DVT and PE is essentially the same).

3. When vascular ultrasound is unrevealing, the next step in the evaluation is determined by the presence or absence of lung disease (see Figure 4.1).

C. CT Angiography

For patients with lung disease (i.e., most patients in the ICU), the most reliable test for the detection of PE is computed tomographic angiography (CTA). This test combines spiral CT scanning (where the scanner rotates around the patient to produce a volumetric, two-dimensional view of the lungs) with injection of a contrast agent, to visualize the central pulmonary arteries.

1. CTA has a sensitivity of 83%, a specificity of 96%, a positive predictive value of 86%, and a negative predictive value of 95% for the diagnosis of PE (25).

2. Although CTA can miss emboli in smaller, subsegmental vessels, withholding anticoagulant therapy based on a negative CTA does adversely affect clinical outcomes (26).

3. CTA carries a risk of nephrotoxicity from the radiocontrast dye, particularly in patients with renal insufficiency, diabetes or volume depletion. These risk factors must be considered in the decision to perform CTA. (See Chapter 26 for more on dye-induced renal injury.)

D. Radionuclide Lung Scan

Ventilation-perfusion lung scans are problematic in the presence of lung disease (particularly infiltrative disease), which produces an abnormal scan in about 90% of cases (27). Lung scans are most reliable in patients with no underlying lung disease (which excludes most ICU patients). If the decision is made to proceed with a lung scan, the results can be used as follows (27):

1. A normal lung scan excludes the presence of a pulmonary embolus, whereas a high-probability lung scan carries a 90% probability that a pulmonary embolus is present.

2. A low-probability lung scan does not reliably exclude the presence of a PE. However, when combined with a negative ultrasound evaluation of the legs, a low-probability scan is sufficient reason to stop the diagnostic workup and observe the patient.

3. An intermediate-probability or indeterminate lung scan has no value in predicting the presence or absence of a pulmonary embolus. In this situation, the options include spiral CT angiography or conventional pulmonary angiography (see next).

E. Angiography

Conventional pulmonary angiography is the "gold standard" method for the diagnosis of PE, but is reserved only for the very few cases where other diagnostic testing is not sufficient *and* there is a high clinical suspicion of PE.

IV. MANAGEMENT

A. Anticoagulation

The initial management of VTE that is not immediately life-threatening is anticoagulation with heparin.

1. **Unfractionated Heparin**

   Intravenous heparin (bolus, then infusion) is preferred for initial management because it achieves rapid anticoagulation, and monitoring is easily available to ensure therapeutic anticoagulation is achieved.

   a. Heparin dosing based on body weight, like the regimen in Table 4.4, achieves more rapid anticoagulation than fixed-dosing regimens (28).

   b. The anticoagulant effect is monitored with the activated partial thromboplastin time (PTT); the target PTT is 46–70 seconds, or a PTT ratio (test/control) of 1.5–2.5 (6).

Table 4.4	Weight-based Heparin Dosing Regimen

1. Give initial bolus dose of 80 IU/kg and follow with continuous infusion of 18 IU/kg/hr. (Use actual body weight.)

2. Check PTT 6 hrs after start of infusion, and adjust heparin dose as indicated below.

PTT (sec)	PTT Ratio	Bolus Dose	Continuous Infusion
<35	<1.2	80 IU/kg	Increase by 4 IU/kg/hr
35–45	1.3–1.5	40 IU/kg	Increase by 2 IU/kg/hr
46–70	1.5–2.3	—	—
71–90	2.3–3.0	—	Decrease by 2 IU/kg/hr
>90	>3	—	Stop infusion for 1 hr then decrease by 3 IU/kg/hr

3. Check PTT 6 hrs after each dose adjustment. When in the desired range (46–70 sec), monitor daily.

From Reference 28.

2. **Low–Molecular-Weight Heparin**

   LMWH is an effective alternative to unfractionated heparin for treating VTE (29), but is not preferred for initial management for reasons stated previously.

   a. Enoxaparin is favored because it is the LMWH studied most extensively in acute PE. The dose for therapeutic anticoagulation is 1 mg/kg by subcutaneous injection every 12 hours. Half of this dose is recommended when the creatinine clearance is <30 mL/min (6).

   b. If anticoagulant monitoring for LMWH is desired (e.g., in patients with renal failure), the laboratory test of choice is the heparin-Xa (anti-Xa) level in plasma. This should be measured 4 hours after an LMWH dose, and the desired anti-Xa level is 0.6–1.0 units/ml for twice-daily enoxaparin dosing, and >1 unit/mL for once-daily enoxaparin dosing (6).

3. **Warfarin**

   a. Oral anticoagulation with warfarin should be started on the first day of heparin anticoagulation. The initial dose is usually 5 mg daily, with subsequent dosing tailored to the international normalized ratio (INR).

   b. The target INR is 2–3; when this is achieved, heparin anticoagulation can be discontinued.

B. Thrombolytic Therapy

1. The general features of thrombolytic therapy for VTE are summarized in Table 4.5.

2. The usual indication for thrombolytic therapy is acute PE with hemodynamic deterioration or right ventricular dysfunction. Although hemodynamics are improved in both conditions, there is no survival benefit (29,30).

Table 4.5	Thrombolytic Therapy in Acute Pulmonary Embolism

When Used:

1. Pulmonary embolism with hemodynamic instability
2. Pulmonary embolism with right ventricular dysfunction

Therapeutic Regimens:

1. Continuous infusion heparin is used in conjunction with lytic therapy.
2. Standard thrombolytic regimen:
   Alteplase: 100 mg infused over 2 hrs
3. Regimens aimed at accelerated clot lysis:
   Alteplase: 0.6 mg/kg infused over 15 min.
   Reteplase: 10 U by IV bolus and repeat in 30 min.

Complications:

1. Major hemorrhage: 10–12%
2. Intracranial hemorrhage: 1–2%

From References 29–32.

3. The standard thrombolytic regimen is a 2-hour infusion of alteplase (recombinant tissue plasminogen activator) (29). However, other drug regimens can achieve more rapid clot lysis, and these are included in Table 4.5 (31,32).

4. Continuous-infusion heparin is used in conjunction with thrombolytic therapy. Heparin is particularly advantageous after thrombolysis because clot dissolution releases thrombin, which can lead to thrombotic reocclusion of the involved vessel.

5. About 10–12 % of patients experience a major bleeding episode after thrombolytic therapy, and 1–2 % develop intracranial hemorrhage (29,30).

C. Embolectomy

If immediately available, embolectomy (either surgical or catheter-based) should be considered for life-threatening PE. Survival rates of 83% have been reported with emergency embolectomy (33).

D. Vena Cava Filter

Filters can be placed (percutaneously) in the inferior vena cava to trap thrombi that break loose from leg veins and prevent them from travelling to the lungs (34).

1. Indications for a vena cava filter include:

   a. Acute PE despite therapeutic anticoagulation.

   b. Evidence of VTE with an absolute contraindication to anticoagulation.

   c. Proximal DVT in the legs, with a free-floating thrombus (i.e., the leading edge of the thrombus is not adherent to the vessel wall), or with limited cardiopulmonary reserve (i.e., unlikely to tolerate a pulmonary embolus).

REFERENCES

1. Shojania KG, Duncan BW, McDonald KM, et al, eds. Making healthcare safer: a critical analysis of patient safety practices. Evidence report/technology assessment No. 43. AHRQ Publication No. 01-E058. Rockville, MD: Agency for Healthcare Research and Quality, July, 2001.

2. Geerts WH, Bergqvist D, Pineo GF, et al. Prevention of venous thromboembolism. American College of Chest Physicians evidence-based clinical practice guideline (8th edition). Chest 2008; 133(Suppl):381S–453S.

3. Guyatt GH, Aki EA, Crowther M, et al. Executive summary: Antithrombotic Therapy and Prevention of Thrombosis, 9th ed: American College of Chest Physicians Evidence-Based Clinical Practice Guidelines. Chest 2012; 141(Suppl):7S–47S.

4. McLeod AG, Geerts W. Venous thromboembolism prophylaxis in critically ill patients. Crit Care Clin 2011; 27:765–780.

5. Heit JA, Silverstein MD, Mohr DM, et al. Risk factors for deep vein thrombosis and pulmonary embolism: a population-based case-control study. Arch Intern Med 2000; 160:809–815.

6. Garcia DA, Baglin TP, Weitz JI, Samama MM. Parenteral anticoagulants. Antithrombotic Therapy and Prevention of Thrombosis, 9th ed: American College of Chest Physicians Evidence-Based Clinical Practice Guidelines. Chest 2012; 141(Suppl):e24S–e43S.

7. King CS, Holley AB, Jackson JL, et al. Twice vs three times daily heparin dosing for thromboembolism prophylaxis in the general medical population. A meta-analysis. Chest 2007; 131:507–516.

8. Cade JF. High risk of the critically ill for venous thromboembolism. Crit Care Med 1982; 10:448–450.

9. Collins R, Scrimgeour A, Yusuf S. Reduction in fatal pulmonary embolism and venous thrombosis by perioperative administration of subcutaneous heparin: overview of results of randomized trials in general, orthopedic, and urologic surgery. N Engl J Med 1988; 318:1162–1173.

10. Medico CJ, Walsh P. Pharmacotherapy in the critically ill obese patient. Crit Care Clin 2010; 26:679–688.

11. Martel N, Lee J, Wells PS. The risk of heparin-induced thrombocytopenia with unfractionated and low-molecular-weight heparin thromboprophylaxis: a meta-analysis. Blood 2005; 106:2710–2715.

12. The PROTECT Investigators. Dalteparin versus unfractionated heparin in critically ill patients. N Engl J Med 2011; 364:1304–1314.

13. Enoxaparin. AHFS Drug Information, 2012. Bethesda, MD: American Society of Health System Pharmacists, 2012:1491–1501.

14. Rondina MT, Wheeler M, Rodgers GM, et al. Weight-based dosing of enoxaparin for VTE prophylaxis in morbidly obese medical patients. Thromb Res 2010; 125:220–223.

15. Dalteparin. AHFS Drug Information, 2012. Bethesda, MD: American Society of Health System Pharmacists, 2012:1482–1491.

16. Douketis J, Cook D, Meade M, et al. Prophylaxis against deep vein thrombosis in critically ill patients with severe renal insufficiency with the low-molecular-weight heparin dalteparin: an assessment of safety and pharmacokinetics. Arch Intern Med 2008; 168:1805–1812.

17. Goldhaber SZ, Marpurgo M, for the WHO/ISFC Task Force on Pulmonary Embolism. Diagnosis, treatment and prevention of pulmonary embolism. JAMA 1992; 268:1727–1733.

18. Sachdeva A, Dalton M, Amarigiri SV, Lees T. Graduated compression stockings for prevention of deep vein thrombosis. Cochrane Database Syst Rev 2010; 7: CD001484

19. Kabrhel C, Camargo CA, Goldhaber SZ. Clinical gestalt and the diagnosis of pulmonary embolism. Chest 2005; 127:1627–1630.

20. Hoellerich VL, Wigton RS. Diagnosing pulmonary embolism using clinical findings. Arch Intern Med 1986; 146:1699–1704.

21. Kollef MH, Zahid M, Eisenberg PR. Predictive value of a rapid semiquantitative D-dimer assay in critically ill patients with suspected thromboembolism. Crit Care Med 2000; 28:414–420.

22. Hyers TM. Venous thromboembolism. Am J resp Crit Care Med 1999; 159:1–14.

23. Tracey JA, Edlow JA. Ultrasound diagnosis of deep venous thrombosis. Emerg Med Clin N Am 2004; 22:775–796.

24. Girard P, Sanchez O, Leroyer C, et al. Deep venous thrombosis in patients with acute pulmonary embolism. Prevalence, risk factors, and clinical significance. Chest 2005; 128:1593–1600.

25. Stein PD, Fowler SE, Goodman LR, et al. Multidetector computed tomography for acute pulmonary embolism. N Engl J Med 2006; 354:2317–2327.

26. Quiroz R, Kucher N, Zou KH, et al. Clinical validity of a negative computed tomography scan in patients with suspected pulmonary embolism. JAMA 2005; 293:2012–2017.

27. The PIOPED Investigators. Value of the ventilation/perfusion scan in acute pulmonary embolism. Results of the prospective investigation of pulmonary embolism diagnosis (PIOPED). JAMA 1990; 263:2753–2759.

28. Raschke RA, Reilly BM, Guidry JR, et al. The weight-based heparin dosing nomogram compared with a "standard care" nomogram. Ann Intern Med 1993; 119:874–881.

29. Tapson VF. Treatment of pulmonary embolism: anticoagulation, thrombolytic therapy, and complications of therapy. Crit Care Clin 2011; 27: 825–839.

30. Meyer G, Vicaut E, Danays T, et al. Fibrinolysis for patients with inter-mediate-risk pulmonary embolism. N Engl J Med 2014; 370:1402–1411.

31. Goldhaber SZ, Agnelli G, Levine MN. Reduced-dose bolus alteplase vs. conventional alteplase infusion for pulmonary embolism throm-bolysis: an international multicenter randomized trial: the Bolus Alteplase Pulmonary Embolism Group. Chest 1994; 106:718–724.

32. Tebbe U, Graf A, Kamke W, et al. Hemodynamic effects of dou-ble bolus reteplase versus alteplase infusion in massive pul-monary embolism. Am Heart J 1999; 138:39–44.

33. Sareyyupoglu B, Greason KL, Suri RM, et al. A more aggressive approach to emergency embolectomy for acute pulmonary embolism. Mayo Clin Proc 2010; 85:785–790.

34. Fairfax LM, Sing RF. Vena cava interruption. Crit Care Clin 2011; 27:781–804.

Chapter 5

The Pulmonary Artery Catheter

This chapter presents the spectrum of hemodynamic parameters that can be monitored with pulmonary artery catheters. The clinical applications of these parameters are described in future chapters.

I. CATHETER BASICS

A. The Principle

The pulmonary artery (PA) catheter is equipped with a small inflatable balloon at the distal end. When inflated, the balloon allows the flow of venous blood to carry the catheter through the right side of the heart and into one of the pulmonary arteries. This *balloon flotation* principle allows catheterization of the right heart and pulmonary arteries without fluoroscopic guidance.

B. The Catheter

1. The PA catheter is 110 cm in length (about 5–6 times longer than a central venous catheter), and has an outside diameter of 2.3 mm (about 7 French).

2. There are two internal channels: one channel emerges at the tip of the catheter, and the other channel emerges 30 cm proximal to the catheter tip (and should be situated in the right atrium when the catheter is properly positioned).

3. The tip of the catheter has an inflatable balloon (1.5 mL capacity) that helps to carry the catheter to its final destination.

4. A small thermistor (a temperature-sensing transducer) is placed near the tip of the catheter, and this allows measurement of the cardiac output by the thermodilution method (described later).

C. Placement

The PA catheter is inserted through a large-bore (8–9 French) introducer sheath that has been placed in the subclavian vein or internal jugular vein. The distal lumen of the catheter is attached to a pressure transducer to guide catheter placement. When the catheter emerges from the introducer sheath and enters the superior vena cava, a venous pressure waveform appears. The balloon is then inflated and the catheter is advanced, using pressure tracings to determine the location of the catheter tip, as shown in Figure 5.1.

1. The pressure in the superior vena cava shows small amplitude oscillations. This pressure remains unchanged when the catheter tip enters the right atrium.

2. When the catheter tip is advanced across the tricuspid valve and into the right ventricle, a pulsatile waveform appears. The peak (systolic) pressure is a function of the strength of right ventricular contraction, and the lowest (diastolic) pressure is equivalent to the pressure in the right atrium.

3. When the catheter moves across the pulmonic valve and enters a main pulmonary artery, the pressure waveform shows a sudden rise in diastolic pressure with no change in the systolic pressure. The rise in diastolic pressure is caused by resistance to flow in the pulmonary circulation.

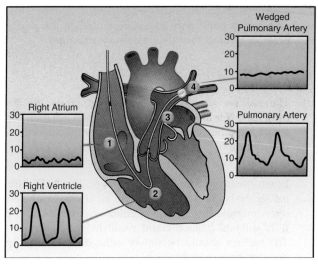

FIGURE 5.1 The pressure waveforms encountered during placement of a pulmonary artery catheter. See text for explanation.

4. As the catheter is advanced along the pulmonary artery, the pulsatile waveform eventually disappears, leaving a nonpulsatile pressure (which is typically at the same level as the diastolic pressure of the pulsatile waveform). This is the *pulmonary artery occlusion pressure*, also called the *wedge pressure*, and it is a reflection of the filling pressure of the left side of the heart (see the next section).

5. When the wedge pressure tracing first appears, the catheter is held in place (not advanced further). The balloon is then deflated, and the pulsatile pressure waveform should reappear. The catheter is then secured in place.

6. In about 25% of cases, the pulsatile PA pressure never disappears despite advancing the PA catheter maximally (1). When this occurs, the PA diastolic pressure can be used as

a surrogate measure of the wedge pressure, except in the presence of pulmonary hypertension (when the wedge pressure is lower than the PA diastolic pressure).

D. The Balloon

1. The balloon should remain deflated while the PA catheter is left in place (sustained balloon inflation can result in pulmonary artery rupture or pulmonary infarction). Balloon inflation is permitted only when it is desirable to measure the wedge pressure.

2. When measuring the wedge pressure, DO NOT fully inflate the balloon with 1.5 mL air all at once (catheters often migrate into smaller pulmonary arteries, and a fully inflated balloon could result in vessel rupture). The balloon should be slowly inflated until a wedge pressure tracing is obtained.

3. Once the wedge pressure is recorded, the balloon should be fully deflated. Detaching the syringe from the balloon injection port will help prevent inadvertent balloon inflation while the catheter is in place.

II. THE WEDGE PRESSURE

A. The Principle

The principle of the wedge pressure measurement is illustrated in Figure 5.2.

1. Inflation of the balloon on the PA catheter obstructs blood flow (Q) in the pulmonary artery, and this creates a static column of blood between the tip of the catheter and the left atrium. In this situation, the "wedged" pressure at the tip of the catheter (P_W) is the same as the pulmonary capillary pressure (P_C) and the pressure in

the left atrium (P_{LA}); i.e., if $Q = 0$, then $P_W = P_C = P_{LA}$.

2. The wedge pressure will reflect left atrial pressure only if the pulmonary capillary pressure is greater than the alveolar pressure ($P_C > P_A$). This condition is not satisfied when the wedge pressure varies with the respiratory cycle (2) (see later).

3. If the mitral valve is behaving normally, the left atrial pressure (wedge pressure) is equivalent to the end-diastolic pressure (the filling pressure) of the left ventricle. Therefore, in the absence of mitral valve disease, the wedge pressure is a measure of left ventricular filling pressure.

B. Wedge vs. Pulmonary Capillary Pressure

1. The wedge pressure is often mistaken as a measure of the physiological pressure in the pulmonary capillaries,

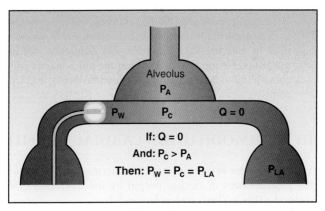

FIGURE 5.2 The principle of the wedge pressure measurement. When flow ceases because of balloon inflation ($Q=0$), the wedge pressure (P_W) is the same as the pulmonary capillary pressure (P_C) and the pressure in the left atrium (P_{LA}), but this relationship occurs only when the pulmonary capillary pressure exceeds the alveolar pressure ($P_C > P_A$).

but this is not the case (3,4) because the wedge pressure is measured in the absence of blood flow. When the balloon is deflated and flow resumes, *the pressure in the pulmonary capillaries must be higher than the pressure in the left atrium (the wedge pressure); otherwise, there would be no pressure gradient for flow in the pulmonary veins.*

2. The difference between pulmonary capillary pressure (P_C) and left atrial pressure (P_{LA}) is determined by the rate of blood flow (Q) and the resistance to flow in the pulmonary veins (R_V); i.e.,

$$P_C - P_{LA} = Q \times R_V \qquad (5.1)$$

Since the wedge pressure (P_W) is equivalent to the left atrial pressure, Equation 5.1 can be restated as follows:

$$P_C - P_W = Q \times R_V \qquad (5.2)$$

3. Therefore, *in the presence of blood flow, the wedge pressure will always underestimate the pulmonary capillary pressure.* The magnitude of the (P_C-P_W) difference is not possible to determine in individual patients because it is not possible to measure R_V. However, this difference will be magnified by conditions that promote pulmonary venoconstriction, such as hypoxemia, endotoxemia, and the acute respiratory distress syndrome (ARDS) (5,6).

III. THERMODILUTION CARDIAC OUTPUT

The PA catheter is equipped with a thermistor that allows the measurement of cardiac output by the thermodilution method. This is illustrated in Figure 5.3.

A. The Method

1. A dextrose or saline solution that is colder than blood is

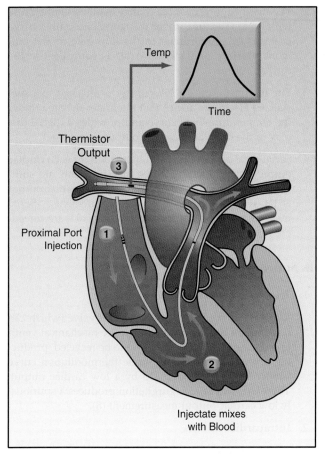

FIGURE 5.3 The thermodilution method of measuring cardiac output. See text for explanation.

injected through the proximal port of the PA catheter (usually located in the right atrium). This cools the blood in the right heart chambers, and the cooled blood then flows past the thermistor at the distal end of the PA catheter.

2. The thermistor records the change in blood temperature with time. The area under the temperature-time curve is inversely proportional to the flow rate in the pulmonary artery, and this flow rate is equivalent to the cardiac output.

3. The thermistor on the PA catheter is attached to a specialized electronic device that integrates the area under the temperature–time curve and provides a digital display of the calculated cardiac output.

4. Serial measurements are recommended for each cardiac output determination. Three measurements are sufficient if they differ by 10% or less, and the cardiac output is taken as the average of all measurements. Serial measurements that differ by more than 10% are considered unreliable (7).

B. Sources of Error

1. **Tricuspid Regurgitation**

   Regurgitant flow across the tricuspid valve (which can be common during positive-pressure mechanical ventilation) causes the indicator fluid to be recycled, producing a prolonged, low-amplitude thermodilution curve similar to the one produced by a low cardiac output. Therefore, tricuspid regurgitation produces a spuriously low cardiac output measurement (8).

2. **Intracardiac Shunts**

   Intracardiac shunts produce falsely elevated cardiac output measurements.

   a. In right-to-left shunts, a portion of the cold injectate fluid passes through the shunt, creating an abbreviated thermodilution curve similar to the one produced by a high-cardiac output.

   b. In left-to-right shunts, the thermodilution curve is

also abbreviated, because the shunted blood increases the blood volume in the right heart chambers, and this reduces the change in blood temperature produced by the cold injectate fluid.

IV. CARDIOVASCULAR PARAMETERS

The PA catheter provides a wealth of information about cardiovascular function and systemic oxygen transport. The following parameters provide information on cardiac performance, and the hemodynamic origins of hypotension. These parameters are included in Table 5.1, along with the normal range of values for each parameter.

Table 5.1	Cardiovascular and Oxygen Transport Parameters	
Parameter	**Abbreviation**	**Normal Range**
Central Venous Pressure	CVP	0–5 mm Hg
Pulmonary Artery Wedge Pressure	PAWP	6–12 mm Hg
Cardiac Index	CI	2.4–4.0 L/min/m²
Stroke Index	SI	20–40 mL/m²
Systemic Vascular Resistance Index	SVRI	25–30 Wood Units†
Pulmonary Vascular Resistance Index	PVRI	1–2 Wood Units†
Oxygen Delivery	DO₂	520–570 mL/min/m²
Oxygen Uptake	VO₂	110–160 mL/min/m²
Oxygen Extraction Ratio	O₂ER	0.2–0.3

†mm Hg per L/min per m².

A. Cardiac Filling Pressures

1. **Central Venous Pressure**

   When the PA catheter is properly placed, the proximal port of the catheter should be situated in the right atrium, and the pressure recorded from this port should be the mean right atrial pressure, also known as the *central venous pressure* (CVP). This pressure is equivalent to the right ventricular end-diastolic pressure (RVEDP) when tricuspid valve function is normal.

$$CVP = RVEDP \qquad (5.3)$$

   The CVP is normally a low pressure (0–5 mm Hg), which helps to promote venous return to the right side of the heart.

2. **Pulmonary Artery Wedge Pressure**

   The pulmonary artery wedge pressure (PAWP) is described earlier in the chapter, and is equivalent to the left ventricular end-diastolic pressure (LVEDP) when mitral valve function is normal.

$$PAWP = LVEDP \qquad (5.4)$$

   The normal PAWP (6–12 mm Hg) is slightly higher than the CVP, and this pressure difference keeps the foramen ovale closed (which prevents intracardiac right-to-left shunts).

   VARIABILITY: There is an inherent variability in the wedge pressure, which does not exceed 4 mm Hg in most patients (10). Therefore, *a recorded change in the wedge pressure should exceed 4 mm Hg to be considered a clinically significant change.*

3. **Respiratory Fluctuations**

   Changes in intrathoracic pressure can be transmitted into blood vessels in the thorax, and this can produce respiratory fluctuations in the CVP or wedge pressure, as shown in Figure 5.4. These changes in intrathoracic pressure are misleading because the *transmural pressure* (i.e., the physiologically important pressure) is not changing.

Therefore, *when respiratory variations are evident in the CVP or wedge pressure, the pressure should be measured at the end of expiration,* when intrathoracic pressure is closest to atmospheric (zero reference) pressure.

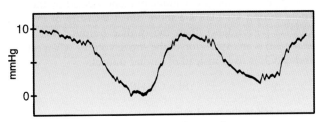

FIGURE 5.4 Respiratory fluctuations in the central venous pressure.

B. Cardiac Index

The thermodilution cardiac output (CO) is expressed in relation to body size using the body surface area (BSA). The size-adjusted cardiac output is called the *cardiac index* (CI).

$$CI = CO/BSA \qquad (5.5)$$

(Size-adjusted hemodynamic parameters typically include the term *index*.)

1. The thermistor on the PA catheter is connected to a cardiac output monitor that will automatically determine the BSA based on the patient's height and weight. The BSA can also be determined with the following simple formula (11):

$$BSA\ (m) = \frac{Ht\ (cm) + Wt\ (kg) - 60}{100} \qquad (5.6)$$

(An average-sized adult has a BSA of 1.7 m².)

2. The normal cardiac index is 2.4–4 L/min/m², and there is an inherent variability of ±10% (10), which means that *a change in the cardiac index must exceed 10% to be considered a clinically significant change.*

C. Stroke Index

The stroke volume (the volume of blood ejected by the ventricle during systole) is a more direct measure of intrinsic cardiac performance than the cardiac output. The *stroke index* (SI) is an expression of the stroke volume when cardiac index (CI) is used instead of cardiac output:

$$SI = CI/HR \qquad (5.7)$$

(where HR is the heart rate).

D. Vascular Resistance

The resistance to flow in the systemic and pulmonary circulations is not a clinically measurable quantity because resistance is flow dependent, and blood vessels are compressible and not rigid. The following measures of vascular resistance are simply expressions of the relationship between averaged flow rates (cardiac output) and intravascular pressure gradients.

1. **Systemic Vascular Resistance Index**

   The *systemic vascular resistance index* (SVRI) is calculated as the difference between mean arterial pressure (MAP) and CVP, divided by the cardiac index (CI).

   $$SVRI = (MAP - CVP)/CI \qquad (5.8)$$

   The SVRI is expressed in Wood units (mm Hg/L/min/m²), which can be multiplied by 80 to convert to conventional units of resistance (dynes•sec⁻¹•cm⁻⁵/m²) (12). However, this conversion offers no advantage.

2. **Pulmonary Vascular Resistance Index**

The *pulmonary vascular resistance index* (PVRI) is calculated as the difference between the mean pulmonary artery pressure (MPAP) and the mean left atrial pressure. or pulmonary artery wedge pressure (PAWP), divided by the cardiac index (CI).

$$PVRI = (MPAP - PAWP)/CI \qquad (5.9)$$

The PVRI has the the the same units (mm $Hg/L/min/m^2$) as the SVRI, and has the same limitations just described for the SVRI.

V. OXYGEN TRANSPORT PARAMETERS

Oxygen transport parameters are global measures of systemic oxygen supply and oxygen consumption, and they provide an indirect assessment of tissue oxygenation (as demonstrated in the next chapter). These parameters are expressed in relation to body size, and the normal range for each parameter is shown in Table 5.1.

A. Oxygen Delivery

The rate of oxygen transport in arterial blood is known as *oxygen delivery* (DO_2), and is equivalent to the product of the cardiac index (CI) and the O_2 content in arterial blood (CaO_2).

$$DO_2 = CI \times CaO_2 \times 10 \qquad (5.10)$$

1. The CaO_2 is expressed as mL O_2 per 100 mL blood (mL/100 mL), and the multiplier of 10 is used to convert the units to mL/L.

2. CaO_2 is equivalent to the product of the hemoglobin concentration [Hb] (g/100 mL), the O_2 binding capacity of Hb (1.34 mL/g/100 mL), and the saturation of Hb

with O_2 in arterial blood (SaO_2). Therefore, Equation 5.10 can be restated as follows:

$$DO_2 = CI \times (1.34 \times [Hb] \times SaO_2) \times 10 \qquad (5.11)$$

3. DO_2 is expressed as $mL/min/m^2$, and the normal range is 520–600 $mL/min/m^2$.

B. Oxygen Uptake

Oxygen uptake (VO_2) is the rate at which O_2 is taken up from the systemic capillaries into the tissues. Since O_2 is not stored in tissues, VO_2 *is equivalent to O_2 consumption.* The VO_2 is calculated as the product of the cardiac index (CI) and the difference in O_2 content between arterial and venous blood ($CaO_2 - CvO_2$).

$$VO_2 = CI \times (CaO_2 - CvO_2) \times 10 \qquad (5.12)$$

(The multiplier of 10 is included for the same reason as explained for the DO_2.) This equation is a modified version of the Fick equation for cardiac output ($CO = VO_2/(CaO_2 - CvO_2)$.

1. If the CaO_2 and CvO_2 are each broken down into their component parts, Equation 5.12 can be rewritten as:

$$VO_2 = CI \times 1.34 \times [Hb] \times (SaO_2 - SvO_2) \times 10 \qquad (5.13)$$

where SaO_2 and SvO_2 are the oxyhemoglobin saturations in arterial and venous blood, respectively. (Venous blood in this instance is "mixed" venous blood in the pulmonary arteries.)

2. VO_2 is expressed as $mL/min/m^2$, and the normal range is 110–160 $mL/min/m^2$. A subnormal VO_2 in critically ill patients (who rarely have a low metabolic rate) is reasonable evidence of impaired tissue oxygenation.

3. The inherent variability of the calculated VO_2 is high ($\pm18\%$) because it represents the summed variability of the 4 component measurements (10,13,14).

4. The calculated VO_2 from the modified Fick equation is not the whole body VO_2 because it does not include the O_2 consumption of the lungs. The VO_2 of the lungs normally accounts for less than 5% of the whole body VO_2 (1), but it can make up 20% of the whole body VO_2 when there is inflammation in the lungs (which is common in ICU patients) (16).

C. Oxygen Extraction Ratio

The balance between O_2 delivery (DO_2) and O_2 uptake (VO_2) is expressed by the oxygen extraction ratio (O_2ER), which is equivalent to the VO_2/DO_2 ratio (often multiplied by 100 to express it as a percent).

$$O_2ER = VO_2/DO_2 \qquad (5.14)$$

1. The normal O_2ER is 0.2–0.3, which means that only 20–30% of the O_2 delivered to the systemic capillaries is taken up into the tissues. The O_2ER can increase up to 0.5–0.6 when O_2 delivery is reduced, and this helps to maintain tissue oxygenation despite a declining O_2 supply.

2. The next chapter describes how the O_2ER can be used to evaluate tissue oxygenation.

REFERENCES

1. Swan HJ. The pulmonary artery catheter. Dis Mon 1991; 37:473–543.

2. O'Quin R, Marini JJ. Pulmonary artery occlusion pressure: clinical physiology, measurement, and interpretation. Am Rev Respir Dis 1983; 128:319–326.

3. Cope DK, Grimbert F, Downey JM, et al. Pulmonary capillary pressure: a review. Crit Care Med 1992; 20:1043–1056.

4. Pinsky MR. Hemodynamic monitoring in the intensive care unit. Clin Chest Med 2003; 24:549–560.

5. Tracey WR, Hamilton JT, Craig ID, Paterson NAM. Effect of endothelial injury on the responses of isolated guinea pig pulmonary venules to reduced oxygen tension. J Appl Physiol 1989; 67:2147–2153.

6. Kloess T, Birkenhauer U, Kottler B. Pulmonary pressure–flow relationship and peripheral oxygen supply in ARDS due to bacterial sepsis. Second Vienna Shock Forum, 1989:175–18.

7. Nadeau S, Noble WH. Limitations of cardiac output measurement by thermodilution. Can J Anesth 1986; 33:780–784.

8. Konishi T, Nakamura Y, Morii I, et al. Comparison of thermodilution and Fick methods for measurement of cardiac output in tricuspid regurgitation. Am J Cardiol 1992; 70:538–540.

9. Nemens EJ, Woods SL. Normal fluctuations in pulmonary artery and pulmonary capillary wedge pressures in acutely ill patients. Heart Lung 1982; 11:393–398.

10. Sasse SA, Chen PA, Berry RB, et al. Variability of cardiac output over time in medical intensive care unit patients. Chest 1994; 22:225–232.

11. Mattar JA. A simple calculation to estimate body surface area in adults and its correlation with the Dubois formula. Crit Care Med 1989; 846–847.

12. Bartlett RH. Critical Care Physiology. New York: Little, Brown & Co, 1996:36.

13. Schneeweiss B, Druml W, Graninger W, et al. Assessment of oxygen-consumption by use of reverse Fick-principle and indirect calorimetry in critically ill patients. Clin Nutr 1989; 8:89–93.

14. Bartlett RH, Dechert RE. Oxygen kinetics: Pitfalls in clinical research. J Crit Care 1990; 5:77-80.

15. Nunn JF. Non respiratory functions of the lung. In: Nunn JF (ed). Applied Respiratory Physiology. Butterworth, London, 1993:306–317.

16. Jolliet P, Thorens JB, Nicod L, et al. Relationship between pulmonary oxygen consumption, lung inflammation, and calculated venous admixture in patients with acute lung injury. Intensive Care Med 1996; 22:277–285.

Chapter 6

Systemic Oxygenation

One of the fundamental goals of critical care management is to promote tissue oxygenation, yet it is not possible to monitor tissue oxygen levels in a clinical setting. This chapter describes the measures of "systemic" oxygenation that are available, and how they can be used to evaluate tissue oxygenation.

I. MEASURES OF SYSTEMIC OXYGENATION

A. Oxygen Content of Blood

The concentration of O_2 in blood (called the O_2 *content*) is the summed contribution of the O_2 that is bound to hemoglobin (Hb) and the O_2 that is dissolved in plasma.

1. **Hemoglobin–Bound O_2**

   The concentration of hemoglobin-bound O_2 (HbO_2) is determined as follows (1):

   $$HbO_2 = 1.34 \times Hb \times SO_2 \quad \text{(mL/dL)} \qquad (6.1)$$

   where Hb is the hemoglobin concentration in g/dL (grams per 100 mL), 1.34 is the O_2 binding capacity of hemoglobin (mL/g), and SO_2 is the O_2 saturation of Hb, expressed as a ratio (HbO_2/Total Hb).

   a. Equation 6.1 states that, when Hb is fully saturated with oxygen ($SO_2 = 1$), each gram of Hb binds 1.34 mL O_2.

2. **Dissolved O_2**

The concentration of dissolved O_2 in plasma is determined as follows (2):

$$\text{Dissolved } O_2 = 0.003 \times PO_2 \quad \text{(mL/dL)} \quad (6.2)$$

where PO_2 is the partial pressure of O_2 in blood (in mm Hg), and 0.003 is the solubility coefficient of O_2 in plasma (mL/dL/mm Hg) at normal body temperature.

   a. Equation 6.2 states that, at normal body temperature (37°C), each 1 mm Hg increment in PO_2 will increase the concentration of dissolved O_2 by 0.003 mL/dL (or 0.03 mL/L) (2). This highlights *the poor solubility of oxygen in plasma* (which is why hemoglobin is needed as a carrier molecule).

3. **Total O_2 Content**

   . The total O_2 content in blood (mL/dL) is determined by combining Equations 6.1 and 6.2:

$$O_2 \text{ Content} = (1.34 \times Hb \times SaO_2) + (0.003 \times PaO_2) \quad (6.3)$$

   . Table 6.1 shows the normal concentrations of O_2 (bound, dissolved, and total O_2) in arterial and venous blood. Note that the contribution of dissolved O_2 is very small; as a result, *the O_2 content of blood is considered equivalent to the Hb-bound fraction.*

$$O_2 \text{ Content} = 1.34 \times Hb \times SO_2 \quad \text{(mL/dL)} \quad (6.4)$$

B. Oxygen Delivery

1. The rate of O_2 transport in arterial blood, also known as *oxygen delivery* (DO_2), is a function of the cardiac output (CO) and the O_2 content of arterial blood (CaO_2) (3).

$$DO_2 = CO \times CaO_2 \times 10 \quad \text{(mL/min)} \quad (6.5)$$

(The multiplier of 10 is used to convert the CaO_2 from mL/dL to mL/L.) If the CaO_2 is broken down into its components, Equation 6.5 can be rewritten as:

$$DO_2 = CO \times (1.34 \times Hb \times SaO_2) \times 10 \qquad (6.6)$$

Note: The SaO_2 is monitored continuously with pulse oximeters, and the cardiac output can be measured with a pulmonary artery catheter (described in pages 88–91), or it can be measured noninvasively using techniques described in Reference 4.

Table 6.1	Normal Measures of Blood Oxygenation	
Measure	**Arterial Blood**	**Venous Blood**
Partial Pressure of O_2	90 mm Hg	40 mm Hg
% Oxygenated Hb	98%	73%
Hb-bound O_2	19.7 mL/dL	14.7 mL/dL
Dissolved O_2	0.3 mL/dL	0.1 mL/dL
Total O_2 Content	20 mL/dL	14.8 mL/dL
Blood Volume†	1.25 L	3.75 L
Total Volume of O_2	250 mL	555 mL

Values shown are for a body temperature of 37°C and a hemoglobin concentration of 15 g/dL.

†Volume estimates based on a total blood volume (TBV) of 5 Liters, arterial blood volume = 25% of TBV, and venous blood volume = 75% of TBV.

Abbreviations: Hb = hemoglobin; dL = deciliter (100 mL).

3. The normal range of values for DO_2 are shown in Table 6.2. Note that the DO_2 (and VO_2) are expressed in absolute and size-adjusted terms; the body size adjustment is based on body surface area in square meters (m^2).

Table 6.2	Measures of Systemic Oxygen Balance	
Measure	**Normal**	**Tissue Hypoxia**
DO_2	900–1100 mL/min or 520–600 mL/min/m²	Variable
VO_2	200–270 mL/min or 110–160 mL/min/m²	<200 mL/min or <110 mL/min/m²
O_2ER	20–30%	≥50%
SvO_2	65–75%	≤50%
$ScvO_2$	70–80%	?
Lactate	1–2.2 mmol/L[1]	>1–2.2 mmol/L[1]

[1]Normal lactate levels vary from 1.0 to 2.2 mmol/L in individual laboratories.

Abbreviations: DO_2 = O_2 delivery; VO_2 = O_2 consumption; O_2ER = O_2 extraction ratio; SvO_2 = mixed venous O_2 saturation; $ScvO_2$ = central venous O_2 saturation.

C. Oxygen Consumption

The rate of O_2 uptake into tissues is equivalent to the *oxygen consumption* (VO_2) because O_2 is not stored in tissues There are two methods for determining the VO_2.

1. **Calculated VO_2**

   The VO_2 can be calculated as the product of the cardiac output (CO) and the difference between arterial and venous O_2 contents ($CaO_2 - CvO_2$).

   $$VO_2 = CO \times (CaO_2 - CvO_2) \times 10 \quad \text{(mL/min)} \quad (6.7)$$

   (The multiplier of 10 is explained for the DO_2.) The CaO_2 and CvO_2 share a common term ($1.34 \times Hb$), so Equation 6.7 can be rewritten as:

   $$VO_2 = CO \times 1.34 \times Hb \times (SaO_2 - SvO_2) \times 10 \quad (6.8)$$

Note: Three of the four measurements used to calculate the VO_2 are also used to calculate the DO_2. The one additional measurement is the SvO_2, which is described later in the chapter.

a. The normal range of values for VO_2 is shown in Table 6.2. Note that the VO_2 is much smaller than the DO_2; the significance of this discrepancy is described later.

b. Each of the measurements used to calculate the VO_2 has an inherent variability, and the summed variability of the 4 measurements is $\pm 18\%$ (5-7). Therefore, *the calculated VO_2 must change by at least 18% for the change to be considered significant.*

2. **Calculated vs. Whole Body VO_2**

   The calculated VO_2 is not the whole body VO_2 because it does not include the O_2 consumption of the lungs. Normally, the VO_2 of the lungs represents $<5\%$ of the whole body VO_2 (8), but it can account for as much as 20% of the whole body VO_2 when there is an inflammatory process in the lungs (9).

3. **Measured VO_2**

   The whole body VO_2 can be measured with an O_2 analyzer that measures the fractional concentration of O_2 in inhaled and exhaled gas. The VO_2 is then derived as follows:

   $$VO_2 = V_E \times (F_IO_2 - F_EO_2) \qquad (6.9)$$

   where F_IO_2 and F_EO_2 are the fractional concentrations of O_2 in inhaled and exhaled gas, respectively, and V_E is the volume of gas exhaled each minute.

   a. The metabolic carts used by nutrition support services can measure whole body VO_2 at the bedside (see Section IB in Chapter 36).

   b. The inherent variability of the measured VO_2 is $\pm 5\%$ (5,7), which is much less than the inherent variability ($\pm 18\%$) of the calculated VO_2.

D. Oxygen Extraction

1. The relationship between O_2 delivery and O_2 consumption is expressed as the *oxygen extraction ratio* (O_2ER); i.e.,

$$O_2ER = VO_2/DO_2 \qquad (6.10)$$

   (This ratio is commonly multiplied by 100 and expressed as a percentage.) This expresses the fraction of the O_2 delivered to tissues that is used by aerobic metabolism.

2. The normal range for the O_2ER is 0.2–0.3 (20–30%), which means that *in healthy adults at rest, only 20–30% of the O_2 delivered to tissues is used by aerobic metabolism.*

3. The VO_2 and DO_2 in Equation 6.10 share common terms ($Q \times 1.34 \times Hb \times 10$), so the equation can be reduced to the following terms:

$$O_2ER = (SaO_2 - SvO_2)/SaO_2 \qquad (6.11)$$

   Since the traditional practice is to keep the SaO_2 above 90%, (close to an $SaO_2 = 1$), Equation 6.11 can be rewritten as:

$$O_2ER = SaO_2 - SvO_2 \qquad (6.12)$$

   or

$$O_2ER = 1 - SvO_2 \qquad (6.13)$$

   Thus, *the balance between O_2 delivery and O_2 consumption can be monitored using a single variable; i.e., the venous O_2 saturation (SvO_2), which is described next.*

E. Mixed Venous O_2 Saturation

1. The global (whole-body) measure of venous O_2 saturation (SvO_2) is obtained from venous blood in the pulmonary arteries, and is called the *mixed venous O_2 satu-*

ration. This measurement requires a pulmonary artery catheter (described in Chapter 5), and is not routinely available.

2. The determinants of SvO_2 can be identified by rearranging the terms in Equation 6.8; i.e.,

$$SvO_2 = SaO_2 - (VO_2/CO \times 1.34 \times Hb) \qquad (6.14)$$

If arterial blood is fully oxygenated ($SaO_2 \sim 1$), the denominator in the parentheses is equivalent to the DO_2 (see Equation 6.6), and Equation 6.14 can be rewritten as:

$$SvO_2 = 1 - VO_2/DO_2 \qquad (6.15)$$

(This is equivalent to Equation 6.13 with the terms rearranged.)

3. Equation 6.15 predicts that the SvO_2 will decrease if there is an increase in VO_2 (increased metabolic rate) or a decrease in DO_2 (e.g., from anemia or a low cardiac output).

4. The normal SvO_2 is 65–75% (10).

F. Central Venous O_2 Saturation

1. The O_2 saturation in the superior vena cava, known as the *central venous O_2 saturation* ($ScvO_2$), has become a popular surrogate for the SvO_2 because it is more readily available.

2. The $ScvO_2$ can be measured in blood samples withdrawn through a central venous catheter, or it can be monitored continuously using fiberoptic catheters (PreSep Catheters, Edwards Life Sciences, Irvine, CA).

3. The $ScvO_2$ is higher than the SvO_2 by an average of 5% in critically ill patients (11), and this translates to a normal $ScvO_2$ of 70–80% (i.e., 5% higher than the normal range for SvO_2). However, there can be large discrepan-

cies between the $ScvO_2$ and SvO_2, in hemodynamically unstable patients.

4. Changes in $ScvO_2$ correlate closely with changes in SvO_2 (11,12). As a result, trends in the $ScvO_2$ are considered more reliable than single measurements.

II. SYSTEMIC OXYGEN BALANCE

A. Control of VO_2

1. The aerobic support system operates to maintain a constant rate of aerobic metabolism (VO_2) despite variations in O_2 supply (DO_2). This is possible because changes in DO_2 are accompanied by reciprocal changes in O_2 extraction (O_2ER). These relationships are shown by rearranging Equation 6.10; i.e.,

$$VO_2 = DO_2 \times O_2ER \qquad (6.16)$$

2. Equation 6.16 predicts that the VO_2 will remain constant if changes in DO_2 are accompanied by equal and opposite changes in O_2ER. However, if the O_2ER is fixed and invariant, changes in DO_2 will result in equivalent changes in VO_2. Therefore, *the adjustability of O_2 extraction allows VO_2 to remain independent of changes in O_2 supply.*

B. The DO_2–VO_2 Curve

1. The response to a progressive decline in O_2 supply is shown in Figure 6.1 (13). The equation at the top of the figure is similar to Equation 6.16, but O_2 extraction is represented by the (SaO_2 – SvO_2), as in Equation 6.12.

   a. As the DO_2 decreases (arrows indicating movement to the left along the curve), the VO_2 remains constant

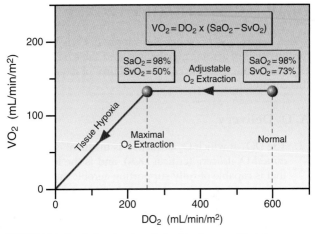

FIGURE 6.1 Graph showing the relationships between O_2 delivery (DO_2), O_2 consumption (VO_2), and O_2 extraction ($SaO_2 - SvO_2$) when DO_2 is progressively decreased. See text for explanation.

until a point is reached where the SvO_2 has decreased from 73% to 50%, and the corresponding O_2 extraction ($SaO_2 - SvO_2$) has increased from 25% to 48%. This point is the maximum O_2 extraction that can be achieved in response to decreases in O_2 delivery.

b. When O_2 extraction is maximal, further decreases in DO_2 are accompanied by equivalent decreases in VO_2. When this occurs, aerobic metabolism is restricted by the supply of oxygen, and there is a switch to anaerobic glycolysis and the subsequent accumulation of lactic acid.

c. Therefore, *the point where O_2 extraction is maximal is the anaerobic threshold*, and this point can be detected clinically, as described next.

III. DETECTING TISSUE HYPOXIA

Tissue hypoxia occurs when the supply of O_2 is inadequate for the needs of aerobic metabolism, and Table 6.2 shows the expected changes in the clinical measures of oxygenation in this condition.

A. O_2 Delivery

1. The DO_2 at which O_2 extraction is maximal is called the *critical O_2 delivery* (critical DO_2), and is the lowest DO_2 that is capable of fully supporting aerobic metabolism.

2. The critical DO_2 has varied widely in studies of critically ill patients (13,14), and it is not possible to identify the critical DO_2 in any individual patient.

B. O_2 Consumption

1. A subnormal VO_2 can be the result of hypometabolism or tissue hypoxia.

2. Hypometabolism is uncommon in critically ill patients, so a low VO_2 (<200 mL/min or <110 mL/min/m²) can be used as evidence of tissue hypoxia.

C. O_2 Extraction $(SaO_2 - SvO_2)$

1. As indicated in Figure 6.1, an increase in $(SaO_2 - SvO_2)$ to approximately 50% represents the maximum O_2 extraction (i.e., the anaerobic threshold).

2. Therefore, an $(SaO_2 - SvO_2) \geq 50\%$ can be used as evidence of threatened or impaired tissue oxygenation.

D. Venous O_2 Saturation $(SvO_2, ScvO_2)$

1. The curve in Figure 6.1 shows that the mixed venous O_2

saturation (SvO_2) decreases to 50% at the point where O_2 extraction is maximum (i.e., the anaerobic threshold).

2. Therefore, an $SvO_2 \leq 50\%$ can be used as evidence of threatened or impaired tissue oxygenation.

3. A central venous O_2 saturation ($ScvO_2$) <70% is considered abnormal, and an $ScvO_2$ >70% has been recommended as a goal of therapy aimed at increasing O_2 delivery (15,16). However, the $ScvO_2$ that identifies tissue hypoxia has not been defined.

E. Blood Lactate

Note: There are several conditions unrelated to tissue oxygenation that promote lactate accumulation in blood, and these are described in Chapter 24. The following pertains only to hyperlactatemia from derangements in tissue oxygenation.

1. Lactic acid is the end-product of anaerobic glycolysis, and the accumulation of lactate in blood is the most widely used marker of tissue hypoxia.

2. Lactate levels can be measured in venous or arterial blood, with equivalent results (17).

3. The upper limit of normal for the serum lactate concentration varies from 1.0 to 2.2 mmol/L in individual laboratories (17), but 2 mmol/L seems to be a common cut-off point.

4. The serum lactate level is not only a diagnostic tool, but also has predictive value; i.e., *the probability of survival is related to both the initial lactate level (prior to treatment), and the time required for normalization of lactate levels* (called *lactate clearance*). These relationships are demonstrated in Figure 6.2.

   a. The graph on the left in Figure 6.2 is from a study of septic patients (18), and shows a direct relationship

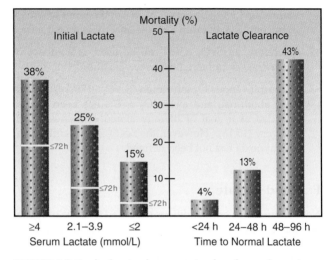

FIGURE 6.2 Graphs showing the prognostic value of serum lactate levels. Graph on the left (from Reference 18) shows the association between initial lactate levels and in-hospital mortality, including the mortality rate in the first 3 days after presentation. Graph on the right (from Reference 20) shows the association between the time for elevated lactate levels to return to normal (lactate clearance) and in-hospital mortality rate.

between initial lactate levels and in-hospital mortality. It also shows that mortality rates in the first 72 hours increase dramatically when the initial lactate level exceeds 4 mmol/L. Other studies have also noted that *the greatest increase in ICU mortality rates occur when serum lactate levels rise above 4 mmol/L* (19).

b. The graph on the right in Figure 6.2 is from a study involving hemodynamically unstable patients (20), and shows that mortality was lowest when lactate levels were normalized within 24 hours, while the mortality rate increased dramatically when lactate levels remained elevated after 48 hours.

5. Studies involving patients with septic shock show that *the rate of lactate clearance has greater prognostic value than the initial lactate level* (20,21). As a result, serial lactate measurements are advised for all patients with elevated lactate levels at presentation.

F. Cytopathic Hypoxia

Oxygen-restricted aerobic metabolism can also be the result of a defect in O_2 utilization in mitochondria. This condition is known as *cytopathic hypoxia* (22), and it is the presumed *mechanism for cellular dysfunction in septic shock.* Cytopathic hypoxia (in septic shock) differs from tissue hypoxia in the following ways.

1. Tissue O_2 levels may not be reduced in patients with cytopathic hypoxia. This is supported by studies showing that tissue PO_2 is *increased* in patients with systemic sepsis (23), and that a majority of patients with septic shock have a normal (rather than reduced) $ScvO_2$ (24).

2. Lactate elevation has the same diagnostic and prognostic implications in septic shock (18,21). However, lactate accumulation in sepsis may not be the result of an inadequate O_2 supply, but instead may be related to inhibition of pyruvate dehydrogenase (the enzyme that converts pyruvate to acetyl coenzyme A) (25).

3. The notion that tissue O_2 levels are not deficient in patients with cytopathic hypoxia (septic shock) has important implications for the management of these patients (which is described in Chapter 9).

REFERENCES

1. Zander R. Calculation of oxygen concentration. In: Zander R, Mertzlufft F, eds. The oxygen status of arterial blood. Basel: S. Karger, 1991:203–209.

2. Christoforides C, Laasberg L, Hedley-Whyte J. Effect of temperature on solubility of O_2 in plasma. J. Appl Physiol 1969; 26: 56–60.

3. Hameed S, Aird W, Cohn S. Oxygen delivery. Crit Care Med 2003; 31(Suppl): S658–S667.

4. Mohammed I, Phillips C. Techniques for determining cardiac output in the intensive care unit. Crit Care Clin 2010; 26:353–364.

5. Schneeweiss B, Druml W, Graninger W, et al. Assessment of oxygen-consumption by use of reverse Fick-principle and indirect calorimetry in critically ill patients. Clin Nutr 1989; 8:89–93.

6. Sasse SA, Chen PA, Berry RB, et al. Variability of cardiac output over time in medical intensive care unit patients. Chest 1994; 22:225–232.

7. Bartlett RH, Dechert RE. Oxygen kinetics: Pitfalls in clinical research. J Crit Care 1990; 5:77–80.

8. Nunn JF. Non respiratory functions of the lung. In Nunn JF (ed). Applied Respiratory Physiology. Butterworth, London, 1993:306–317.

9. Jolliet P, Thorens JB, Nicod L, et al. Relationship between pulmonary oxygen consumption, lung inflammation, and calculated venous admixture in patients with acute lung injury. Intensive Care Med 1996; 22:277–285.

10. Maddirala S, Khan A. Optimizing hemodynamic support in septic shock using central venous and mixed venous oxygen saturation. Crit Care Clin 2010; 26:323–333.

11. Reinhart K, Kuhn H-J, Hartog C, Bredle DL. Continuous central venous and pulmonary artery oxygen saturation monitoring in the critically ill. Intensive Care Med 2004; 30: 1572–1578.

12. Dueck MH, Kilmek M, Appenrodt S, et al. Trends but not individual values of central venous oxygen saturation agree with mixed venous oxygen saturation during varying hemodynamic conditions. Anesthesiology 2005; 103:249–257.

13. Leach RM, Treacher DF. Relationship between oxygen delivery and consumption. Disease-a-Month 1994; 30:301–368.

14. Ronco J, Fenwick J, Tweedale M, et al. Identification of the critical oxygen delivery for anaerobic metabolism in critically ill septic and nonseptic humans. JAMA 1993; 270:1724–1730.

15. Vallet B, Robin E, Lebuffe G. Venous oxygen saturation as a transfusion trigger. Crit Care 2010; 14:213–217.

16. Dellinger RP, Levy MM, Rhodes A, et al. Surviving sepsis campaign: international guidelines for management of severe sepsis and septic shock: 2012. Intensive Care Med 2013; 39:165–228.

17. Kraut JA, Madias NE. Lactic acidosis. N Engl J Med 2014; 371:2309–2319.

18. Trzeciak S, Dellinger RP, Chansky ME, et al. Serum lactate as a predictor of mortality in patients with infection. Intensive Care Med 2007; 33:970–977.

19. Aduen J, Bernstein WK, Khastgir T, et al. The use and clinical importance of a substrate-specific electrode for rapid determination of blood lactate concentrations. JAMA 1994; 272:1678–1685.

20. McNelis J, Marini CP, Jurkiewicz A, et al. Prolonged lactate clearance is associated with increased mortality in the surgical intensive care unit. Am J Surg 2001; 182:481–485.

21. Okorie ON, Dellinger P. Lactate: biomarker and potential therapeutic target. Crit Care Clin 2011; 27:299–326.

22. Fink MP. Cytopathic hypoxia. Mitochondrial dysfunction as a mechanism contributing to organ dysfunction in sepsis. Crit Care Clin 2001; 17:219–237.

23. Sair M, Etherington PJ, Winlove CP, Evans TW. Tissue oxygenation and perfusion in patients with systemic sepsis. Crit Care Med 2001; 29:1343–1349.

24. Vallee F, Vallet B, Mathe O, et al. Central venous-to-arterial carbon dioxide difference: an additional target for goal-directed therapy in septic shock? Intensive Care Med 2008; 34:2218–2225.

25. Thomas GW, Mains CW, Slone DS, et al. Potential dysregulation of the pyruvate dehydrogenase complex by bacterial toxins and insulin. J Trauma 2009; 67:628–633.

Chapter 7

Hemorrhage and Hypovolemia

The circulatory system operates with a relatively small volume and a volume-responsive pump. This is an energy-efficient design, but it quickly falters when volume is lost. While most internal organs like the lungs, liver, and kidneys can lose as much as 75% of their functional mass without life-threatening organ failure, loss of less than 50% of the blood volume can be fatal. This intolerance to blood loss is the dominant concern in the bleeding patient.

I. BODY FLUIDS & BLOOD LOSS

A. Distribution of Body Fluids

The volume of selected body fluids in adults is shown in Table 7.1 (1). The following points deserve mention:

1. Total body fluid (in liters) accounts for about 60% of the lean body weight in males (600 mL/kg) and 50% of the lean body weight in females (500 mL/kg).

2. Blood volume represents only 11–12% of the total body fluids.

3. Plasma volume is about 25% of interstitial fluid volume. This relationship is important for understanding the volume effects of sodium-rich crystalloid fluids, which is described later in the chapter.

Table 7.1	Volume of Selected Body Fluids in Adults			
Body Fluid	**Men**		**Women**	
	mL/kg	75 kg†	mL/kg	60 kg†
Total Body Fluid	600	45 L	500	30 L
Interstitial Fluid	150	11.3 L	125	7.5 L
Whole Blood	66	5 L	60	3.6 L
Red Blood Cells	26	2. L	24	1.4 L
Plasma	40	3 L	36	2.2 L

†Lean body weight for an average adult male and female. Volume of blood, red blood cells, and plasma (in mL/kg) from Reference 1.

B. Severity of Blood Loss

The American College of Surgeons has proposed the following classification system for acute blood loss (2).

1. **Class I**

   a. Loss of <15% of the blood volume (or <10 mL/kg).

   b. This degree of blood loss is usually fully compensated by interstitial fluid shifts (transcapillary refill), so that blood volume is maintained and clinical findings are minimal or absent.

2. **Class II**

   a. Loss of 15–30% of the blood volume (or 10–20 mL/kg).

   b. This represents the compensated phase of hypovolemia, where blood pressure is maintained by systemic vasoconstriction. Postural changes in pulse rate and blood pressure may be evident, but these findings are inconsistent.

   c. The extremities become cool at this stage, and urine output falls, but does not reach oliguric levels (<0.5 ml/kg/hr).

3. **Class III**

   a. Loss of 30–40% of the blood volume (or 20–30 mL/kg).

   b. This stage marks the onset of decompensated blood loss or *hemorrhagic shock*, where the vasoconstrictor response is no longer able to sustain blood pressure and organ perfusion.

   c. Clinical findings can include supine hypotension, cold extremities, confusion, oliguria (urine output <0.5 mL/kg/hr) and increased lactate levels in blood.

4. **Class IV**

   a. Loss of $>40\%$ of blood volume (or >30 mL/kg).

   b. This degree of blood loss results in progressive hemorrhagic shock, and includes *massive blood loss*; i.e., loss of $>50\%$ of the blood volume in 3 hours.

   c. Clinical findings include limb cyanosis, evidence of multiorgan dysfunction (e.g., lethargy, oliguria, increased liver enzymes, etc.) and progressive lactic acidosis.

II. CLINICAL EVALUATION

The clinical detection of hypovolemia is so flawed that is has been called a *comedy of errors* (3).

A. Vital Signs

The reliability of vital signs in the detection of acute blood loss is shown in Table 7.2 (4,5). Note the following:

1. Supine tachycardia and supine hypotension are absent

(i.e., low sensitivity) in a majority of patients with blood volume deficits up to 1.1 liters (i.e., up to a 25% loss of blood volume in average sized males).

2. Postural pulse increments (≥30 beats/min) and postural hypotension (decrease in systolic pressure ≥20 mm Hg) are uncommon when blood loss is less than 630 mL, but with greater blood loss, postural pulse increments are a sensitive and specific marker of hypovolemia.

Table 7.2	Accuracy of Vital Signs in Detecting Hypovolemia	
Abnormal Finding	**Sensitivity/Specificity**	
	Blood Loss (450–630 mL)†	**Blood Loss (630–1150 mL)§**
Supine Tachycardia[1]	0 / 96%	12% / 96%
Supine Hypotension[2]	13% / 97%	33% / 97%
Postural Pulse Increment[3]	22% / 98%	97% / 98%
Postural Hypotension[4] Age <65 yrs Age ≥65 yrs	9% / 94% 27% / 86%	Not studied Not studied

[1]Pulse rate >100 beats/min. [2]Systolic pressure <95 mm Hg. [3]Increase in pulse rate >30 beats/min. [4]Decrease in systolic pressure >20 mm Hg.
†Equivalent to loss of 10–12% of blood volume in an average-sized male.
§Equivalent to loss of 12–25% of blood volume in an average-sized male.
From References 4 and 5.

B. Central Venous Pressure

1. The central venous pressure (CVP) has traditionally played a prominent role in the evaluation of intravascular volume. However, clinical studies have consistently shown a poor correlation between the CVP and objective measures of blood volume (6). This is demonstrated in Figure 7.1 (7).

2. The consistent lack of correlation between CVP and blood volume measurements has prompted the recommendation that the *CVP should never be used to evaluate blood volume* (6).

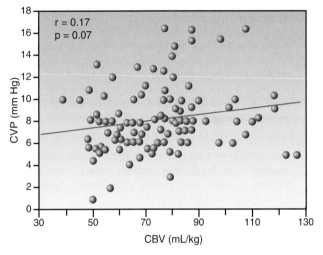

FIGURE 7.1 Scatter plot showing paired measurements of circulating blood volume (CBV) and central venous pressure (CVP) in a group of postoperative patients. Correlation coefficient (r) and p value indicate no significant relationship between the two measurements. Redrawn from Reference 7.

C. Venous O_2 Saturation

1. The O_2 saturation in the superior vena cava ($ScvO_2$) is a surrogate measure of the mixed venous O_2 saturation in the pulmonary arteries (SvO_2), and is a marker of the balance between systemic O_2 delivery (DO_2) and O_2 consumption (VO_2) (see Equation 6.15).

2. Hypovolemia will prompt a decrease in cardiac output and a subsequent decrease in DO_2, which will result in

a decrease in $ScvO_2$. The normal $ScvO_2$ is 70–80%, so in a patient with suspected hypovolemia, an $ScvO_2$ <70% will help to confirm the diagnosis (for more on the $ScvO_2$, see Chapter 6, Sections I-F and III-D).

D. Hemoglobin/Hematocrit

1. Acute hemorrhage involves the loss of whole blood, which is not expected to alter the hemoglobin concentration or hematocrit. This is supported by studies showing a poor correlation between changes in hematocrit and blood volume deficits (or erythrocyte deficits) in acute hemorrhage (8).

2. Any decrease in hemoglobin or hematocrit in acute hemorrhage is a reflection of volume resuscitation with asanguinous fluids (e.g., saline), which expands the plasma volume and causes a dilutional decrease in hemoglobin and hematocrit (9).

3. For the reasons stated above, the hemoglobin and hematocrit should NEVER be used to evaluate the extent of acute blood loss (2).

E. Serum Lactate

1. In the setting of acute blood loss, an elevated serum lactate level (generally >2 mmol/L) is evidence of *hemorrhagic shock*, even in the absence of hypotension. (See Chapter 6, Section III-E for information on lactate as a marker of tissue hypoxia.)

2. Lactate levels also have prognostic value; i.e.,

   a. The magnitude of elevation in lactate levels has a close correlation with the risk of a fatal outcome (10).

   b. The rate of decline in lactate levels (*lactate clearance*) is also related to outcome (see Chapter 6, Figure 6.2).

In one study of trauma victims with hemorrhagic shock, there were no deaths when lactate levels returned to normal within 24 hours, while 86% of the patients died when lactate levels remained elevated after 48 hours (11). Therefore, *normalization of lactate levels within 24 hours can be used as an end-point of resuscitation for hemorrhagic shock* (see later).

F. Arterial Base Deficit

1. The base deficit is the amount (in millimoles) of base needed to titrate one liter of whole blood to a pH of 7.40 (at a PCO_2 of 40 mm Hg); it is considered a more specific marker of metabolic acidosis than the serum bicarbonate (12).

2. The normal range for base deficit is +2 to -2 mmol/L. Increases in base deficit are classified as mild (-3 to -5 mmol/L), moderate (-6 to -14 mmol/L), or severe (≥ -15 mmol/L).

3. In the bleeding patient, there is a direct correlation between the severity of the base deficit and the magnitude of blood loss, and rapid correction of the base deficit is associated with more favorable outcomes (13).

4. Monitoring the base deficit has been a popular practice in trauma resuscitation, but the base deficit is essentially a surrogate measure of lactic acidosis, and it has less predictive value than serum lactate levels in trauma patients (14). Since lactate levels are easily obtained, there is no justification for monitoring the base deficit.

G. Measuring Blood Volume

1. Blood volume measurements have traditionally been too labor intensive and time consuming to be useful in a clinical setting, but this has changed with the introduction of a semiautomated blood volume analyzer (Daxor

Corporation, New York, NY) that provides blood volume measurements is less than an hour.

2. The potential value of this new technology is illustrated by a study of shock resuscitation in surgical patients (15), where 53% of the blood volume measurements led to a change in fluid management, and this was associated with a significant decline in mortality rate (from 24% to 8%).

III. FLUID RESPONSIVENESS

The evaluation of fluid responsiveness is designed to uncover *functional hypovolemia*, and is intended for patients who are hemodynamically unstable or have a declining urine output. The aim of this approach is to limit volume resuscitation to those who are likely to benefit, and thereby reduce the risk of fluid overload, which has an adverse effect on outcomes in critically ill patients (16).

A. Fluid Challenge

1. The goal of a fluid challenge is to increase ventricular end-diastolic volume, and *rapid infusion* is the most important factor in achieving this goal (17).

2. There is no universal standard for a fluid challenge, and *recommendations include 200 mL or 3 mL/kg of a colloid fluid, or 500 mL of a crystalloid fluid, infused over 5–10 minutes* (17,18).

3. Fluid responsiveness is evaluated by monitoring the change in stroke volume or cardiac output (invasively or noninvasively).

   a. An increase in stroke volume or cardiac output of at least 10% indicates fluid responsiveness (18).

   b. The response is short lived, and can disappear 30 minutes after the fluid challenge (18).

4. Parameters that are more easily measured than cardiac output have been studied in relation to fluid challenges, and the following responses have shown a good correlation with a positive cardiac output response:

    a. An increase in pulse pressure >23% by invasive blood pressure recordings (19).

    b. An increase in central venous O_2 saturation ($ScvO_2$) of >4% (20).

    c. An increase in end-tidal PCO_2 of ≥5% (21).

B. Passive Leg Raising

1. Elevating the legs to 45° above the horizontal plane while in the supine position will move 150–750 mL of blood out of the legs and towards the heart (22), thereby serving as an "intrinsic" fluid challenge. The autotransfusion effect can be enhanced by starting with the patient's head in a semirecumbent position (45° above the horizontal plane); placing the head supine with the legs elevated can then mobilize blood from the mesenteric circulation (23).

2. The pooled results from 21 studies shows that a positive response to passive leg raising (i.e., an increase in cardiac output of ≥10%) shows a very good correlation with a similar response to fluid challenges (24).

3. Passive leg raising is a thus a reliable alternative to a fluid challenge, and may be preferred when volume restriction is desirable. It is not advised in patients with increased intraabdominal pressure because the hemodynamic effects are attenuated or lost (25).

C. Predicting Fluid Responsiveness

Respiratory variations in selected parameters have been proposed as methods of predicting fluid responsiveness without the need for a fluid challenge. Despite serious flaws, these methods have become popular, so they are briefly reviewed here.

1. **Inferior Vena Cava Diameter**

   a. The diameter of the inferior vena cava (IVCD) is measured about 2 cm before the junction with the right atrium using a long-axis ultrasound image in the subcostal area. (Some prefer the M mode for the IVCD measurement.)

   b. In spontaneously breathing patients, the collapsibility of the IVC during inspiration shows a close correlation with the central venous pressure (CVP); i.e., the greater the inspiratory decrease in IVCD, the lower the CVP (26). This observation led to the proposal that respiratory changes in IVCD could be used to identify fluid responsiveness. However, as demonstrated in Table 7.3, there is no consistent relationship between respiratory changes in IVCD and fluid responsiveness.

2. **Stroke Volume Variation**

   During a positive-pressure breath, there is an increase in left ventricular (LV) stroke volume during lung inflation (caused, in part, by pulmonary venous blood that is squeezed into the left atrium, which increases LV preload), and a decrease in LV stroke volume during the lung deflation (caused by an empty pulmonary venous system, which decreases LV preload). This *stroke volume variation (SVV) is a measure of the preload (fluid) responsiveness of the left ventricle.*

   a. The pooled results of 12 clinical studies shows that an SVV > 12% predicts fluid responsiveness with 72% certainty (27).

   b. Monitoring SVV requires all of the following:

      1) Invasive blood pressure monitoring.

      2) An electronic system that derives the stroke volume

from the arterial pressure waveform (FloTrac sensor and Vigileo monitor, Edwards Lifesciences).

3) Volume-cycled mechanical ventilation with NO spontaneous breathing efforts, and a tidal volume ≥8 mL/kg predicted body weight (to magnify the respiratory changes in stroke volume).

4) A regular cardiac rhythm.

Table 7.3	Lack of Consistency in Predicting Fluid Responsiveness from Respiratory Changes in Inferior Vena Cava Diameter
Condition	**Observations**
Spontaneous Breathing	1. ΔIVCD ≥40–42% predicts fluid responsiveness, but ΔIVCD <40–42% does not exclude fluid responders. *(Crit Care 2012; 16:R188; 2015; 19:400)*
	2. No correlation between ΔIVCD and fluid response. *(Emerg Med Australas 2012; 24:534)*
Mechanical Ventilation†	1. ΔIVCD >12% predicts fluid responsiveness. *(Intensive Care Med 2004; 30:1834)*
	2. ΔIVCD >12% is not specific for fluid responsiveness. *(J Intensive Care Med 2011; 26:116)*
	3. ΔIVCD >18% predicts fluid responsiveness. *(Intensive Care Med 2004; 30:1740)*
	4. No correlation between ΔIVCD and fluid response. *(J Cardiothorac Vasc Anesth 2015; 29:663)*

†Volume-cycled ventilation with tidal volume ≥8 mL/kg (predicted body weight) and no spontaneous breathing efforts.

c. The multiple requirements and expense of SVV monitoring limit its applicability. Furthermore, there are sources of inaccuracy in the use of the arterial pressure waveforms to determine stroke volume (e.g., changes in arterial compliance).

3. **Pulse Pressure Variation**

The respiratory changes in stroke volume during positive pressure ventilation are accompanied by similar changes in the pulse pressure. As a result, *the pulse pressure variation (PPV) is also a measure of preload (fluid) responsiveness.*

a. The pooled results of 22 clinical studies shows that a PPV >13% predicts fluid responsiveness with 78% certainty (greater than that for stroke volume variation) (27). False positive results have been reported in patients with right ventricular dysfunction (28).

b. Monitoring the PPV requires everything listed for the SVV except the electronic system for determining the stroke volume. The pulse pressure can be measured directly from the arterial pressure waveform.

c. The multiple requirements for PPV monitoring (like SVV monitoring) limit its applicability; e.g., in one study, only 2% of ICU patients satisfied the criteria for PPV monitoring (29). However, when appropriate, PPV should be preferred to SVV (more accurate, easier to obtain) for evaluating fluid responsiveness.

IV. INFUSING FLUIDS

The steady flow of fluids through small, rigid tubes is described by the *Hagen-Poiseuille equation* shown below (30).

$$Q = \Delta P \, (\pi r^4 / 8 \mu L) \qquad (7.1)$$

This equation states that steady flow (Q) through a rigid tube is directly related to the driving pressure (ΔP) for flow and the fourth power of the inner radius (r) of the tube, and is inversely related to the length (L) of the tube and the viscosity (μ) of the infusate. These relationships also describe the infusion of resuscitation fluids through vascular catheters.

A. Central vs. Peripheral Catheters

1. The Hagen-Poiseuille equation predicts that infusion rates will be highest in short, large-bore catheters. This is demonstrated in Figure 7.2, which shows that the gravity-driven flow of water is far greater in short (1.2 inch) peripheral catheters than in longer (8 inch) central venous catheters of equivalent bore size.

2. Figure 7.2 demonstrates why *short, large-bore peripheral catheters are preferred to central venous catheters for aggressive volume resuscitation.*

B. Introducer Sheaths

The resuscitation of trauma victims can require infusion of more than 5 liters in the first hour, and infusion of more than 50 liters in one hour has been reported (31).

1. Very rapid flow rates can be achieved with large-bore *introducer sheaths* (normally used as conduits for pulmonary artery catheters), which can be used as stand-alone infusion devices, and are available in sizes of 8.5 and 9 French (2.7 and 3 mm outside diameter, respectively).

2. Flow through introducer sheaths can reach 15 mL/sec (54 L/hr), which is slightly less than the maximum flow (18 mL/sec or 65 L/hr) through standard (3 mm diameter) intravenous tubing (32).

3. Some introducer sheaths have a side infusion port on the hub, but the flow capacity of this port is only 25% of

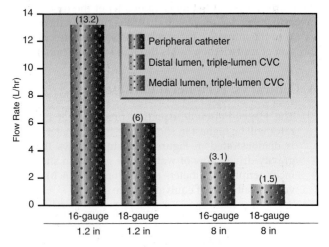

FIGURE 7.2 Gravity-driven flow of water through short (1.2 inch) peripheral catheters and a longer (20 cm or 8 inch) triple-lumen central venous catheter (CVC). Flow rates for peripheral catheters from Ann Emerg Med 1983; 12:149, and Emergency Medicine Updates (www.emupdates.com). Flow rates for triple-lumen CVC from manufacturer (Arrow International).

that in the introducer sheath (32), so the side infusion port should not be used for rapid infusions.

C. Infusing Packed Red Blood Cells

1. Whole blood is not available for replacement of blood loss, and erythrocyte losses are replaced with stored units of concentrated erythrocytes called *packed red blood cells* (PRBCs).

2. Each unit of PRBCs has a hematocrit of 55–60% and a viscosity about 6 times that of water (33). As a result, PRBCs flow sluggishly through catheters (as predicted by the Hagen-Poiseuille equation), and dilution with crystalloid fluids is often necessary.

3. The following demonstrates the influence of dilution on the gravity-driven flow rate of packed RBCs through an 18-gauge peripheral catheter (34):

    a. When infused alone, the flow rate of PRBCs is 5 mL/min (or one hour for infusion of one unit of PRBCs, which has a volume of about 350 mL).

    b. When one unit of PRBCs is diluted with 100 ml saline, the flow rate increases to 39 mL/min (about an 8-fold increase).

    c. When one unit of PRBCs is diluted with 250 mL isotonic saline, the flow rate is 60 mL/min (a 12-fold increase over the undiluted flow rate). At this rate, one unit of PRBCs can be infused in 5–6 minutes.

    d. Pressurized infusions of PRBCs achieve twice the flow rate of gravity-driven infusions (34).

4. Remember that Ringer's solutions should NOT be used to dilute PRBCs because they contain calcium, which can bind to the citrate anticoagulant in PRBCs and promote clumping (see Chapter 10 for more on Ringer's solutions).

V. RESUSCITATION PRACTICES

The following practices pertain to the resuscitation of active hemorrhage or hemorrhagic shock. The general goals and end-points are summarized in Figure 7.3.

A. Standard Resuscitation Practices

1. Despite the superiority of colloid fluids over crystalloid fluids for expanding the plasma volume (see Figure 10.1), crystalloid fluids are preferred for volume resuscitation.

2. The standard practice for trauma victims who present with active bleeding or hypotension is to infuse 2 liters of crystalloid fluid over 15 minutes (35).

3. If hypotension or bleeding continue, PRBCs are infused along with crystalloid fluids to achieve the following goals:

   a. Mean arterial pressure ≥65 mm Hg.

   b. Urine output >0.5 ml/kg/hr.

   c. Hemoglobin concentration ≥7 g/dl in otherwise healthy subjects, or ≥9 g/dL in patients with active coronary artery disease (36).

   d. Central venous O_2 saturation ($ScvO_2$) >70%.

   e. Normal blood lactate (usually <2 mmol/L).

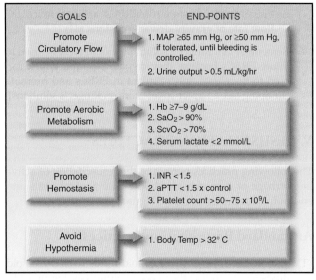

GOALS	END-POINTS
Promote Circulatory Flow	1. MAP ≥65 mm Hg, or ≥50 mm Hg, if tolerated, until bleeding is controlled. 2. Urine output >0.5 mL/kg/hr
Promote Aerobic Metabolism	1. Hb ≥7–9 g/dL 2. SaO_2 > 90% 3. $ScvO_2$ >70% 4. Serum lactate <2 mmol/L
Promote Hemostasis	1. INR <1.5 2. aPTT <1.5 x control 3. Platelet count >50–75 x 10⁹/L
Avoid Hypothermia	1. Body Temp > 32° C

FIGURE 7.3 The general goals and associated end-points of resuscitation for hemorrhagic shock. MAP = mean arterial pressure, Hb = hemoglobin concentration in blood, SaO_2 = arterial O_2 saturation, $ScvO_2$ = central venous O_2 saturation, INR = international normalized ratio, aPTT = activated partial thromboplastin time.

B. Damage Control Resuscitation

Because uncontrolled hemorrhage is the leading cause of death in hemorrhagic shock, the following practices are being adopted to limit the extent of bleeding in cases of *massive blood loss* (defined as the loss of one blood volume within 24 hours). These practices are collectively known as *damage control resuscitation* (37).

1. **Hypotensive Resuscitation**

   a. Observations with penetrating trauma have shown that aggressive volume replacement can exacerbate bleeding (37-39).

   b. This observation has led to an emphasis on permitting low blood pressures (i.e., systolic BP of 90 mm Hg or mean BP of 50 mm Hg) in trauma patients with hemorrhagic shock until the bleeding is controlled (37).

   c. This strategy has been shown to reduce resuscitation volumes (38,39), and has been associated with improved survival rates (38).

   d. Low blood pressures are maintained only if there is evidence of adequate organ perfusion (e.g., patient is awake and follows commands).

2. **Hemostatic Resuscitation**

   a. FRESH FROZEN PLASMA: For the resuscitation of massive blood loss, the traditional practice has been to give one unit of fresh frozen plasma (FFP) for every 6 units of packed RBCs (34), to prevent a dilutional coagulopathy. However, the discovery that severely injured trauma victims often have a coagulopathy on presentation (40) has led to the practice of *giving one unit of FFP for every one or two units of PRBCs,* and several studies have shown improved survival rates with this practice (34,37,41). Transfusion of FFP is aimed at maintaining an INR <1.5 and an activated PTT <1.5 times normal (42).

b. CRYOPRECIPITATE: Although FFP is a good source of fibrinogen (2–5 g/L), cryoprecipitate provides equivalent amounts of fibrinogen in a much smaller volume (3.2–4 grams in 150–200 mL, which is two "pools" of cryoprecipitate) (42). Cryoprecipitate can be used to maintain serum fibrinogen levels >1 g/L if volume control is desirable.

c. PLATELETS: The standard practice of giving one unit of platelets for every 10 units of PRBCs has been questioned, and improved survival rates have been recorded when one unit of platelets is given for every 2–5 units of PRBCs (34). The optimal ratio of platelets to PRBCs has yet to be determined, and platelet transfusions can be guided by the platelet count. The standard goal is to maintain a platelet count >50,000/μL when bleeding is active, but some advocate a platelet count >75,000/μL until bleeding is controlled (42).

3. **Avoiding Hypothermia**

a. Severe trauma is accompanied by loss of thermoregulation, and trauma-related hypothermia (temp <32°C) is associated with increased mortality, possibly from reduced activity of coagulation factors and platelets (37).

b. Since the infusion of blood products (stored at 4°C) promotes hypothermia, in-line fluid warmers are used routinely for the resuscitation of massive blood loss.

c. The use of warming blankets and in-line fluid warmers has reduced the incidence of hypothermia to <1% in combat-support hospitals (37).

VI. POSTRESUSCITATION INJURY

The restoration of blood pressure and hemoglobin levels in

hemorrhagic shock does not ensure a satisfactory outcome because it can be followed in 48–72 hours by progressive multiorgan failure (43).

A. Features

1. Postresuscitation injury is the result of *reperfusion injury* (44), believed to originate in the splanchnic circulation, where reperfusion of ischemic bowel releases proinflammatory cytokines into the systemic circulation.

2. The earliest manifestation is progressive respiratory failure from the acute respiratory distress syndrome (ARDS, described in Chapter 17), and this can be followed by progressive dysfunction involving the kidneys, liver, heart, and central nervous system.

3. The mortality rate is determined by the number of organs involved, and averages 50–60% (43).

B. Predisposing Factors

1. Several factors predispose to postresuscitation injury, including the time required to reverse tissue ischemia (e.g., lactate clearance >24 hrs), the number of units of PRBCs transfused (>6 units in 12 hrs), and the age of the transfused blood (>3 weeks) (43).

2. Infection may be involved if the onset is longer than 3 days after the resuscitation (43).

C. Management

1. Management involves general supportive measures, but attention to rapid reversal of ischemia (i.e., lactate clearance <24 hrs) could reduce the risk of postresuscitation injury.

2. In late-onset (>72 hrs) postresuscitation injury, prompt recognition and treatment of an underlying infection is essential.

REFERENCES

1. Walker RH (ed). Technical Manual of the American Association of Blood Banks. 10th ed., Arlington, VA: American Association of Blood Banks, 1990:650.

2. American College of Surgeons. Advanced Trauma Life Support for Doctors (ATLS): Student Course Manual. 8th ed. Chicago, IL: American College of Surgeons, 2008.

3. Marik PE. Assessment of intravascular volume: A comedy of errors. Crit Care Med 2001; 29:1635.

4. McGee S, Abernathy WB, Simel DL. Is this patient hypovolemic. JAMA 1999; 281:1022–1029.

5. Sinert R, Spektor M. Clinical assessment of hypovolemia. Ann Emerg Med 2005; 45:327–329.

6. Marik PE, Baram M, Vahid B. Does central venous pressure predict fluid responsiveness? Chest 2008; 134:172–178.

7. Oohashi S, Endoh H. Does central venous pressure or pulmonary capillary wedge pressure reflect the status of circulating blood volume in patients after extended transthoracic esophagectomy? J Anesth 2005; 19:21–25.

8. Cordts PR, LaMorte WW, Fisher JB, et al. Poor predictive value of hematocrit and hemodynamic parameters for erythrocyte deficits after extensive vascular operations. Surg Gynecol Obstet 1992; 175:243–248.

9. Stamler KD. Effect of crystalloid infusion on hematocrit in non-bleeding patients, with applications to clinical traumatology. Ann Emerg Med 1989; 18:747–749.

10. Okorie ON, Dellinger P. Lactate: biomarker and potential therapeutic agent. Crit Care Clin 2011; 27:299–326.

11. Abramson D, Scalea TM, Hitchcock R, et al. Lactate clearance and survival following injury. J Trauma 1993; 35:584–589.

12. Severinghaus JW. Case for standard-base excess as the measure of non-respiratory acid-base imbalance. J Clin Monit 1991; 7:276–277.

13. Davis JW, Shackford SR, Mackersie RC, Hoyt DB. Base deficit as a guide to volume resuscitation. J Trauma 1998; 28:1464–1467.

14. Martin MJ, Fitzsullivan E, Salim A, et al. Discordance between lactate and base deficit in the surgical intensive care unit: which one do you trust? Am J Surg 2006; 191:625–630.

15. Yu M, Pei K, Moran S, et al. A prospective randomized trial using blood volume analysis in addition to pulmonary artery catheter, compared with pulmonary artery catheter alone to guide shock resuscitation in critically ill surgical patients. Shock 2011; 35:220–228.

16. Boyd JH, Forbes J, Nakada TA, et al. Fluid resuscitation in septic shock: A positive fluid balance and elevated central venous pressure are associated with increased mortality. Crit Care Med 2011; 39:259–265.

17. Cecconi M, Parsons A, Rhodes A. What is a fluid challenge? Curr Opin Crit Care 2011; 17:290–295.

18. Marik PE. Fluid responsiveness and the six guiding principles of fluid resuscitation. Crit Care Med 2016; DOI 10.1097/CCM.0000000000001483.

19. Lakhal K, Ehrmann S, Perrotin S, et al. Fluid challenge: tracking changes in cardiac output with blood pressure monitoring (invasive or non-invasive). Intensive Care Med 2013; 39:1953–1962.

20. Giraud R, Siegenthaler N, Gayet-Ageron A, et al. ScvO(2) as a marker to define fluid responsiveness. J Trauma 2011; 70:802–807.

21. Monnet X, Bataille A, Magalhaes E, et al. End-tidal carbon dioxide is better than arterial pressure for predicting volume responsiveness by the passive leg raising test. Intensive Care Med 2013; 39:93–100.

22. Enomoto TM, Harder L. Dynamic indices of preload. Crit Care Clin 2010; 26:307–321.

23. Monnet X, Teboul JL. Passive leg raising: five rules, not a drop of fluid. Crit Care 2015, Jan 14 (Epub). Free article available on PubMed (PMID 25658678).

24. Monnet X, Marok P, Teboul JL. Passive leg raising for predicting fluid responsiveness: a systematic review and meta-analysis. Intensive Care Med 2016, Jan 29 (Epub ahead of print). Abstract available at PubMed (PMID: 26825952).

25. Mahjoub Y, Touzeau J, Airapetian N, et al. The passive leg-raising maneuver cannot accurately predict fluid responsiveness in patients with intra-abdominal hypertension. Crit Care Med 2010; 36:1824–1829.

26. Rudski LG, Lai WW, Afialo J, et al. Guidelines for the echocardiographic assessment of the right heart in adults: A report from the American Society of Echocardiography. J Am Soc Echocardiogr 2010; 23:685–687.

27. Marik PE, Cavallazzi R, Vasu T, Hirani A. Dynamic changes in arterial waveform derived variables and fluid responsiveness in mechanically ventilated patients: A systematic review of the literature. Crit Care Med 2009; 37:2642–2647.

28. Mahjoub Y, Pila C, Frigerri A, et al. Assessing fluid responsiveness in critically ill patients: False-positive pulse pressure variation is detected by Doppler echocardiographic evaluation of the right ventricle. Crit Care Med 2009; 37:2570–2575.

29. Mahjoub Y, Lejeune V, Muller L, et al. Evaluation of pulse pressure variation validity criteria in critically ill patients: a prospective, observational multicentre point-prevalence study. Br J Anesth 2014; 112:681–685.

30. Chien S, Usami S, Skalak R. Blood flow in small tubes. In Renkin EM, Michel CC (eds). Handbook of Physiology. Section 2: The cardiovascular system. Volume IV. The microcirculation. Bethesda: American Physiological Society, 1984:217–249.

31. Barcelona SL, Vilich F, Cote CJ. A comparison of flow rates and warming capabilities of the Level 1 and Rapid Infusion Systems with various-size intravenous catheters. Anesth Analg 2003; 97:358–363.

32. Hyman SA, Smith DW, England R, et al. Pulmonary artery catheter introducers: Do the component parts affect flow rate? Anesth Analg 1991; 73:573–575.

33. Documenta Geigy Scientific Tables, 7th ed. Basel: Documenta Geigy, 1966:557.

34. de la Roche MRP, Gauthier L. Rapid transfusion of packed red blood cells: effects of dilution, pressure, and catheter size. Ann Emerg Med 1993; 22:1551–1555.

35. American College of Surgeons. Shock. In Advanced Trauma Life Support Manual, 7th ed. Chicago: American College of Surgeons, 2004: 87–107.

36. Napolitano LM, Kurek S, Luchette FA, et al. Clinical practice guideline: red blood cell transfusion in adult trauma and critical care. Crit Care Med 2009; 37:3124–3157.

37. Beekley AC. Damage control resuscitation: a sensible approach to the exsanguinating surgical patient. Crit Care Med 2008; 36:S267–S274.

38. Bickell WH, Wall MJ Jr, Pepe PE, et al. Immediate versus delayed fluid resuscitation for hypotensive patients with penetrating torso injuries. N Engl J Med 1994; 331:1105–1109.

39. Morrison CA, Carrick M, Norman MA, et al. Hypotensive resuscitation strategy reduces transfusion requirements and severe postoperative coagulopathy in trauma patients with hemorrhagic shock: preliminary results of a randomized controlled trial. J Trauma 2011; 70:652–663.

40. Brohi K, Singh J, Heron M, Coats T. Acute traumatic coagulopathy. J Trauma 2003; 54:1127–1130.

41. Magnotti LJ, Zarzaur BL, Fischer PE, et al. Improved survival after hemostatic resuscitation: does the emperor have no clothes? J Trauma 2011; 70:97–102.

42. Stainsby D, MacLennan S, Thomas D, et al, for the British Committee for Standards in Hematology. Guidelines on the management of massive blood loss. Br J Haematol 2006; 135:634–641.

43. Dewar D, Moore FA, Moore EE, Balogh Z. Postinjury multiorgan failure. Injury 2009; 40:912–918.

44. Eltzschig HK, Collard CD. Vascular ischaemia and reperfusion injury. Br Med Bull 2004; 70:71–86.

Chapter 8

Acute Heart Failure(s)

Heart failure is not a single entity, and is classified according to the portion of the cardiac cycle that is affected (systolic or diastolic heart failure) and the side of the heart that is involved (right-sided or left-sided heart failure). This chapter describes the different types of heart failure, and focuses on the advanced stages of heart failure that require management in an ICU.

I. TYPES OF HEART FAILURE

A. Systolic vs. Diastolic Heart Failure

Early descriptions of heart failure attributed most cases to contractile failure during systole (*systolic heart failure*). However, about 50% of hospital admissions for heart failure are the result of diastolic dysfunction (*diastolic heart failure*) (1).

1. **Pressure–Volume Relationship**

   The pressure-volume curves in Figure 8.1 will be used to demonstrate the similarities and differences between systolic and diastolic heart failure.

   a. The curves in the top panel of Figure 8.1 (called *ventricular function curves*) show that heart failure is associated with a decrease in stroke volume and an increase in end-diastolic pressure (EDP). These changes occur in both types of heart failure.

   b. The curves in the lower panel of Figure 8.1 (called *ventricular compliance curves*) show that the increase in EDP in systolic heart failure is associated with an *increase* in end-diastolic volume, while the increase in EDP in diastolic heart failure is associated with a *decrease* in end-diastolic volume.

c. The difference in end-diastolic volume (EDV) in systolic and diastolic heart failure is the result of differences in ventricular distensibility or *compliance* (C), which is defined by the following relationships:

$$C = \Delta EDV / \Delta EDP \qquad (8.1)$$

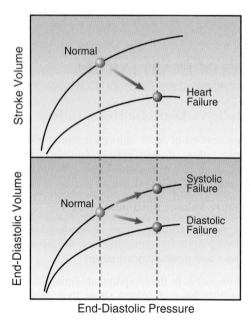

FIGURE 8.1 Pressure-volume curves showing the influence of systolic and diastolic dysfunction on measures of cardiac performance. Upper panel shows ventricular function curves, and lower panel shows diastolic compliance curves. See text for explanation.

The slope of the lower curves in Figure 8.1 is a reflection of ventricular compliance; the decreased slope in diastolic heart failure indicates a decreased compliance. Thus, *the functional disorder in diastolic heart failure is a decrease in ventricular distensibility that impairs ventricular filling during diastole.*

d. Figure 8.1 demonstrates that the EDV (not the EDP) is a distinguishing feature that identifies systolic or diastolic heart failure (see Table 8.1). However, the EDV is not easily measured, so the ejection fraction (described next) is used to identify the type of heart failure.

Table 8.1	Measures of LV Performance in Systolic and Diastolic Heart Failure	
Measure	**Systolic Heart Failure**	**Diastolic Heart Failure**
End-Diastolic Pressure	Increased	Increased
End-Diastolic Volume	Increased	Decreased
Ejection Fraction[†]	≤40%	≥50%

[†]From Reference 1.

2. **Ejection Fraction**

The fraction of the end-diastolic volume that is ejected during systole, known as the *ejection fraction* (EF), is equivalent to the ratio of stroke volume (SV) to end-diastolic volume (EDV):

$$EF = SV/EDV \qquad (8.2)$$

The EF is directly related to the strength of ventricular contraction, and is used a measure of systolic function.

Transthoracic echocardiography is the most frequently used method of measuring the ejection fraction (1).

a. CRITERIA: Heart failure with a left ventricular (LV) EF ≤40% is systolic heart failure, and heart failure with an LVEF ≥50% is diastolic heart failure (see Table 8.1) (1). Heart failure with an LVEF of 41–49% is in an intermediate category, but this type of heart failure behaves very much like diastolic failure (1).

3. **Terminology**

Many cases of heart failure involve some degree of systolic and diastolic dysfunction, so the following terms have been proposed for the different types of heart failure (1):

a. Heart failure that is predominantly the result of systolic dysfunction is called *heart failure with reduced ejection fraction*.

b. Heart failure that is predominantly the result of diastolic dysfunction is called *heart failure with preserved ejection fraction*.

Because these terms are lengthy, and offer no advantage in identifying the primary problem in ventricular performance, the terms "systolic heart failure" and "diastolic heart failure" are retained in this chapter, and throughout the book.

4. **Etiologies**

a. The causes of systolic heart failure are broadly classified as ischemic and dilated cardiomyopathies; the latter term including a heterogeneous group of disorders that includes toxic (e.g., ETOH), metabolic (e.g., thiamine deficiency), and infectious (e.g., HIV) conditions (1).

b. The most common cause of diastolic heart failure is hypertension with left ventricular hypertrophy, which is responsible for up to 90% of cases (1).

B. Right Heart Failure

Right-sided heart failure is more prevalent than suspected in ICU patients (2,3). Most cases are the result of pulmonary hypertension (e.g., from pulmonary emboli, acute respiratory distress syndrome, or chronic obstructive lung disease) and inferior wall myocardial infarction.

1. **Right Ventricular Function**

   a. Right heart failure is a contractile (systolic) failure that results in an increase in right ventricular end-diastolic volume (RVEDV).

   b. Despite the increase in RVEDV, the central venous pressure (CVP), which is a measure of right ventricular end-diastolic pressure, is normal in about one-third of cases of right heart failure (2).

   c. The CVP does not rise until the increase in RVEDV is restricted by the pericardium (pericardial constraint). The delayed rise in venous pressure hampers the clinical detection of right heart failure.

2. **Echocardiography**

   Cardiac ultrasound is an invaluable tool for detecting right heart failure in the ICU. Although the transesophageal approach provides better views of the right ventricle, transthoracic echocardiography can provide the following important measurements (see Table 8.2) (3):

   a. The *RV:LV area ratio* is measured by tracing the area of the two chambers at end-diastole. A ratio >0.6 indicates an enlarged RV chamber.

   b. The *right ventricular fractional area change* (RVFAC) is the ratio of the change in RV area during systole to the RV area at end-diastole, and is a surrogate measure of the RV ejection fraction. An RVFAC <32% indicates RV systolic dysfunction.

For a more comprehensive description of the ultrasound evaluation of the right ventricle, see References 3 and 4.

Table 8.2	Detecting Right Heart Failure with TTE	
Measurement	**View**	**Abnormal Value**
RV/LV Area Ratio	Apical Four Chamber	>0.6
RV Fractional Area Change	Apical Four Chamber	<32%

From Reference 3. TTE = Transthoracic Echocardiography.

C. Acute Heart Failure

1. Most (80–85%) cases of acute heart failure are exacerbations of chronic heart failure, often as a result of noncompliance with medications, uncontrolled hypertension, or rapid atrial fibrillation (5).

2. About 15–20% of cases are new-onset heart failure, and acute coronary syndromes are the major culprit (5).

3. *Stress-induced cardiomyopathy* deserves mention as an emerging cause of acute heart failure. This condition is attributed to catecholamine excess, and typically occurs in postmenopausal women with emotional stress, and in patients with acute neurologic injuries such as subarachnoid hemorrhage and traumatic brain injury (6).

   a. The clinical presentation includes dyspnea and chest pain, and is often mistaken as an acute coronary syndrome. ECG changes can include ST segment changes and T-wave inversions (6).

   b. Cardiac ultrasound typically shows apical ballooning or hypokinesis involving the apex of the left ventricle.

c. The associated heart failure can be severe, with hemodynamic instability, but the condition resolves in several days to weeks (6).

d. Catecholamine drugs (e.g., dobutamine) are NOT advised for hemodynamic support in this condition.

II. CLINICAL EVALUATION

Acute heart failure is a clinical diagnosis based on the patient's history, the presence of edema (pulmonary and/or peripheral) and evidence of cardiac dysfunction (by ECG and echocardiography). The following tests are also useful.

A. B-Type Natriuretic Peptide

1. Stretch of the atrial and ventricular walls triggers the release of four *natriuretic peptides* from cardiac myocytes. These peptides "unload" the ventricles by promoting sodium excretion in the urine (which reduces ventricular preload) and dilating systemic blood vessels (which reduces ventricular afterload).

2. One of these natriuretic peptides is brain-type or *B-type natriuretic peptide* (BNP), which is released as a precursor or prohormone (proBNP), which is then cleaved to form BNP (the active hormone) and N-terminal (NT)-proBNP, which is metabolically inactive.

3. NT-proBNP has a longer half-life than BNP, resulting in plasma levels that are 3–5 times higher than BNP levels.

4. Clinical Use

a. Plasma levels of BNP and NT-proBNP are used to evaluate the presence and severity of heart failure. The predictive value of these peptide levels is shown in Table 8.3 (7-9).

b. Note that advancing age and renal insufficiency can elevate peptide levels. Other conditions that can elevate peptide levels include critical illness, bacterial sepsis, anemia, obstructive sleep apnea, and severe pneumonia (1).

c. Since the conditions other than heart failure that raise peptide levels (including critical illness) are almost universal in ICU patients, the clinical utility of peptide levels in the ICU is questionable.

Table 8.3	B-Type Natriuretic Peptide in Acute Heart Failure		
Peptide Assay	**Likelihood of Acute Heart Failure**		
	Unlikely	**Uncertain**	**Likely**
BNP (pg/mL):			
Age ≥18 yrs	<100	100–500	>500
GFR < 60 mL/min	<200	200–500	>500
NT-proBNP (pg/mL):			
Age 18–49 yrs	<300	300–450	>450
Age 50–75 yrs	<300	300–900	>900
Age >75 yrs	<300	300–1800	>1800

From References 7–9.

B. Measuring Blood Volume

The introduction of a clinically useful technique for measuring blood volume using radiolabeled albumin (Daxor Corp, New York, NY) has important implications for the diagnosis and management of acute heart failure. A preliminary study utilizing this technique in patients with decompensated heart failure (10) found that not all patients were hypervolemic, and further that diuretic therapy did not substantially reduce blood volume even though body weight was significantly reduced. These results show the potential value of blood volume measurements in the evaluation and management of heart failure.

III. MANAGEMENT STRATEGIES

The management described here is primarily directed at decompensated, left-sided, systolic heart failure, and involves intravenous (rather than oral) drugs. The approach is organized according to the presenting blood pressure.

A. High Blood Pressure

About 25% of patients with acute heart failure have hypertension on presentation (5).

1. **Recommendation**

   Management should include vasodilator therapy with *nitroglycerin or nitroprusside*, combined with diuretic therapy (using *furosemide*) if there is evidence of volume overload (1). Nitroglycerin and nitroprusside are described in detail in Chapter 45 (see Sections V and VI), and dosing recommendations for these drugs are shown in Table 8.4. Furosemide dosing is described later in the chapter.

2. **Which Vasodilator is Preferred?**

   Nitroglycerin is the safer choice. Nitroprusside not only creates the risk of cyanide and thiocyanate toxicity (described in Chapter 45), it can also produce a *coronary steal syndrome* in acute coronary syndromes by diverting blood flow away from non-dilating blood vessels in ischemic regions of the myocardium (11).

3. **Caveat**

   Although the standard practice is to initiate therapy for acute heart failure with a diuretic, *intravenous furosemide produces an acute vasoconstrictor response* (12) by stimulating renin release, which leads to the formation of angiotensin II, a potent vasoconstrictor. Because this response can aggravate hypertension, aggressive furosemide dosing should delayed, if possible, until the blood pressure is controlled with vasodilator therapy.

B. Normal Blood Pressure

Over half of patients with acute heart failure have a normal blood pressure (5).

1. **Recommendations**

   a. Management should include vasodilator therapy with *nitroglycerin* or *nesiritide*, combined with diuretic therapy (using *furosemide*) if there is evidence of volume overload.

   b. For cases of vasodilator intolerance (i.e., hypotension) or signs of systemic hypoperfusion (e.g., decreased urine output), inodilator therapy with *dobutamine, milrinone, or levosimendan* is appropriate.

   c. For cases of acute heart failure with pulmonary edema, *positive pressure breathing* can be used as an adjunctive measure.

2. **Nesiritide**

   Nesiritide (Natrecor) is a recombinant human B-type natriuretic peptide that has a potential advantage over other vasodilators by promoting diuresis as well as vasodilation (see Table 8.4 for dosing recommendations). However, clinical studies have shown that nesiritide has little diuretic effect, and does not improve clinical outcomes (13). At the present time, there is no reason to favor nesiritide over nitroglycerin.

Table 8.4	Intravenous Vasodilator Therapy in Acute Heart Failure
Vasodilator	**Dosing Recommendations**
Nitroglycerin	1. Do NOT infuse through polyvinylchloride tubing (drug binds to PVC).
	2. Start infusion at 5–10 µg/min, and increase by 5–10 µg/min every 5 min to achieve the desired effect. The effective dose is ≤ 100 µg/min, in most cases.
	3. Nitrate tolerance can develop after 24 hrs.
Nitroprusside	1. Add thiocyanate (550 mg per 50 mg of drug) to infusate to bind the cyanide released by nitroprusside.
	2. Start infusion at 0.2–0.3 µg/kg/min and titrate upward every 5 min, to achieve the desired effect. The effective dose is 2–5 µg/kg/min in most cases, but avoiding dose rates >3 µg/kg/min will reduce the risk of cyanide toxicity.
	3. To limit the risk of thiocyanate toxicity, avoid using the drug in patients with renal failure.
Nesiritide	1. Do NOT infuse through heparin-bonded catheters (drug binds to heparin).
	2. Start with a bolus dose of 2 µg/kg, and infuse at 0.01 µg/kg/min. If necessary, give a second bolus dose of 1 µg/kg and increase the infusion rate by 0.005 µg/kg/min. This can be repeated every 3 hrs to a maximum rate of 0.03 µg/kg/min.

3. **Inodilators**

Inodilators are drugs with positive inotropic and vasodilator effects. The drugs in this class include dobutamine, milrinone, and levosimendan, and dosing recommendations for these drugs are shown in Table 8.5.

Table 8.5	Intravenous Inodilator Therapy in Acute Heart Failure	
Inodilator	**Dosing Recommendations**	
Dobutamine	1. Do NOT infuse with alkaline solutions.	
	2. Start infusion at 5 μg/kg/min, and increase in increments of 3–5 μg/kg/min, if necessary. Usual dose range is 5–20 μg/kg/min.	
Levosimendan	1. Initial dose is 12 μg/kg (over 10 min), followed by an infusion rate of 0.1 μg/kg/min. After 1 hr, infusion rate can be increased to 0.2 μg/kg/min, if necessary.	
	2. Infusions are usually limited to 24 hrs because a long-acting metabolite produces salutary effects for at least 7 days.	
Milrinone	1. Initial dose is 50 μg/kg (over 10 min), followed by an infusion rate of 0.375–0.75 μg/kg/min. Daily dose should not exceed 1.13 mg/kg.	
	2. Dose adjustments are recommended for creatinine clearance (CrCL) ≤50 mL/min:	

CrCL (mL/min)	50	40	30	20	10	5
Dose (μg/kg/min)	0.43	0.38	0.33	0.28	0.23	0.20

DOBUTAMINE: Dobutamine is a synthetic catecholamine that has positive inotropic effects (β_1-receptor stimulation), and mild vasodilator effects (β_2-receptor stimulation). This drug is described in detail in Chapter 45 (Section I). Because dobutamine is a catecholamine, it can produce unwanted cardiac stimulation, including an increase in myocardial O_2 consumption (14), which is deleterious in both the ischemic myocardium (where oxygen supply is impaired) and the failing myocardium (where O_2 consumption is already increased).

MILRINONE: Milrinone is a phosphodiesterase inhibitor that acts via the same pathway as dobutamine (i.e., cyclic AMP-mediated calcium influx into cardiac myocytes). When compared to dobutamine, milrinone is less likely to produce unwanted cardiac stimulation, but more likely to produce hypotension (15). Dose reduction is advised when the creatinine clearance is ≤50 mL/min (14), as shown in Table 8.5.

LEVOSIMENDAN: Levosimendan (Simdax) is a novel inotropic agent that: (a) enhances contractility by sensitizing cardiac myofilaments to calcium, (b) promotes vasodilation by facilitating potassium influx into vascular smooth muscle, and (c) has cardioprotective effects (reduces apoptosis) (16). Levosimendan *does not increase myocardial O$_2$ consumption* (16), and it is *the only inotropic agent with a proven survival benefit* (17). Infusions of levosimendan are usually limited to 24 hrs because it has a long-acting, active metabolite with peak effects 72 hours after the onset of therapy. Adverse effects include tachycardia and hypotension, which can be prolonged because of the active metabolite. Despite the appeal of levosimendan, it has not gained recognition in the United States.

4. **Caveat**

In diastolic heart failure, vasodilators should be used cautiously (because of the risk of hypotension), and positive inotropic agents should not be used at all (because systolic function is not abnormal).

5. **Positive Pressure Breathing**

   a. Positive pressure breathing (PPB) reduces left ventricular afterload by decreasing the transmural wall pressure during systole (18), and this enhances the stroke output of the left ventricle (19).

   b. Clinical studies in patients with cardiogenic pulmonary edema have shown that PPB hastens clinical improvement when added to conventional therapy (20,21).

c. The PPB modalities studied include continuous positive airway pressure (CPAP) and noninvasive pressure-support ventilation. (See Chapter 20 for a description of these modalities.)

C. Low Blood Pressure (Cardiogenic Shock)

Acute heart failure with hypotension (about 10% of cases) is a life-threatening condition that often *represents cardiogenic shock when accompanied by systemic hypoperfusion* (i.e., reduced urine output) *and elevated blood lactate levels.* This condition is most often the result of acute myocardial infarction. Less common causes include pericardial tamponade, massive pulmonary embolism, and acute mitral or aortic regurgitation.

1. **Recommendation**

   a. Echocardiography is essential for selecting the appropriate management (e.g., if pericardial tamponade is identified, then pericardiocentesis is most appropriate).

   b. When contractile failure is the problem, use the combination of *dobutamine and norepinephrine* to achieve a mean arterial pressure ≥65 mm Hg (22), and follow this with *mechanical circulatory support* in selected cases.

2. **Pharmacologic Support**

   a. There are two hemodynamic goals in cardiogenic shock: (a) increase ventricular stroke volume (SV), and (b) increase mean arterial pressure (MAP).

   b. Dobutamine provides inotropic support to increase SV, but the vasodilator effects of dobutamine often prevent a significant rise in MAP, so norepinephrine is added to promote vasoconstriction and increase MAP.

c. Norepinephrine is given by continuous infusion without a loading dose. The initial infusion rate is 2–3 μg/min and the usual dose range is 2–20 μg/min. (For more information on norepinephrine, see Chapter 45, Section VII.)

3. **Mechanical Circulatory Support**

Mechanical circulatory support is used primarily in cases of acute myocardial infarction with planned coronary revascularization. Mechanical support is described later in the chapter.

D. Diuretic Therapy

1. **Diuresis and Cardiac Output**

Although diuretic therapy is the cornerstone of therapy for fluid retention, it has the following disadvantages:

a. Several studies in patients with acute heart failure have shown that diuretic therapy (with IV furosemide) is accompanied by a *decrease* in cardiac output (23-25), which is the result of a decrease in venous return. For this reason, diuretic therapy should never be used alone in the treatment of acute heart failure, and should always be combined with vasodilator or inodilator therapy.

b. In patients with diastolic heart failure, where the problem is inadequate cardiac filling, the tendency of diuretics to reduce cardiac output can be magnified. Therefore, diuretics should be used cautiously in patients with diastolic heart failure (e.g., hypertensive heart failure).

2. **Bolus Dosing of Furosemide**

a. Following an IV bolus dose of furosemide, diuresis normally begins within 15 minutes, peaks at one hour, and lasts 2 hours (26).

b. For patients with normal renal function, the initial furosemide dose should be 40 mg IV. If the diuresis is not adequate (at least 1 liter) after 2 hours, the dose is doubled (80 mg). The dose that produces a satisfactory response is then given twice daily. Failure to respond to an IV dose of 80 mg is evidence of diuretic resistance, and is managed as described in the next section.

c. For patients with renal insufficiency, the initial furosemide dose should be 100 mg IV, which can be increased to 200 mg if necessary. The dose that produces a satisfactory response is then given twice daily. Failure to respond to an IV dose of 200 mg is evidence of diuretic resistance.

d. The goal of diuresis is a minimum weight loss of 5–10% of body weight (27).

3. **Diuretic Resistance**

Attenuated responses to furosemide are common in advanced heart failure, and can be the result of rebound sodium retention, reduced renal blood flow, or *diuretic braking* (i.e., decreased responsiveness as hypervolemia resolves) (28). The following measures can enhance furosemide responsiveness.

a. ADD A THIAZIDE: Thiazide diuretics block sodium reabsorption in the distal tubules, and can enhance the diuretic response to furosemide (which blocks sodium reabsorbtion in the loop of Henle). The favored thiazide is *metolazone*, which retains its efficacy in renal insufficiency (28). Metolazone is given orally, in a single daily dose of 2.5–10 mg; the diuretic response begins at one hour and peaks at 9 hours, so it should be given hours before furosemide is given.

b. CONTINUOUS-INFUSION FUROSEMIDE: The diuretic effect of furosemide is a function of its urinary excretion rate (not the plasma concentration), and thus continuous infusions of the drug produce a more vigorous diuresis than intermittent bolus doses (29). The dosing regimen for continuous-infusion furosemide is influenced by renal function (27,28):

Creatinine Clearance	Loading Dose	Initial Infusion Rate
> 75 mL/min	100 mg	10 mg/hr
25–75 mL/min	100–200 mg	10–20 mg/hr
< 25 mL/min	200 mg	20–40 mg/hr

The infusion rate is titrated to achieve the desired urine output (e.g., ≥100 mL/hr). The maximum recommended infusion rate is 240–360 mg/hr (28), or 170 mg/hr in elderly patients (30).

IV. MECHANICAL CIRCULATORY SUPPORT

There are 3 types of mechanical circulatory support: (a) pressure unloading of the left ventricle (intra-aortic balloon pump), (b) volume unloading of the left ventricle (left-ventricular assist device), and (c) biventricular volume unloading with extracorporeal membrane oxygenation (ECMO). Unfortunately, *none of these modalities has a proven survival benefit* (31,32). The following presentation focuses on the intra-aortic balloon pump, the most frequently used method of mechanical cardiac support.

A. Intra-aortic Balloon Counterpulsation

In cases of acute myocardial infarction complicated by cardiogenic shock, the intra-aortic balloon pump (IABP) is used for temporary support when coronary revascularization (either percutaneous or surgical) is planned (31). It is contraindicated in the presence of aortic valve insufficiency or aortic dissection.

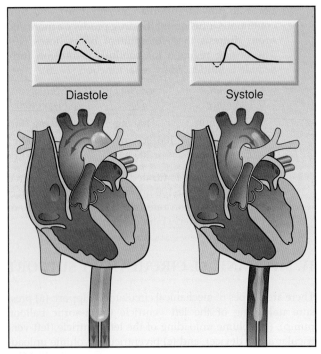

FIGURE 8.2 Intra-aortic balloon counterpulsation showing balloon inflation during diastole (left panel), and balloon deflation during systole (right panel). The arrows indicate the direction of blood flow. The effects on the aortic pressure waveform are shown by the dotted lines.

1. **Method**

   a. The intra-aortic balloon is an elongated polyurethane balloon that is inserted percutaneously into the femoral artery and advanced up the aorta until the tip lies just below the origin of the left subclavian artery (see Figure 8.2).

   b. A pump attached to the balloon uses helium (a low

density gas) to rapidly inflate and deflate the balloon. Inflation begins at the onset of diastole, just after the aortic valve closes (using the R wave on the ECG as a trigger), and deflation begins at the onset of ventricular systole, just before the aortic valve opens.

2. **Effects**

The hemodynamic effects of IABP support are demonstrated in Figure 8.2.

a. The aortic pressure waveform on the left shows that balloon inflation during diastole increases the peak diastolic pressure, and subsequently increases the mean arterial pressure (equivalent to the integrated area under the aortic pressure tracing).

b. The increase in peak diastolic pressure increases coronary blood flow (which occurs predominantly during diastole). The increase in mean arterial pressure obviates the need for a vasopressor, but is not accompanied by an increase in systemic blood flow (31).

c. The aortic pressure tracing on the right shows that balloon deflation creates a suction effect that decreases aortic pressure when the aortic valve opens. This reduces the impedance to left ventricular outflow (i.e., afterload) and augments ventricular stroke output. The decrease in LV afterload is accompanied by a decrease in cardiac work and myocardial O_2 consumption.

d. In summary, the IABP increases cardiac stroke output while increasing myocardial O_2 delivery (via increased coronary blood flow) and reducing myocardial O_2 consumption. Despite these beneficial effects, *numerous studies have shown no consistent survival benefit with IABP support* (31,32).

3. **Complications**

a. Limb ischemia is reported in 3–20% of patients

(33,34), and can appear while the balloon is in place or shortly after removal. Most cases are the result of in-situ thrombosis at the balloon insertion site.

b. Loss of distal pulses alone does not warrant removal of the balloon as long as sensorimotor function in the legs is intact (35). Loss of sensorimotor function in the legs should always prompt immediate removal of the device.

c. Surgical intervention is required in 30–50% of cases of limb ischemia (35).

d. Fever is reported in 50% of patients during IABP support, but bacteremia is reported in only 15% of patients (36).

REFERENCES

1. Yancy CW, Jessup MJ, Bozkurt B, et al. 2013 ACCF/AHA guideline for the management of heart failure. Report of the American College of Cardiology Foundation /American Heart Association Task Force on Practice Guidelines. Circulation 2013; 128:e240–e327.

2. Isner JM. Right ventricular myocardial infarction. JAMA 1988; 259:712–718.

3. Acute right ventricular dysfunction. Real-time management with echocardiography. Chest 2015; 147:835–846.

4. Rudski LG, Lai WW, Afilalo J, et al. Guidelines for the echocardiographic assessment of the right heart in adults: A report from the American Society of Echocardiography. J Am Soc Echocardiogr 2010; 23:685–713.

5. Gheorghiade M, Pang PS. Acute heart failure syndromes. JACC 2009; 53:557–573.

6. Boland TA, Lee VH, Bleck TP. Stress-induced cardiomyopathy. Crit Care Med 2015; 43:686–693.

7. Maisel AS, Krishnaswamy P, Nomak RM, et al. Rapid measurement of B-type natriuretic peptide in the emergency diagnosis of heart failure. N Engl J Med 2002; 347:161–167.

8. Maisel AS, McCord J, Nowak J, et al. Bedside B-type natriuretic peptide in the emergency diagnosis of heart failure with reduced or preserved ejection fraction. JACC 2003; 41:2010–2017.

9. Januzzi JL, van Kimmenade R, Lainchbury J, et al. NT-proBNP testing for diagnosis and short-term prognosis in acute destabilized heart failure: an international pooled analysis of 1256 patients. Europ Heart J 2006; 27:330–337.

10. Miller WL, Mullan BP. Understanding the heterogeneity in volume overload and fluid distribution in decompensated heart failure is key to optimal volume management. JACC Heart Fail 2014; 2:298–305.

11. Mann T, Cohn PF, Holman LB, et al. Effect of nitroprusside on regional myocardial blood flow in coronary artery disease. Results in 25 patients and comparison with nitroglycerin. Circulation 1978; 57:732–738.

12. Francis GS, Siegel RM, Goldsmith SR, et al. Acute vasoconstrictor response to intravenous furosemide in patients with chronic congestive heart failure. Ann Intern Med 1986; 103:1–6.

13. O'Connor CM, Starling RC, Hernanadez PW, et al. Effect of nesiritide in patients with acute decompensated heart failure. N Engl J Med 2011; 365:32–43.

14. Milrinone Lactate. In: McEvoy GK, ed. AHFS Drug Information, 2014. Bethesda, MD: American Society of Health System Pharmacists, 2014:1753–55.

15. Bayram M, De Luca L, Massie B, Gheorghiade M. Reassessment of dobutamine, dopamine, and milrinone in the management of acute heart failure syndromes. Am J Cardiol 2005; 96(Suppl): 47G–58G.

16. Nieminen MS, Fruhwald S, Heunks LMA, et al. Levosimendan: current data, clinical use and future development. Heart Lung Vessel 2013; 5:227–245.

17. Belletti A, Castro ML, Silvetti S, et al. The effects of inotropes and vasopressors on mortality. A meta-analysis of randomized clinical trials. Br J Anaesth 2015; 115: 656–675.

18. Naughton MT, Raman MK, Hara K, et al. Effect of continuous positive airway pressure on intrathoracic and left ventricular transmural pressures in patients with congestive heart failure. Circulation 1995; 91:1725–1731.

19. Bradley TD, Holloway BM, McLaughlin PR, et al. Cardiac output response to continuous positive airway pressure in congestive heart failure. Am Rev Respir Crit Care Med 1992; 145:377–382.

20. Nouira S, Boukef R, Bouida W, et al. Non-invasive pressure support ventilation and CPAP in cardiogenic pulmonary edema: a multicenter randomized study in the emergency department. Intensive Care Med 2011; 37:249–256.

21. Ducros L, Logeart D, Vicaut E, et al. CPAP for acute cardiogenic pulmonary edema from out-of-hospital to cardiac intensive care unit: a randomized multicenter study. Intensive Care Med 2011; 37:1501–1509.

22. Levy P, Perez P, Perny J, et al. Comparison of norepinephrine-dobutamine to epinephrine for hemodynamics, lactate metabolism, and organ function variables in cardiogenic shock. A prospective, randomized pilot study. Crit Care Med 2011; 39:450–455.

23. Kiely J, Kelly DT, Taylor DR, Pitt B. The role of furosemide in the treatment of left ventricular dysfunction associated with acute myocardial infarction. Circulation 1973; 58:581–587.

24. Mond H, Hunt D, Sloman G. Haemodynamic effects of frusemide in patients suspected of having acute myocardial infarction. Br Heart J 1974; 36:44–53.

25. Nelson GIC, Ahuja RC, Silke B, et al. Haemodynamic advantages of isosorbide dinitrate over frusemide in acute heart failure following myocardial infarction. Lancet 1983a; i:730–733.

26. Furosemide. In: McEvoy GK, ed. AHFS Drug Information, 2014. Bethesda, MD: American Society of Health System Pharmacists, 2014:2822–2825.

27. Jenkins PG. Diuretic strategies in acute heart failure. N Engl J Med 2011; 364:21

28. Asare K, Lindsey K. Management of loop diuretic resistance in the intensive care unit. Am J Health Syst Pharm 2009; 66:1635–1640.

29. Amer M, Adomaityte J, Qayyum R. Continuous infusion versus intermittent bolus furosemide in ADHF: an updated meta-analysis of randomized control trials. J Hosp Med 2012; 7:270–275.

30. Howard PA, Dunn MI. Aggressive diuresis for severe heart failure in the elderly. Chest 2001; 119:807–810.

31. Werden K, Gielen S, Ebelt H, Hochman JS. Mechanical circulatory support in cardiogenic shock. Eur Heart J 2014; 35:156–167.

32. Ahmad Y, Sen S, Shun-Sin MJ, et al. Intra-aortic balloon pump therapy for acute myocardial infarction. A meta-analysis. JAMA Intern Med 2015; 175:931–939.

33. Boehner JP, Popjes E. Cardiac failure: mechanical support strategies. Crit Care Med 2006; 34(Suppl):S268–S277.

34. Arafa OE, Pedersen TH, Svennevig JL, et al. Vascular complications of the intra-aortic balloon pump in patients undergoing open heart operations: 15-year experience. Ann Thorac Surg 1999; 67:645–651.

35. Baldyga AP. Complications of intra-aortic balloon pump therapy. In Maccioli GA, ed. Intra-aortic balloon pump therapy. Philadelphia: Williams & Wilkins, 1997, 127–162.

36. Crystal E, Borer A, Gilad J, et al. Incidence and clinical significance of bacteremia and sepsis among cardiac patients treated with intra-aortic balloon counterpulsation pump. Am J Cardiol 2000; 86:1281–1284.

Chapter 9

Systemic Infection and Inflammation

The most significant discovery in critical care in the past 20–30 years is the prominent role played by inflammation in the pathogenesis of multiorgan dysfunction in critically ill patients. This chapter presents four disorders that involve inflammatory injury in major organs: sepsis, septic shock, anaphylaxis, and anaphylactic shock.

I. CLINICAL SYNDROMES

A. Systemic Inflammatory Response Syndrome

1. The inflammatory response is a complex process that is triggered by conditions that threaten the functional integrity of the host. Examples of such conditions include physical injury (trauma), chemical injury (e.g., gastric acid aspiration), oxidant injury (e.g., radiation), thermal injury (burns), and microbial invasion.

2. The clinical manifestations of the inflammatory response are listed in Table 9.1; the presence of at least two of these findings has been called the *systemic inflammatory response syndrome* (SIRS) (1).

3. The diagnosis of SIRS has two limitations that deserve emphasis:

   a. *The presence of SIRS does not indicate the presence of infection;* i.e., infection is identified in only 25–50% of patients with SIRS (2,3).

b. The presence of SIRS does not always indicate the presence of inflammation; e.g., anxiety can produce tachycardia and tachypnea, which qualifies for the diagnosis of SIRS despite the absence of an inflammatory response.

4. SIRS is essentially a signal to search for the responsible condition (primarily infection).

Table 9.1	Systemic Inflammatory Response Syndrome (SIRS)

The diagnosis of SIRS requires at least 2 of the following:

1. Temperature >38°C or <36°C

2. Heart rate >90 beats/min

3. Respiratory rate >20 breaths/min, or $PaCO_2$ <32 mm Hg (<4.3 kPa)

4. WBC count >12,000/mm³ or <4000/mm³, or 10% immature neutrophils (band forms)

From Reference 2.

B. Sepsis

Sepsis is defined as life-threatening organ dysfunction caused by a dysregulated host response to infection (4). The organ dysfunction is attributed to inflammatory injury, which is the result of uncontrolled inflammation and/or inadequate host defenses against inflammatory injury.

1. SOFA Score

In patients with a suspected or documented infection, the *Sepsis-related Organ Failure Assessment (SOFA) score* is recommended for identifying organ dysfunction (4,5). (See Appendix 4 for the SOFA scoring method.)

a. A change in the baseline SOFA score of ≥2 points is evidence of organ dysfunction, and this condition has a mortality rate that is 2- to 25-fold higher than the mortality with uncomplicated infections (4).

b. The baseline SOFA score is assumed to be zero unless the patient has pre-existing organ dysfunction.

2. **Quick SOFA Criteria**

The SOFA score requires laboratory measurements, which can delay recognition of organ dysfunction, but rapid recognition of organ dysfunction is possible with the Quick SOFA (qSOFA) criteria shown in Table 9.2 (4).

a. The presence of any two of the qSOFA criteria is presumptive evidence of organ dysfunction (4).

b. The qSOFA criteria should be used as a screening tool, and a positive result should prompt further evaluation of organ dysfunction (e.g., with the full SOFA score).

Table 9.2	Quick SOFA (qSOFA) Criteria

Sepsis is likely if an infection is accompanied by any 2 of the following conditions:

1. Respiratory Rate ≥22 breaths/min
2. Altered Mentation (Glasgow Coma Score ≤13)
3. Systolic Blood Pressure ≤100 mm Hg

From Reference 4.

C. Septic Shock

1. Septic shock is a subset of sepsis that is characterized by the following conditions (4):

a. Hypotension that is not corrected by volume resuscitation.

b. Sustained requirement for a vasopressor to maintain a mean arterial pressure ≥65 mm Hg.

c. A serum lactate level >2 mmol/L.

2. The mortality rate in septic shock is 35–55%, which is much higher than the mortality rate of 10–20% in sepsis (4).

II. MANAGEMENT OF SEPTIC SHOCK

The management of septic shock requires an understanding of the associated changes in hemodynamics and energy metabolism as described next.

A. Pathophysiology

1. **Hemodynamic Alterations**

   a. Septic shock is characterized by systemic *vasodilation* involving both arteries and veins, which reduces ventricular preload (from venodilation) and ventricular afterload (from arterial vasodilation). The vascular changes are attributed to the enhanced production of nitric oxide (a vasodilator) in vascular endothelial cells (6).

   b. Injury in the vascular endothelium (from neutrophil attachment and degranulation) leads to fluid extravasation and hypovolemia (6), which adds to the reduced cardiac filling from venodilation.

   c. Proinflammatory cytokines promote cardiac dysfunction (both systolic and diastolic dysfunction), however the cardiac output is usually increased as a result of tachycardia and decreased afterload (7).

   d. Despite the increased cardiac output, splanchnic blood flow is typically reduced in septic shock (6). This can lead to disruption of the intestinal mucosa and "translocation" of enteric pathogens and endotoxins across the mucosa and into the systemic circulation.

This, then, can be a source of progressive and unregulated systemic inflammation (which is the source of organ dysfunction in sepsis and septic shock).

e. In the advanced stages of septic shock, cardiac output begins to decline, eventually resulting in a hemodynamic pattern that resembles cardiogenic shock (i.e., high cardiac filling pressures, low cardiac output, and increased systemic vascular resistance).

2. **Cytopathic Hypoxia**

a. As mentioned at the end of Chapter 6 (see Section III-F), the impaired energy metabolism in septic shock is the result of a defect in oxygen utilization in mitochondria (8); a condition known as *cytopathic hypoxia* (9). Tissue O_2 levels are not reduced, and can actually be increased (10).

b. Since tissue O_2 levels are not impaired in septic shock, *efforts to improve tissue oxygenation* (e.g., with blood transfusions) *are not justified*.

B. Early Management

The management of septic shock described here is based on the most recent guidelines from the Surviving Sepsis Campaign (11). The early management (in the first 6 hours after diagnosis) is outlined in Table 9.3.

1. **Volume Resuscitation**

Volume infusion is the first priority in septic shock because cardiac filling is expected to be reduced as a result of: (a) venodilation, and (b) a decrease in intravascular volume from fluid extravasation through "leaky capillaries".

a. Crystalloid fluids are preferred because of their lower cost. (See Chapter 10, Section IV, for the colloid-crystalloid debate.)

b. The recommended infusion volume is 30 mL/kg (11), which should be given within 3 hours.

c. After the initial volume resuscitation, the infusion rate of maintenance fluids should be adjusted to avoid unnecessary fluid accumulation, because a positive fluid balance is associated with increased mortality in septic shock (12).

Table 9.3	Early (First 6 hrs) Management of Septic Shock
Category	**Components**
Interventions	1. Administer a crystalloid fluid challenge using 30 mL/kg.
	2. If hypotension persists, add a vasopressor (norepinephrine preferred).
	3. Insert a central venous catheter to monitor CVP and $ScvO_2$.
	4. Obtain blood cultures and administer broad spectrum antibiotics.
Goals	1. CVP = 8 mm Hg for spontaneous breathing, or 12–15 mm Hg for mechanical ventilation.
	2. MAP ≥65 mm Hg.
	3. Urine output ≥0.5 mL/kg/hr.
	4. $ScvO_2$ ≥70%.
	5. Reduced or normal serum lactate level.

Adapted from Reference 11. CVP = central venous pressure; $ScvO_2$ = central venous O_2 saturation; MAP = mean arterial pressure.

2. **Vasopressor Therapy**

Volume resuscitation does not correct hypotension in septic shock, and vasopressor therapy is needed to achieve a mean arterial pressure (MAP) ≥65 mm Hg.

a. *Norepinephrine* is the preferred vasopressor in septic shock (11). The usual dose range is 2–20 µg/min. (For more information on norepinephrine, see Chapter 45, Section VII.)

b. *Vasopressin* can be added to norepinephrine for resistant or refractory hypotension, but should never be used alone as a vasopressor. The recommended dose in this situation is 0.03–0.04 U/min (11). Although vasopressin may help in raising the blood pressure, the accumulated experience with vasopressin shows no influence on outcomes in septic shock (28).

c. *Epinephrine* is also recommended as an additional vasopressor in cases of refractory hypotension (11), but the enhanced lactate production associated with epinephrine can interfere with lactate clearance (a goal of early management), so this recommendation seems ill-advised. (For information on epinephrine dosing and adverse effects, see Chapter 45, Section III.)

d. Because of the risk of tachyarrhythmias, *dopamine* is recommended as an alternative vasopressor only in patients with absolute or relative bradycardia (11). (For information on dopamine dosing and adverse effects, see Chapter 45, Section II.)

4. **Inotropic Therapy**

When the central venous O_2 saturation ($ScvO_2$) is low (<70%) despite correction of the blood pressure with vasopressors, then O_2 delivery is inadequate, and infusion of the positive inotropic agent dobutamine is indicated. (See Chapter 45, Section I for dosing information on dobutamine.) At this point, monitoring the cardiac output (invasively or noninvasively) is advised.

5. **Antimicrobial Therapy**

Delays in initiating appropriate antibiotic therapy can

adversely affect outcomes in septic shock, which is the basis for the recommendation that *antimicrobial therapy should be started within the first hour after the diagnosis of septic shock* (11). This is operationally difficult to achieve because of the time involved to obtain blood cultures, and to order, dispense, and deliver antimicrobial agents. Nevertheless, antimicrobial therapy should be started as soon as feasible. (See Chapter 35 for recommendations on empiric antibiotic coverage for suspected sepsis.)

6. **Blood Cultures**

   One dose of an intravenous antibiotic can sterilize blood cultures within a few hours, so blood cultures should be obtained prior to administering antibiotics.

   a. At least 2 sets of blood cultures are recommended, one drawn percutaneously and one drawn through a vascular access device (11).

   b. If a central venous catheter has been in place longer than 48 hrs, one blood culture should be drawn through each lumen of the catheter and compared to a percutaneous blood culture using quantitative culture techniques (described in Chapter 2, Section III-D).

   c. The yield from blood cultures is influenced by the volume of blood that is cultured, and a volume of 10 mL is recommended for each culture bottle (11).

C. Goals of Early Management

The Surviving Sepsis Campaign recommends that the goals listed in Table 9.3 should be reached within 6 hours after the diagnosis of septic shock. However, there are limitations associated with these goals that deserve mention.

1. **Central Venous Pressure**

   The use of the central venous pressure (CVP) as a goal

of management is contrary to the evidence that the CVP is not an accurate reflection of the circulating blood volume (see Figure 7.1), and thus should not be used to guide fluid management.

2. **Central Venous O$_2$ Saturation**

The use of the central venous O$_2$ saturation (ScvO$_2$) as a goal of management is based on the assumption that the tissue O$_2$ levels are reduced in septic shock. This is contrary to the results of studies showing that tissue O$_2$ levels are not reduced in septic shock (10), and that a majority of patients with septic shock have a normal ScvO$_2$ (14).

3. **Survival Value**

The value of the early goals of management in Table 9.3 has been challenged by the results of three large, randomized studies from separate countries (USA, Great Britain, and Australia) showing no survival benefit associated with achievement of these goals (15).

D. Corticosteroids

Despite a large body of evidence showing that steroids do not improve outcomes in septic shock (16), steroids continued to be recommended in selected cases of septic shock. The following statements reflect the current recommendations (11).

1. Steroids should be considered when hypotension is refractory to vasopressors. Evidence of adrenal insufficiency (by the rapid ACTH stimulation test) is not required.

2. The recommended steroid regimen is *IV hydrocortisone in a daily dose of 200 mg, delivered by continuous infusion* (to limit the risk of hyperglycemia from bolus doses).

3. Steroids should be continued as long as vasopressor therapy is required.

E. Supportive Care

1. As mentioned earlier, careful attention to avoiding fluid accumulation is important because of evidence that a positive fluid balance is associated with increased mortality in septic shock (12). Daily reviews of fluid balance are essential in this regard.

2. Blood glucose levels should be ≤180 mg/dL (11), which is above the standard upper limit of 110 mg/dL used for glycemic control. This recommendation is based on a large study showing a lower mortality rate when glycemic control was based on an upper limit of 180 mg/dL instead of 110 mg/dL (17). Although there is no lower limit of blood glucose in this recommendation, hypoglycemia may be more dangerous than hyperglycemia in critically ill patients (18), so careful attention to avoiding hypoglycemia is essential.

3. Red blood cell (RBC) transfusions have an immunosuppressive effect (see Chapter 11, Section V-E), so it is important to avoid unnecessary RBC transfusions in patients with septic shock. In the absence of active bleeding, RBC transfusions are not advised until the Hb falls below 7 g/dL (11).

III. ANAPHYLAXIS

Anaphylaxis is an acute multiorgan dysfunction syndrome produced by the immunogenic release of inflammatory mediators from basophils and mast cells. The characteristic feature is an exaggerated immunoglobulin E (IgE) response to an external antigen; i.e., a hypersensitivity reaction. Common triggers include food, antimicrobial agents, and insect bites.

A. Clinical Features

1. Anaphylactic reactions are typically abrupt in onset,

and appear within minutes of exposure to the external trigger. However, some reactions can appear as late as 72 hours after exposure (19).

2. A characteristic feature of anaphylactic reactions is edema and swelling in the involved organ, caused by increased vascular permeability and fluid extravasation.

3. The clinical manifestations of anaphylaxis are shown in Table 9.4.

   a. The most common manifestations are urticaria and sub-cutaneous angioedema (typically involving the face).

   b. Troublesome manifestations include angioedema of the upper airway (e.g., laryngeal edema), bronchospasm, and hypotension.

   c. The most feared manifestation is hypotension with evidence of systemic hypoperfusion (e.g., depressed consciousness), which represents *anaphylactic shock*.

Table 9.4	Clinical Manifestations of Anaphylaxis
Manifestation	**Frequency of Occurrence**
Urticaria	85–90%
Subcutaneous angioedema	85–90%
Upper airway angioedema	50–60%
Bronchospasm and wheezing	45–50%
Hypotension	30–35%
Abdominal cramping, diarrhea	25–30%
Substernal chest pain	4–6%
Pruritis without rash	2–5%

From Reference 19.

B. Management of Anaphylaxis

1. **Epinephrine**

   Epinephrine blocks the release of inflammatory mediators from sensitized basophils and mast cells, and is the drug of choice for severe anaphylactic reactions. The drug is available in a (confusing) variety of aqueous solutions, and these are shown in Table 9.5.

   a. The usual treatment for anaphylactic reactions is 0.3–0.5 mg of epinephrine (0.3–0.5 mL of 1:1,000 epinephrine solution) administered by deep intramuscular (IM) injection in the lateral thigh, and repeated every 5 minutes if necessary (19).

   b. Epinephrine can be nebulized for laryngeal edema using the dosing regimen in Table 9.5, but the efficacy of this regimen is unclear.

Table 9.5	Aqueous Epinephrine Solutions and Their Clinical Uses	
Aqueous Dilution	**Condition**	**Dosing Regimen**
1:100 (10 mg/mL)	Laryngeal Edema	0.25 mL (2.5 mg) in 2 mL saline and administer by nebulizer
1:1,000 (1 mg/mL)	Anaphylaxis	0.3–0.5 mL (mg) by deep IM injection in the thigh every 5 min as needed
1:10,000 (0.1 mg/mL)	Asystole or PEA	10 mL (1 mg) IV every 3–5 min as needed
1:100,000 (10 μg/mL)	Anapylactic Shock	Add 1 mL of 1:1,000 solution to 100 mL saline (1 mg/100 mL or 10 μg/mL) and infuse at 30–100 mL/hr (5–15 μg/min)

From Reference 19.

c. GLUCAGON: Epinephrine inhibits degranulation of inflammatory cells by stimulating β-adrenergic receptors, and ongoing therapy with β-receptor antagonists can attenuate or eliminate the response. Glucagon can restore epinephrine responsiveness (see Chapter 46, Section III-B for the mechanism). The dose of glucagon is 1–5 mg by slow intravenous injection, followed by a continuous infusion at 5–15 µg/min (19). Glucagon can induce vomiting, and patients with depressed consciousness should be placed on their side to reduce the risk of aspiration.

2. **Second-Line Agents**

The following drugs are used to treat the consequences of anaphylaxis, and will not hasten the resolution of the underlying process.

a. ANTIHISTAMINES: Histamine receptor antagonists can be used to relieve pruritis in cutaneous reactions. The histamine-H_1 blocker *diphenhydramine* (25–50 mg PO, IM, or IV) and the histamine-H_2 blocker *ranitidine* (50 mg IV or 150 mg PO) should be given together because they are more effective in combination.

b. BRONCHODILATORS: Inhaled β-2 receptor agonists like *albuterol* are used to relieve bronchospasm, and are administered by nebulizer (2.5 mL or a 0.5% solution) or by metered-dose inhaler.

c. NO STEROIDS: Despite the popularity of steroids for hypersensitivity reactions, there is no evidence that steroids are effective in reversing, slowing, or preventing recurrences of anaphylactic reactions (19). As a result, the most recent guideline on treating anaphylaxis does not include a recommendation for steroid therapy (19).

C. Management of Anaphylactic Shock

Anaphylactic shock is an immediate threat to life, with profound hypotension from systemic vasodilation and fluid loss through leaky capillaries. The hemodynamic alterations are similar to those in septic shock, but are more pronounced.

1. **Epinephrine**

   There is no standardized dosing regimen for epinephrine in anaphylactic shock, but the intravenous regimen in Table 9.5 (5–15 µg/min), has been cited for its efficacy (19). A bolus dose (5–10 µg) can precede the continuous infusion (20).

2. **Volume Resuscitation**

   Aggressive volume resuscitation is essential in anaphylactic shock because *35% of the intravascular volume can be lost through leaky capillaries* (19). The initial volume resuscitation should include 1–2 liters of crystalloid fluid (or 20 mL/kg), or 500 mL of 5% albumin, given over 5–10 minutes (19). Thereafter, the infusion rate of fluids should be tailored to the hemodynamic status of the patient.

3. **Refractory Hypotension**

   Persistent hypotension despite epinephrine infusion and volume resuscitation can be managed by adding *glucagon* or another vasopressor (e.g., *norepinephrine*).

REFERENCES

1. American College of Chest Physicians/Society of Critical Care Medicine Consensus Conference Committee. Definitions of sepsis and organ failure and guidelines for the use of innovative therapies in sepsis. Chest 1992; 101:1644–1655.

2. Pittet D, Range-Frausto S, Li N, et al. Systemic inflammatory response syndrome, sepsis, severe sepsis, and septic shock: incidence, morbidities and outcomes in surgical ICU patients. Intensive Care Med 1995; 21:302–309.

3. Rangel-Frausto MS, Pittet D, Costigan M, et al. Natural history of the systemic inflammatory response syndrome (SIRS). JAMA 1995; 273:117–123.

4. Singer M, Deutschman CS, Seymore CW, et al. The Third International Consensus Definitions for Sepsis and Septic Shock (Sepsis-3). JAMA 2016; 315:801–810.

5. Vincent JL, de Moreno R, Takala J, et al. The SOFA (Sepsis-related Organ Failure Assessment) score to describe organ dysfunction/failure. Intensive Care Med 1996; 22:707–710.

6. Abraham E, Singer M. Mechanisms of sepsis-induced organ dysfunction. Crit Care Med 2007; 35:2409–2416.

7. Snell RJ, Parillo JE. Cardiovascular dysfunction in septic shock. Chest 1991; 99:1000–1009.

8. Ruggieri AJ, Levy RJ, Deutschman CS. Mitochondrial dysfunction and resuscitation in sepsis. Crit Care Clin 2010; 26:567–575.

9. Fink MP. Cytopathic hypoxia. Mitochondrial dysfunction as mechanism contributing to organ dysfunction in sepsis. Crit Care Clin 2001; 17:219–237.

10. Sair M, Etherington PJ, Winlove CP, Evans TW. Tissue oxygenation and perfusion in patients with systemic sepsis. Crit Care Med 2001; 29:1343–1349.

11. Dellinger RP, Levy MM, Rhodes A, et al. Surviving Sepsis Campaign: International guidelines for management of severe sepsis and septic shock, 2012. Intensive Care Med 2013; 39:165–228.

12. Boyd JH, Forbes J, Nakada T-A, et al. Fluid resuscitation in septic shock: a positive fluid balance and elevated central venous pressure are associated with increased mortality. Crit Care Med 2011; 39:259–265.

13. Polito A, Parisini E, Ricci Z, et al. Vasopressin for treatment of vasodilatory shock: an ESICM systematic review and meta-analysis. Intensive Care Med 2012; 38:9–19.

14. Vallee F, Vallet B, Mathe O, et al. Central venous-to-arterial carbon dioxide difference: an additional target for goal-directed therapy[y in septic shock? Intensive Care Med 2008; 34:2218–2225.

15. Angus DC, Barnato AE, Bell D, et al. A systematic review and meta-analysis of early goal-directed therapy for septic shock: the ARISE, ProCESS, and ProMISe Investigators. Intensive Care Med 2015; 41:1549–1560.

16. Volbeda M, Wetterslev J, Gluud C, et al. Glucocorticoids for sepsis: systematic review with meta-analysis and trial sequential analysis. Intensive Care Med 2015; 41:1220–1234.

17. NICE-SUGAR Study Investigators. Intensive versus conventional glucose control in critically ill patients. N Engl J Med 2009; 360:1283–1297.

18. Marik PE, Preiser J-C. Toward understanding tight glycemic control in the ICU. Chest 2010; 137:544–551.

19. Lieberman P, Nicklas RA, Oppenheimer J, et al. The diagnosis and management of anaphylaxis practice parameter: 2010 update. J Allergy Clin Immunol 2010; 126:480.e1–480.e42.

20. Sampson HA, Munoz-Furlong A, Campbell RL, et al. Second symposium on the definition and management of anaphylaxis: summary report. Ann Emerg Med 2006; 47:373–380.

Chapter 10

Colloid and Crystalloid Resuscitation

This chapter presents the variety of crystalloid and colloid fluids available for use, and describes the salient features of these fluids, both individually and as a group.

I. CRYSTALLOID FLUIDS

Crystalloid fluids are electrolyte solutions that move freely from the plasma to the interstitial fluid. The principal ingredient in crystalloid fluids is the inorganic salt, sodium chloride.

A. Volume Distribution

Crystalloid fluids distribute uniformly in extracellular fluid: i.e., plasma and interstitial fluid. Since plasma volume is 25% of the interstitial fluid volume (see Table 7.1), then 25% of an infused crystalloid fluid will expand the plasma volume, and 75% of the infused volume will expand the interstitial fluid (1). Thus, *the principal effect of crystalloid fluids is to expand the interstitial fluid volume, not the plasma volume.*

B. Isotonic Saline

The most widely used crystalloid fluid is 0.9% sodium chloride (0.9% NaCL), better known as *normal saline* (a misnomer, as will be demonstrated).

1. **Features**

   The notable features of 0.9% NaCL are shown in Table 10.1 (2). When compared to plasma (also included in the table), 0.9% NaCL has a higher sodium concentration (154 vs. 141 mEq/L), a much higher chloride concentration (154 vs. 103 mEq/L), and a lower pH (5.7 vs. 7.4). The only feature of 0.9% NaCL that matches plasma is the measured osmolality. These comparisons show that *normal saline is not normal* chemically, *but it is isotonic with plasma*. Therefore, *the appropriate name for this fluid is isotonic saline*, not normal saline.

   Note: The measured osmolalities in Table 10.1 (measured by freezing point depression) provide a more accurate reflection of in vivo osmotic activity than the calculated osmolarities (which are the summed concentrations of all osmotically active species in a fluid). Note that the measured osmotic activities are lower than the calculated (predicted) activities. This discrepancy is caused by electrostatic interactions between ions in the fluid, which reduces the number of osmotically active particles. This deserves mention because the manufacturers of crystalloid fluids use the calculated osmotic activity to describe the in vivo behavior of the fluid.

2. **Volume Effects**

   The volume effects of 0.9% NaCL in plasma and interstitial fluid are illustrated in Figure 10.1.

   a. Infusion of one liter of 0.9% NaCL adds 275 mL to the plasma volume and 825 mL to the interstitial fluid volume (1). This is the volume distribution expected from a crystalloid fluid.

   b. Note that the total increase in extracellular volume in Figure 10.1 (1,100 mL) is slightly greater than the infused volume. The additional 100 mL of extracellular fluid is the result of a fluid shift from intracellular to extracellular fluid compartments, prompted by the excess sodium in 0.9% NaCL.

Table 10.1	Comparison of Crystalloid Fluids and Plasma			
Components	Plasma	0.9% NaCL	Ringer's Lactate	Normosol, Plasma-Lyte
Sodium (mEq/L)	135-145	154	130	140
Chloride (mEq/L)	98-106	154	109	98
Potassium (mEq/L)	3.5-5.0	—	4	5
Ionized Calcium (mg/dL)	3.0-4.5	—	4	—
Magnesium (mg/dL)	1.8-3.0	—	—	3
Buffer (mmol/L)	HCO_3 (22-28)	—	Lactate (28)	Acetate (27) Gluconate (23)
pH	7.36-7.44	5.7	6.5	7.4
Calculated osmolarity (mosm/L)	291	308	273	295
Measured osmolality† (mosm/kg H_2O)	287	286	256	271

†More accurate reflection of osmotic activity in vivo. See text for explanation.
From Reference 2.

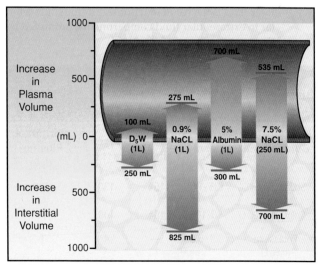

FIGURE 10.1 The effects of selected intravenous fluids on plasma volume and interstitial fluid volume. The infusion volume of each fluid is shown in parentheses. Data from Reference 1.

3. Adverse Effects

a. Interstitial edema is a risk with all crystalloid fluids, but the risk is greatest with isotonic saline (3) because the sodium load exceeds that in other crystalloid fluids (and sodium is the principal determinant of extracellular volume).

b. Rapid or large-volume infusions of isotonic saline are often accompanied by a *hyperchloremic metabolic acidosis* (4), which is attributed to the excess chloride in isotonic saline. The pathological significance of this condition has been debated, but there is evidence that hyperchloremia is associated with increased mortality in critically ill patients (5).

c. Infusions of isotonic saline are accompanied by a decrease in renal perfusion, presumably as a result of chloride-mediated renal vasoconstriction (6). This has raised concern about the potential for isotonic saline to promote acute kidney injury (AKI). However, at least 12 clinical trials have shown no evidence of a causal link between isotonic saline and AKI (4,6).

C. Ringer's Lactate

Ringer's solution (introduced in 1880 by Sydney Ringer, a British physician) is a 0.9% NaCL solution that contains potassium and calcium (which were added to promote the viability of frog heart preparations, a research interest of Dr. Ringer). Lactate was later added as a buffer (by Alexis Hartmann, an American pediatrician) to create *Ringer's lactate solution* (also known as *Hartmann's solution*).

1. **Features**

   The chemical features of Ringer's lactate are included in Table 10.1. The following comparisons with 0.9% NaCL are significant:

   a. The addition of potassium and calcium (in concentrations that approximate the free or ionized levels in plasma) is balanced by a reduction in the sodium concentration (to 130 mEq/L) to maintain electrical neutrality.

   b. Lactate is added (as sodium lactate) as a buffer, and is metabolized to bicarbonate in the liver. The chemical reaction is as follows:

   $$CH_2\text{-}CHOH\text{-}COO^- + 3O_2 \rightarrow 2CO_2 + 2H_2O + HCO_3^- \quad (10.1)$$

   Note that oxygen is required for this reaction, which means that *lactate will not act as a buffer source when tissue hypoxia is present* (i.e., in circulatory shock) (2).

c. The addition of lactate requires a reduction in chloride concentration for electrical neutrality. *The chloride concentration in Ringer's lactate is close to that in plasma*, which *minimizes the risk of hyperchloremic metabolic acidosis.*

d. The osmolality of Ringer's lactate is significantly lower than plasma, and is the lowest of the crystalloid fluids. This hypotonicity makes Ringer's lactate the least desirable crystalloid fluid for patients with cerebral edema, or those at risk for cerebral edema (e.g., traumatic head injuries).

2. **Adverse Effects**

a. The calcium in Ringer's lactate can bind to the citrated anticoagulant in blood products. For this reason, *Ringer's solutions are contraindicated as diluent fluids for the transfusion of packed red blood cells* (2). However, clot formation does not occur if the volume of Ringer's solution does not exceed 50% of the volume of packed RBCs, or if the fluid is infused rapidly (7).

b. The lactate content in Ringer's lactate (28 mmol/L) creates the risk of hyperlactatemia, especially when lactate metabolism is impeded (i.e., in liver failure or circulatory shock). This risk was evident in a study of burn patients, where hyperlactatemia was common when Ringer's lactate was used for fluid management, but not when a lactate-free Ringer's fluid was used (8).

c. Considering this risk of hyperlactatemia, and the diagnostic and prognostic value of serum lactate levels in critically ill patients (see Figure 6.2), *it seems wise to avoid Ringer's lactate solution in patients with elevated lactate levels, liver failure, or circulatory shock.*

d. *Note:* Blood samples withdrawn through catheters being used for Ringer's lactate infusions can yield spuriously high lactate levels (9).

D. Normal pH Fluids

There are two crystalloid fluids with a pH in the normal, physiological range: *Normosol* and *Plasma-Lyte*. The composition of these fluids is identical, and is shown in Table 10.1.

1. **Features**

   a. The chloride concentration in these fluids (98 mEq/L) is within the normal, physiological range, and they contain magnesium (3 mg/dL) instead of calcium.

   b. These fluids contain both acetate (27 mmol/L), and gluconate (23 mmol/L) as buffers. Gluconate is a weak alkalinizing agent that adds little to the buffer capacity (2), but acetate is rapidly metabolized to bicarbonate in skeletal muscle via the following oxidation reaction:

   $$CH_3\text{-}COO^- + 2O_2 \;\rightarrow\; CO_2 + H_2O + HCO_3^- \qquad (10.2)$$

   Note that O_2 is required for this reaction, which means that acetate may not serve as a buffer source when tissues are hypoxic (e.g., in circulatory shock), similar to lactate (see Equation 10.1).

   c. According to the measured osmolality of these fluids (271 mosm/kg H_2O), they are hypotonic to plasma, but not as hypotonic as Ringer's lactate (256 mosm/kg H_2O).

2. **Advantages**

   These fluids offer the following advantages over other crystalloid fluids:

   a. The physiological chloride concentration eliminates the risk of hyperchloremic metabolic acidosis.

   b. The absence of lactate eliminates the risk of spurious hyperlactatemia in patients with liver failure or circulatory shock. In addition, acetate is considered superior to lactate as a buffer source because it is more rapidly converted to bicarbonate (2).

c. The absence of calcium makes these fluids suitable for use with blood transfusions.

d. In studies comparing isotonic saline and Plasma-Lyte, the latter showed less tendency for interstitial edema, and was associated with improved outcomes (3,10).

E. Hypertonic Saline

Concentrated NaCL (hypertonic saline) solutions have been used in the management of traumatic shock, traumatic brain injury, and symptomatic hyponatremia. The most widely used hypertonic saline solutions are shown in Table 10.2.

Table 10.2	Hypertonic Saline			
Solution	Sodium (mEq/L)	Chloride (mEq/L)	Osmolarity† (mosm/L)	pH
3% NaCL	513	513	1026	5
5% NaCL	856	856	1712	5
7.5% NaCL	1283	1283	2566	5.7

3% and 5% NaCL is available in 500 mL unit sizes from Baxter International. 7.5% NaCL is not commercially available, but is prepared on request by hospital pharmacies.

†Calculated as the sum of the Na and CL concentrations.

1. **Volume Effects**

a. Small volumes of hypertonic saline are more effective for expanding the plasma volume than larger volumes of isotonic saline. This is demonstrated in Figure 10.1. Note that 250 ml of 7.5% NaCL produces a 535 ml increment in plasma volume and a 700 ml increase in interstitial fluid (total volume increment = 1,235 ml), whereas one liter of 0.9% NaCL produces only a 275 ml increase in plasma volume.

b. Intracellular fluid shifts are responsible for the extra-cellular volume expansion, with RBCs and endothelial cells contributing to the increment in plasma volume.

2. **Traumatic Shock**

Despite numerous physiological benefits (11), resuscitation of trauma-related hemorrhagic shock with hypertonic saline (500 ml of 5% saline or 250 ml of 7.5% saline) has demonstrated no consistent survival benefit over resuscitation with isotonic fluids (12). Nevertheless, small-volume resuscitation with hypertonic saline has a continuing appeal for early resuscitation of combat injuries in the field (where large volumes of resuscitation fluids are not immediately available).

3. **Traumatic Brain Injury**

a. In cases of post-traumatic intracranial hypertension, hypertonic saline has proven effective in reducing intracranial pressure (ICP), and offers some advantages over conventional therapy with mannitol (i.e., greater magnitude of ICP reduction, longer duration of action, and no rebound increase in ICP) (13).

b. Effective hypertonic regimens include (14):

1) 250 ml of 3% or 5% saline, given as needed, to keep the ICP below 20–25 mm Hg.

2) 3% saline as a continuous infusion at 1 ml/kg/hr.

3) Plasma sodium should be monitored, and should not exceed 160 mEq/L.

II. 5% DEXTROSE SOLUTIONS

A. Protein-Sparing Effect

1. Prior to the standard use of enteral tube feedings and total

parenteral nutrition (TPN), 5% dextrose solutions were used to provide calories in patients who were unable to eat.

2. One gram of dextrose provides 3.4 kilocalories (kcal) when fully metabolized, so a 5% dextrose solution (50 grams per liter) provides 170 kcal per liter.

3. Daily infusion of 3 liters of a 5% dextrose (D_5) solution provides about 500 kcal per day, which is enough non-protein calories to limit the breakdown of endogenous proteins to meet daily caloric requirements. This protein-sparing effect is responsible for the early popularity of dextrose-containing fluids.

4. The current availability of enteral and parenteral nutrition regimens obviates the need for dextrose-containing fluids.

B. Volume Effects

1. The addition of dextrose to intravenous fluids increases osmolality; i.e., 50 g of dextrose adds 278 mosm/L to an intravenous fluid.

2. For a 5% dextrose-in-water solution (D_5W), the added dextrose brings the osmolality close to that of plasma. However, since the dextrose is taken up by cells and metabolized, this osmolality effect rapidly wanes, and the added water then moves into cells. This is shown in Figure 10.1, in the arrow marked D_5W, where the combined increments in plasma volume (100 mL) and interstitial fluid volume (250 mL) are far less than the volume infused (1,000 mL). This difference (650 mL) is the result of fluid movement into cells, which means that *D_5W primarily expands the intracellular volume, and should never be used as a plasma volume expander.*

C. Adverse Effects

1. **Enhanced Lactate Production**

a. In healthy subjects, only 5% of an infused glucose load will be metabolized to lactate, but in critically ill patients with tissue hypoperfusion, as much as 85% of glucose metabolism is diverted to lactate production (15).

b. Studies in patients with compromised circulatory flow have shown that infusion of 5% dextrose solutions produces significant increases in serum lactate levels (16).

2. **Hyperglycemia**

Infusion of D_5W increases the risk of hyperglycemia, which has several undesirable effects in critically ill patients, including immune suppression (17), aggravation of ischemic brain injury (see Chapter 42), and an association with increased mortality (18).

D. Recommendation

Considering that dextrose-containing fluids offer no benefit, but can be harmful, *the routine use of these fluids should be abandoned.*

III. COLLOID FLUIDS

The behavior of colloid fluids is determined by a force that is described briefly in the next section.

A. Colloid Osmotic Pressure

1. Colloid fluids contain large molecules that do not readily move out of the vascular compartment. These molecules create an osmotic force called the *colloid osmotic pressure* (or *oncotic pressure*) that promotes the retention of water in the vascular compartment.

2. The following relationship identifies the role of the colloid osmotic pressure in capillary fluid exchange.

$$Q \sim (P_c - COP) \qquad (10.3)$$

a. Q is the flow rate across the capillaries.

b. P_c is the hydrostatic pressure in the capillaries.

c. COP is the colloid osmotic pressure of plasma. About 80% of the COP is attributed to the albumin concentration in plasma.

3. The two pressures (P_c and COP) act in opposition: P_c favors the movement of fluid out of the capillaries, and COP favors movement into the capillaries.

4. In the supine position, the normal P_c averages 25 mm Hg, and the normal COP is about 28 mm Hg (19), so the two forces are roughly matched.

5. The volume distribution of both crystalloid and colloid fluids can be explained by their effect on the COP of plasma.

a. Crystalloid fluids reduce the plasma COP (dilutional effect), which favors the movement of these fluids out of the bloodstream.

b. Colloid fluids tend to preserve the plasma COP, which favors the retention of these fluids in the bloodstream.

B. Volume Effects

1. The effect of colloid fluid resuscitation on plasma and interstitial fluid volumes is shown in Figure 10.1. The colloid fluid in this case is a 5% albumin solution; infusion of one liter adds 700 mL to the plasma and 300 mL to the interstitial fluid. Thus, 70% of the infused colloid fluid is retained in the vascular compartment.

2. Comparing the effects of the colloid and crystalloid fluid on plasma volume in Figure 10.1 reveals that *colloid fluids are about three times more effective than crystalloid fluids for increasing the plasma volume* (1,20,21).

C. Albumin Solutions

Albumin solutions are heat-treated preparations of human serum albumin that are available as a 5% solution (50 g/L) and a 25% solution (250 g/L) in 0.9% NaCL. The salient features of these fluids are shown in Table 10.3.

1. **Volume Effects**

   a. The 5% albumin solution is a *hypooncotic* fluid (i.e., the COP is 20 mm Hg, which is less than the COP of plasma). It is given in aliquots of 250 mL, and the volume effect (at least 70% retention in plasma, as indicated in Table 10.3) begins to dissipate at 6 hours, and is lost after 12 hours (1,20).

   b. The 25% albumin solution is a *hyperoncotic* fluid (i.e., the COP is 70 mm Hg, about 2.5 times that of plasma). It is given in aliquots of 50 or 100 mL, and the increment in plasma volume is about 3–4 times the infused volume, as shown in Table 10.3. (This volume is drawn from interstitial fluid.) The duration of effect is similar to 5% albumin.

   c. Because 25% albumin does not replace lost volume, but instead shifts fluid from one compartment to another, it *should not be used for volume resuscitation in cases of acute blood loss*. The principal role for 25% albumin is in patients with hypoalbuminemia and edema who are either hypotensive or resistant to diuretic therapy. (In both instances, 25% albumin can increase plasma volume in an attempt to correct the problem without infusing relatively large volumes of isotonic crystalloid fluids.)

2. **Safety**

a. Early claims of increased mortality attributed to albumin solutions have not been corroborated in more recent studies (22,23).

b. The consensus opinion at the present time is that 5% albumin is safe to use as a resuscitation fluid, with the possible exception of patients with traumatic head injury; i.e., one large study has shown a higher mortality rate in patients with traumatic brain injury who were resuscitated with albumin instead of isotonic saline (24).

Table 10.3	Colloid Fluid Comparisons		
Fluid	**COP (mm Hg)**	**ΔPlasma Infusate Volume**	**Duration of Effect**
5% Albumin	20	0.7–1.3	12 hr
6% Hetastarch	30	1.0–1.3	24 hr
10% Dextran-40	40	1.0–1.5	6 hr
25% Albumin	70	3.0–4.0	12 hr

Data from References 1, 20, 21, 25.

D. Hetastarch

Hydroxyethyl starch (hetastarch) is a chemically modified starch polymer that is available as a 6% solution in isotonic saline.

1. **Features**

Hetastarch has a higher COP than 5% albumin, and is slightly more effective as a plasma volume expander (see Table 10.3) (20,25). The volume effects of hetastarch also last longer (up to 24 hours) than those of 5% albumin (25).

2. **Safety**

   a. There is convincing evidence that critically ill patients who receive hetastarch have an increased risk of renal failure requiring hemodialysis, and an increased mortality rate (26,27). Hetastarch is also associated with an increased risk of bleeding, especially following cardiopulmonary bypass (28).

   b. Because of the poor safety profile, *the FDA issued a warning in 2013 advising against the use of hetastarch in critically ill patients* (29).

E. Dextrans

The dextrans are glucose polymers that were first introduced as plasma volume expanders in the 1940s. The two most common dextran preparations are 10% dextran-40 and 6% dextran-70.

1. **Features**

   Both dextran preparations have a COP of 40 mm Hg (i.e., hyperoncotic fluids), and produce a greater increase in plasma volume than either 5% albumin or 6% hetastarch (see Table 10.3). Dextran-70 may be preferred because the duration of action (12 hours) is longer than that of dextran-40 (6 hours) (20).

2. **Disadvantages**

   a. Dextrans produce a dose-related bleeding tendency that involves impaired platelet aggregation, decreased levels of Factor VIII and von Willebrand factor, and enhanced fibrinolysis (30,31). The hemostatic defects are minimized by limiting the daily dextran dose to 20 mL/kg.

   b. Dextrans coat the surface of red blood cells and can interfere with the ability to cross-match blood. Red cell preparations must be washed to eliminate this problem. Another consequence of this interaction with red blood cells is an increase in the erythrocyte sedimentation rate (30).

c. Dextrans have been associated with a hyperoncotic renal injury similar to that reported with hetastarch (32). However, this is a rare occurrence.

d. Anaphylactic reactions were once common with dextrans, but are now reported in only 0.03% of infusions (30).

IV. THE COLLOID-CRYSTALLOID DEBATE

A. The Debate

There is a longstanding debate concerning which type of fluid (colloid or crystalloid) is most appropriate for correcting hypovolemia. The essential arguments are as follows:

1. Proponents of crystalloid resuscitation cite the lack of a proven survival benefit with colloid resuscitation (33), and the lower cost of crystalloid fluids.

2. Proponents of colloid resuscitation cite the relatively large volume of crystalloid fluids needed to expand the plasma volume (at least 3 times the volume of colloid fluids), thereby promoting edema formation and a positive fluid balance, both of which are associated with increased morbidity and mortality in critically ill patients (10,34).

As in all longstanding debates, the truth is somewhere in the middle.

B. A Resolution

The fallacy in the colloid-crystalloid debate is the assumption that one type of fluid is best for all the conditions associated with hypovolemia. The following examples demonstrate that *tailoring the type of resuscitation fluid to the specific cause of hypovolemia is a more logical approach than using the same type of fluid for all cases of hypovolemia.*

1. In cases of hypovolemic shock (where prompt restoration of intravascular volume is a priority), a colloid fluid like 5% albumin (which is much more effective for increasing plasma volume than crystalloid fluids) is physiologically the best choice.

2. In cases of hypovolemia due to dehydration (where there is uniform loss of interstitial fluid and plasma), a crystalloid fluid like Ringer's lactate solution (which is distributed uniformly throughout the extracellular fluid) is most appropriate.

3. In cases of hypovolemia where hypoalbuminemia is implicated (causing fluid shifts from plasma to interstitial fluid) small volumes of a hyperoncotic colloid fluid like 25% albumin (which will shift fluid back from interstitium to plasma) is an appropriate choice.

REFERENCES

1. Imm A, Carlson RW. Fluid resuscitation in circulatory shock. Crit Care Clin 1993; 9:313–333.

2. Reddy S, Weinberg L, Young P. Crystalloid fluid therapy. Crit Care 2016; 20:59.

3. Chowdhury AH, Cox EF, Francis ST, Lobo DN. A randomized, controlled, double-blind crossover study on the effects of 2-L infusions of 0.9% saline and Plasma-Lyte 148 on renal blood flow and renal cortical tissue perfusion in healthy volunteers. Ann Surg 2012; 256:18–24.

4. Orbegozo Cortes D, Rayo Bonor A, Vincent JL. Isotonic crystalloid solutions: a structured review of the literature. Br J Anesth 2014; 112:968–981.

5. Neyra JA, Canepa-Escaro F, Li X, et al. Association of hyper-chloremia with hospital mortality in critically ill septic patients. Crit Care Med 2015; 43:1938–1944.

6. Young P, Bailey M, Beasely R, et al. Effect of buffered crystalloid solution vs saline on acute kidney injury among patients in the intensive care unit. The SPLIT randomized clinical trial. JAMA 2015; 314:1701–1710.

7. King WH, Patten ED, Bee DE. An in vitro evaluation of ionized calcium levels and clotting in red blood cells diluted with lactated Ringer's solution. Anesthesiology 1988; 68:115–121.

8. Klezcewski GJ, Malcharek M, Raff T, et al. Safety of resuscitation with Ringer's acetate solution in severe burn (VolTRAB) – an observational trial. Burns 2014; 40:871–880.

9. Jackson EV Jr, Wiese J, Sigal B, et al. Effects of crystalloid solutions on circulating lactate concentrations. Part 1. Implications for the proper handling of blood specimens obtained from critically ill patients. Crit Care Med 1997; 25:1840–1846.

10. Shaw AD, Bagshaw SM, Goldstein SL, et al. Major complications, mortality, and resource utilization after open abdominal surgery: 0.9% saline compared to Plasma-Lyte. Ann Surg 2012; 255:821–829.

11. Galvagno SM, Mackenzie CF. New and future resuscitation fluids for trauma patients using hemoglobin and hypertonic saline. Anesthesiology Clin 2013; 31: 1–19.

12. Bunn F, Roberts I, Tasker R, et al. Hypertonic versus near isotonic crystalloid for fluid resuscitation in critically ill patients. Cochrane Database Syst Rev 2004; 3:CD002045.

13. Mangat HS, Hartl R. Hypertonic saline for the management of raised intracranial pressure after severe traumatic brain injury. Ann NY Acad Sci 2015; 1345:83–88.

14. Patanwala AE, Amini A, Erstad BL. Use of hypertonic saline injection in trauma. Am J Health Sys Pharm 2010; 67:1920–1928.

15. Gunther B, Jauch W, Hartl W, et al. Low-dose glucose infusion in patients who have undergone surgery. Arch Surg 1987; 122:765–771.

16. DeGoute CS, Ray MJ, Manchon M, et al. Intraoperative glucose infusion and blood lactate: endocrine and metabolic relationships during abdominal aortic surgery. Anesthesiology 1989; 71;355–361.

17. Turina M, Fry D, Polk HC, Jr. Acute hyperglycemia and the innate immune system: Clinical, cellular, and molecular aspects. Crit Care Med 2005; 33:1624–1633.

18. Van Den Berghe G, Wouters P, Weekers F, et al. Intensive insulin therapy in critically ill patients. New Engl J Med 2001; 345:1359–1367.

19. Guyton AC, Hall JE. Textbook of Medical Physiology. 10th ed., Philadelphia: W.B. Saunders, Co, 2000, pp. 169–170.

20. Griffel MI, Kaufman BS. Pharmacology of colloids and crystalloids. Crit Care Clin 1992; 8:235–254.

21. Kaminski MV, Haase TJ. Albumin and colloid osmotic pressure: implications for fluid resuscitation. Crit Care Clin 1992; 8:311–322.

22. Wilkes MN, Navickis RJ. Patient survival after human albumin administration: A meta-analysis of randomized, controlled trials. Ann Intern Med 2001; 135:149–164.

23. SAFE Study Investigators. A comparison of albumin and saline for fluid resuscitation in the Intensive Care Unit. N Engl J Med 2004; 350:2247–2256.

24. The SAFE Study Investigators. Saline or albumin for fluid resuscitation in patients with severe head injury. N Engl J Med 2007; 357:874–884.

25. Treib J, Baron JF, Grauer MT, Strauss RG. An international view of hydroxyethyl starches. Intensive Care Med 1999; 25:258–268.

26. Gattas DJ, Dan A, Myburgh J, et al. Fluid resuscitation with 6% hydroxyethyl starch (130/0.4 and 130/0.42) in acutely ill patients: systemic review of effects on mortality and treatment with renal replacement therapy. Intensive Care Med 2013; 39:558–568.

27. Zarychanski R, Abou-Setta AM, Turgeon AF, et al. Association of hydroxyethyl starch administration with mortality and acute kidney injury in critically ill patients requiring volume resuscitation: a systemic review and meta-analysis. JAMA 2013; 309:678–688.

28. Navickis RJ, Haynes GR, Wilkes MM. Effect of hydroxyethyl starch on bleeding after cardiopulmonary bypass: a meta-analysis of randomized trials. J Thorac Cardiovasc Surg 2012:144:223–30.

29. U.S. Food and Drug Administration. FDA Safety Communication: Boxed Warning on increased mortality and severe renal injury, and additional warning on risk of bleeding, for use of hydroxyethyl starch solutions in some settings. Available at www.fda.gov/BiologicsBloodVaccines/SafetyAvailability/ucm 358271.htm#professionals. Accessed 3/2016.

30. Nearman HS, Herman ML. Toxic effects of colloids in the intensive care unit. Crit Care Clin 1991; 7:713–723.

31. de Jonge E, Levi M. Effects of different plasma substitutes on blood coagulation: A comparative review. Crit Care Med 2001; 29:1261–1267.

32. Drumi W, Polzleitner D, Laggner AN, et al. Dextran-40, acute renal failure, and elevated plasma oncotic pressure. N Engl J Med 1988; 318:252–254.

33. Annane D, Siami S, Jaber S, et al. Effects of fluid resuscitation with colloids vs crystalloids on mortality in critically ill patients presenting with hypovolemic shock. The CRISTAL randomized trial. JAMA 2013; 310:1809–1817.

34. Boyd JH, Forbes J, Nakada TA, et al. Fluid resuscitation in septic shock: A positive fluid balance and elevated central venous pressure are associated with increased mortality. Crit Care Med 2011; 39:259–265.

Chapter 11

Anemia and Erythrocyte Transfusions

Anemia is almost universal in patients who spend a few days in the ICU (1), and about 50% of ICU patients receive erythrocyte transfusions to alleviate anemia (1-3). These transfusions can do harm, yet they are given without physiological evidence of need or benefit.

I. ANEMIA IN THE ICU

A. Definition

1. Anemia is defined as a *decrease in the oxygen carrying capacity of blood*. The most accurate measure of this is the red cell mass, which is not easily obtained. As a result, the hemoglobin (Hb) and hematocrit (Hct) are used as surrogate measures of the O_2 carrying capacity of blood. (The reference ranges for Hb, Hct, and other erythrocyte-related measurements are shown in Table 11.1.)

2. There is one problem with Hb and Hct as measures of O_2 carrying capacity; i.e., they are influenced by the plasma volume. For example, an increase in plasma volume will decrease the Hb and Hct (dilution effect), thereby creating the false impression of a drop in the O_2 carrying capacity of blood (pseudoanemia). Clinical studies have confirmed that the *Hb and Hct are unreliable as markers of anemia in critically ill patients* (4-6).

Table 11.1	Reference Ranges for Red Cell Parameters in Adults

Red Cell Count	**Mean Cellular Volume (MCV)**
Males: 4.6×10^{12}/L	Males: $80-100 \times 10^{-15}$/L
Females: 4.2×10^{12}/L	Females: same
Reticulocyte Count	**Hematocrit**
Males: $25-75 \times 10^{9}$/L	Males: 40–54%
Females: same	Females: 38–47%
Red Cell Volume	**Hemoglobin**
Males: 26 mL/kg	Males: 14–18 g/dL
Females: 24 mL/kg	Females: 12–16 g/dL

Sources: (1) Walker RH (ed.). Technical Manual of the American Association of Blood Banks, 10th ed., VA: American Association of Blood Banks, 1990: 649-650; (2) Billman RS, Finch CA. Red cell manual. 6th ed. Philadelphia, PA: Davis, 1994: 46.

B. Contributing Factors

ICU-associated anemia is attributed to two conditions: systemic inflammation, and repeated phlebotomy for laboratory studies.

1. Inflammation

   a. Inflammation is responsible for the *anemia of chronic disease*, which *is now called the anemia of inflammation* (3-6).

   b. The hematologic effects of inflammation include inhibition of erythropoietin release from the kidneys, reduced marrow responsiveness to erythropoietin, iron sequestration in macrophages, and increased destruction of RBCs (3,7).

c. The resulting anemia is hypochromic and microcytic, with a low plasma iron level. Inflammatory anemia can be confused with iron-deficiency anemia. However, the plasma ferritin level (a marker of tissue iron stores) is increased in inflammatory anemia, and decreased in iron-deficiency anemia.

2. **Phlebotomy**

a. The volume of blood withdrawn for laboratory tests averages 40–70 mL daily in ICU patients (8), and the cumulative loss of blood in one week can reach 500 mL (one unit of whole blood).

b. A significant percentage of blood loss for laboratory testing is related to technique; i.e., when a blood sample is obtained from a vascular catheter, an initial aliquot of blood is withdrawn first and discarded, to eliminate interference from intravenous fluids in the catheter. The discarded volume is about 5 mL per blood draw, and returning this blood to the patient can reduce daily phlebotomy loss by 50% (9).

C. Physiological Effects of Anemia

Anemia elicits two responses that help to preserve tissue oxygenation: (a) an increase in cardiac output, and (b) an increase in O_2 extraction from capillary blood.

1. **Cardiac Output**

The influence of anemia on cardiac output is explained by the Hagen-Poiseuille equation (see Equation 7.1 in Chapter 7), which shows that the flow rate of a fluid is inversely related to the viscosity of the fluid. Since Hct is the principal determinant of blood viscosity, a decrease in Hct will decrease blood viscosity, which will result in an increase in blood flow (cardiac output).

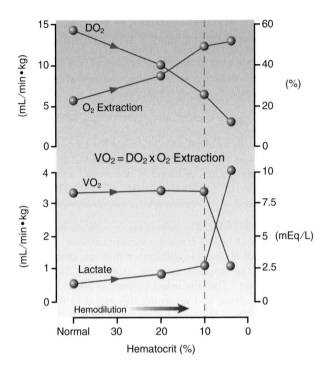

FIGURE 11.1 The influence of progressive isovolemic anemia on measures of systemic oxygenation. $DO_2 = O_2$ delivery, $VO_2 = O_2$ consumption. Data from Reference 10.

2. **O_2 Extraction**

   As described in Chapter 6, Section I-D, O_2 extraction is the ratio of O_2 consumption (VO_2) to O_2 delivery (DO_2); i.e.,

   $$O_2 \text{ Extraction } = VO_2 / DO_2 \qquad (11.1)$$

   Rearranging terms in this relationship yields the following:

   $$VO_2 = DO_2 \times O_2 \text{ Extraction} \qquad (11.2)$$

This relationship predicts that a decrease in O_2 delivery (e.g., from anemia), will not impair aerobic metabolism (VO_2) if there is a proportional increase in O_2 extraction. This type of response is demonstrated in Figure 11.1 (10); i.e.,

a. The progressive decrease in Hct is accompanied by a similar decrease in O_2 delivery (DO_2). However, the decrease in DO_2 is initially accompanied by an increase in O_2 extraction, and this keeps the O_2 consumption (VO_2) constant.

b. When the Hct falls below 10%, the increase in O_2 extraction is no longer able to match the decrease in DO_2, and the VO_2 begins to fall. This is the *anaerobic threshold*.

c. Thus, aerobic metabolism is maintained during progressive anemia because of an increase in O_2 extraction, and the Hct and Hb must fall to extremely low levels before aerobic metabolism is affected.

3. **Tolerance to Anemia**

   Animal studies have shown that when the intravascular volume is maintained, a decrease in Hct to as low as 5 to 10% (Hb = 1.5 to 3 g/dL) does not adversely affect aerobic metabolism (10-12). In other words, *severe anemia is tolerated when the intravascular volume is maintained.*

II. TRANSFUSION TRIGGERS

A. Hemoglobin

Surveys indicate that 90% of erythrocyte transfusions in ICU patients are given to alleviate anemia (13), and thus are guided by the Hb concentration in blood.

1. The first transfusion trigger, which dates back to 1942, was a Hb concentration of 10 g/dL and a corresponding

Hct of 30% (14). This "10/30" rule became the standard for over half a century.

2. More recent clinical studies have demonstrated that adopting a lower transfusion trigger (i.e., Hb <7 g/dL) has no adverse consequences, and decreases the transfusion burden considerably (13,15).

3. However, *the use of the Hb concentration in blood as a "transfusion trigger" is a flawed practice* for two reasons:

   a. The Hb concentration in blood provides no information about the state of tissue oxygenation.

   b. The Hb concentration in blood is influenced by changes in plasma volume, which means that changes in the Hb concentration in blood do not always reflect changes in the O_2 carrying capacity of blood.

4. The most recent guidelines on erythrocyte transfusions in critically ill patients state that the use of the Hb concentration as a "trigger" for transfusions *should be avoided* (4). Despite this statement, the guidelines recommend that transfusion *should be considered* when the Hb is <7 g/dL in critically ill patients, and <8 g/dL in acute coronary syndromes (4).

B. Oxygen Extraction

1. As described earlier (and shown in Figure 11.1), anemia elicits a compensatory increase in O_2 extraction from capillary blood, which serves to maintain a constant rate of aerobic metabolism. However, the increase in O_2 extraction reaches a maximum at about 50%, whereupon further decreases in Hb are accompanied by proportional decreases in O_2 consumption.

2. Therefore, *an O_2 extraction of 50% identifies the anaerobic threshold, and can serve as a physiologic transfusion trigger* (16,17).

3. CENTRAL VENOUS O_2 SATURATION: When the arterial O_2 saturation is close to 100%, the O_2 extraction is roughly equivalent to the difference between the arterial and central venous O_2 saturations $(SaO_2 - ScvO_2)$:

$$O_2 \text{ Extraction } = \ SaO_2 - ScvO_2 \qquad (11.3)$$

(See Chapter 6, Section I-D for the derivation of this relationship), or to simplify further:

$$O_2 \text{ Extraction } = \ 1 - ScvO_2 \qquad (11.4)$$

An $ScvO_2$ <70% has been proposed as a transfusion trigger (20), although a lower $ScvO_2$ (i.e., closer to 50%) would be more appropriate for identifying the anaerobic threshold.

III. ERYTHROCYTE PRODUCTS

The red blood cell (RBC) preparations available for transfusion are listed in Table 11.2.

A. Packed RBCs

1. The RBC fraction of donated blood is placed in a preservative fluid and stored at $1-6°C$. Newer preservative solutions contain adenine, which helps to maintain ATP levels in stored RBCs, and allows storage of donor RBCs for up to 42 days (18).

2. Each unit of donor RBCs, known as packed RBCs (PRBCs), has a Hct of about 60% and a volume of about 350 mL.

3. PRBCs also contain 30–50 mL of residual plasma, and a considerable number of leukocytes (1–3 billion leukocytes per unit of PRBCs) (18).

Table 11.2	Erythrocyte Transfusion Preparations
Preparation	**Features**
Packed RBCs	1. Each unit has a volume of 350 mL and hematocrit of about 60%. 2. Contains leukocytes and residual plasma (15–30 mL per unit). 3. Can be stored for 42 days with appropriate additives.
Leukocyte-Poor RBCs	1. Donor RBCs are passed through specialized filters to remove most of the leukocytes. This reduces the risk of febrile reactions to RBC transfusions. 2. Indicated for patients with a history of febrile transfusion reactions.
Washed RBCs	1. Saline washing of packed RBCs removes residual plasma, which reduces the risk of hypersensitivity reactions. 2. Used in patients with a history of transfusion-related allergic reactions, and in patients with IgA deficiency, who are at risk for transfusion-related anaphylaxis.

From Reference 20.

B. Leukocyte-Reduced RBCs

1. The leukocytes in PRBCs can trigger an antibody response in the recipient after repeated transfusions, and this is responsible for *febrile non-hemolytic transfusion reactions* (see later).

2. To reduce the risk of this reaction, donor RBCs are passed through specialized filters to remove most of the leukocytes. This is performed routinely in many blood banks, but universal leukocyte reduction has yet to be adopted in the United States.

3. Leukocyte-reduced RBCs are recommended for patients with prior febrile non-hemolytic transfusion reactions (18).

C. Washed RBCs

1. Donor RBCs can be washed with isotonic saline to remove residual plasma. This reduces the risk of hypersensitivity reactions caused by prior sensitization to plasma proteins in donor blood.

2. Washed RBCs are recommended for patients with a history of hypersensitivity reactions to blood transfusions, and for patients with immunoglobulin A deficiency, who have an increased risk of transfusion-related anaphylaxis (18).

3. Saline washing does not effectively remove leukocytes.

IV. ERYTHROCYTE TRANSFUSIONS

A. RBC Compatibility

1. **Blood Groups**

   a. There are four major blood groups, based on the presence or absence of two antigens (A and B) on the surface of red blood cells (A, B, AB, and no antigens, designated O). Each blood group is classified further by the presence or absence of another surface antigen, the *Rhesus* (Rh) factor.

   b. Plasma contains antibodies to antigens that are absent on the RBCs. For example, type O blood has no A or B antigens on the RBCs, and the plasma contains anti-A and anti-B antibodies.

2. **Universal Donor RBCs**

   a. Life-threatening hemolytic transfusion reactions are

the result of anti-A, anti-B, or anti-Rh antibodies in the recipient that react with their corresponding antigens on donor RBCs.

b. Transfusing antigen-free PRBCs (i.e., type-O, Rh-negative) eliminates the risk of hemolytic transfusion reactions. Therefore, type-O, Rh-negative blood is called the *universal red cell donor.*

c. Uncrossmatched type-O Rh-positive RBCs are often used in cases of acute hemorrhage. In a study of over five hundred transfusions of type-O Rh-positive RBCs, only one Rh-negative patient developed anti-Rh antibodies after transfusion (18).

3. **Rh Immunoglobulin**

a. If an Rh-negative woman receives Rh-positive RBCs, anti-Rh antibodies may be formed, and these antibodies can cross the placenta during pregnancy and cause hemolysis in an Rh-positive fetus. Rh immunoglobulin (RhoGAM, Kedrion Biopharma, Fort Lee, NJ) can prevent the formation of anti-Rh antibodies in response to an Rh-positive transfusion.

b. In women of childbearing age who are Rh-negative, an injection of Rh immunoglobulin should be given within 72 hours of a transfusion with Rh-positive PRBCs (19).

B. Blood Filters

Standard blood filters (pore size 170–260 microns) are required for the transfusion of all blood products (20). These filters trap blood clots and other debris, but they do not trap leukocytes, and are not effective for leukocyte reduction (20). These filters can become an impediment to flow as they collect trapped debris, and sluggish infusion rates should prompt replacement of the filter.

C. Physiologic Effects

1. In an average sized adult, one unit of PRBCs is expected to raise the Hb concentration and Hct by 1 g/dL and 3%, respectively (20).

2. The effects of RBC transfusions on measures of systemic oxygenation are shown in Figure 11.2. The data in this figure is from a group of postoperative patients with severe normovolemic anemia (Hb <7 g/dL) who were transfused with 1–2 units of PRBCs to raise the Hb above 7 g/dL. The RBC transfusions increased the mean Hb concentration from 6.4 to 8 g/dL (25% increase), and there was a similar increase in O_2 delivery (DO_2). However, systemic O_2 consumption (VO_2) was unchanged, indicating that RBC transfusions did not enhance tissue oxygenation.

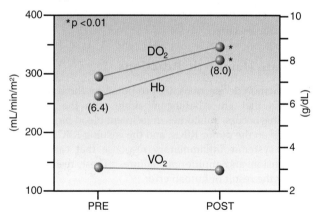

FIGURE 11.2 Effects of erythrocyte transfusions (1–2 units PRBCs) on hemoglobin concentration (Hb), O_2 delivery (DO_2), and O_2 consumption (VO_2) in 11 postoperative patients with severe anemia (Hb <7 g/dL). Data points represent mean values for each parameter. Numbers in parentheses are the mean Hb concentrations before and after transfusion. Data from personal observations.

3. Failure of RBC transfusions to enhance tissue oxygenation has been confirmed in several clinical studies (21-23), and prolonged storage of RBCs can actually impair tissue oxygenation after transfusion (24). These studies have prompted the following statement in the guidelines for RBC transfusions (4): *"RBC transfusion should not be considered an absolute method to improve tissue oxygenation in critically ill patients."*

V. TRANSFUSION RISKS

The spectrum of adverse events associated with blood transfusions are shown in Table 11.3, along with the incidence of each event expressed in relation to the number of units transfused (20,25-27). Note that transfusion errors are much more frequent than the feared transmission of HIV or the hepatitis B virus. The following is a brief description of the principal transfusion reactions.

A. Acute Hemolytic Reactions

Acute hemolytic reactions are prompted by the transfusion of RBCs that are ABO-incompatible with the recipient. When this occurs, antibodies in recipient blood bind to ABO antigens on the donor RBCs, and the ensuing RBC lysis triggers a systemic inflammatory response that can lead to hypotension and multiorgan failure. These reactions are usually the result of human error.

1. Clinical Features

The hallmark of acute hemolytic reactions is the abrupt onset of fever, dyspnea, chest pain, low back pain, and hypotension, within minutes after starting the transfusion. Severe reactions are accompanied by a consumptive coagulopathy and progressive multiorgan dysfunction.

Table 11.3	Adverse Events Associated with RBC Transfusions (per units transfused)
Immune Reactions	**Other Risks**
Nonhemolytic fever (1 in 200)	Transmitted Infections:
Hypersensitivity Reactions:	Bacterial (1 in 500,000)
Urticaria (1 in 100)	Hepatitis B virus (1 in 220,000)
Anaphylaxis (1 in 1,000)	Hepatitis C virus (1 in 1.6 million)
Anaphylactic shock (1 in 50,000)	HIV (1 in 1.6 million)
Acute lung injury (1 in 12,000)	Transfusion Errors:
Nosocomial Infections (?)	Wrong person transfused (1 in 15,000)
Acute hemolytic reaction (1 in 35,000)	Incompatible transfusion (1 in 33,000)
Fatal hemolytic reaction (1 in 1 million)	

From References 20, 25-27.

2. **Management**

a. If a hemolytic reaction is suspected, STOP the transfusion immediately and verify that the correct blood was given to the correct patient. It is imperative to stop the transfusion as soon as possible because the severity of hemolytic reactions is a function of the volume of blood transfused (25).

b. If the donor blood is correctly matched to the patient, an acute hemolytic reaction is unlikely. However, the blood bank must be notified, and they will ask for blood samples to perform a plasma free hemoglobin determination (for evidence of intravascular hemolysis) and a direct Coomb's test (for evidence of the anti-ABO antibodies).

c. If an acute hemolytic reaction is confirmed, support blood pressure and ventilation as needed. The management of severe hemolytic reactions is similar to septic shock (i.e., volume resuscitation and a vasopressor, if necessary). Most patients should survive the illness.

B. Febrile Nonhemolytic Reactions

1. **Clinical Features**

   a. A febrile, nonhemolytic transfusion reaction is defined as a temperature elevation >1°C (1.8°F) that occurs during transfusion or up to 6 hours after transfusion, and is not attributed to another cause (20).

   b. The fever typically does not appear in the first hour after the start of transfusion (unlike the fever associated with acute hemolytic reactions), but it can be accompanied by rigors.

   c. The culprit is the presence of antileukocyte antibodies in recipient blood that react with antigens on donor leukocytes. This triggers the release of endogenous pyrogens from phagocytes, which is the source of the fever.

   d. This reaction is reported in 0.5% of RBC transfusions and occurs in patients who have received prior transfusions, and in multiparous women.

   e. Transfusion of leukocyte-reduced RBCs reduces, but does not eliminate, the risk of this reaction (20).

2. **Management**

   The initial approach to transfusion-related fever is the same as described for hemolytic transfusion reactions. The diagnosis is confirmed by excluding the presence of hemolysis with the tests described previously.

a. The blood bank will perform a gram stain on the donor blood, and may request blood cultures on the recipient. This is usually unrewarding because microbial contamination in stored blood is rare (1 per 5,000,000 units).

3. **Future Transfusions**

a. More than 75% of patients with a nonhemolytic fever will not experience a similar reaction to subsequent transfusions (27). Therefore, no special precautions are needed for future transfusions.

b. If a second febrile reaction occurs, leukocyte-reduced RBCs are advised for all subsequent transfusions.

C. Hypersensitivity Reactions

Hypersensitivity reactions are the result of sensitization to plasma proteins in donor blood from prior transfusions. Patients with IgA deficiency are prone to hypersensitivity transfusion reactions, and prior exposure to plasma products is not required.

1. **Clinical Features**

a. The most common hypersensitivity reaction is urticaria, which is reported in one of every 100 units transfused (27), and appears during the transfusion.

b. The abrupt onset of dyspnea during a transfusion could represent laryngeal edema or bronchospasm from anaphylaxis, and hypotension from anaphylactic shock can be mistaken for an acute hemolytic reaction.

2. **Management**

a. Mild urticaria without fever does not require interruption of the transfusion. However, the popular practice is to stop the transfusion temporarily and administer an antihistamine for symptom relief (e.g., *diphenhydramine*, 25–50 mg PO, IM, or IV).

b. Anaphylactic reactions should be managed as described in Chapter 9, Section III. The transfusion should be stopped immediately if anaphylaxis is suspected.

c. Washed RBCs should be used for all future transfusions in patients with hypersensitivity reactions. However, in patients with anaphylactic reactions, future transfusions are risky, even with washed RBCs, and should be avoided unless absolutely necessary.

d. Patients who develop hypersensitivity reactions should be tested for an underlying IgA deficiency.

D. Acute Lung Injury

Transfusion-related acute lung injury (TRALI) is an inflammatory lung injury associated with RBC and platelet transfusions (28), and resembles the acute respiratory distress syndrome or ARDS (described in Chapter 17). The incidence is 1 per 12,000 transfusions (28), and the mortality rate is 6% (26,28). *TRALI is the leading cause of transfusion-related deaths* (28).

1. **Etiology**

   TRALI is believed to be the result of antileukocyte antibodies in donor blood that bind to antigens on circulating neutrophils in the recipient. This triggers neutrophil activation, and the activated neutrophils become sequestered in pulmonary capillaries and migrate into the lungs to produce the inflammatory injury.

2. **Clinical Features**

   a. Signs of respiratory compromise (dyspnea, tachypnea, hypoxemia, etc.) can appear for up to 6 hours after the start of a transfusion, but they usually appear within the first hour after the transfusion begins (28).

b. Fever is common, and the chest x-ray typically shows diffuse infiltrates in both lungs.

c. TRALI can be severe at the outset, and often requires mechanical ventilation, but the condition typically resolves within a week (28).

3. **Management**

a. If the transfusion is not completed, it should be stopped at the first signs of respiratory difficulty. The blood bank should be notified for all cases of TRALI. (Assays for antileukocyte antibodies are available, but are not currently used in the diagnostic evaluation of TRALI.)

b. The management of TRALI is supportive, and is very similar to the management of ARDS described in Chapter 17 (see Sections II and III).

4. **Future Transfusions**

There are no firm recommendations regarding future transfusions in patients who develop TRALI. Some recommend using washed RBCs to remove antibodies from donor blood, but the effectiveness of this measure is not known.

E. Nosocomial Infections

RBC transfusions have an immunosuppressant effect (29), and several clinical studies have shown that patients who receive blood transfusions have a higher incidence of nosocomial infections (30,31). Furthermore, at least 22 studies have shown that blood transfusion is an independent risk factor for nosocomial infections (32).

F. More Risk than Benefit

A review of 45 clinical studies evaluating RBC transfusions in critically ill patients, which included 272,596 patients, revealed the following findings (32):

1. In 42 of the 45 studies, the adverse effects of RBC transfusions outweighed any benefits.

2. Only 1 of 45 studies showed that the benefits of RBC transfusions outweighed the adverse effects.

3. Eighteen studies evaluated the relationship between RBC transfusions and survival, and 17 of the 18 studies showed that RBC transfusions were an independent risk factor for death. The likelihood of a fatal outcome was, on average, 70% higher in patients who received an RBC transfusion.

REFERENCES

1. Hebert PC, Tinmouth A, Corwin HL. Controversies in RBC transfusions in the critically ill. Chest 2007; 131:1583–1590.

2. Hayden SJ, Albert TJ, Watkins TR, Swenson ER. Anemia in critical illness. Am J Respir Crit Care Med 2012; 185(10):1049–1057.

3. Vincent JL, Baron JF, Reinhart K, et al. Anemia and blood transfusion in critically ill patients. JAMA 2002; 288:1499–1507.

4. Napolitano LM, Kurek S, Luchette FA, et al. Clinical practice guideline: Red blood cell transfusion in adult trauma and critical care. Crit Care Med 2009; 37:3124–3157.

5. Ferraris VA, Ferraris SP, Saha SP, et al. Perioperative blood transfusion and blood conservation in cardiac surgery; the Society of Thoracic Surgeons and the Society of Cardiovascular Anesthesiologists Clinical Practice Guideline. Ann Thorac Surg 2007; 83 (Suppl):S27–S86.

6. Jones JG, Holland BM, Wardrop CAJ. Total circulating red cells versus hematocrit as a primary descriptor of oxygen transport by the blood. Br J Hematol 1990; 76:228–232.

7. Hebert PC, Van der Linden P, Biro G, Hu LQ. Physiologic aspects of anemia. Crit Care Clin 2004; 20:187–212.

8. Smoller BR, Kruskall MS. Phlebotomy for diagnostic laboratory tests in adults: Pattern of use and effect on transfusion requirements. N Engl J Med 1986; 314:1233–1235.

9. Silver MJ, Li Y-H, Gragg LA, et al. Reduction of blood loss from diagnostic sampling in critically ill patients using a blood-conserving arterial line system. Chest 1993; 104:1711–1715.

10. Wilkerson DK, Rosen AL, Gould SA, et al. Oxygen extraction ratio: a valid indicator of myocardial metabolism in anemia. J Surg Res 1987; 42:629–634.

11. Levine E, Rosen A, Sehgal L, et al. Physiologic effects of acute anemia: implications for a reduced transfusion trigger. Transfusion 1990; 30:11–14.

12. Weiskopf RB, Viele M, Feiner J, et al. Human cardiovascular and metabolic response to acute, severe, isovolemic anemia. JAMA 1998; 279:217–221.

13. Hebert PC, Yetisir E, Martin C, et al. Is a low transfusion threshold safe in critically ill patients with cardiovascular disease. Crit Care Med 2001; 29:227–234.

14. Adam RC, Lundy JS. Anesthesia in cases of poor risk: Some suggestions for decreasing the risk. Surg Gynecol Obstet 1942: 74:1011–1101.

15. Hebert PC, Wells G, Blajchman MA, et al. A multicenter, randomized, controlled clinical trial of transfusion requirements in critical care. N Engl J Med 1999; 340:409–417.

16. Levy PS, Chavez RP, Crystal GJ, et al. Oxygen extraction ratio: a valid indicator of transfusion need in limited coronary vascular reserve? J Trauma 1992; 32:769–774.

17. Vallet B, Robin E, Lebuffe G. Venous oxygen saturation as a physiologic transfusion trigger. Crit Care 2010; 14:213–217.

18. Dutton RP, Shih D, Edelman BB, Hess J, Scalea TM. Safety of uncrossmatched type-O cells for resuscitation from hemorrhagic shock. J Trauma 2005; 59:1445–1449.

19. Qureshi H, Massey E, Kirwan D, Davies T, Robson S, White J, Jones J, Allard S. BCSH guideline for the use of anti-D immunoglobulin for the prevention of haemolytic disease of the fetus and newborn. Transfusion Medicine 2014; 24:8–20.

20. King KE (ed). Blood Transfusion Therapy: A Physician's Handbook. 9th ed. Bethesda, MD: American Association of Blood Banks, 2008:1–18.

21. Conrad SA, Dietrich KA, Hebert CA, Romero MD. Effects of red cell transfusion on oxygen consumption following fluid resuscitation in septic shock. Circ Shock 1990; 31:419–429.

22. Dietrich KA, Conrad SA, Hebert CA, et al. Cardiovascular and metabolic response to red blood cell transfusion in critically ill volume-resuscitated nonsurgical patients. Crit Care Med 1990; 18:940–944.

23. Marik PE, Sibbald W. Effect of stored-blood transfusion on oxygen delivery in patients with sepsis. JAMA 1993; 269:3024–3029.

24. Kiraly LN, Underwood S, Differding JA, Schreiber MA. Transfusion of aged packed red blood cells results in decreased tissue oxygenation in critically ill trauma patients. J Trauma 2009; 67:29–32.

25. Kuriyan M, Carson JL. Blood transfusion risks in the intensive care unit. Crit Care Clin 2004; 237–253.

26. Goodnough LT. Risks of blood transfusion. Crit Care Med 2003; 31:S678–686.

27. Sayah DM, Looney MR, Toy P. Transfusion reactions: newer concepts on the pathophysiology, incidence, treatment, and prevention of transfusion-related acute lung injury. Crit Care Clin 2012; 28:363–372.

28. Toy P, Gajic O, Bachetti P, et al. Transfusion-related acute lung injury: incidence and risk factors. Blood 2012; 119:1757–1767.

29. Vamvakas EC, Blajchman MA. Transfusion-related immunomodulation (TRIM): an update. Blood Rev 2007; 21:327–348.

30. Agarwal N, Murphy JG, Cayten CG, Stahl WM. Blood transfusion increases the risk of infection after trauma. Arch Surg 1993; 128:171–177.

31. Taylor RW, O'Brien J, Trottier SJ, et al. Red blood cell transfusions and nosocomial infections in critically ill patients. Crit Care Med 2006; 34:2302–2308.

32. Marik PE, Corwin HL. Efficacy of red blood cell transfusion in the critically ill: A systematic review of the literature. Crit Care Med 2008; 36:2667–2674.

Chapter 12

Platelets and Plasma

This chapter begins with a description of thrombocytopenia and platelet therapy in critically ill patients, and then focuses on the transfusion of plasma products, including recommendations for the rapid reversal of warfarin anticoagulation.

I. THROMBOCYTOPENIA

Thrombocytopenia is the most common hemostatic disorder in critically ill patients, with a reported incidence of up to 60% (1,2). Although thrombocytopenia is defined as a platelet count <150,000/μL, the ability to form a hemostatic plug is retained until the platelet count falls below 100,000/μL (2), so a platelet count <100,000/μL is more appropriate for identifying clinically significant thrombocytopenia.

A. Bleeding Risk

1. The risk of major bleeding is not determined by the platelet count alone, but also requires a structural lesion that is prone to bleeding.

2. In the absence of a structural lesion, platelet counts as low as 5,000/μL can be tolerated, without evidence of major bleeding (3).

3. The principal risk with a platelet counts <10,000/μL is spontaneous intracerebral hemorrhage, which is uncommon (2).

B. Etiologies

1. The most likely causes of thrombocytopenia in the ICU setting are listed in Table 12.1.

2. *Sepsis is the most common cause of thrombocytopenia in ICU patients* (4), and is the result of increased platelet destruction by macrophages.

Table 12.1	Potential Sources of Thrombocytopenia in the ICU
Nonpharmacological	**Pharmacological**
Cardiopulmonary Bypass	Anticonvulsants:
Disseminated Intravascular Coagulation (DIC)	Phenytoin
	Valproic Acid
HELLP Syndrome	Antimicrobial Agents:
	β-Lactams
Hemolytic-Uremic Syndrome	Linezolid
	TMP/SMX
HIV Infection	Vancomycin
Intra-aortic Balloon Pump	Antineoplastic Agents
Liver Disease/Hypersplenism	Antithrombotic Agents
	Heparin
Massive Transfusion	IIb/IIIa Inhibitors
Renal Replacement Therapy	Histamine H_2 Blockers
Sepsis	Miscellaneous Drugs
	Amiodarone
	Furosemide
Thrombotic thrombocytopenia	Thiazides
purpura (TTP)	Morphine

C. Pseudothrombocytopenia

1. Pseudothrombocytopenia is a condition where antibodies to EDTA (the anticoagulant in blood collection tubes) produce clumping of platelets *in vitro*, resulting in spuriously low platelet counts.

2. This phenomenon has been reported in 2% of platelet counts performed by hospital laboratories (5).

3. If suspected (e.g., by sudden, unexpected thrombocytopenia), blood collection tubes that use citrate or heparin as an anticoagulant should be used to measure the platelet count.

II. HEPARIN AND THROMBOCYTOPENIA

There are two types of thrombocytopenia associated with heparin.

1. The first is a nonimmune response that results in mild thrombocytopenia (platelet counts often 100,000–150,000/μL) in the first few days after starting heparin. This reaction is reported in 10–30% of patients receiving heparin (6), and it resolves spontaneously without interruption of heparin, and without adverse consequences.

2. The second (*heparin-induced thrombocytopenia*, or HIT) is an immune-mediated response that typically appears 5–10 days after starting heparin (6). This reaction is much less common (incidence = 1–3%) but can have serious consequences, with a mortality rate as high as 30% when unrecognized (6).

3. HIT is the result of heparin binding to a protein (platelet factor 4) on platelets, to form an antigenic complex that induces the formation of IgG antibodies, which bind to

the antigen complex and form cross-bridges between contiguous platelets. This promotes platelet aggregation, which can lead to symptomatic thrombosis (not bleeding) and a consumptive thrombocytopenia. Heparin-associated antibodies usually disappear within 3 months after discontinuing heparin (5).

A. Risk Factors

1. *HIT is not a dose-dependent reaction*, and can be triggered by the small amounts of heparin used to flush intravascular catheters, or even heparin-coated pulmonary artery catheters (7).

2. The type of heparin preparation influences the risk of HIT; i.e., *the risk of HIT is ten times greater with unfractionated heparin than with low-molecular-weight heparin* (8).

3. The risk of HIT also varies by patient population; it is highest in patients undergoing orthopedic and cardiac surgical procedures, and lowest in medical patients (6,8).

B. Clinical Features

1. HIT typically appears 5–10 days after the first exposure to heparin, but it can appear within 24 hours in patients exposed to heparin within the preceding 3 months (8).

2. Platelet counts are usually between 50,000–150,000/µL, and are rarely below 20,000/µL (6,8).

3. The major complication of HIT is *thrombosis*, which *precedes the thrombocytopenia in up to 25% of cases* (8).

   a. Venous thrombosis is much more common than arterial thrombosis. Up to 55% of patients with HIT develop deep vein thrombosis in the legs and/or pulmonary embolism, whereas only 1–3% of patients develop arterial thromboses (which can result in limb ischemia, ischemic stroke, or acute coronary syndromes) (8).

C. Diagnosis

1. Multiple assays are available for detecting HIT antibodies. The most popular is an enzyme-linked immunosorbent assay (ELISA) for antibodies to the platelet factor 4-heparin complex.

2. A negative antibody assays helps to exclude the diagnosis of HIT, but a positive assay does not confirm the diagnosis because HIT antibodies do not always produce thrombocytopenia or thrombosis (8).

3. The diagnosis of HIT requires a positive antibody assay and a high index of clinical suspicion.

D. Acute Management

Heparin must be discontinued immediately (don't forget to discontinue heparin flushes and remove heparin-coated catheters). Therapeutic anticoagulation with one of the direct thrombin inhibitors shown in Table 12.2 should be started immediately, *even in cases where HIT is not accompanied by thrombosis* (8).

1. Argatroban

    Argatroban is a synthetic analogue of L-arginine that reversibly binds to the active site on thrombin. It has a rapid onset of action, and is given by continuous infusion using the dosing regimen in Table 12.2. The therapeutic goal is an activated partial thromboplastin time (aPTT) of 1.5–3 times control values.

    a. The drug is cleared primarily by the liver, and a dose adjustment is required in hepatic insufficiency.

    b. Argatroban is *recommended in patients with renal insufficiency* (8) because a dose adjustment is not necessary.

Table 12.2	Direct Thrombin Inhibitors for Anticoagulation in HRT			
Drug	**Dosing Recommendations**			

Argatroban	Normal:	Infuse at 2 μg/kg/min, and titrate dose to achieve aPTT = 1.5–3 x control. Max dose is 10 μg/kg/min.		
	Liver Failure:	Start infusion at 0.5 μg/kg/min.		

Lepirudin	Normal:	Start with IV bolus of 0.4 mg (for life-threatening thrombosis). Begin infusion at 0.15 mg/kg/h and titrate to achieve aPTT = 1.5–3 x control.
	Renal Failure:	Reduce IV bolus to 0.2 mg/kg (if needed), and decrease infusion rate as follows:

Serum Creat (mg/dL)	1.6–2.0	2.1–3.0	3.1–6.0	>6.0
% Decrease in Infusion Rate	50%	70%	85%	Avoid

From References 10, 11, and 14. HIT = heparin-induced thrombocytopenia.

2. **Lepirudin**

Lepirudin is a recombinant form of hirudin, an anticoagulant that binds irreversibly to thrombin. Lepirudin is given by continuous infusion, which can be preceded by a bolus injection in cases of life-threatening thrombosis. The therapeutic goal is the same as with argatroban (aPTT = 1.5–3 × control).

a. Lepirudin is cleared by the kidneys, and a dose adjustment is necessary when renal function is impaired (see Table 12.2).

b. Re-exposure to lepirudin can produce life-threatening anaphylactic reactions (8), so treatment with lepirudin is a one-time affair.

3. **Duration of treatment**

   Full anticoagulation with argatroban or lepirudin is recommended until the platelet count rises above 150,000/µL (8). Thereafter, coumadin can be used for long-term anticoagulation if HIT is associated with thrombosis, but there are 2 caveats: 1) coumadin should NOT be started until the platelet count increases beyond 150,000/µL, and 2) the initial coumadin dose should not exceed 5 mg (8). These precautions are intended to reduce *the risk of limb gangrene associated with coumadin therapy during the active phase of HIT*. The antithrombin agents should be continued until coumadin achieves full anticoagulation.

III. THROMBOTIC MICROANGIOPATHIES

The following conditions are characterized by a "consumptive" thrombocytopenia with microvascular thrombosis and dysfunction in one or more vital organs. The hematologic features of these conditions are shown in Table 12.3.

A. Disseminated Intravascular Coagulation

Disseminated intravascular coagulation (DIC) is a secondary disorder that is triggered by widespread tissue injury (e.g., multisystem trauma) and obstetric emergencies (i.e., amniotic fluid embolism, abruptio placentae, eclampsia, retained fetus syndrome). These conditions promote the release of *tissue factor* from the endothelium, which activates a series of clotting factors in the bloodstream, culminating with the formation of fibrin. This leads to widespread microvascular thrombosis and secondary depletion of platelets and clotting factors, resulting in a *consumptive coagulopathy* (9).

1. **Clinical Features**

   a. The microvascular thrombosis in DIC can lead to

multiorgan failure, most often involving the lungs, kidneys, and central nervous system, while depletion of platelets and coagulation factors can promote bleeding, particularly from the GI tract.

b. DIC can also be accompanied by symmetrical necrosis and ecchymoses involving the limbs. This condition (known as *purpura fulminans*) is usually seen with overwhelming sepsis, most notably with meningococcemia (4).

2. **Laboratory Studies**

    a. In addition to thrombocytopenia, DIC is usually (but not always) associated with prolongation of the prothrombin time and the activated partial thromboplastin time (aPTT); both abnormalities being the result of consumption of clotting factors in blood (10-11).

    b. The widespread thrombosis is accompanied by enhanced fibrinolysis, which elevates the fibrin degradation products in plasma (i.e., plasma d-dimers) (10-11).

    c. There is a *microangiopathic hemolytic anemia* that is identified by the presence of fragmented erythrocytes (*schistocytes*) in the peripheral blood smear (10).

3. **Management**

    There is no specific treatment for DIC other than supportive care (10).

    a. Replacement therapy with platelets and coagulation factors (plasma products) rarely helps, and can be deleterious by "adding fuel" to the microvascular thrombosis.

    b. In severe cases of DIC with multiorgan failure, the mortality rate is ≥80% (4,10).

B. Thrombotic Thrombocytopenic Purpura

Thrombotic thrombocytopenia purpura (TTP) is a thrombotic microangiopathy that is caused by platelet binding to abnormal von Willebrand factor on the microvascular endothelium (2). This can be a devastating condition that is fatal within 24 hours of onset. There is often no predisposing condition, although it seems to follow a nonspecific viral illness in some cases.

Table 12.3	Hematologic Features of Thrombotic Microangiopathies		
Feature	**DIC**	**TTP**	**HELLP**
Schistocytes	Present	Present	Present
Platelets	↓	↓	↓
INR, aPTT	↑	Normal	Normal
Fibrinogen	↓	Normal	Normal
Plasma D–dimer	↑	Normal	Normal

From Reference 4. DIC = disseminated intravascukar coagulation; TTP = thrombotic thrombocytopenia purpura; HELLP = hemolysis, elevated liver enzymes, low platelets.

1. **Clinical Features**

   TTP presents with a characteristic *pentad* of clinical manifestations that includes: (a) fever, (b) altered mental status, (c) acute renal failure, (d) thrombocytopenia, and (e) microangiopathic hemolytic anemia. The presence of all 5 conditions is not necessary for the diagnosis of TTP, but the diagnosis requires thrombocytopenia and evidence of a microangiopathic hemolytic anemia (i.e., schistocytes in the peripheral blood smear).

   a. TTP can be distinguished from DIC because clotting factors are not depleted in TTP, so the INR, aPTT, and fibrinogen levels are normal in TTP (see Table 12.3).

2. **Management**

   a. Platelet transfusions are contraindicated in TTP because they can aggravate the underlying thrombosis.

b. *The treatment of choice for TTP is plasma exchange* (12), where blood from the patient is diverted to a device that separates and discards the patient's plasma and reinfuses plasma from a healthy donor. This is continued until 1.5 times the normal plasma volume is exchanged, and this process is repeated daily for 3–7 days.

c. Acute, fulminant TTP is almost always fatal if untreated, but if plasma exchange is started early (with 48 hours of symptom onset), as many as 90% of patients can survive the illness (12).

C. HELLP Syndrome

HELLP (**H**emolysis, **E**levated **L**iver enzymes, **L**ow **P**latelets) syndrome is a thrombotic microangiopathy that occurs late in pregnancy or in the early postpartum period (13). The culprit in the HELLP syndrome is unexplained activation of clotting factors and platelets, leading to a consumptive thrombocytopenia, microvascular thrombosis, and a microangiopathic hemolytic anemia.

1. **Clinical Features**

    a. HELLP is characterized by the triad of hemolysis, thrombocytopenia, and elevated liver enzymes.

    b. The most common clinical presentation is abdominal pain.

    c. HELLP can be confused with DIC (which can have the same predisposing conditions), but the INR, aPTT, and fibrinogen levels are usually normal in HELLP (see Table 12.3).

2. **Management**

    The HELLP syndrome is an obstetric emergency, and a detailed description of the management of this condition is beyond the scope of this text. For more information on this topic, pertinent reviews are included in the bibliography at the end of the chapter (13,14).

IV. PLATELET TRANSFUSIONS

A. Indications

1. **Active Bleeding**

   In the presence of active bleeding (other than ecchymoses or petechiae), platelet transfusions are recommended for platelet counts <50,000/μL (15). For intracranial hemorrhage, higher platelet counts (>100,000/μL) should be maintained (15).

2. **No Active Bleeding**

   For cases of drug-induced hypoproliferative thrombocytopenia, platelet transfusions are recommended when platelet counts drop to 10,000/μL or lower (16).

3. **Procedures**

   Platelet transfusions are advised for each of the following (16):

   a. For elective insertion of a central venous catheter, when the platelet count is less than 20,000/μL.

   b. For elective lumbar puncture, when the platelet count is <50,000/μL.

   c. For major, elective nonneuraxial surgery, when the platelet count is <50,000/μL.

B. Platelet Products

1. **Pooled Platelets**

   a. Platelets are separated from fresh whole blood by differential centrifugation, and the platelet concentrates from 5 donors are pooled together prior to storage.

   b. The "pooled" platelet concentrate contains about

38×10^{10} platelets in 260 mL plasma, which is equivalent to a platelet count of about $130 \times 10^9/\mu L$ (which is six orders of magnitude higher than the normal platelet count of $150-400 \times 10^3/\mu L$).

2. **Apheresis Platelets**

   a. Apheresis platelets are collected from a single donor, and have a platelet count and volume that is equivalent to the pooled platelet concentrate from 5 donors.

   b. The proposed benefits of single-donor platelet transfusions include a lower risk of transmitted infections, and a lower risk of platelet *alloimmunization* (i.e., developing antibodies to donor platelets, which reduces the effect of platelet transfusions). However, these proposed benefits have not been validated in clinical trials (17).

3. **Leukoreduction**

   a. Platelet concentrates are not free of leukocytes, and leukocyte reduction has the following advantages (17): a lower incidence of cytomegalovirus transmission (because this organism is transmitted in leukocytes), fewer febrile reactions, and a lower incidence of platelet alloimmunization.

   b. Because of these advantages, leukocyte reduction is becoming a routine practice for platelet transfusions.

C. Response to Transfused Platelets

1. In an average-sized adult with no ongoing blood loss, *a platelet concentrate from one unit of whole blood should increase the circulating platelet count by 7,000 to 10,000/μL at one hour post-transfusion* (17). Since an average of 5 platelet concentrates are pooled together for each platelet transfusion, the expected (or ideal) increase in platelet count is 35,000 to 50,000/μL one-hour post-transfusion.

2. The increment in platelet count declines with multiple trans-
    fusions (18). This is the result of antiplatelet antibodies in
    the recipient directed at ABO antigens on donor platelets.
    Transfusing ABO-matched platelets mitigates this effect.

D. Adverse Effects

The risks associated with platelet transfusions are listed in
Table 12.4 (16).

Table 12.4	Risks Associated with Platelet Transfusions
Adverse Event	**Odds per Transfusion**
Febrile reaction	1 in 14
Allergic reaction	1 in 50
Bacterial sepsis	1 in 75,000
Acute lung injury	1 in 138,000
HBV infection	1 in 2,652,580
HCV infection	1 in 3,315,729
HIV infection	0–1 in 1,461,888

From Reference 16.

1. **Nonhemolytic Fever**

    Febrile nonhemolytic reactions are the most common
    adverse events associated with platelet transfusions,
    and are much more common than reported with ery-
    throcyte transfusions (see Chapter 11, Table 11.3).
    Leukoreduction reduces the risk of this reaction.

2. **Allergic Reactions**

    Allergic reactions (urticaria, anaphylaxis, anaphylactic
    shock) are also more more common with platelet transfu-
    sions than with erythrocyte transfusions (see Table 11.3).

Since these are reactions to proteins in donor plasma, removing the plasma from platelet concentrates will reduce the risk of these reactions.

3. **Bacterial Transmission**

Bacteria are much more likely to flourish in platelet concentrates than in packed red blood cells (PRBCs) because platelets are stored at room temperature (22°C) while PRBCs are refrigerated at 4°C.

4. **Acute Lung Injury**

Transfusion-related acute lung injury is described in Chapter 11, Section V-D. This condition is most often associated with erythrocyte transfusions, but is also a risk with platelet transfusions (16,19).

V. PLASMA PRODUCTS

A. Fresh Frozen Plasma

Plasma is separated from donor blood and frozen at -18°C within 8 hours of blood collection. This *fresh frozen plasma* (FFP) has a volume of about 230 mL, and can be stored for one year. Once thawed, FFP can be stored at 1–6°C for up to 5 days.

1. **Indications**

FFP is used to replace clotting factors, and *should never be used for volume resuscitation*. The principal indications for FFP include the following:

a. MASSIVE BLOOD LOSS: As described in Chapter 7, Section V-B, the resuscitation of massive blood loss is optimal when one unit of FFP is transfused for every 1–2 units of packed RBCs, with the goal being an INR < 1.5 (20).

b. REVERSING WARFARIN: FFP (10–15 mL/kg) has been

used to replace vitamin K-dependent clotting factors (II, VII, IX, X) in cases of major bleeding associated with warfarin anticoagulation (21). However, FFP is no longer favored in this setting (22,23), primarily because: (a) the time required to correct the prothrombin time can be 12 hours or longer (24), and the volume of fluid required can aggravate the bleeding, or promote pulmonary edema. (See Section B for the preferred method of rapidly reversing warfarin anticoagulation.)

c. LIVER FAILURE: FFP can be used to correct the prothrombin time in patients with hepatic failure and uncontrolled bleeding. Therapy is guided by the prothrombin time, and the response is erratic (22).

Table 12.5	Risks Associated with Fresh Frozen Plasma
Adverse Event	**Odds per Transfusion**
Urticaria	1 in 30–100
Anaphylaxis	1 in 20,000
Acute lung injury	1 in 5,000
HIV infection	1 in 10,000,000
HBV infection	1 in 12,000,000
HCV infection	1 in 50,000,000

From References 22, 23, and 25.

2. **Adverse Effects**

The adverse effects associated with FFP are listed in Table 12.5 (22,23,25).

a. Urticaria is the most common adverse effect of FFP transfusions (22). Anaphylaxis is rare.

b. Freezing eliminates the risk of bacterial contamination (22), but does not eliminate the risk of transmitting hepatitis and human immunodeficiency viruses. However, as shown in Table 12.5, the risk of transmitting these viruses is miniscule.

B. Prothrombin Complex Concentrate

Prothrombin complex concentrate (Kcentra, CSL Behring), or PCC, contains all four vitamin K-dependent clotting factors (II, VII, IX, and X), and is favored over FFP for rapid reversal of warfarin anticoagulation in patients with life-threatening hemorrhage (22,23). The advantages of PCC over FFP are as follows:

1. PCC is a lyophilized powder that is quickly reconstituted in a relatively small volume (usually <150 mL) of IV fluid. This avoids the time delays involved in thawing FFP, and greatly decreases the volume of infusion.

2. PCC can reverse the anticoagulant effects of warfarin in less than half the time required with FFP (24), and this can occur within 30 minutes after PCC is administered (26).

3. The more rapid response and limited volume associated with PCC makes this product particularly well suited for warfarin-associated intracranial hemorrhage.

4. The recommended dosing of PCC is shown in Table 12.6 (26). Note that the dosing regimen is determined by the factor IX potency (in units), which varies in individual PCC preparations (26).

5. PCC is costly (about $5,000 for a dose of 50 units/kg in an 80 kg adult, compared to about $300 for 4 units of FFP) (26), and thus should be used only for cases of major or life-threatening (especially intracranial) hemorrhage associated with warfarin anticoagulation.

Table 12.6	Rapid Reversal of Warfarin Anticoagulation

Use Only for Life-Threatening Hemorrhage

1. **Vitamin K:** 10 mg IV over 10 minutes (dilute in 50 mL IV fluid).

AND

2. **Prothrombin Complex Concentrate:** Dosing regimen per factor IX potency (units), body weight, and pretreatment INR:

INR	2.0–3.9	4.0–6.0	>6.0
IV Dose	25 units/kg	35 units/kg	50 units/kg
Max Dose	2,500 units	3,500 units	5,000 units

From References 23 and 26.

C. Cryoprecipitate

1. Preparation

When FFP is allowed to thaw at 4°C, a milky residue forms that is rich in cold-insoluble proteins (cryoglobulins) like fibrinogen, von Willebrand factor, and factor VIII. This *cryoprecipitate* can be separated from plasma and stored at -18°C for up to one year. The storage volume is 10 to 15 mL.

2. Indications

Cryoprecipitate use in the ICU is generally reserved for cases of uncontrolled bleeding associated with hypofibrinogenemia (serum fibrinogen <100 mg/dL). Most cases involve massive bleeding, or bleeding associated with liver failure.

a. One unit of cryoprecipitate contains about 200 mg of fibrinogen, and infusion of 10 units of cryoprecipitate (2 grams of fibrinogen) should raise the serum fibrinogen level by about 70 mg/dL in an average-sized adult (27). The goal is a serum fibrinogen level above 100 mg/dL.

VI. HEMOSTATIC ADJUNCTS

A. Desmopressin

Desmopressin is a vasopressin analogue (deamino-arginine vasopressin or DDAVP) that does not have the vasoconstrictor or antidiuretic effects of vasopressin, but is capable of elevating plasma levels of von Willebrand factor and correcting the abnormal bleeding time in 75% of patients with renal failure (28). However, the effects on uremic bleeding are unclear.

1. **Dosing**

   The recommended dose is *0.3 µg/kg IV or by subcutaneous injection, or 30 µg/kg by intranasal spray* (26). The effect lasts only 6 to 8 hours, and repeat dosing leads to tachyphylaxis.

B. Antifibrinolytic Agents

Antifibrinolytic agents (*tranexamic acid* and *aminocaproic acid*) inhibit the lysis of fibrin by blocking the conversion of plasminogen to plasmin.

1. **Indications**

   Antifibrinolytics are used for selected cases of bleeding associated with fibrinolysis (e.g., identified by >3% lysis at 30 minutes using conventional thromboelastography). They have been studied in cardiac surgery, trauma, orthopedic surgery, and liver surgery, and the available evidence shows a reduction in blood loss without an increase in thromboembolic complications (29).

2. **Dosing**

    a. *Tranexamic Acid*: 1 gram IV over 10 minutes, then infuse 1 gram over 8 hours (27).

    b. *Aminocaproic Acid*: 50 mg/kg IV as a loading dose, then infuse at 25 mg/kg/hr until bleeding and/or fibrinolysis has subsided (27).

3. **Adverse Effects**

These agents are relatively safe when used in the recommended doses. Seizures have been reported with tranexamic doses that exceed 1 gram (27).

REFERENCES

1. Parker RI. Etiology and significance of thrombocytopenia in critically ill patients. Crit Care Clin 2012; 28:399–411.

2. Rice TR, Wheeler RP. Coagulopathy in critically ill patients. Part 1: Platelet disorders. Chest 2009; 136:1622–1630.

3. Slichter SJ, Harker LA. Thrombocytopenia: mechanisms and management of defects in platelet production. Clin Haematol 1978; 7:523–527.

4. DeLoughery TG. Critical care clotting catastrophies. Crit Care Clin 2005; 21:531–562.

5. Payne BA, Pierre RV. Pseudothrombocytopenia: a laboratory artifact with potentially serious consequences. Mayo Clin Proc 1984; 59:123–125.

6. Shantsila E, Lip GYH, Chong BH. Heparin-induced thrombocytopenia: a contemporary clinical approach to diagnosis and management. Chest 2009; 135:1651–1664.

7. Laster J, Silver D. Heparin-coated catheters and heparin-induced thrombocytopenia. J Vasc Surg 1988; 7:667–672.

8. Linkins L-A, Dans AL, Moores LK, et al. Treatment and prevention of heparin-induced thrombocytopenia. Antithrombotic Therapy and Prevention of Thrombosis, 9th ed: American College of Chest Physicians Evidence-Based Clinical Practice Guidelines. Chest 2012; 141(Suppl):495S–530S.

9. Senno SL, Pechet L, Bick RL. Disseminated intravascular coagulation (DIC). Pathophysiology, laboratory diagnosis, and management. J Intensive Care Med 2000; 15:144–158.

10. Levy M. Disseminated intravascular coagulation. Crit Care Med 2007; 35:2191–2195.

11. Taylor FBJ, Toh CH, Hoots WK, et al. Towards definition, clinical and laboratory criteria, and a scoring system for disseminated intravascular coagulation. Thromb Haemost 2001; 86:1327–1330.

12. Rock GA, Shumack KH, Buskard NA, et al. Comparison of plasma exchange with plasma infusion in the treatment of thrombotic thrombocytopenia purpura. N Engl J Med 1991; 325:393–397.

13. Kirkpatrick CA. The HELLP syndrome. Acta Clin Belg 2010; 65:91–97.

14. Sibai BM. Diagnosis, controversies, and management of the syndrome of hemolysis, elevated liver enzymes, and low platelet count. Obstet Gynecol 2004; 103:981.

15. Slichter SJ. Evidence-based platelet transfusion guidelines. Hematol 2007; 2007:172–178.

16. Kaufman RM, Djulbegovic B, Gernsheimer T, et al. Platelet transfusion: A clinical practice guideline from the AABB. Ann Intern Med 2015; 162:205–213.

17. Slichter SJ. Platelet transfusion therapy. Hematol Oncol Clin N Am 2007; 21:697–729.

18. Slichter SJ, Davis K, Enright H, et al. Factors affecting post-transfusion platelet increments, platelet refractoriness, and platelet transfusion intervals in thrombocytopenic patients. Blood 2005; 105:4106–4114.

19. Sayah DM. Looney MR, Toy P. Transfusion reactions. Newer concepts on the pathophysiology, incidence, treatment, and prevention of transfusion-related acute lung injury. Crit Care Clin 2012; 28:363–372.

20. Holcomb JB, Tilley BC, Baraniuk S, Fox EE, et al. for the PROPPR Study Group. Transfusion of plasma, platelets, and red blood cells in a 1:1:1 vs. a 1:1:2 ratio and mortality in patients with severe trauma: the PROPPR randomized clinical trial. JAMA 2015; 313(5):471–82.

21. Zareh M, Davis A, Henderson S. Reversal of warfarin-induced hemorrhage in the emergency department. West J Emerg Med 2011; 12:386–392.

22. British Committee for Standards in Haematology, Blood Transfusion Task Force. Guidelines for the use of fresh-frozen plasma, cryoprecipitate, and cryosupernatant. Br J Haematol 2004; 126:11–28.

23. Ageno W, Gallus AS, Wittkowsky A, et al. Oral anticoagulant therapy: antithrombotic therapy and prevention of thrombosis, 9th ed: American College of Chest Physicians evidence-based clinical practice guidelines. Chest 2012; 141(Suppl 2):e44S–e88S.

24. Hickey M, Gatien M, Taljaard M, et al. Outcomes of urgent warfarin reversal with fresh frozen plasma versus prothrombin complex concentrate in the emergency department. Circulation 2013; 128:360–364.

25. Popovsky MA. Transfusion-Related Acute Lung Injury: Incidence, pathogenesis and the role of multicomponent apheresis in its prevention. Transfus Med Hemother. 2008; 35:76–79.

26. Kcentra package insert. CSL Behring GmbH, Marburg, Germany.

27. Callum JL, Karkouti K, Lin Y. Cryoprecipitate: the current state of knowledge. Transfus Med Rev 2009; 23:177–184.

28. Salman S. Uremic bleeding: pathophysiology, diagnosis, and management. Hosp Physician 2001; 37:45–76.

29. Ortmann E, Besser MW, Klein AA. Antifibrinolytic agents in current anaesthetic practice. Br J Anaesth 2013; 111: 549–563.

Chapter 13

Tachyarrhythmias

A rapid heart rate or *tachycardia* in a critically ill patient is usually evidence of a problem, but the tachycardia may not be the problem (e.g., sinus tachycardia). This chapter describes tachycardias that are a problem (i.e., *tachyarrhythmias*), and require prompt recognition and management. Many of the recommendations in this chapter are based on the most recent clinical practice guidelines on the subject (1,2).

I. RECOGNITION

The diagnostic evaluation of tachycardias (heart rate >100 beats/min) is based on 3 findings on the ECG: (a) the duration of the QRS complex, (b) the uniformity of the R-R intervals, and (c) the characteristics of the atrial activity. This scheme is outlined in Figure 13.1.

A. Narrow-QRS-Complex Tachycardias

Tachycardias with a narrow QRS complex (≤0.12 sec) originate from a site above the AV conduction system, and are also known as *supraventricular tachycardias*. These include sinus tachycardia, atrial tachycardia, AV nodal re-entrant tachycardia (also called paroxysmal supraventricular tachycardia), atrial flutter, and atrial fibrillation. The specific arrhythmia can be identified using the uniformity of the R-R interval (i.e., the regularity of the rhythm), and the characteristics of the atrial activity, as described next.

1. **Regular Rhythm**

   If the R-R intervals are uniform in length (indicating a

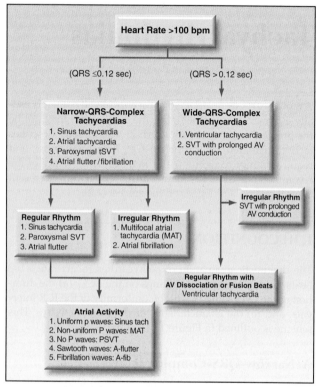

FIGURE 13.1 Flow diagram for the evaluation of tachycardias.

regular rhythm), the possible arrhythmias include sinus tachycardia, AV nodal re-entrant tachycardia, or atrial flutter with a fixed (2:1, 3:1) AV block. The atrial activity on the ECG can identify each of these rhythms using the following criteria:

a. Uniform P waves and P–R intervals are evidence of sinus tachycardia.

b. The absence of P waves suggests an AV nodal re-entrant tachycardia (see Figure 13.2).

   c. Sawtooth waves are evidence of atrial flutter.

2. **Irregular Rhythm**

If the R-R intervals are not uniform in length (indicating an irregular rhythm), the most likely arrhythmias are multifocal atrial tachycardia and atrial fibrillation. Once again, the atrial activity on the ECG helps to identify each of these rhythms; i.e.,

   a. Multiple P wave morphologies and variable PR intervals are evidence of multifocal atrial tachycardia (see Panel A, Figure 13.3).

   b. The absence of P waves with highly disorganized atrial activity (fibrillation waves) is evidence of atrial fibrillation (see Panel B, Figure 13.3).

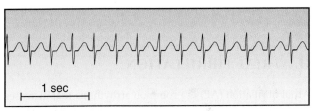

FIGURE 13.2 Narrow-QRS-complex tachycardia with a regular rhythm. Note the absence of visible P waves (which are hidden in the QRS complex). This is an AV nodal re-entrant tachycardia, also called a "paroxysmal supraventricular tachycardia" because it has an abrupt onset.

B. Wide-QRS-Complex Tachycardias

Tachycardias with a wide QRS complex (>0.12 sec) can originate from a site below the AV conduction system (i.e., ventricular tachycardia), or they can represent a supraventricular tachycardia (SVT) with prolonged AV conduction (e.g., from a bundle branch block). The distinction between these two arrhythmias is described later in the chapter.

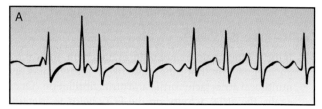

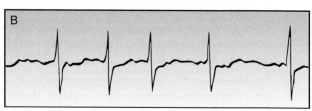

FIGURE 13.3 Narrow-QRS-complex tachycardias with an irregular rhythm. Panel A shows a multifocal atrial tachycardia, identified by multiple P wave morphologies and variable PR intervals. Panel B is atrial fibrillation, identified by the highly disorganized atrial activity (fibrillation waves).

II. ATRIAL FIBRILLATION

Atrial fibrillation (AF) is a common arrhythmia that increases in prevalence with advancing age; the reported prevalence is 2% with age <65 years, and 9% with age ≥65 years (1).

A. Etiologies

1. Most patients with AF have underlying heart disease, including valvular disease.

2. Potentially reversible causes of AF include binge drinking, major surgery, myocardial infarction, myocarditis, pericarditis, pulmonary embolism, and hyperthyroidism.

3. Postoperative AF is reported in up to 45% of cardiac surgeries, up to 30% of non-cardiac thoracic surgeries, and up to 8% of other major surgeries (3).

B. Adverse Consequences

The adverse consequences of AF are impaired cardiac performance and thromboembolism.

1. **Cardiac Performance**

   The principal threat from AF is reduced ventricular filling from loss of atrial contractions (which normally contribute 25% of the ventricular end-diastolic volume) and the rapid heart rate (which reduces the time for diastolic filling). Reduced ventricular compliance (e.g., from ventricular hypertrophy) and mitral stenosis will magnify the problem. The effect on cardiac stroke output will depend on the rate and the type and severity of underlying cardiac disease.

2. **Thromboembolism**

   a. AF predisposes to thrombus formation in the left atrium, and these thrombi can dislodge and embolize in the cerebral circulation to produce an acute ischemic stroke.

   b. The risk of thromboembolic stroke is increased when AF is accompanied by certain risk factors (e.g., heart failure, advanced age). The methods used to determine the risk of stroke are described later in the chapter.

   c. The increased risk of embolic stroke pertains to all types of AF (paroxysmal, etc.), except first episodes of AF that are <48 hrs in duration (1).

C. Acute Rate Control

In patients with rapid AF who are hemodynamically stable, the immediate goal is to slow the ventricular rate to ≤80 beats/min using drugs that prolong AV conduction. These drugs are shown in in Table 13.1, along with the intravenous and oral (maintenance) dosing regimens. (*Note:* These drugs should not be used in cases of AF due to re-entry of impulses through an accessory pathway, as described later.)

Table 13.1	Drug Regimens for Rate Control in Atrial Fibrillation
Drug	**Dosing Regimens**
Diltiazem	IV: 0.25 mg/kg over 2 min, then infuse at 5–15 mg/hr. If heart rate >90 bpm after 15 min, give second bolus of 0.35 mg/kg.
	Oral: 120–360 mg (extended release) daily.
Metoprolol	IV: 2.5–5 mg over 2 min, and repeat every 5–10 min if needed to a total of 3 doses.
	Oral: 25–100 mg BID.
Esmolol	IV: 500 µg/kg bolus, then infuse at 50 µg/kg/min. Increase dose in increments of 25 µg/kg/min every 5 min if needed to a maximum rate of 200 µg/kg/min.
	Oral: N/A.
Amiodarone	IV: 150 mg over 10 min, and repeat if needed, then infuse at 1 mg/min for 6 hr and 0.5 mg/min for 18 hr. Total dose should not exceed 2.2 grams in 24 hr.
	Oral: 100–200 mg daily.
Digoxin	IV: 0.25 mg every 2 hr to a total of 1.5 mg over 24 hr.
	Oral: 0.125–0.25 mg daily.

From Reference 1.

1. **Diltiazem**

   a. Diltiazem is a calcium receptor antagonist that achieves *satisfactory rate reduction in about 85% of cases of AF* (1). The drug is given as an intravenous bolus followed by a continuous infusion (see Table 13.1), and the response is superior to that seen with IV amiodarone or digoxin (4).

b. Adverse effects include hypotension and cardiac depression (negative inotropic effect). Because of the latter effect, diltiazem is not recommended for patients with decompensated systolic heart failure (1).

2. **β-Receptor Antagonists**

a. β-blockers achieve *successful rate control in 70% of cases of acute AF* (11), and they are preferred for rate control when AF is associated with hyperadrenergic states (e.g., acute MI and post-cardiac surgery) (1,3).

b. Two cardioselective β-blockers that have proven efficacy in AF are *esmolol* and *metoprolol*, and their dosing regimens are shown in Table 13.1. Esmolol is an ultra-short-acting drug (with a serum half-life of 9 minutes) and is given by continuous infusion, which allows rapid dose titration to the desired effect (unlike metoprolol) (12).

c. Adverse effects are similar to those of diltiazem, and these agents are not advised in the setting of decompensated systolic heart failure (1).

3. **Amiodarone**

a. Amiodarone prolongs conduction in the AV node, and is an effective agent for acute rate control in critically ill patients with AF (1).

b. Amiodarone causes less cardiac depression than diltiazem (6), and is a preferred agent for rate control in patients with systolic heart failure (1,7). Otherwise, because of the toxic effects associated with long-term use, amiodarone is usually reserved for cases of AF that are refractory to rate control with other agents (1).

c. The dosing regimen for amiodarone is shown in Table 13.1. The IV regimen usually lasts only 24 hrs before a change to oral maintenance therapy.

d. Amiodarone is also an antiarrhythmic agent (Class III), and is *capable of converting AF to a sinus rhythm.* Conversion is uncommon with persistent AF (present for more than one year) (1), but the success rate for converting recent-onset AF is 55–95% when a loading dose and continuous infusion are used, and the daily dose exceeds 1500 mg (7). Unanticipated cardioversion can be problematic when patients are not adequately anticoagulated (see later).

e. Adverse effects of short-term IV amiodarone include hypotension (15%), bradycardia (5%), and elevated liver enzymes (3%) (8,9). (*Note:* IV amiodarone is available in 2 formulations: one contains polysorbate 80, a vasoactive solvent that promotes hypotension, and one contains captisol, which has no vasoactive effects.)

f. Amiodarone has several drug interactions by virtue of its metabolism by the cytochrome P450 enzyme system in the liver (9). These interactions include *inhibition of digoxin and warfarin metabolism*, which requires attention if amiodarone is continued for oral maintenance therapy.

4. **Digoxin**

Digoxin prolongs conduction in the AV node, and is a popular drug for long-term rate control in AF. However, the response to intravenous digoxin is slow, and the peak response can take over 6 hours to develop (1). Because of this delayed response, digoxin is not recommended alone for acute rate control in AF, but it can be used in combination with β-blockers in patients with compensated heart failure (1).

D. Electrical Cardioversion

1. Direct-current cardioversion is indicated when AF is associated with hypotension, pulmonary edema, or

myocardial ischemia, or when AF is a re-entrant rhythm involving an accessory pathway (see later).

2. Biphasic shocks are recommended, and are synchronized to the QRS complex of the ECG to avoid triggering ventricular fibrillation. An energy of 100 J is usually successful using biphasic shocks, but 200 J is typically used for the initial shocks.

3. When immediate cardioversion is required and the duration of AF is >48 hrs or is unknown, anticoagulation (with heparin) should be started as soon as possible and continued (with oral agents) for at least 4 weeks (1).

E. Anticoagulation

The following recommendations for the prevention of thromboembolic stroke are taken from the most recent guidelines on AF (1). These recommendations pertain to all cases of AF except first episodes that are less than 48 hrs in duration.

1. **Indications**

   a. Long-term anticoagulation is recommended for all patients with AF who have mechanical or bioprosthetic heart valves, rheumatic mitral stenosis, or mitral valve repair.

   b. For patients with nonvalvular AF, an assessment of the yearly risk for stroke is recommended using the CH_2DS_2-VASc scoring system (see Appendix 4). Long-term anticoagulation is indicated for patients with a prior stroke, TIA, or a CH_2DS_2-VASc score ≥2.

2. **Oral Anticoagulants**

   a. Warfarin is recommended for patients with prosthetic heart valves, and the target INR is 2.0–3.0.

   b. For nonvalvular AF, the options for oral anticoagulation include warfarin, the direct thrombin inhibitor *dabigatran* (Pradaxa), and the factor Xa inhibitors *rivaroxaban* (Xarelto) and *apixaban* (Eliquis).

c. Dosing of the newer oral anticoagulants (dabigatran, rivaroxaban, and apixaban) is influenced by renal function, as shown in Table 13.2. Note that *dabigatran and rivaroxaban are contraindicated in renal failure* (creatinine clearance <15 mL/min), while no recommendations are available for apixaban in renal failure.

Warfarin dosing is not influenced by renal function.

Table 13.2	Renal Dosing for Oral Anticoagulants		
Cr CL	**Dabigatran**	**Rivaroxiban**	**Apixaban**
>50	150 mg BID	20 mg QD	2.5–5 mg BID†
31–50	150 mg BID	15 mg QD	2.5–5 mg BID†
15–30	75 mg	15 mg QD	?
<15	Do Not Use	Do Not Use	?

†Use 2.5 mg BID for patients with any 2 of the following: Cr CL ≥1.5 mg/dL, Age ≥80 yrs, Weight ≤60 kg. Cr CL = creatinine clearance. Question mark indicates no recommendations are available. From Reference 1.

F. Wolff-Parkinson-White Syndrome

1. The Wolff-Parkinson-White (WPW) syndrome (short P–R interval and delta waves before the QRS) is characterized by recurrent supraventricular tachycardias that are triggered by re-entry of impulses through an accessory pathway in the AV node.

2. When AF is the result of such a mechanism, drugs that block conduction in the AV node will not slow the ventricular rate because the accessory pathway is not blocked. Furthermore, selective block of the AV node

can trigger ventricular fibrillation. Therefore (as mentioned earlier) *drugs that block the AV node* (e.g., calcium channel blockers, β-blockers) *should NOT be used when AF is a re-entrant tachycardia.* The preferred management in this situation is electrical cardioversion.

III. MULTIFOCAL ATRIAL TACHYCARDIA

Multifocal atrial tachycardia or MAT is an irregular supraventricular tachycardia with numerous (≥3) P-wave morphologies and an irregular atrial activation pattern (see Panel A in Figure 13.3).

A. Etiologies

1. MAT is a disorder of the elderly, and over half of the cases occur in patients with chronic lung disease and pulmonary hypertension (10).

2. Other predisposing conditions include magnesium and potassium depletion, theophylline toxicity, and coronary artery disease (1,11).

B. Acute Management

MAT can be difficult to control.

1. Identify and correct hypomagnesemia and hypokalemia, if present.

2. Since serum magnesium levels can be normal despite total body magnesium depletion (see Chapter 29), intravenous magnesium can be given when serum magnesium levels are normal.

   a. Start with *2 grams MgSO₄ (in 50 mL saline) IV over 15 minutes, then infuse 6 grams MgSO₄ (in 500 mL saline) over 6 hours.*

b. In one study, this regimen had a remarkable 88% success rate in converting MAT to a sinus rhythm, and the effect was independent of serum magnesium levels (11).

3. If the prior measures fail, the following two drugs can be successful (although neither is recommended for patients with decompensated systolic heart failure):

a. *Metoprolol* in the doses shown in Table 13.1 *has a reported 89% success rate in slowing or converting MAT to sinus rhythm* (12).

b. If metoprolol is a concern in patients with bronchospastic COPD, the calcium channel blocker *verapamil* has a reported success rate of 44% in slowing or converting MAT (12). The dose is *0.25–5 mg IV over 2 min, which can be repeated every 15–30 min, if necessary, to a total dose of 20 mg* (4). The major risks with verapamil are cardiac depression and hypotension.

IV. PAROXYSMAL SUPRAVENTRICULAR TACHYCARDIAS

Paroxysmal supraventricular tachycardias (PSVT) are narrow-QRS-complex tachycardias that are second only to atrial fibrillation as the most prevalent rhythm disturbances in the general populace.

A. Mechanism

These arrhythmias occur when impulse transmission in one pathway of the AV conduction system is slowed. This creates a difference in the refractory period for impulse transmission in the abnormal and normal conduction pathways, which allows impulses travelling down one pathway to travel back through the other pathway. The retrograde transmission of impulses is called *re-entry*, and it results in a circular pattern of impulse transmission that is self-sustaining; i.e., a *re-entrant tachycardia*. Re-entry is triggered by an ectopic atrial impulse in one of the two conduction pathways, which results in the *abrupt onset* that is *characteristic of re-entrant tachycardias*.

1. **AV Nodal Re-Entrant Tachycardia**

   There are 5 different types of PSVT, based on the location of the re-entrant pathway. The most common PSVT is *AV nodal re-entrant tachycardia* (AVNRT), where the re-entrant pathway is located in the AV node. AVNRT accounts for 50–60% of cases of PSVT (13), and is the focus of the this section.

B. Clinical Features

1. AVNRT typically appears in young adults without structural heart disease, and >60% of cases are in women (2).

2. The onset is abrupt, and the heart rate is typically 180–200 bpm, but can range from 110 to >250 bpm in individual patients (2). Hemodynamic compromise is uncommon.

3. The ECG shows a narrow-QRS-complex tachycardia with a regular rhythm and the absence of visible P waves (see Figure 13.2).

C. Vagal Maneuvers

1. Maneuvers that increase vagal tone (carotid sinus massage and the Valsalva maneuver) are recommended as the initial attempt to terminate AVNRT. These should be performed with the patient supine (2).

2. The reported success rate is 18% for the Valsalva maneuver and 12% for carotid sinus massage (14).

D. Adenosine

1. When vagal maneuvers are ineffective, adenosine is the drug of choice for terminating AVNRT (2,15,16). Adenosine is an endogenous nucleotide that relaxes vascular smooth muscle and slows conduction in the AV node.

2. When given by *rapid* IV injection, adenosine has a rapid onset of action (<30 sec) and produces a transient AV block that can terminate AVNRTs. Adenosine is quickly cleared from the bloodstream, and the effects last only 1–2 minutes.

3. The dosing regimen for adenosine is shown in Table 13.3. This regimen *successfully terminates over 90% of re-entrant tachycardias* (2).

4. Note that the drug should be injected through a peripheral vein. Injection of standard doses of adenosine through central venous catheters can produce ventricular asystole, so a 50% dose reduction is recommended for injection through a central venous catheter (17).

5. The adverse effects of adenosine (see Table 13.3) are short-lived. The most frequent adverse effect is post-conversion bradycardia, including AV block that is refractory to atropine, but resolves spontaneously within 60 seconds (16).

6. Dipyridamole enhances the AV block produced by adenosine, while methylxanthines (e.g., caffeine, theophylline) block adenosine receptors and reduce efficacy (2,16).

E. Other Therapies

1. For cases where adenosine is contraindicated or ineffective and the patient is hemodynamically stable, intravenous β-blockers, diltiazem, or verapamil (in doses mentioned previously) can be used to terminate AVNRT (2). Amiodarone can be used when all other pharmacotherapies fail (2).

Table 13.3	Intravenous Adenosine for Paroxysmal SVT
Feature	**Recommendations**
Dosing Regimen	1. Administer through a peripheral vein.
	2. Give 6 mg by rapid IV injection followed by a 20 mL saline flush.
	3. If no response after 2 min, double the dose (12 mg).
	4. If still no response after 2 min, the 12 mg dose can be repeated.
Dose Adjustments	Decrease dose by 50% for:
	1. Drug injection into the superior vena cava
	2. Ongoing therapy with calcium antagonists, β-blockers, or dipyridamole
Drug Interactions	1. Dipyridamole (blocks adenosine uptake)
	2. Theophylline (blocks adenosine receptors)
Contra-indications	1. Asthma
	2. 2nd or 3rd degree AV block
	3. Sick sinus syndrome
Adverse Effects	1. Bradycardia, AV block (50%)
	2. Facial flushing (20%)
	3. Dyspnea (12%)
	4. Chest pressure (7%)

From References 15 and 16.

2. Synchronized cardioversion is recommended for cases that are hemodynamically unstable, or refractory to pharmacologic agents (2).

V. VENTRICULAR TACHYCARDIA

Ventricular tachycardia (VT) is a wide-QRS-complex tachycardia that has an abrupt onset, a regular rhythm, and a rate above 100 bpm (usually 140–200 bpm) (18,19). The appearance can be *monomorphic* (uniform QRS complexes) or *polymorphic* (multiple QRS morphologies). Monomorphic VT rarely occurs in the absence of structural heart disease.

A. VT versus SVT

Monomorphic VT can be difficult to distinguish from an SVT with prolonged AV conduction. There are two abnormalities on an ECG that will identify VT.

1. The presence of *AV dissociation* (i.e., no fixed relationship between P waves and QRS complexes) is evidence of VT. This may not be evident on a single-lead tracing, and is more likely to be discovered on a 12-lead ECG. (P waves are most visible in the inferior limb leads and the anterior precordial leads.)

2. The presence of *fusion beats* like the one in Figure 13.4 is evidence of ventricular ectopic activity. A fusion beat is produced by the retrograde transmission of a ventricular ectopic impulse that collides with a supraventricular (e.g., sinus node) impulse. The result is a hybrid QRS complex that is a mixture of the normal QRS complex and the ventricular ectopic impulse.

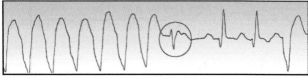

FIGURE 13.4 An example of a fusion beat (circled in red), which is a hybrid QRS complex produced by the collision of a supraventricular impulse and a ventricular ectopic impulse. The presence of fusion beats is evidence of ventricular ectopic activity.

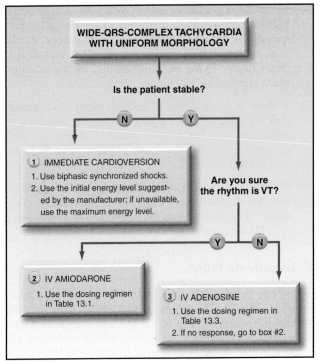

FIGURE 13.5 Flow diagram for the management of patients with wide-QRS-complex tachycardias.

B. Management

The management of patients with a wide-QRS-complex tachycardia is organized in a flow diagram in Figure 13.5.

1. If there is evidence of hemodynamic compromise, *electrical cardioversion* is the appropriate intervention, regardless of whether the rhythm is VT or SVT with aberrant conduction. The shocks should be synchronized, and biphasic shocks are preferred (20) because they are effective at lower energy levels. According to

the updated guidelines on ACLS (20), the energy of the initial shock should be according to the manufacturers suggestion; if not available, maximum-energy shocks (e.g., 200 J with biphasic shocks) should be considered. (See Chapter 15 for recommendations on the management of pulseless VT.)

2. If there is no evidence of hemodynamic compromise and the diagnosis of VT is uncertain, the response to adenosine can be helpful because adenosine will abruptly terminate most cases of paroxysmal SVT, but will not terminate VT.

3. If there is no evidence of hemodynamic compromise and the diagnosis of VT is certain, intravenous *amiodarone is the favored drug for suppression of monomorphic VT* (20); the dosing regimen is shown in Table 13.1.

C. Torsade de Pointes

Torsade de pointes ("twisting around the points") is a polymorphic VT with QRS complexes that appear to be twisting around the isoelectric line of the ECG, as shown in Figure 13.6. This arrhythmia is associated with a prolonged QT interval, and it can be congenital or acquired (the latter being much more common).

1. **Predisposing Factors**

   The acquired form of torsade de pointes (TdP) is caused by a variety of drugs and electrolyte abnormalities that prolong the QT interval (21,22).

   a. The drugs most frequently implicated in TdP are listed in Table 13.4 (22).

   b. The electrolyte disorders that prolong the QT interval include hypokalemia, hypocalcemia, and hypomagnesemia.

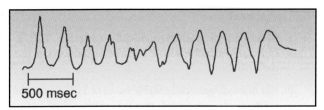

FIGURE 13.6 Torsade de pointes, a polymorphic ventricular tachycardia described as "twisting around the (isoelectric) point". Tracing courtesy of Dr. Richard M. Greenberg, M.D.

Table 13.4	Drugs That Can Induce Torsade de Pointes		
Antiarrhythmics	**Antimicrobials**	**Neuroleptics**	**Others**
IA { Quinidine Disopyramide Procainamide	Clarithromycin Erithromycin Pentamidine	Chlorpromazine Thioridazine Droperidol Haloperidol	Cisapride Methadone
III { Ibutilide Sotalol			

From Reference 22. For a complete list of drugs, go to www.torsades.org

2. **Measuring the QT Interval**

The QT interval (from the onset of the QRS complex to the end of the T wave) varies inversely with heart rate, so a rate-corrected QT interval (QTc) provides a more accurate assessment of QT prolongation. The QTc is calculated by dividing the QT interval by the square root of the R-R interval (23,24); i.e.,

$$QTc = QT / \sqrt{R\text{-}R} \qquad (13.1)$$

A normal QTc is ≤0.44 seconds, and *a QTc >0.5 seconds represents an increased risk of TdP* (24).

3. Management

    a. Sustained or hemodynamically unstable TdP requires nonsynchronized electric cardioversion (i.e., defibrillation).

    b. For hemodynamically stable cases of TdP, IV magnesium is the preferred therapy, even when serum magnesium levels are normal. The recommended regimen is *2 grams MgSO₄ over 1–2 min, followed by an infusion of 2–4 mg/min* (22).

    c. IV potassium can also be used, even in normokalemic patients. The goal is to raise the serum potassium by 0.5 mEq/L (22).

    d. For cases of TdP that are refractory to magnesium, overdrive transvenous pacing with a target rate of 90–110 (which reduces the duration of the QT interval) should be considered (22).

REFERENCES

1. January CT, Wann LS, Alpert JS, et al. 2014 AHA/ACC/HRS guideline for the management of patients with atrial fibrillation. Circulation 2014; 130:e199–e267.

2. Page RL, Joglar JA, Al-Khatib SM, et al. 2015 ACC/AHA/HRS guideline for the management of adult patients with supraventricular tachycardia: executive summary. Circulation 2015; 132:000-000 (available at www.acc.org, accessed 3/2/2016).

3. Mayson SE, Greenspon AJ, Adams S, et al. The changing face of postoperative atrial fibrillation: a review of current medical therapy. Cardiol Rev 2007; 15:231–241.

4. Siu C-W, Lau C-P, Lee W-L, et al. Intravenous diltiazem is superior to intravenous amiodarone or digoxin for achieving ventricular rate control in patients with acute uncomplicated atrial fibrillation. Crit Care Med 2009; 37:2174–2179.

5. Gray RJ. Managing critically ill patients with esmolol. An ultrashort-acting β-adrenergic blocker. Chest 1988; 93:398–404.

6. Karth GD, Geppert A, Neunteufl T, et al. Amiodarone versus diltiazem for rate control in critically ill patients with atrial tachyarrhythmias. Crit Care Med 2001; 29:1149–1153.

7. Khan IA, Mehta NJ, Gowda RM. Amiodarone for pharmacological cardioversion of recent-onset atrial fibrillation. Int J Cardiol 2003; 89:239–248.

8. VerNooy RA, Mounsey P. Antiarrhythmic drug therapy in atrial fibrillation. Cardiol Clin 2004; 22:21–34.

9. Chow MSS. Intravenous amiodarone: pharmacology, pharmacokinetics, and clinical use. Ann Pharmacother 1996; 30:637–643.

10. Kastor J. Multifocal atrial tachycardia. N Engl J Med 1990; 322:1713–1720.

11. Iseri LT, Fairshter RD, Hardeman JL, Brodsky MA. Magnesium and potassium therapy in multifocal atrial tachycardia. Am Heart J 1985; 312:21–26.

12. Arsura E, Lefkin AS, Scher DL, et al. A randomized, double-blind, placebo-controlled study of verapamil and metoprolol in treatment of multifocal atrial tachycardia. Am J Med 1988; 85:519–524.

13. Trohman RG. Supraventricular tachycardia: implications for the internist. Crit Care Med 2000; 28 (Suppl):N129–N135.

14. Lim SH, Anantharaman V, Teo WS, et al. Comparison of treatment of supraventricular tachycardia by Valsalva maneuver and carotid sinus massage. Ann Emerg Med 1998; 31:30–35.

15. Rankin AC, Brooks R, Ruskin JM, McGovern BA. Adenosine and the treatment of supraventricular tachycardia. Am J Med 1992; 92:655–664.

16. Chronister C. Clinical management of supraventricular tachycardia with adenosine. Am J Crit Care 1993; 2:41–47.

17. McCollam PL, Uber W, Van Bakel AB. Adenosine-related ventricular asystole. Ann Intern Med 1993; 118:315–316.

18. Gupta AK, Thakur RK. Wide QRS complex tachycardias. Med Clin N Am 2001; 85:245–266.

19. Akhtar M, Shenasa M, Jazayeri M, et al. Wide QRS complex tachycardia. Ann Intern Med 1988; 109:905–912.

20. Link MS, Berkow LC, Kudenchuk PJ, et al. Part 7: Adult advanced cardiovascular life support. 2015 American Heart

Association Guidelines Update for Cardiopulmonary Resuscitation and Emergency Cardiovascular Care. Circulation 2015; 132 (Suppl 2):S444–S464.

21. Vukmir RB. Torsades de pointes: a review. Am J Emerg Med 1991; 9:250–262.

22. Nachimuthu S, Assar MD, Schussler JM. Drug-induced QT-interval prolongation: mechanisms and clinical management. Ther Adv Drug Saf 2012; 3:241–253.

23. Sadanaga T, Sadanaga F, Yoo H, et al. An evaluation of ECG leads used to assess QT prolongation. Cardiology 2006; 105:149–154.

24. Trinkley KE, Page RL 2nd, Lien H, et al. QT interval prolongation and the risk of torsades de pointes: essentials for clinicians. Curr Med Res Opin 2013; 29:1719–1726.

Chapter 14

Acute Coronary Syndromes

This chapter describes the management of patients with acute, occlusive coronary artery thrombosis (acute coronary syndromes, or ACS). The importance of this disorder is shown by the claim that *a fatal coronary event occurs once every minute in the United States* (1). The focus of this chapter is on the early management of ACS, and not the diagnostic evaluation, and the recommendations are based on clinical practice guidelines from the American Heart Association (2,3).

I. PROTECTIVE MEASURES

The following measures are aimed at protecting the myocardium from ischemic injury and limiting the extent of myocardial damage.

A. Oxygen Therapy

1. INDICATIONS: Oxygen therapy is recommended for an arterial O_2 saturation <90%, and for patients with respiratory distress (2,3).

2. COMMENT: Supplemental O_2 is no longer recommended as a routine measure in ACS because O_2 promotes coronary artery vasoconstriction (4), and toxic O_2 metabolites have been implicated in reperfusion injury (5). The potential for harm from O_2 therapy was confirmed in a randomized study of patients with acute myocardial infarction in which patients who received supplemental

O_2 developed larger infarctions and more frequent arrhythmias than patients allowed to breathe room air (6).

B. Nitroglycerin

1. INDICATIONS: Sublingual nitroglycerin (NTG) is recommended for immediate relief of ischemic chest pain. NTG is also given by continuous IV infusion for recurrent chest pain, hypertension, or decompensated heart failure associated with ACS.

2. DOSE: The sublingual dose of NTG is 0.4 mg, which can be repeated every 5 minutes for a total of 3 doses, if needed. The IV dose is a continuous infusion, starting at a rate of 5–10 μg/min, and titrating upward to achieve the desired effect. Dose rates above 100 μg/min are usually not necessary.

3. CONTRAINDICATIONS: NTG is not recommended for right ventricular infarction (because the venodilator effects of NTG are counterproductive), and in patients who have taken a phosphodiesterase inhibitor for erectile dysfunction within the past 24 hours (because of the risk of hypotension) (2,3).

4. NOTE: For more information on NTG, including adverse effects and NTG tolerance, see Chapter 45, Section V.

C. Morphine

1. INDICATIONS: Intravenous morphine is the drug of choice for ischemic chest pain that is refractory to nitroglycerin, and is also used for hydrostatic pulmonary edema (because of its venodilating and sedating effects).

2. DOSE: The effective dose of morphine can vary widely in individual patients. The initial dose is usually 4–8 mg as an IV bolus, followed by doses of 2–8 mg IV every 5 or 10 minutes, as needed (2,3).

3. NOTE: For information on the adverse effects of opioids, see Chapter 43, Section I-C.

D. Aspirin

1. INDICATIONS: Aspirin is an antiplatelet agent that is recommended for all patients with ACS who are not aspirin-sensitive or intolerant, and should be given as soon as possible (decreases mortality and re-infarction rate) (2,3).

2. DOSE: The initial dose is 162–320 mg, as a chewable tablet (enhances absorption), and the maintenance dose is 81 mg PO daily, using enteric-coated tablets (2,3).

3. NOTE: For patients who are aspirin-sensitive or intolerant, *clopidogrel* (Plavix) is a suitable alternative (2,3). (The dosing regimen for clopidogrel is presented later in the chapter.)

E. β-Receptor Antagonists

1. INDICATIONS: β-receptor blockade is recommended for all patients with ACS who do not have a contraindication, and should be started within 24 hrs after presentation (2,3). Oral therapy is suitable for most cases; IV therapy is reserved for patients with persistent chest pain or troublesome tachycardia or hypertension.

2. CONTRAINDICATIONS: β-blockers are contraindicated in cases of high-grade AV block, decompensated systolic heart failure, hypotension, and reactive airway disease (2,3), and in cases of ACS associated with cocaine or amphetamine intoxication (risk of aggravated coronary vasospasm from unopposed α-receptor activity) (3).

3. DOSING REGIMENS: Metoprolol (a selective β_1-antagonist) is a preferred β-blocker for ACS. The oral dosing regimen is 25–50 mg PO every 6 hrs for 48 hrs, then 100 mg PO BID for maintenance therapy. (Longer-acting

metoprolol succinate can be used for maintenance therapy at a dose of 200 mg once daily.) The IV dosing regimen is 5 mg as a bolus dose every 5 minutes, as tolerated, to a total of 3 doses (2).

F. RAA Inhibitors

Drugs that inhibit the renin-angiotensin-aldosterone (RAA) system include angiotensin-converting enzyme (ACE) inhibitors and angiotensin-receptor blockers (ARBs).

1. INDICATIONS: ACE inhibitors are recommended for all cases of ACS that do not have a contraindication. They are especially beneficial in patients with anterior infarction or systolic dysfunction (ejection fraction ≤40%), and are recommended in the first 24 hrs after presentation in these patients (2). ARBs are reserved for patients who do not tolerate ACE inhibitors.

2. CONTRAINDICATIONS: These agents are contraindicated in patients with hypotension, bilateral renal artery stenosis, renal failure, or hyperkalemia.

3. DOSING REGIMENS: ACE inhibitors are given orally (risk of hypotension with IV ACE inhibitors post-MI), and several drugs can be used. One of the popular ACE inhibitors is *lisinopril*, which is started at a dose of 2.5 to 5 mg once daily, and gradually increased to 10 mg daily, as tolerated (2). For ACE inhibitor-intolerant patients the ARB *valsartan* has equivalent efficacy in acute MI (7). The initial dose is 20 mg PO BID, which is gradually increased to 160 mg PO BID, as tolerated (2).

G. Statins

1. INDICATIONS: High-intensity statin therapy is recommended for all cases of ACS that have been stabilized, including those with LDL cholesterol levels <70 mg/dL

(2,3). Of the available statins, only high-dose *atorvastatin* has a proven survival benefit in ACS (8).

2. DOSE: Atorvastatin, 80 mg PO daily (2,3).

3. COMMENT: The troublesome side effects of statins, such as myopathy and hepatotoxicity, occur with chronic therapy, and are not a concern when initiating statin therapy for ACS. There are drug interactions that deserve mention; i.e., statins are metabolized by the cytochrome P450 system (CYP3A4), and drugs that inhibit this enzyme (e.g., amiodarone, omeprazole) can increase the risk of toxic reactions.

II. REPERFUSION

A. The Approach

1. The fundamental goal in ACS is to relieve the obstruction and restore flow in the infarct-related coronary artery. There are three methods for achieving this goal: (a) percutaneous coronary intervention or PCI (coronary angiography, angioplasty, and stent placement), (b) thrombolytic therapy, and (c) coronary artery bypass surgery.

2. The approach to reperfusion is determined by the presence or absence of ST elevation on the ECG, as described next.

B. ACS with ST Elevation

ACS with ST elevation ≥0.1 mv in at least 2 contiguous leads usually indicates a transmural infarction, from complete obstruction of the infarct-related artery. This condition, *ST-elevation myocardial infarction or STEMI*, requires emergent intervention.

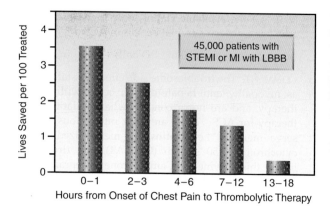

FIGURE 14.1 The survival benefit of thrombolytic therapy in relation to the time elapsed from the onset of chest pain. STEMI = ST-elevation myocardial infarction, LBBB = left bundle branch block. Data from Reference 9.

1. **Time-Dependence**

    There is convincing evidence that reperfusion with either PCI or thrombolytic therapy can restore flow in occluded arteries and decrease the mortality rate (2). However, the benefit from reperfusion therapy is time-dependent, and diminishes as the time progresses from the onset of chest pain. This is demonstrated in Figure 14.1 for thrombolytic therapy (9); note that the survival benefit is negligible after 12 hours from symptom onset.

2. **Indications for Reperfusion Therapy**

    The major indications for reperfusion in patients with STEMI (or a new left bundle branch block) are as follows (2):

    a. Time from onset of symptoms <12 hrs.

    b. Evidence of ongoing ischemia 12–24 hours after symptom onset.

c. Acute, severe heart failure, or cardiogenic shock, regardless of the time from symptom onset.

3. **Percutaneous Coronary Intervention**

Percutaneous coronary intervention (PCI) is superior to thrombolytic therapy for restoring flow in occluded arteries and improving outcomes (see Figure 14.2) (10-12). Unfortunately, PCI is not available in many hospitals. The recommendations for providing PCI to eligible STEMI patients (i.e., symptom onset <12 hrs, etc.) are as follows (2):

a. If the patient is at a PCI-capable hospital, the procedure should be performed within 90 minutes of the first patient contact (in the field).

b. If the patient is at a hospital that is not capable of per-

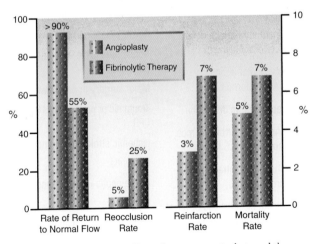

FIGURE 14.2 Comparative effects of coronary angioplasty and thrombolytic therapy on vascular events (graph on the left) and clinical outcomes (graph on the right) in patients with ST-elevation myocardial infarction. Data from References 10-12.

forming PCI, the recommended strategy is transfer to a PCI-capable hospital, with the goal of performing the PCI within 2 hours of the initial patient contact.

4. **Thrombolytic Therapy**

Thrombolytic therapy is the alternative to PCI when the latter is not available, or cannot be performed in a timely manner. For optimal results, therapy should begin no later than 30 minutes after the patient arrives at the hospital (2). The major restriction to thrombolytic therapy is a long list of contraindications, as shown in Table 14.1.

Table 14.1	Contraindications to Thrombolytic Therapy
Absolute Contraindications	**Relative Contraindications**
Active bleeding other than menses	Systolic BP >180 mm Hg or diastolic BP >110 mm Hg
Malignant intracranial neoplasm (primary or metastatic)	Active bleeding in past 4 weeks
Cardiovascular anomaly (e.g., AV malformation)	Noncompressible vascular punctures
Suspected aortic dissection	Major surgery in past 3 weeks
Ischemic stroke within 3 mos. (but not within 4.5 hrs)	Traumatic or prolonged (>10 min) CPR
Prior history of intracranial hemorrhage	Ischemic stroke over 3 mos. ago
	Dementia
Significant closed-head or facial trauma in past 3 months	Active peptic ulcer disease
	Pregnancy
	Ongoing therapy with warfarin

From Reference 2.

a. LYTIC AGENTS: Fibrinolytic drugs act by converting plasminogen to plasmin, which then breaks fibrin strands into smaller subunits. The drugs in Table 14.2 act on plasminogen that is bound to fibrin (clot-specific fibrinolysis), which limits the extent of systemic fibrinolysis and reduces the risk of bleeding. The success rate in restoring flow is equivalent (about 85%) for all fibrinolytic drugs (2).

Table 14.2	Fibrinolytic Drugs				
Drug	**Dosing Regimen**				
Alteplase (tPA)	1. 15 mg IV initially, then 2. 0.75 mg/kg (but not >50 mg) over 30 min, then 3. 0.5 mg/kg (but not >35 mg) over 60 min 4. Maximum dose is 100 mg over 90 min.				
Reteplase (rPA)	10 Units IV, with a repeat dose in 30 min.				
Tenecteplase (TNK-tPA)	1. A single IV dose, based on body weight:				

Wt (kg)	<60	60–69	70–79	80–89	>90
Dose (mg)	30	35	40	45	50

From Reference 2.

b. BLEEDING RISK: The risk of major bleeding, such as intracerebral hemorrhage (0.5–1%), and extracranial hemorrhage that requires blood transfusions (5–15%), is equivalent for all the fibrinolytic drugs (13,14).

c. Major bleeding from thrombolysis can be treated with cryoprecipitate (10 to 15 bags) followed by fresh frozen plasma (up to 6 units) if necessary, to achieve a serum fibrinogen ≥100 mg/mL. The use of antifibrinolytic agents such as *epsilon-aminocaproic acid* (5 grams IV over 15–30 min) is reserved for refractory cases of bleeding (because of the risk of thrombosis) (14).

C. ACS without ST Elevation

The absence of ST elevation on the ECG indicates less extensive myocardial injury than a transmural MI, or ischemia with threatened myocardial injury(troponin levels can help distinguish between these two). This condition, called *non-ST-elevation MI*, or *nonSTEMI*, is the result of partial coronary occlusion, or transient complete occlusion with spontaneous revascularization. As such, it may not require emergent reperfusion. The approach to reperfusion therapy in these cases is summarized below.

1. The timing of PCI in nonSTEMI is determined by the severity of the patient's clinical condition (3);

   a. Indications for emergent PCI include refractory or recurrent angina, severe heart failure, hemodynamic instability, and cardiogenic shock.

   b. In clinically stable patients, clinical scoring systems are used to predict the likelihood of a poor outcome, and the results of these tests are used to determine the need, and timing, of PCI (3).

2. Thrombolytic therapy is not used in nonSTEMI cases.

III. ADJUNCTIVE ANTITHROMBOTIC THERAPY

Anticoagulation and dual antiplatelet therapy are standard practices for the early management of ACS. The following is a brief summary of the preferred agents and dosing regimens.

A. Anticoagulation

1. For STEMI patients who undergo PCI, unfractionated heparin (UFH) is preferred for anticoagulation.

   a. The dosing regimen involves IV bolus doses of 70–100 Units/kg, or 50–70 Units/kg if a glycoprotein receptor antagonist (described later) is planned, to achieve a therapeutic activated clotting time (250–350 sec) (2).

2. Following PCI and thrombolytic therapy, UFH is recommended for short-term (48 hrs) anticoagulation, using the following regimen (2).

   a. 60 Units/kg IV bolus (maximum 4,000 Units) followed by an infusion at 12 Units/kg/hr (maximum 1,000 Units/hr), and adjusted to achieve an activated PTT of 1.5 to 2 times control (2).

3. Low-molecular-weight heparin (LMWH) is preferred for long-term (one week) anticoagulation after thrombolytic therapy. The recommended LMWH is enoxaparin, in the following dosing regimen (2).

   a. For age <75 yrs, 30 mg IV initially, followed in 15 min by 1 mg/kg subQ every 12 hrs (maximum 100 mg for first 2 doses).

   b. For age ≥75 yrs, the dose is 0.75 mg/kg subQ (maximum 75 mg for first 2 doses) without an IV loading dose.

   c. Regardless of age, if the creatinine clearance is <30 mL/min, the dose is 1 mg/kg subQ every 24 hrs.

4. For nonSTEMI, enoxaparin (LMWH) can be used for the duration of the hospitalization or until PCI is performed.

   a. The recommended dose in this setting is 1 mg/kg subQ every 12 hrs, or 1 mg/kg subQ every 24 hrs if the creatinine clearance is <30 mL/min (3).

B. P2Y$_{12}$ Inhibitors

1. The P2Y$_{12}$ inhibitors are oral antiplatelet agents that block surface receptors involved in ADP-induced platelet aggregation. This mechanism of action differs from that of aspirin, so the antiplatelet effects of aspirin and P2Y$_{12}$ inhibitors are additive.

2. Three P2Y$_{12}$ inhibitors are approved for use in ACS: *clopidogrel, prasugrel,* and *ticagrelor*. Clopidogrel and prasugrel are prodrugs that require activation in the liver, and their effects are irreversible. Prasugrel has the most potent antiplatelet effects, and the highest risk of bleeding; as a result, *prasugrel is not recommended in patients with prior stroke or TIA* (2,3).

3. P2Y$_{12}$ inhibitors are routinely used in combination with aspirin, and their dosing regimens are shown in Table 14.3. When PCI is anticipated, the loading dose of P2Y$_{12}$ inhibitors should be given as early as possible, or at the time of the procedure.

C. Glycoprotein Receptor Antagonists

When platelets are activated, glycoprotein receptors (IIb and IIIa) on the platelet surface begin to bind fibrinogen, and the fibrinogen molecules form bridges between adjacent platelets, which promotes platelet aggregation.

1. Glycoprotein receptor antagonists (also called IIb/IIIa inhibitors) block the binding of fibrinogen to activated platelets, which inhibits platelet aggregation. These drugs are the most potent antiplatelet agents available, and are known as *superaspirins*.

2. The available IIb/IIIa inhibitors include *abciximab* (ReoPro), *eptifibatide* (Integrilin), and *tirofiban* (Aggrastat). All three are given by IV infusion using the dosing regimens in Table 14.3.

3. These drugs are used in high-risk patients who receive emergent PCI, and are given just before or at the start of the procedure.

4. Abciximab is the most potent, most expensive, and longest-acting IIb/IIIa inhibitor. After discontinuing this drug, bleeding times can take 12 hours to normalize (15). Eptifibatide and tirofiban are short-acting agents; after

discontinuing these drugs, bleeding times return to normal in 15 minutes for eptifibatide and 4 hours for tirofiban (15).

Table 14.3	Antiplatelet Drugs
Drug	**Dosing Regimen**
P2Y$_{12}$ Inhibitors	
Clopidogrel	300 mg PO initially (600 mg for PCI), then 75 mg PO daily.
Prasugrel	60 mg PO initially, then 10 mg PO daily.
Ticagrelor	60 mg PO initially, then 90 mg PO BID.
IIb/IIIa Inhibitors	
Abciximab	0.25 mg/kg IV bolus, then 0.125 µg/kg/min (max 10 µg/min) for up to 12 hr.
Eptifibatide	180 µg/kg IV bolus, then 2 µg/kg/min for 12–18 hr For PCI in STEMI, repeat bolus dose in 10 min if renal function is normal. Reduce infusion rate by 50% when Cr CL <50 mL/min.
Tirofiban	25 µg/kg IV bolus, then 0.1 µg/kg/min for 12–24 hr. Reduce infusion rate by 50% when Cr CL <30 mL/min.

From References 2 and 3.

IV. COMPLICATIONS

The complications of ACS can be classified as electrical or mechanical. The former are presented in Chapters 13 and 15, and the latter are briefly described here.

A. Structural Defects

Structural defects are the result of transmural (ST-elevation) infarctions. They can appear at any time in the first week, but most occur in the first 24 hrs (2). Diagnosis is usually by transthoracic ultrasound. Temporary support with intra-aortic balloon counterpulsation is often necessary, and emergency surgical repair is required in most cases.

1. ACUTE MITRAL REGURGITATION is the result of papillary muscle rupture or postinfarction LV remodeling, and presents with the sudden onset of pulmonary edema and the characteristic holosystolic murmur. Diagnosis is by echocardiography, and should prompt emergent surgical consultation; as delays to surgery diminish the prognosis (16). Temporary support with arterial vasodilators (e.g., hydralazine) and the intra-aortic balloon pump can be used as a bridge to surgery. The mortality rate with mitral valve repair is 20% (2) vs. 70% without surgery (17).

2. RUPTURE OF THE VENTRICULAR SEPTUM often occurs in the first 24 hrs, and is more common following thrombolytic therapy (18). The presentation can mimic acute mitral regurgitation, with acute heart failure and a prominent systolic murmur. Transthoracic ultrasound will identify the problem. Some patients may be hemodynamically stable, but the condition can progress, and emergent surgical repair is required. The reported mortality rate is 20 to 80% with surgery (the higher mortality rates are in patients with shock) (2).

3. LEFT VENTRICULAR FREE-WALL RUPTURE presents with the return of chest pains and new ST-segment abnormalities on the ECG. Accumulation of blood in the pericardium often leads to rapid deterioration from pericardial tamponade. Diagnosis is by cardiac ultrasound, and pericardiocentesis can be life-saving. Immediate surgery is the only course of action, and mortality rates as low as 12% have been reported with a new "patch and glue" surgical technique (19).

B. Cardiac Pump Failure

1. About 10% of cases of ST-elevation MI (STEMI) are associated with cardiac pump failure and cardiogenic shock (20). About 15% of cases occur at presentation, and the remainder develop during the hospitalization (2).

2. Management involves emergent PCI (or thrombolysis if PCI is not available) and coronary bypass surgery, if necessary. In one multicenter study, revascularization with PCI or bypass surgery within 6 hours was associated with a 13% absolute decrease in mortality when compared with medical management and delayed surgery (21).

3. The hemodynamic management of cardiogenic shock is described in Chapter 8 (see Sections III-C and IV). An important consideration in postinfarction cardiogenic shock is providing hemodynamic support without producing undesirable increases in myocardial O_2 consumption. Table 14.4 shows the superiority of the intra-aortic balloon pump over pharmacologic support in that regard.

Table 14.4	Hemodynamic Support and Myocardial VO$_2$	
Parameter	**IABP**	**Dobut/Norepi**
Preload	↓	↑
Contractility	—	↑↑
Afterload	↓	↑
Heart Rate	—	↑↑
Summed effect on myocardial VO$_2$	↓↓	↑↑↑↑↑↑

IABP = intra-aortic balloon pump; Dobut = dobutamine; Norepi = norepi-nephrine; VO$_2$ = oxygen consumption.

V. ACUTE AORTIC DISSECTION

Aortic dissection involving the ascending aorta can be mistaken as ACS, and can also be a cause of ACS. However unlike ACS, aortic dissection is a surgical emergency that is often fatal if not managed appropriately.

A. Pathophysiology

Aortic dissection occurs when a tear in the aortic intima allows blood to dissect between the intimal and medial layers of the aorta, creating a false lumen. When the dissection involves the ascending aorta, retrograde propagation can result in coronary insufficiency, aortic insufficiency, and pericardial tamponade (22).

B. Clinical Manifestations

1. The most common complaint is the abrupt onset of chest pain, which is often sharp, and can be substernal (ascending aortic dissection) or in the back (descending aortic dissection). Most importantly, *the chest pain can subside spontaneously for hours to days* (23,24), and this can be a source of missed diagnoses. About 5% of patients have no pain (22).

2. The most common clinical findings are hypertension (50% of patients) and aortic insufficiency (50% of patients) (23,24). Unequal pulses in the upper extremities (from obstruction of the left subclavian artery in the aortic arch) are found in only 15% of patients (24).

3. The chest x-ray can show mediastinal widening (60% of cases) (24), or can be normal (20% of cases) (22). The ECG can show ischemic changes (15% of cases) or evidence of MI (5% of cases), but the ECG is normal in 30% of cases (22).

C. Imaging Studies

1. The diagnosis of aortic dissection requires one of four

imaging modalities: magnetic resonance imaging (MRI) (sensitivity and specificity 98%), transesophageal echocardiography (sensitivity 98%, specificity 77%), contrast-enhanced computed tomography (sensitivity 94%, specificity 87%), and aortography (sensitivity 88%, specificity 94%) (25). As indicated *MRI is the most sensitive and specific imaging modality for the diagnosis aortic dissection.*

D. Management

The goals of management in aortic dissection are control of hypertension and surgical intervention.

1. Antihypertensive Therapy

   Antihypertensive therapy should NOT increase cardiac stroke output because increased flow in the aorta will augment the shear forces that promote further dissection. For this reason, *β-receptor antagonists are preferred* because they decrease the force of ventricular contraction (negative inotropic effect). The drug regimens that are used for blood pressure control in aortic dissection are presented in Table 14.5.

Table 14.5	Antihypertensive Agents for Acute Aortic Dissection
Drug	**Dosing Regimen and Comments**
Esmolol	500 μkg IV bolus, then infuse at 50 μg/kg/min. Increase in increments of 25 μg/kg/min every 5 min until systolic BP is 120 mm Hg or heart rate is 60 bpm. Maximum dose is 200 μg/kg/min.
Labetalol	20 mg IV over 2 min, then 20–40 mg IV every 10 min if needed, or infuse at 1–2 mg/min to same end-points as esmolol. Maximum cumulative dose is 300 mg.

Dosing regimens are manufacturer's recommendations.

   a. The β-blocker that is most favored is *esmolol* (Brevibloc), which has a short duration of action (9 minutes) and can be rapidly titrated to achieve the desired end-point.

b. An alternative drug is labetalol, a combined α–β–blocker that can be given in IV bolus doses or by continuous infusion.

2. Outcomes

With medical management alone, the mortality in acute aortic dissection increases 1–2% per hour after the onset of symptoms (22). Surgical repair reduces the mortality rate to 10% at 24 hours and 12% at 48 hours (22).

REFERENCES

1. Roger V, Go AS, Lloyd-Jones D, et al. Heart disease and stroke statistics—2012 update: a report from the American Heart Association. Circulation 2012; 125:e2–e220.

2. Ogara PT, Kushner FG, Ascheim DD, et al. 2013 ACCF/AHA guideline for the management of ST-elevation myocardial infarction. J Am Coll Cardiol 2013; 61:e78–e140..

3. Amsterdam EA, Wenger NK, Brindis RG, et al. 2014 AHA/ACC guideline for the management of patients with non-ST-elevation myocardial acute coronary syndromes. Circulation 2014; 130:e344–e426.

4. McNulty PH, King N, Scott S, et al. Effects of supplemental oxygen administration on coronary blood flow in patients undergoing cardiac catheterization. Am J Physiol Heart Circ Physiol. 2005; 288:H1057–1062.

5. Bulkley GB. Reactive oxygen metabolites and reperfusion injury: aberrant triggering of reticuloendothelial function. Lancet 1994; 344:934–936.

6. Stub D, Smith K, Bernard S, et al; AVOID Investigators. Air versus oxygen in ST-segment elevation myocardial infarction. Circulation 2015; 131:2143–2150.

7. Pfeffer MA, McMurray JJV, Velazquez EJ, et al. Valsartan, captopril, or both in myocardial infarction complicated by heart fail-

ure, left ventricular dysfunction, or both. N Engl J Med. 2003; 349:1893–96.

8. Cannon CP, Braunwald E, McCabe CH, et al. Intensive versus moderate lipid lowering with statins after acute coronary syndromes. N Engl J Med. 2004; 350:1495–504.

9. Fibrinolytic Therapy Trialists Collaborative Group. Indications for fibrinolytic therapy in suspected acute myocardial infarction: collaborative overview of early mortality and major morbidity results from all randomized trials of more than 1000 patients. Lancet 1994; 343:311–322.

10. The GUSTO IIb Angioplasty Substudy Investigators. A clinical trial comparing primary coronary angioplasty with tissue plasminogen activator for acute myocardial infarction. New Engl J Med 1997; 336:1621–1628.

11. Keeley EC, Boura JA, Grines CL. Primary angioplasty versus intravenous thrombolytic therapy for acute myocardial infarction: a quantitative review of 23 randomized trials. Lancet 2003; 361:13–20.

12. Stone GW, Cox D, Garcia E, et al. Normal flow (TIMI-3) before mechanical reperfusion therapy is an independent determinant of survival in acute myocardial infarction. Circulation 2001; 104:636–641.

13. Llevadot J, Giugliano RP, Antman EM. Bolus fibrinolytic therapy in acute myocardial infarction. JAMA 2001; 286:442–449.

14. Young GP, Hoffman JR. Thrombolytic therapy. Emerg Med Clin 1995; 13:735–759.

15. Patrono C, Coller B, Fitzgerald G, et al. Platelet-active drugs: the relationship among dose, effectiveness, and side effects. Chest 2004; 126:234S–264S.

16. Tepe NA, Edmunds LH Jr. Operation for acute postinfarction mitral insufficiency and cardiogenic shock. J Thorac Cardiovasc Surg. 1985; 89:525–30.

17. Thompson CR, Buller CE, Sleeper LA, et al. Cardiogenic shock due to acute severe mitral regurgitation complicating acute myocardial infarction: a report from the SHOCK trial registry. J Am Coll Cardiol 2000; 36:1104–1109.

18. Prêtre R, Ye Q, Grünenfelder J, et al. Operative results of "repair" of ventricular septal rupture after acute myocardial infraction. Am J Cardiol. 1999; 84:785–8.

19. Haddadin S, Milano AD, Faggian G, et al. Surgical treatment of postinfarction left ventricular free wall rupture. J Card Surg 2009; 24:624–631.

20. Samuels LF, Darze ES. Management of acute cardiogenic shock. Cardiol Clin 2003; 21:43–49.

21. Hochman JS, Sleeper LA, While HD, et al. One-year survival following early revascularization for cardiogenic shock. JAMA 2001; 285:190–192.

22. Tsai TT, Nienaber CA, Eagle KA. Acute aortic syndromes. Circulation 2005; 112:3802–3813.

23. Khan IA, Nair CK. Clinical, diagnostic, and management perspectives of aortic dissection. Chest 2002; 122:311–328.

24. Knaut AL, Cleveland JC. Aortic emergencies. Emerg Med Clin N Am 2003; 21:817–845.

25. Zegel HG, Chmielewski S, Freiman DB. The imaging evaluation of thoracic aortic dissection. Appl Radiol 1995; (June):15–25.

Chapter 15

Cardiac Arrest

This chapter presents the essential elements of cardiopulmonary resuscitation (CPR) and post-CPR care, including criteria for predicting a poor neurologic outcome after cardiac arrest. The material in this chapter is based on the most recent clinical practice guidelines on CPR from the American Heart Association (1-3).

I. BASIC LIFE SUPPORT

The essential components of basic life support (BLS) are: (a) chest compressions, (b) airway opening (i.e., establishing a patent oropharynx), and (c) periodic lung inflations.

A. Chest Compressions

1. The original mnemonic ABC (_A_irway, _B_reathing, _C_irculation) for the components of BLS has been rearranged to CAB (_C_irculation, _A_irway, _B_reathing), reflecting the shift in emphasis to chest compressions in the resuscitation effort. The rationale for this shift was the realization that cardiac arrest is primarily a circulatory (not ventilatory) disorder.

2. The recommendations for chest compressions in the BLS guidelines are shown in Table 15.1. Early and uninterrupted chest compressions are a major emphasis of the guidelines.

B. Airway Opening

Airway opening refers to the act of establishing a patent

oropharynx, which can become obstructed by a flaccid tongue in comatose patients who are supine. The "head tilt/chin up" maneuver (which hyperextends the neck and moves the lower jaw forward) is designed to pull the tongue away from the posterior oropharynx and relieve any obstruction from a floppy tongue.

Table 15.1	Chest Compressions

From the BLS Guidelines:

1. Chest compressions should be delivered to the lower half of the sternum at a rate of 100–120/min.

2. Each chest compression should achieve a depth of at least 2 inches (5 cm) but no greater than 2.4 inches (6 cm), and the chest should be allowed to recoil completely, to allow the heart to fill before the next compression.

3. First responders should begin CPR with a series of 30 chest compressions, followed by a brief pause for 2 rescue breaths. This compression-ventilation ratio (30:2) should be continued until an advanced airway is placed.

4. Once an advanced airway is in place, chest compressions should continue uninterrupted, with no pause for lung inflations.

5. Chest compressions should only be interrupted when absolutely necessary (e.g., to deliver electric countershocks).

From Reference 1.

C. Ventilation

1. Prior to endotracheal intubation, ventilation can be delivered with a face mask that is connected to a self-inflating ventilation bag (e.g., Ambu Respirator) that fills with oxygen. The bag is compressed by hand to deliver the breath, and 2 breaths are provided for every 30 chest compressions (as in Table 15.1).

2. After an endotracheal tube is in place, lung inflations should be delivered at 6-second intervals (10 breaths/min)

while chest compressions continue uninterrupted.

3. **Inflation Volumes**

   a. Large inflation volumes are common during CPR, resulting in hyperinflation of the lungs (4), which can impede cardiac filling and diminish the effectiveness of chest compressions.

   b. The recommended inflation volume during "bagged breathing" is 6–7 mL/kg (5), or about 500 mL for an average-sized adult. However, the volume of lung inflations is not monitored during CPR, so adhering to this recommendation does not seem possible.

   c. One method of avoiding large inflation volumes is based on the volume capacity of the inflation bag (which is 1–2 liters in most bags). For example, if the inflation bag has a capacity of 1 liter, then compressing the bag until it is about half full will deliver about 500 mL to the lungs. Another approach is "one-handed bagging"; i.e., squeezing the bag with one hand expels a volume of 600–800 mL (personal observation), which is unlikely to produce serious hyperinflation.

4. **Rapid Inflations**

   Rapid lung inflation rates are common during CPR (4,6), with average rates of 30 inflations/min in one report (6). Rapid breathing is problematic because there is insufficient time for the lungs to empty, and the extra volume in the lungs at the end of expiration creates a positive pressure; i.e., positive end-expiratory pressure, or PEEP. This self-generated or "intrinsic PEEP" increases intrathoracic pressure, which reduces venous return to the heart, and can restrict expansion of the ventricles during diastole; both of these effects diminish the ability of chest compressions to augment cardiac output. Intrinsic PEEP is described in more detail in Chapter 21.

II. ADVANCED LIFE SUPPORT

Advanced cardiovascular life support, or ACLS, includes a variety of interventions, such as airway intubation, mechanical ventilation, defibrillation, and the administration of circulatory-support drugs (2). This section will focus on defibrillation and circulatory-support drugs, and how these interventions are used in cardiac arrests associated with ventricular fibrillation (VF) or pulseless ventricular tachycardia (VT), and cardiac arrests associated with asystole or pulseless electrical activity (PEA).

A. VF or Pulseless VT

The outcomes in cardiac arrest are most favorable when the initial rhythm is VF or pulseless VT, which are "shockable" arrhythmias.

1. **Defibrillation**

   Electrical cardioversion using asynchronous shocks (i.e., not timed to the QRS complex), which is called *defibrillation*, is the most effective resuscitation measure for cardiac arrest associated with VF or pulseless VT. However, the survival benefit from defibrillation is *time-dependent*, as shown in Figure 15.1 (7).

   a. IMPULSE ENERGY: Modern defibrillators use biphasic waveforms to deliver the shocks (because they are effective at lower energy levels than monophasic waveforms), but there are 3 different biphasic waveforms, and each delivers a different current at the same energy setting. This creates difficulty in recommending a single energy level for defibrillation, and the current ACLS guidelines recommend using the manufacturer's suggested energy level for the initial shock (2). If this is not available, the maximum effective energy level (about 200 J for biphasic and 360 J for monophasic shocks) should be selected for the

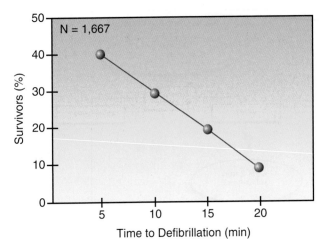

FIGURE 15.1 Relationship between survival and elapsed time from cardiac arrest to initial defibrillation attempt in out-of-hospital cardiac arrest
with VF or pulseless VT. N = number of cases studied. Data from
Reference 7.

initial shock (2). (Automated external defibrillators,
or AEDs, use a preselected energy level.)

2. **Protocol**

The flow diagram in Figure 15.2 is the ACLS algorithm
for cardiac arrest in adults, and the defibrillation protocol for pulseless VT and VF is shown in the left half of
the diagram.

a. Three defibrillation attempts are allowed, if needed,
using the same impulse energy.

b. After each shock is delivered, 2 minutes of uninterrupted chest compressions are advised before check-
ing the post-shock rhythm (to prevent repeat shocks
in rapid succession, which prolongs the interruption
of chest compressions) (2).

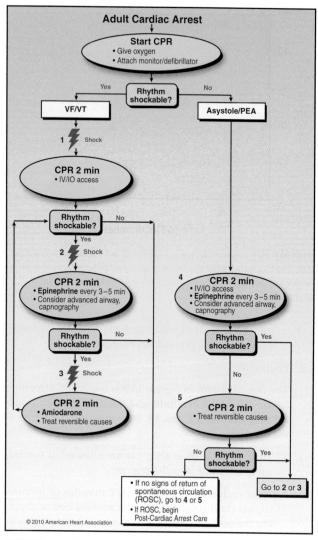

FIGURE 15.2 The ACLS algorithm for adult cardiac arrest. IO = intra-osseous. From Reference 2.

c. If a second defibrillation attempt is required, bolus injections of *epinephrine* are started (1 mg IV, or intraosseous, every 3–5 min, for the duration of the resuscitation effort).

d. If a third defibrillation attempt is required, *amiodarone* is administered IV or IO using a dose of 300 mg, which can be followed by a second dose of 150 mg, if needed.

e. Failure to terminate VF/VT with two defibrillation attempts carries a poor prognosis.

B. Asystole or PEA

The resuscitation of cardiac arrests associated with asystole or PEA ("nonshockable" arrhythmias) is notoriously unsuccessful. The resuscitation scheme is shown on the right half of the flow diagram in Figure 15.2. The major intervention is epinephrine injections (same regimen as used for VF and pulseless VT), and there are no defibrillation attempts unless the rhythm changes to VF or VT.

1. **Reversible Causes of PEA**

There are four potentially reversible causes of PEA, each sharing the letter T: i.e., Tension pneumothorax, pericardial Tamponade, pulmonary Thromboembolism, and Thrombotic occlusion of the coronary arteries. Two of these (pericardial tamponade and tension pneumothorax) can be identified at the bedside with ultrasound imaging, which is readily available in most ERs and ICUs.

C. ACLS Drugs

There are only a few drugs in the ACLS algorithm for adults, and these are shown in Table 15.2. None of these drugs has a proven survival benefit in cardiac arrest (2). (So why do we use them?)

Table 15.2	ACLS Drugs
Drug	**Dosing Regimen and Comments**

Vasopressor

Epinephrine	Dosing:	1 mg IV/IO every 3–5 minutes.
	Comment:	Vasopressor effect can increase coronary perfusion pressure, but cardiac stimulation is counterproductive.

Antiarrhythmic Agents

Amiodarone	Dosing:	300 mg IV/IO, then another 150 mg if needed.
	Comment:	Antiarrhythmic drug of choice for VF/VT that is refractory to defibrillation and vasopressors.
Lidocaine	Dosing:	1–1.5 mg/kg IV/IO, then 0.5–0.75 mg/kg every 5–10 min, as needed, to total of 3 mg/kg. Can use a 1–4 mg/min for maintenance.
	Comment:	Alternative to amiodarone, but much less effective.

From Reference 2. IO = intraosseous.

1. **Epinephrine**

   Epinephrine is a vasopressor that is given in a dose of 1–15 µg/min for the management of circulatory shock (see Chapter 45, Section III). In the doses used for cardiac arrest (1 mg IV bolus every 3–5 min), the systemic vasoconstriction it produces is intense enough to increase coronary perfusion pressure (the difference between aortic and right atrial relaxation pressures, which occur between chest compressions) (8). However, epinephrine also produces β-receptor-mediated cardiac stimulation, which could erase the benefit of the increased coronary perfusion. Epinephrine use is associated with an increased rate of *return to spontaneous circulation (ROSC)*, but the mortality rate is unchanged (2,9).

    a. INJECTION: In the rare instance when intravenous or intraosseous access is not available, epinephrine can be injected into the upper airway through an endotracheal tube. The dose for endotracheal injection is 2–2.5 times the IV dose (2).

2. **Amiodarone**

Amiodarone is the preferred antiarrhythmic agent for VF/pulseless VT that is refractory to defibrillation and epinephrine (2). This preference is based on clinical studies showing increased survival to hospital admission with amiodarone compared to placebo (10) or lidocaine (11). However, amiodarone did not increase survival to hospital discharge in these studies.

3. **Lidocaine**

Lidocaine is the original antiarrhythmic agent used for shock-resistant VF and pulseless VT, but it is now recommended as an alternative to amiodarone.

D. End-Tidal PCO_2

The CO_2 in exhaled gas is a metabolic end-product that is transported to the airways by flow in the pulmonary arteries (i.e., cardiac output). When alveolar ventilation is constant, a decrease in cardiac output results in a similar decrease in exhaled PCO_2 (measured at the end of expiration, and called *end-tidal PCO_2*) (12). This relationship is the basis for the use of end-tidal PCO_2 as a noninvasive marker of changes in cardiac output (13).

1. **Predictive Value**

Monitoring the end-tidal PCO_2 during CPR provides valuable information about the effectiveness of the resuscitation effort, and the likely outcome. This is demonstrated in Figure 15.3, which shows the serial changes in

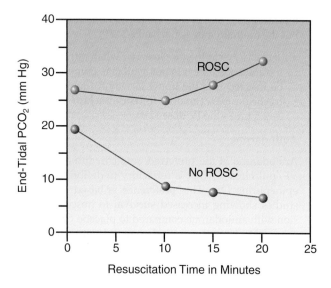

FIGURE 15.3 Serial changes in end-tidal PCO_2 during CPR in relation to return of spontaneous circulation (ROSC). Data points represent mean values for each group of patients. From Reference 14.

end-tidal PCO_2 during 20 minutes of CPR in relation to return of spontaneous circulation (ROSC) (14). Patients who achieved ROSC showed a progressive increase in end-tidal PCO_2, while patients who did not achieve ROSC showed a progressive decline in end-tidal PCO_2.

a. There is convincing evidence that *ROSC is unlikely if the end-tidal PCO_2 is not higher than 10 mm Hg after 20 minutes of CPR* (2,14-16).

III. POST-RESUSCITATION PERIOD

The return of spontaneous circulation does not ensure a satisfactory outcome; i.e., in one survey of 24,000 ICU admissions after successful CPR, 71% of the patients did not survive to hospital discharge (17).

A. Post-Cardiac Arrest Syndrome

The post-cardiac arrest syndrome has 3 major features: (a) brain injury, (b) cardiac dysfunction, and (c) systemic inflammation (18).

1. Brain injury is the *leading cause of death and disability in survivors of cardiac arrest* (18), and is the result of both ischemic and reperfusion injury.

   a. Brain injury *can be aggravated by hypotension, hyperglycemia, and fever*, and these conditions require prompt attention.

2. Cardiac dysfunction is both systolic and diastolic ("stunned" myocardium), and can cause hemodynamic instability. However, it is often reversible, and can resolve within 72 hrs (18).

   a. Acute MI is responsible for at least 50% of cardiac arrests (18), and immediate coronary angiography with angioplasty can improve outcomes (19).

3. Systemic inflammation (fever, leukocytosis) is prominent, is triggered by reperfusion, and can lead to multiorgan dysfunction.

B. Targeted Temperature Management

Targeted temperature management (TTM) involves lowering the body temperature to a preselected level to limit the extent of reperfusion injury, primarily in the brain. When used appropriately, TTM reduces the extent of neurologic injury, and increases survival rates (20). The general features of TTM are shown in Table 15.3, and are summarized below.

1. Candidates for TTM are patients who have survived a

cardiac arrest but have not regained consciousness, regardless of the location of the arrest or the associated rhythm (2).

2. TTM should be started as soon as possible after the cardiac arrest.

3. The use of cold intravenous fluids to initiate cooling can increase the re-arrest rate (21), and should be considered carefully.

4. Cooling is optimal with automated devices that use surface cooling or endovascular cooling. The latter method requires insertion of a specialized central venous catheter, but avoids erratic surface cooling caused by cold-induced vasoconstriction in the skin.

5. The recommended target temperature is 32°C to 36°C (2), but *the highest target temperature (36°C) is advisable* because it easier to achieve, and has equivalent outcomes when compared to lower target temperatures (22,23).

6. The target temperature is maintained for 24 hours.

7. Slow rewarming (0.25–0.5°C/hr) is recommended (24), and is managed by the automated cooling systems.

8. Complications of TTM include shivering, bradycardia, cardiac depression, hypotension, diuresis, hypokalemia, hyperglycemia, impaired coagulation, nonconvulsive status epilepticus, and infection (18,25).

9. Shivering is common during the cooling phase, and is counterproductive because it increases the body temperature. Shivering can be controlled with *propofol* (0.1–0.2 mg/kg/min IV) or *midazolam* (0.02–0.1 mg/kg/hr IV), while *magnesium* (5 grams IV over 5 hours) can also be effective (18). Refractory shivering is managed with neuromuscular blockade (e.g., *cisatracurium*, 0.15–0.2 mg/kg IV bolus, then 1–2 µg/kg/min, if needed).

10. If available, continuous EEG monitoring is advised during TTM because nonconvulsive status epilepticus is reported in 10% of patients (25).

11. Hypothermia slows the metabolism of sedative agents, so it is important to discontinue sedation as soon as possible after rewarming, to avoid delays in evaluating the patient's level of consciousness.

Table 15.3	Targeted Temperature Management
Feature	**Description**
Candidates	Patients with post-cardiac arrest coma
Contraindications	Temp ≤36°C, major bleeding, cryoglobulinemia
Target Temperature	32–36°C
Duration	24 hr
Rewarming Rate	0.25–0.5°C/hr
Complications	Shivering, bradycardia, cardiac depression, hypotension, diuresis, hypokalemia, coagulopathy, nonconvulsive seizures, infection

C. Predicting Neurologic Outcome

1. When patients do not regain consciousness after CPR or TTM, at least 3 days should be allowed to pass before predicting the likelihood of a poor neurologic outcome (i.e., failure to regain consciousness or independent living).

2. For patients who remain comatose 72 hours after CPR with no TTM, or 72 hours after TTM, any one of the following conditions can be used as evidence of a poor neurologic outcome (3).

    a. Absence of pupillary light reflexes.

    b. Status myoclonus (repetitive, irregular movements of the face, trunk, and extremities).

    c. Presence of burst suppression on EEG, or absence of EEG reactivity to external stimuli.

3. For patients who do not have conditions a, b, or c above, persistent coma for 7 days after CPR with no TTM can be used as evidence of a poor neurologic outcome (26). The predictive value of persistent coma 7 days after TTM has not been reported, but there is evidence that TTM does not prolong the time to awaken when compared to CPR without TTM (27), so it is reasonable to assume that persistent coma 7 days after TTM can be used as evidence of a poor neurologic outcome.

4. Abnormal extensor responses to a painful stimulus (decerebrate posturing) are not considered reliable evidence of a poor neurologic outcome after CPR or TTM (3).

REFERENCES

1. Kleinman ME, Brennan EE, Goldberger ZD, et al. Part 5: Adult basic life support and cardiopulmonary resuscitation quality: 2015 American Heart Association Guidelines Update for Cardiopulmonary Resuscitation and Emergency Cardiovascular Care. Circulation 2015; 132(Suppl 2):S414–S435.

2. Link MS, Berkow LC, Kudenchuk PJ, et al. Part 7: Adult advanced cardiovascular life support: 2015 American Heart Association Guidelines Update for Cardiopulmonary Resuscitation and Emergency Cardiovascular Care. Circulation 2015; 132 (Suppl 2):S444–S464.

3. Callaway CW, Donnino MW, Fink EL, et al. Part 8: Post–cardiac arrest care: 2015 American Heart Association Guidelines Update for Cardiopulmonary Resuscitation and Emergency Cardiovascular Care. Circulation 2015; 132 (Suppl 2):S465–S482.

4. Aufderheide TP, Lurie KG. Death by hyperventilation: A common and life-threatening problem during cardiopulmonary resuscitation. Crit Care Med 2004; 32 (Suppl):S345–S351.

5. Berg RA, Hemphill R, Abella BS, et al. Part 5: Adult basic life support: 2010 American Heart Association Guidelines for Cardiopulmonary Resuscitation and Emergency Cardiovascular Care. Circulation 2010; 122 (Suppl 3):S685–S705.

6. Abella BS, Alvarado JP, Mykelbust H, et al. Quality of cardiopulmonary resuscitation during in-hospital cardiac arrest. JAMA 2005; 293:305–310.

7. Larsen MP, Eisenberg M, Cummins RO, Hallstrom AP. Predicting survival from out of hospital cardiac arrest: a graphic model. Ann Emerg Med 1993; 22:1652–1658.

8. Sun S, Tang W, Song F, et al. The effects of epinephrine on outcomes of normothermic and therapeutic hypothermic cardiopulmonary resuscitation. Crit Care Med 2010; 38:2175–2180.

9. Herlitz J, Ekstrom L, Wennerblom B, et al. Adrenaline in out-of-hospital ventricular fibrillation. Does it make any difference? Resuscitation 1995; 29:195–201.

10. Kudenchuk PJ, Cobb LA, Copass MK, et al. Amiodarone for out-of-hospital cardiac arrest due to ventricular fibrillation. New Engl J Med 1999; 341:871–878.

11. Dorian P, Cass D, Schwartz B, et al. Amiodarone as compared to lidocaine for shock-resistant ventricular fibrillation. New Engl J Med 2002; 346:884–890.

12. Nassar BS, Schmidt GA. Capnography during critical illness. Chest 2016; 149:576–585.

13. Monnet X, Bataille A, Magalhaes E, et al. End-tidal carbon dioxide is better than arterial pressure for predicting volume responsiveness by the passive leg raising test. Intensive Care Med 2013; 39:93–100.

14. Kolar M, Krizmaric M, Klemen P, Grmec S. Partial pressure of end-tidal carbon dioxide predicts successful cardiopulmonary resuscitation—a prospective observational study. Crit Care 2008; 12:R115.

15. Sanders AB, Kern KB, Otto CW, et al. End-tidal carbon dioxide monitoring during cardiopulmonary resuscitation. JAMA 1989; 262:1347–1351.

16. Wayne MA, Levine RL, Miller CC. Use of end-tidal carbon dioxide to predict outcome in prehospital cardiac arrest. Ann Emerg Med 1995; 25:762–767.

17. Nolan JP, Laver SR, Welch CA, et al. Outcome following admission to UK intensive care units after cardiac arrest: a secondary analysis of the ICNARC Case Mix Programme Database. Anesthesia 2007; 62:1207–1216.

18. Nolan JP, Neumar RW, Adrie C, et al. Post-cardiac arrest syndrome: epidemiology, pathophysiology, and prognostication. Resuscitation 2008; 79:350–379.

19. Sunde K, Pytte M, Jacobsen D, et al. Implementation of a standard treatment protocol for post-resuscitation care after out-of-hospital cardiac arrest. Resuscitation 2007; 73:29–39.

20. The Hypothermia After Cardiac Arrest Study group. Mild therapeutic hypothermia to improve the neurologic outcome after cardiac arrest. N Engl J Med 2002; 346: 549–556.

21. Kim F, Nichol G, Maynard C, et al. Effect of prehospital induction of mild hypothermia on survival and neurological status among adults with cardiac arrest: a randomized clinical trial. JAMA 2014; 311:45–52.

22. Nielsen N, Wettersley J, Cronberg T, et al. Targeted temperature management at 33°C versus 36°C after cardiac arrest. N Engl J Med 2013; 369:2197–2206.

23. Frydland, Kjaergaard J, Erlinge D, et al. Target temperature management of 33°C and 36°C in patients with out-of-hospital cardiac arrest with non-shockable rhythm—a TTM sub-study. Resuscitation 2015; 89:142–148.

24. Holzer M. Targeted temperature management for comatose survivors of cardiac arrest. N Engl J Med 2010; 363:1256–1264.

25. Rittenberger JC, Popescu A, Brenner RP, et al. Frequency and timing of nonconvulsive status epilepticus in comatose, post-cardiac arrest subjects treated with hypothermia. Neurocrit Care 2012; 16:114–122.

26. Levy DE, Caronna JJ, Singer BH, et al. Predicting outcome from hypoxicischemic coma. JAMA 1985; 253:1420–1426.

27. Fugate JE, Wijdicks EFM, White RD, Rabinstein AA. Does therapeutic hypothermia affect time to awakening in cardiac arrest survivors? Neurology 2011; 77:1346–1350.

Chapter 16

Ventilator-Associated Pneumonia

The clinical approach to pneumonia can be characterized by one word: *problematic*. Fundamental problems include a limited ability to detect parenchymal lung infections, and the lack of a standardized method for identifying responsible pathogen(s).

This chapter presents the current state of affairs regarding pneumonias that appear after 72 hours of mechanical ventilation (i.e., *ventilator-associated pneumonias*), and includes recommendations from clinical practice guidelines (1-3) and recent reviews of this condition (4,5).

I. GENERAL INFORMATION

The following statements summarize some of the relevant observations about ventilator-associated pneumonia (VAP).

1. Pneumonia is the most common nosocomial infection in ICU patients (6), and more than 90% of these pneumonias occur during mechanical ventilation (2). However, the prevalence of VAP is overstated, because post-mortem studies have shown that over half of the cases of VAP are false-positive diagnoses (7).

2. Unlike community-acquired pneumonias, where the predominant pathogens are pneumococci, atypical organisms, and viruses, three-quarters of the responsible pathogens in VAP are gram-negative aerobic bacilli and *Staphylococcus aureus* (see Table 16.1) (8).

3. The mortality rate associated with VAP varies widely, from 0% to 65% (3,9), and there are claims that VAP is not a life-threatening illness (9). However, VAP-associated mortality rates must be viewed with caution because of the tendency for overdiagnosis of VAP (as mentioned earlier) (7).

Table 16.1	Pathogenic Isolates in Ventilator-Associated Pneumonia	
Organisms	**Frequency**
Gram-negative Bacilli	56.5%
Pseudomonas aeruginosa	18.9%
Escherichia coli	9.2%
Hemophilus spp	7.1%
Enterobacter spp	3.8%
Proteus	3.8%
Klebsiella pneumoniae	3.2%
Others	10.5%
Gram-positive Cocci	42.1%
Staphylococcus aureus	18.9%
Streptococcus pneumoniae	13.2%
Hemophilus spp	1.4%
Others	8.6%
Fungal Isolates	1.3%

From Reference 8.

II. PREVENTIVE MEASURES

Aspiration of pathogenic organisms from the oropharynx is believed to be the inciting event in most cases of VAP. The pathogens that most often colonize the oropharynx in ICU patients are gram-negative aerobic bacilli (see Chapter 3, Figure 3.2), and this explains the predominance of these pathogens in VAP.

A. Oral Decontamination

1. The realization that VAP begins with pathogenic colonization of the oropharynx resulted in the introduction of measures to decontaminate the oropharynx as a preventive measure for VAP.

2. The methods of oral decontamination (i.e., with chlorhexidine or topical antibiotics) are described in Chapter 3, Section II, and the benefits of oral decontamination in reducing tracheal colonization and VAP are shown in Figure 3.3.

3. Routine oral care with chlorhexidine (as a mouth rinse or gel, used 2–3 times daily) has become a standard practice in ventilator-dependent patients.

B. Routine Airway Care

The inner surface of artificial airways (endotracheal and tracheostomy tubes) becomes colonized with pathogenic organisms, and passing a suction catheter through the tubes can dislodge these organisms and introduce pathogens into the lower airways (10). Because of this risk, *endotracheal suctioning is not recommended as a routine procedure*, and should be used only when necessary to clear secretions from the airways (11).

C. Clearing Subglottic Secretions

1. Contrary to popular belief, *inflation of the cuff on tracheal tubes to create a seal does not prevent aspiration of mouth secretions into the lower airways*. Aspiration of saliva and liquid tube feedings has been documented in over 50%

of patients with tracheostomies, and the aspiration is clinically silent in most cases (12).

2. Concern about aspiration around inflated cuffs prompted the introduction of specialized endotracheal tubes equipped with a suction port just above the cuff (Mallinckrodt TaperGuard Evac Tube). The suction port is connected to a source of continuous suction (usually not exceeding -20 cm H_2O) to clear the secretions that accumulate in the subglottic region, as illustrated in Figure 16.1.

3. Clinical studies have shown a significant reduction in the incidence of VAP when subglottic secretions are cleared using these specialized endotracheal tubes (13).

III. CLINICAL FEATURES

A. Diagnostic Accuracy

The traditional clinical criteria for the diagnosis of VAP include: (a) fever or hypothermia, (b) leukocytosis or leukopenia, (c) an increase in volume of respiratory secretions or a change in character of the secretions, and (d) a new or progressive infiltrate on the chest x-ray (4).

1. In cases of VAP diagnosed using traditional clinical criteria, the incidence of pneumonia on postmortem exam is only 30% to 40% (7).

2. The accuracy of clinical criteria for the diagnosis of VAP is demonstrated in Table 16.2. This table shows the results of two studies that used autopsy evidence of pneumonia to evaluate the premortem diagnosis of VAP based on clinical findings (14,15). In both studies, the clinical findings were just as likely to occur in the presence or absence of pneumonia. These studies demonstrate that *the diagnosis of VAP is not possible using clinical criteria alone.*

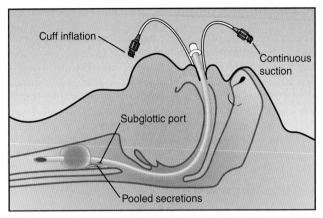

FIGURE 16.1 Endotracheal tube with a suction port placed just above the cuff to clear secretions that accumulate in the subglottic region.

Table 16.2	Predictive Value of Clinical Criteria for Identifying Ventilator-Associated Pneumonia	
Study	**Clinical Criteria**	**Likelihood Ratio for Pneumonia on Autopsy†**
Fagon et al. (14)	Radiographic infiltrate + purulent sputum + fever or leukocytosis	1.03
Timset et al. (15)	Radiographic infiltrate + 2 of the following: fever, leukocytosis, or purulent sputum	0.96

†The likelihood ratio is the likelihood that patients with pneumonia will have the clinical findings compared to the likelihood that patients without pneumonia will have the same clinical findings. A likelihood ratio of 1 indicates that a pneumonia is just as likely to be present or absent based on the clinical findings.

B. Chest Radiography

The performance of portable chest x-rays in detecting pulmonary consolidation is shown in Table 16.3 (16). Note that the poor diagnostic accuracy (49%) is primarily due to a low sensitivity for detecting pulmonary infiltrates. This is demonstrated in Figure 16.2, which shows a portable chest x-ray and CT scan of the lungs in an ICU patient with fever. Note that the chest x-rays shows no apparent infiltrates, while the CT image shows a fine pattern of consolidation in the posterior region of both lungs.

C. Lung Ultrasound

Ultrasound examination of the lungs is a more reliable method for detecting pulmonary consolidation than portable chest x-rays, as demonstrated in Table 16.3. (For a description of the technique involved, see Reference 17.)

Table 16.3	Diagnostic Performance of Portable Chest X-rays and Ultrasound		
	Sensitivity	Specificity	Accuracy
Alveolar Consolidation			
Portable CXR	38%	89%	49%
Ultrasound	100%	78%	95%
Pleural Effusion			
Portable CXR	65%	81%	69%
Ultrasound	100%	100%	100%

Data from Reference 16.

D. Proposed Algorithm

The National Healthcare Safety Network has recently pub-

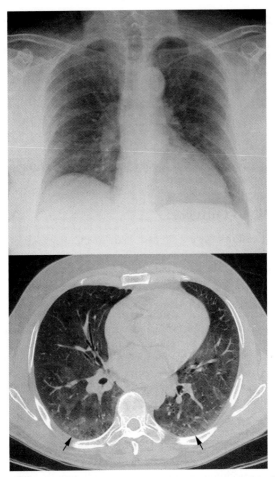

FIGURE 16.2 Demonstration of the limited sensitivity of portable chest radiography in the detection of pulmonary infiltrates. A portable chest x-ray of a patient with fever shows no apparent pulmonary infiltrates, while the CT image from the same patient reveals infiltrates in the posterior region of both lungs (indicated by the arrows).

lished an algorithm for the diagnosis of VAP that does not include findings on a chest x-ray (1). This algorithm is shown in Figure 16.3. Note that the diagnosis of "probable VAP" is not based on clinical criteria, but requires some evidence of a pulmonary infection.

IV. MICROBIOLOGICAL EVALUATION

The diagnosis of VAP rests heavily on identifying a responsible pathogen, and the variety of methods used for this purpose are described next.

A. Blood Cultures

Blood cultures have a limited value in the diagnosis of VAP because they are positive in only 25% of cases (2), and the isolated pathogens are often from extrapulmonary sites of origin (7).

B. Tracheal Aspirates

The traditional approach to suspected VAP involves aspiration of respiratory secretions through an endotracheal or tracheostomy tube. These specimens can be contaminated with mouth secretions that are aspirated into the upper airway, and a screening test (described next) is needed to identify contaminated specimens

1. **Microscopic Analysis**

   a. The presence of more than 10 squamous epithelial cells per low-power field (×100) indicates that the specimen is contaminated with mouth secretions, and is not an appropriate specimen for culture (1).

   b. The presence of neutrophils in tracheal aspirates is not evidence of infection because neutrophils can make up 20% of the cells recovered from a routine mouthwash (18). The neutrophils should be present in abundance to indicate infection; i.e., more than 25 neutrophils per low-power field (×100) can be used as evidence of infection (19).

I. Ventilator-Associated Condition (VAC)

After ≥2 days of stability or improvement on the ventilation, the patient has at least one of the following indications of worsening oxygenation:
1. Increase in daily minimum FiO₂ ≥20% for at least 2 days.
2. Increase in daily minimum PEEP ≥3 cm H₂O for at least 2 days.

⬇

II. Infection-Related Ventilator-Associated Complication (IVAC)

After at least 3 days of mechanical ventilation, and within 2 days of worsening oxygenation, the patient has:
1. Body temperature ≥38° C or <36° OR
2. WBC count ≥12,000/mm³ or ≤4,000/mm³.

⬇

III. Probable Ventilator-Associated Pneumonia

After at least 3 days of mechanical ventilation, and within 2 days of worsening oxygenation, the patient has one of the following:
1. Purulent secretions (≥25 neutrophils and ≤10 squamous cells per low power field AND one of the following:
   a. Positive culture of endotracheal aspirate at 10⁵ CFU/mL.†
   b. Positive culture of broncoalveolar lavage at ≥10⁴ CFU/mL.†
   c. Positive culture of lung tissue at ≥10⁴ CFU/mL.
   d. Positive culture of protected specimen brush at ≥10⁴ CFU/mL.†

2. One of the following (with or without purulent secretions):
   a. Positive pleural fluid culture.
   b. Positive lung histopathology.
   c. Positive diagnostic test for *Legionella* spp.
   d. Positive diagnostic test on respiratory secretions for influenza virus, adenovirus, respiratory syncytial virus, rhinovirus, human metapneumovirus, or coronavirus.

†Excludes the following: (a) normal respiratory flora, (b) *Candida* species or yeast not otherwise specified, (c) coagulase-negative *Staphylococcus* spp., and (d) *Enterococcus* species.

FIGURE 16.3 National Health Safety Network algorithm for the diagnosis of ventilator-associated pneumonia. From Reference 1.

2. **Qualitative Cultures**

The standard culture method for tracheal aspirates provides a qualitative assessment of the presence or absence of organisms.

a. These cultures have a high sensitivity (usually >90%) but a very low specificity (15–40%) for the diagnosis of VAP (20).

b. Thus, *a negative qualitative culture can help to exclude the diagnosis of VAP, but a positive culture is not reliable for detecting the presence of VAP.*

3. **Quantitative Cultures**

a. For quantitative cultures of tracheal aspirates (where growth density is reported), the threshold growth for the diagnosis of VAP is 10^5 colony-forming units per mL (cfu/mL). This threshold has a sensitivity and specificity of about 75% for the diagnosis of VAP (2,20).

b. Comparing the performance of both culture methods for tracheal aspirates (see Table 16.4) indicates that quantitative cultures are more likely to detect the presence of VAP (because of the higher specificity).

C. Bronchoalveolar Lavage

Bronchoalveolar lavage (BAL) is performed by wedging the bronchoscope in a distal airway and performing a lavage with sterile isotonic saline. A minimum lavage volume of 120 mL is recommended for adequate sampling of the lavaged lung segment (21).

1. **Quantitative Cultures**

a. The threshold for a positive BAL culture is 10^4 cfu/mL (1).

b. The reported sensitivity and specificity of BAL cultures are shown in Table 16.4 (2,22). Because BAL cultures have the highest specificity, they are most likely to identify the presence of VAP.

Table 16.4	Culture Methods for the Diagnosis of VAP		
	Tracheal Aspirate		**Bronchoalveolar Lavage**
	Qualitative	**Quantitative**	
Diagnostic Threshold	Any Growth	$\geq 10^5$ cfu/mL	$\geq 10^4$ cfu/mL
Sensitivity	>90%	~75%	~75%
Specificity	<40%	~75%	~80%

From References 2, 20, 22.

2. **Intracellular Organisms**

   a. Inspection of BAL specimens for intracellular organisms can help in guiding initial antibiotic therapy until culture results are available.

   b. *When intracellular organisms are present in more than 3% of the cells in the lavage fluid, the likelihood of pneumonia is over 90%* (23).

   c. This inspection requires special processing and staining, and will require a specific request for the microbiology lab to perform the inspection.

3. **BAL Without Bronchoscopy**

   BAL can also be performed without the aid of bronchoscopy using a sheathed catheter like the one illustrated in Figure 16.4. This catheter (COMBICATH, KOL Bio-Medical, Chantilly, VA) is inserted through a tracheal tube and advanced "blindly" until it wedges in a distal airway. An absorbable polyethylene plug at the tip of the catheter prevents contamination while the catheter is advanced. Once wedged, an inner cannula is advanced for the BAL, which is performed with 20 mL of sterile saline. Only 1 mL of BAL aspirate is required for culture and microscopic analysis.

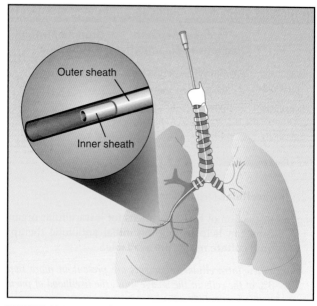

FIGURE 16.4 Protected catheter for performing bronchoalveolar lavage without the aid of bronchoscopy. See text for explanation.

   a. Nonbronchoscopic BAL (also called mini-BAL) is a safe procedure that can be performed by respiratory therapists (24).

   b. Despite the inability to direct the catheter to the region of suspected infection, *the yield from quantitative cultures with mini-BAL is equivalent to the yield with bronchoscopic BAL* (2,25).

V. PARAPNEUMONIC EFFUSIONS

Pleural effusions are present in up to 50% of bacterial pneumonias (26). These *parapneumonic effusions* are more likely to be detected by ultrasound than by portable chest x-rays (see Table 16.3).

A. Thoracentesis

1. Thoracentesis is generally advised for all parapneumonic effusions except small, free-flowing effusions in patients who are not severely ill or are responding to antimicrobial therapy.

2. Ultrasound guidance is advised for aspiration of pleural fluid, especially in ventilator-dependent patients.

3. The following pleural fluid studies are needed to guide decisions regarding drainage of the effusion (27).

   a. Gram stain and culture

   b. pH (measured with a blood gas analyzer)

   c. Glucose concentration (if pH measurement is unavailable)

4. Other pleural fluid studies (e.g., cell count, protein, LDH) are not necessary.

B. Indications for Drainage

The presence of any of the following is an indication for drainage of a parapneumonic effusion (27,28):

1. Effusions that are large (≥ half the hemithorax) or loculated.

2. Purulent pleural aspirate.

3. Presence of organisms on gram stain, or positive culture.

4. Pleural fluid pH <7.2.

5. Pleural fluid glucose <60 mg/dL (if the pH measurement is not available).

C. Drainage

Tube thoracostomy is used for pleural fluid drainage (at least initially). Small-bore chest tubes (10–14 French) are advised, because they are less painful, and they are as effective as large-bore tubes in most cases (28).

1. **Intrapleural Fibrinolysis**

   For loculated pleural effusions or empyema, intrapleural administration of a fibrinolytic agent can facilitate chest tube drainage and reduce the need for surgical drainage (29). The success of intrapleural fibrinolysis has not been consistent, but the following regimen has been shown to facilitate pleural fluid drainage (30):

   a. Administer *tissue plasminogen activator* (5 mg) and *recombinant DNase* (10 mg) via the chest tube twice daily for 3 days, and clamp the chest tube for one hour following each injection. (The DNase is used to break up extracellular DNA, which can increase pleural fluid viscosity.)

   b. Both agents must be used to ensure success (30).

2. **Surgical Drainage**

   Surgical drainage is indicated when other therapies (i.e., antibiotics, chest tube drainage, intrapleural fibrinolysis) fail after 5–7 days (27,28). Video-assisted thoracoscopic surgery (VATS) is preferred because it is minimally invasive, but thoracotomy with pleural decortication is occasionally required.

VI. ANTIMICROBIAL THERAPY

Antimicrobial therapy for pneumonia accounts for half of all antibiotic use in the ICU, and 60% of this antibiotic use is for suspected pneumonias that are not confirmed by bacteriologic studies (31). There is evidence that the mortality rate in VAP is increased by delays in initiating appropriate antibiotic therapy (32), so prompt initiation of empiric antimicrobial therapy is considered essential.

A. Empiric Antibiotic Therapy

1. Empiric antimicrobial therapy for VAP should include coverage for gram-negative aerobic bacilli and *Staphylococcus aureus* (especially methicillin-resistant strains), which are the principal pathogens listed in Table 16.1.

2. Popular regimens include *piperacillin/tazobactam, cefepime*, or a carbapenem (e.g., *meropenem*), plus *vancomycin* (for methicillin-resistant *Staph aureus*). See Chapter 44 for the recommended dosing regimens for these antibiotics.

B. When a Pathogen is Identified

1. When a responsible pathogen is identified, antibiotic therapy will be dictated by the antibiotic susceptibilities of the pathogens at your hospital.

2. One week of antimicrobial therapy is adequate for most cases of VAP, except those caused by non-fermenting gram-negative bacilli (*Pseudomonas aeruginosa* and *Acinetobacter baumannii* account for most of these organisms), in which case 10–15 days of antibiotic therapy is advised (33).

REFERENCES

1. Centers for Disease Control, National Healthcare Safety Network. Device-associated Module: Ventilator-Associated Event Protocol. January, 2013. Available on the National Healthcare Safety Network website (www.cdc.gov/nhsn).

2. American Thoracic Society and Infectious Disease Society of America. Guidelines for the management of adults with hospital-acquired, ventilator-associated, and healthcare-associated pneumonia. Am J Respir Crit Care Med 2005; 171:388–416.

3. Muscedere J, Dodek P, Keenan S, et al. for the VAP Guidelines Committee and the Canadian Critical Care Trials Group.

Comprehensive evidence-based clinical practice guidelines for ventilator-associated pneumonia: Prevention. J Crit Care 2008; 23:126–137.

4. Kollef MH. Ventilator-associated complications, including infection-related complications: The way forward. Crit Care Clin 2013; 29:33–50.

5. Nair GB. Niederman MS. Ventilator-associated pneumonia: present understanding and ongoing debates. Intensive Care Med 2015; 41:34-48.

6. Vincent J-L, Rello J, Marshall J, et al. International study of the prevalence and outcomes of infection in intensive care units. JAMA 2009; 302:2323–2329.

7. Wunderink RG. Clinical criteria in the diagnosis of ventilator-associated pneumonia. Chest 2000; 117:191S–194S.

8. Chastre J, Wolff M, Fagon J-Y, et al. Comparison of 8 vs 15 days of antibiotic therapy for ventilator-associated pneumonia in adults. JAMA 2003; 290:2588–2598.

9. Bregeon F, Cias V, Carret V, et al. Is ventilator-associated pneumonia an independent risk factor for death? Anesthesiology 2001; 94:554–560.

10. Adair CC, Gorman SP, Feron BM, et al. Implications of endotracheal tube biofilm for ventilator-associated pneumonia. Intensive Care Med 1999; 25:1072–1076.

11. AARC Clinical Practice Guideline. Endotracheal suctioning of mechanically ventilated patients with artificial airways 2010. Respir Care 2010; 55:758–764.

12. Elpern EH, Scott MG, Petro L, Ries MH. Pulmonary aspiration in mechanically ventilated patients with tracheostomies. Chest 1994; 105:563–566.

13. Muscedere J, Rewa O, Mckechnie K, et al. Subglottic secretion drainage for the prevention of ventilator-associated pneumonia: a systematic review and meta-analysis. Crit Care Med 2011; 39:1985–1991.

14. Fagon JY, Chastre J, Hance AJ, et al. Detection of nosocomial lung infection in ventilated patients: use of a protected specimen brush and quantitative culture techniques in 147 patients. Am Rev Respir Dis 1988; 138:110–116.

15. Timsit JF. Misset B, Goldstein FW, et al. Reappraisal of distal diagnostic testing in the diagnosis of ICU-acquired pneumonia. Chest 1995; 108:1632–1639.

16. Xirouchaki N, Magkanas E, Vaporidi K, et al. Lung ultrasound in critically ill patients: comparison with bedside chest radiography. Intensive Care Med 2011; 37:1488–1493.

17. Lichtenstein DA, Lascols N, Meziere G, Gepner G. Ultrasound diagnosis of alveolar consolidation in the critically ill. Intensive Care Med 2004; 30:276–281.

18. Rankin JA, Marcy T, Rochester CL, et al. Human airway macrophages. Am Rev Respir Dis 1992; 145:928–933.

19. Wong LK, Barry AL, Horgan S. Comparison of six different criteria for judging the acceptability of sputum specimens. J Clin Microbiol 1982; 16:627–631.

20. Cook D, Mandell L. Endotracheal aspiration in the diagnosis of ventilator-associated pneumonia. Chest 2000; 117:195S–197S.

21. Meduri GU, Chastre J. The standardization of bronchoscopic techniques for ventilator-associated pneumonia. Chest 1992; 102:557S–564S.

22. Torres A, El-Ebiary M. Bronchoscopic BAL in the diagnosis of ventilator-associated pneumonia. Chest 2000; 117:198S–202S.

23. Veber B, Souweine B, Gachot B, et al. Comparison of direct examination of three types of bronchoscopy specimens used to diagnose nosocomial pneumonia. Crit Care Med 2000; 28:962–968.

24. Kollef MH, Bock KR, Richards RD, Hearns ML. The safety and diagnostic accuracy of minibronchoalveolar lavage in patients with suspected ventilator-associated pneumonia. Ann Intern Med 1995; 122:743–748.

25. Campbell CD, Jr. Blinded invasive diagnostic procedures in ventilator-associated pneumonia. Chest 2000; 117:207S–211S.

26. Light RW, Meyer RD, Sahn SA, et al. Parapneumonic effusions and empyema. Clin Chest Med 1985; 6:55–62.

27. Colice GL, Curtis A, Deslauriers J, et al. Medical and surgical treatment of parapneumonic effusions. An evidence-based guideline. Chest 2000; 18:1158–1171.

28. Ferreiro L, San Jose ME, Valdes L. Management of parapneumonic pleural effusion in adults. Arch Bronconeumol 2015; 51:637–646.

29. Cameron R, Davies HR. Intra-pleural fibrinolytic therapy versus conservative management in the treatment of adult parapneu-

monic effusions and empyema. Cochrane Database Syst Rev 2008:CD002312.

30. Rahman NM, Maskell NA, West A, et al. Intrapleural use of tissue plasminogen activator and DNase in pleural infection. N Engl J Med 2011; 365:518–526.

31. Bergmanns DCJJ, Bonten MJM, Gaillard CA, et al. Indications for antibiotic use in ICU patients: a one-year prospective surveillance. J Antimicrob Chemother 1997; 111:676–685.

32. Iregui M, Ward S, Sherman G, et al. Clinical importance of delays in the initiation of appropriate antibiotic treatment for ventilator-associated pneumonia. Chest 2002; 122:262–268.

33. Pugh R, Grant C, Cooke RP, Dempsey G. Short-course versus prolonged-course antibiotic therapy for hospital-acquired pneumonia in critically ill adults. Cochrane Database Syst Rev 2015:CD007577.

Chapter 17

Acute Respiratory Distress Syndrome

The condition described in this chapter, which has the nondescript name *acute respiratory distress syndrome* (ARDS), is a diffuse inflammatory injury of the lungs that is responsible for 10% of ICU admissions and 25% of cases of prolonged mechanical ventilation worldwide (1).

I. FEATURES

A. Pathogenesis

The inciting event in ARDS is activation of circulating neutrophils (as part of the systemic inflammatory response). The activated neutrophils attach to the endothelium in pulmonary capillaries, and subsequently migrate into the lung parenchyma (2). Neutrophil degranulation damages the capillary endothelium, leading to exudation of protein-rich fluid that fills the distal airspaces and impairs pulmonary gas exchange.

B. Predisposing Conditions

1. ARDS is not a primary disorder, but is a consequence of a variety of infectious and noninfectious conditions.

2. The conditions that predispose to ARDS are listed in Table 17.1. The most frequent offenders are pneumonia, extrapulmonary sepsis, and aspiration of gastric secretions (1).

Fewer than 10% of cases have no predisposing condition.

3. The one feature shared by most (but not all) of these conditions is the tendency to trigger a systemic inflammatory response.

Table 17.1	Predisposing Conditions for ARDS
Condition	**Prevalence[1]**
Pneumonia	59.4%
Extrapulmonary Sepsis	16.0%
Aspiration	14.2%
Noncardiogenic Shock	7.5%
Trauma	4.2%
Blood Transfusion	3.9%
Pulmonary Contusion	3.2%
Others[2]	8.6%
No Predisposing Condition	8.3%

[1]From Reference 1, which included 3,022 cases of ARDS from 459 ICUs in 50 countries. The total exceeds 100% because some patients had more than one condition.
[2]Other predisposing conditions include inhalation injury, burns, drug overdose, cardiopulmonary bypass, necrotizing pancreatitis, and intracranial hemorrhage.

C. Clinical Features

The clinical features of ARDS are shown in Table 17.2 (3). The principal features are acute hypoxemic respiratory failure and bilateral, diffuse pulmonary infiltrates that are not explained by left heart failure or volume overload. Most (>90%) cases of ARDS appear within one week of a known predisposing condition, and 80% of cases require mechanical ventilation (1).

Table 17.2	Clinical Features of ARDS[1]
Feature	**Requirements**
Timing	Occurs within one week of a predisposing condition, or one week from symptom onset.
Imaging	Bilateral opacitis (on chest x-ray or CT scan) consistent with alveolar consolidation.
Origin of Edema	No evidence of left heart failure or fluid overload.
Oxygenation[2]	
Mild	$PaO_2/FiO_2 = 201-300$ mm Hg*
Moderate	$PaO_2/FiO_2 = 101-200$ mm Hg
Severe	$PaO_2/FiO_2 \leq 100$ mm Hg
*(PaO_2/FiO_2 measured with PEEP or CPAP ≥ 5 cm H_2O)	

[1]Corresponds to the "Berlin" definition of ARDS, from Reference 3.
[2]For altitudes >1,000 meters, use $PaO_2/FiO_2 \times$ (barometric pressure/760). PaO_2 = arterial PO_2; FiO_2 = fractional concentration of inhaled O_2; PEEP = positive end-expiratory pressure; CPAP = continuous positive airway pressure.

1. **Radiographic Appearance**

   The characteristic appearance of ARDS on a portable chest x-ray is shown in Figure 17.1. The infiltrate has a finely granular or *ground-glass appearance,* and is evenly distributed throughout both lungs. Also note the lack of a prominent pleural effusion, which helps to distinguish ARDS from cardiogenic pulmonary edema.

2. **Oxygenation**

   The impairment in oxygenation in ARDS is assessed using the PaO_2/FiO_2 ratio, measured at a positive end-expiratory pressure (PEEP) of ≥ 5 cm H_2O. (For patients who are not on a ventilator, continuous positive airway pressure, or CPAP, is used instead of PEEP.)

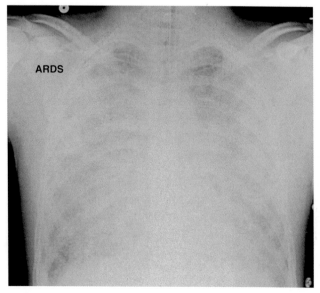

FIGURE 17.1 Portable chest x-ray showing the characteristic appearance of ARDS.

    a. The diagnosis of ARDS requires a PaO_2/FIO_2 ratio <300 mm Hg (with PEEP or CPAP at ≥5 cm H_2O) (3).

    b. Table 17.2 shows a severity of illness classification (mild, moderate, or severe) based on the PaO_2/FIO_2 ratio, which is intended for predicting the likelihood of a fatal outcome. The reported mortality rates for mild, moderate, and severe ARDS are 27%, 32%, and 45% (mean values), respectively (3).

D. Diagnostic Problems

Many clinical features of ARDS are nonspecific, and are shared by other conditions that cause hypoxemic respiratory failure. This creates a tendency for misdiagnosis, as demonstrated by the following observations:

1. In a study of interobserver variability in the radiographic diagnosis of ARDS, a group of 21 experts in ARDS agreed on the diagnosis (ARDS or no ARDS) in only 43% of cases (4).

2. In a large retrospective study designed to identify patients with ARDS based on the clinical criteria in Table 17.2, 40% of the cases of ARDS were not clinically recognized (1).

3. An autopsy study of patients who died with a clinical diagnosis of ARDS showed that only 50% of the patients had postmortem evidence of ARDS (5). This implies that the likelihood of identifying ARDS based on clinical criteria is no greater than the likelihood of predicting heads or tails in a coin toss.

4. **The Wedge Pressure**

   The pulmonary artery occlusion pressure (wedge pressure) has been used to distinguish between ARDS and cardiogenic pulmonary edema; i.e., a wedge pressure ≤18 mm Hg is considered evidence of ARDS (6). This is problematic because the wedge pressure is not a measure of capillary hydrostatic pressure, as explained in Chapter 5, Section II-B. Although the wedge pressure is no longer a required measurement in the diagnosis of ARDS, the limitations of this measurement deserve mention.

II. MECHANICAL VENTILATION

As mentioned earlier, about 80% of patients with ARDS require mechanical ventilation (1). There are two general goals of mechanical ventilation in ARDS: (a) limit the stretch imposed on the distal airspaces during lung inflation, and (b) prevent the distal airspaces from collapsing during lung deflation.

A. Ventilator-Induced Lung Injury

One of the most important discoveries in critical care medicine in the last quarter-century is the role of mechanical ventilation as a *source* of lung injury, particularly in patients with ARDS. This injury is related to excessive stretch of distal air-spaces, as described next.

1. **Inhomogeneity**

   Although portable chest x-rays show an apparent homogeneous pattern of lung infiltration in ARDS, CT images reveal that *the lung infiltration in ARDS is confined to dependent lung regions* (7). This is shown in the CT images in Figure 17.2. Note the dense consolidation in the posterior lung regions (which are the dependent lung regions in the supine position). The uninvolved lung in the anterior portion of the thorax is the functional lung volume, and is the region that receives the inflation volumes from the ventilator.

2. **Volutrauma**

   Because the functional lung volume in ARDS is marked-ly reduced, the usual inflation volumes delivered by mechanical ventilation (10–15 mL/kg) cause *overdistension of alveoli and stress-fractures in the alveolar capillary interface* (8). This volume-related lung injury is known as *volutrauma*.

   a. Volutrauma results in infiltration of the lung with inflammatory cells and proteinaceous material, produc-ing a clinical condition known as *ventilator-induced lung injury* that is strikingly similar to ARDS (8,9).

3. **Atelectrauma**

   The decrease in lung distensibility in ARDS can result in the collapse of small airways at the end of expiration. When this occurs, mechanical ventilation can be associ-ated with cyclic opening and closing of small airways, and this process can be a source of lung injury (10). This type of lung injury is called *atelectrauma* (9), and it may be the result high-velocity shear forces created by the opening of collapsed airways.

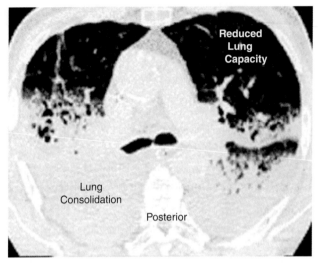

FIGURE 17.2 Computed tomographic images of the lungs in ARDS showing that the consolidation is confined to the posterior lung regions. The uninvolved lung in the anterior one-third of the thorax represents the functional portion of the lung. CT image is from Reference 7 (digitally retouched).

B. Lung Protective Ventilation

Lung protective ventilation employs low tidal volumes (6 mL/kg) to limit the risk of volutrauma, and uses positive end-expiratory pressure (PEEP) to limit the risk of atelectrauma (11).

1. **Protocol**

A protocol for lung protective ventilation has been developed by the ARDS Clinical Network (a network created by the government to evaluate potential therapies for ARDS), and this protocol is shown in Table 17.3. Note that the tidal volume in this protocol (6 mL/kg) is based on the *predicted body weight,* which is the body weight associated with normal lung volumes.

Table 17.3	Protocol for Lung Protective Ventilation

I. FIRST STAGE:

1. Calculate patient's predicted body weight (PBW):

   Males: PBW = 50 + [2.3 x (height in inches − 60)]
   Females: PBW = 45.5 + [2.3 x (height in inches − 60)]

2. Set initial tidal volume (V_T) at 8 mL/kg PBW.

3. Add positive end-expiratory pressure (PEEP) at 5 cm H_2O.

4. Select the lowest FiO_2 that achieves an SpO_2 of 88−95%.

5. Reduce V_T by 1 mL/kg every 2 hrs until V_1 = 6 mL/kg.

II. SECOND STAGE:

1. When V_T = 6 mL/kg measure the end-inspiratory plateau pressure (Ppl).

2. If Ppl >30 cm H_2O, decrease V_T in 1 mL/kg increments until Ppl <30 cm H_2O or V_T = 4 mL/kg.

III. THIRD STAGE:

1. Monitor arterial blood gases for respiratory acidosis.

2. If pH = 7.15−7.30, increase respiratory rate (RR) until pH >7.30 or RR = 35 bpm.

3. If pH <7.15, increase RR to 35 bpm. If pH is still <7.15, increase V_T in 1 mL/kg increments until pH >7.15.

IV. OPTIMAL GOALS:

V_T = 6 mL/kg, Ppl ≤30 cm H_2O, SpO_2 = 88−95%, pH = 7.30−7.45

Adapted from the protocol developed by the ARDS Network, available at www.ardsnet.org.

2. The "Plateau" Pressure

One of the goals of lung protective ventilation is an end-inspiratory "plateau" pressure ≤30 cm H_2O. This pressure is obtained by obstructing the expiratory tubing at the end of inspiration (to hold the tidal volume in the lungs). When this is done, the airway pressure drops to a steady (plateau) level, and because there is no airflow, this pressure is equivalent to the pressure in the alveoli produced by the lung inflation.

a. The plateau pressure is thus a reflection of the alveolar stress produced by positive pressure lung inflations. A plateau pressure >30 cm H_2O can result in alveolar rupture (and ventilator-induced lung injury).

b. The plateau pressure is depicted graphically in Chapter 19, Figure 19.2.

3. **Positive End-Expiratory Pressure**

(For a more detailed description of this pressure, see Chapter 19.) Lung protective ventilation employs a positive end-expiratory pressure (PEEP) of at least 5 cm H_2O to prevent the collapse of small airways at the end of expiration. The goal is to prevent the cyclic opening and closing of small airways (i.e., atelectrauma).

a. PEEP levels are usually kept at 5–7.5 cm H_2O, unless there is an oxygenation problem (see next). The routine use of high PEEP levels does not improve outcomes in ARDS (12).

b. For cases of hypoxemia that require potentially toxic concentrations of inhaled O_2 (FIO_2 >60%), incremental increases in PEEP can help to improve arterial oxygenation and reduce the inhaled O_2 to lower (nontoxic) levels.

c. Increases in PEEP will increase the end-inspiratory plateau (alveolar) pressure, and the maximum "safe" level of PEEP is reached when the plateau pressure reaches 30 cm H_2O.

4. **Permissive Hypercapnia**

One of the potential consequences of low-volume ventilation is a decrease in CO_2 elimination through the lungs, resulting in hypercapnia and respiratory acidosis. This is allowed, as long as there is no evidence of harm (i.e., *permissive hypercapnia*) (13).

a. The limits of tolerance to hypercapnia are unclear, but clinical trials of permissive hypercapnia show that an arterial PCO_2 of 60–70 mm Hg and an arterial pH of 7.2–7.25 are safe for most patients (14).

5. **Impact on Survival**

Lung protective ventilation has been shown to improve survival rates in ARDS (15), although this is not a consistent observation (16). The principal factor that seems to determine the success or failure of this ventilatory method is the ability to keep the end-inspiratory plateau (alveolar) pressure below 30 cm H_2O.

III. OTHER MEASURES

The following measures can influence outcomes in ARDS.

A. Fluid Management

1. Clinical studies have shown that avoiding a positive fluid balance in patients with ARDS can reduce the duration of mechanical ventilation (17), and improve survival rates (18).

2. A simple protocol for fluid management, developed by the ARDS Network, is shown in Table 17.4 (19). This protocol uses the central venous pressure as a reflection of intravascular volume (which is not valid, as shown in Figure 7.1), but it has been effective in achieving a balanced fluid intake and output in patients with ARDS (19).

B. Corticosteroid Therapy

Steroid therapy can be used for the early treatment of moderate-to-severe ARDS, and for unresolving ARDS (20). While there is *no consistent survival benefit* attributed to steroid therapy in ARDS, there are other potential benefits, including a shorter duration of mechanical ventilation, improved gas exchange, and a shorter stay in the ICU (20).

Table 17.4	Protocol for Fluid Management	
Central Venous Pressure (mm Hg)	**Urine Output**	
	<5 mL/kg/hr	**≥5 mL/kg/hr**
>8	Furosemide[†]	Furosemide
4–8	Fluid Bolus	Furosemide
>4	Fluid Bolus	No intervention

Furosemide Dosing:

Begin with 20 mg IV bolus, or 3 mg/hr by infusion, or last known effective dose. Double each subsequent dose, if needed, until goal is achieved. Maximum dose is 160 mg (IV bolus) or 24 mg/hr (IV infusion).

[†]Withhold furosemide when low urine output is associated with renal impairment (serum creatinine >3 mg/dL). From Reference 19.

1. **Moderate-to Severe ARDS**

    The following steroid regimen is recommended for the early treatment of ARDS when the PaO_2/FiO_2 is <200 mm Hg with PEEP of 10 cm H_2O (20).

    a. *Methylprednisolone*: 1 mg/kg (ideal body weight) over 30 minutes, then 1 mg/kg/day by continuous infusion for 14 days, followed by a gradual taper over the next 14 days.

    b. There is no evidence that this regimen increases the risk of infection (20).

2. **Unresolving ARDS**

    ARDS has a fibrinoproliferative phase that begins 7–14

days after the onset of illness, and eventually results in irreversible pulmonary fibrosis (21). High-dose steroid therapy can help to halt the progression to pulmonary fibrosis. When ARDS does not begin to resolve after 7 days, the following steroid regimen is advised (20):

a. *Methylprednisolone:* 2 mg/kg (ideal body weight) over 30 minutes, then 2 mg/kg/day by continuous infusion for 14 days, then 1 mg/kg/day (continuous infusion) for the next 7 days, followed by a gradual taper that ends 2 weeks after extubation.

b. There is no evidence that this regimen increases the risk of infection (20).

C. Prone Positioning

Prone positioning (usually for 12–18 hrs daily) has advantages in patients with severe or refractory hypoxemia.

1. This maneuver improves arterial oxygenation (by increasing blood flow to anterior, better aerated lung regions) and reduces the risk of ventilator-induced lung injury (because lung inflation is more homogeneous) (22).

2. Prone positioning can improve survival if started early (within 48 hrs) in patients with severe hypoxemia (PaO_2/FiO_2 <100 mm Hg with PEEP ≥5 cm H_2O) (23). Prolonged periods of "proning" (≥16 hrs daily) can also have a survival benefit (23).

3. Unstable spine fractures are an absolute contraindication to prone positioning (24). Relative contraindications include pelvic fractures, recent facial trauma or facial surgery, intracranial hypertension, hemodynamic instability, and massive hemoptysis (24).

4. The most noted complications are pressure sores and obstruction of tracheal tubes (23).

D. Things That Don't Work

There is a long list of failed therapies for ARDS, including intratracheal surfactant (in adults), inhaled nitric oxide, intravenous N-acetylcysteine, ibuprofen, prostaglandin E infusions, atrial natriuretic peptide, monoclonal anti-endo-toxin antibodies, neutrophil elastase inhibitors, and immune-modulating feeding formulas (25).

IV. REFRACTORY HYPOXEMIA

About 10 to 15% of patients with ARDS develop severe hypoxemia that is refractory to oxygen therapy and conventional mechanical ventilation (26). Refractory hypoxemia is an immediate threat to life, and the following "rescue therapies" can be used to improve arterial oxygenation.

A. Incremental PEEP

Increases in PEEP to levels above those used for lung protective ventilation can re-expand collapsed alveoli (alveolar recruitment), and thereby improve arterial oxygenation.

1. Using low-volume ventilation (6 mL/kg predicted body weight), PEEP can be increased in increments of 3–5 cm H_2O until the end-inspiratory plateau pressure reaches 30 cm H_2O (the threshold for ventilator-induced lung injury) (27). This method promotes alveolar recruitment and improves arterial oxygenation while limiting the risk of ventilator-induced lung injury.

2. The disadvantage of increased PEEP is the risk for impaired venous return and a subsequent decline in cardiac output. If the blood pressure begins to drop as PEEP is increased, volume infusions will be needed to preserve cardiac filling.

B. Airway Pressure Release Ventilation

1. Airway pressure release ventilation (APRV) involves prolonged periods of spontaneous breathing at relatively high airway pressures (to open collapsed alveoli), interspersed with brief periods of rapid lung deflation (to facilitate CO_2 removal) (28).

2. Because APRV involves spontaneous breathing, high-level continuous positive airway pressure (CPAP) is used instead of PEEP.

3. APRV improves arterial oxygenation gradually, over 24 hours (28), but there is no survival benefit (25).

4. This mode of ventilation is described in detail in Chapter 20.

C. High Frequency Oscillations

1. High frequency oscillatory ventilation (HFOV) delivers small tidal volumes (1–2 mL/kg) using rapid pressure oscillations (300 cycles/min). The small tidal volumes limit the risk of volutrauma, and the rapid pressure oscillations create a mean airway pressure that prevents small airway collapse and thus prevents atelectrauma (29).

2. Like APRV, HFOV often improves arterial oxygenation, but there is no documented survival benefit (25).

3. HFOV is described in detail in Chapter 20.

D. Extracorporeal Membrane Oxygenation

1. Extracorporeal membrane oxygenation (ECMO) is a mode of respiratory support where venous blood is pumped through a membrane oxygenator and returned to the venous system (venovenous ECMO). The membrane oxygenator serves as an adjunct (rather than

replacement) for mechanical ventilation, and ventilation of the lungs is achieved at lower airway pressures to reduce the risk of ventilator-induced lung injury (30).

2. ECMO has rapidly gained in popularity in recent years, but randomized studies evaluating the survival benefit of ECMO have been inconclusive (31).

REFERENCES

1. Bellani G, Laffey JG, Pham T, et al. Epidemiology, patterns of care, and mortality for patients with acute respiratory distress syndrome in intensive care units in 50 countries. JAMA 2016; 315:788–800.

2. Abraham E. Neutrophils and acute lung injury. Crit Care Med 2003; 31(Suppl):S195–S199.

3. The ARDS Definition Task Force. Acute respiratory distress syndrome. The Berlin definition. JAMA 2012; 307:2526–2533.

4. Rubenfeld GD, Caldwell E, Granton J, et al. Interobserver variability in applying a radiographic definition for ARDS. Chest 1999; 116:1347–1353.

5. de Hemptinne Q, Remmelink M, Brimioulle S, et al. ARDS: a clinicopathological confrontation. Chest 2009; 135:944–949.

6. Bernard GR, Artigas A, Brigham KL, et al. The American–European Consensus Conference on ARDS: definitions, mechanisms, relevant outcomes, and clinical trial coordination. Am Rev Respir Crit Care Med 1994; 149:818–824.

7. Rouby J-J, Puybasset L, Nieszkowska A, Lu Q. Acute respiratory distress syndrome: Lessons from computed tomography of the whole lung. Crit Care Med 2003; 31(Suppl):S285–S295.

8. Dreyfuss D, Saumon G. Ventilator-induced lung injury: lessons from experimental studies. Am J Respir Crit Care Med 1998; 157:294–323.

9. Gattinoni L, Protti A, Caironi P, Carlesso E. Ventilator-induced lung injury: the anatomical and physiological framework. Crit Care Med 2010; 38(Suppl):S539–S548.

10. Muscedere JG, Mullen JBM, Gan K, et al. Tidal ventilation at low airway pressures can augment lung injury. Am J Respir Crit Care Med 1994; 149:1327–1334.

11. Brower RG, Rubenfeld GD. Lung-protective ventilation strategies in acute lung injury. Crit Care Med 2003; 31(Suppl):S312–S316.

12. Santa Cruz R, Rojas J, Nervi R, et al. High versus low positive end-expiratory pressure (PEEP) levels for mechanically ventilated adult patients with acute lung injury and acute respiratory distress syndrome. Cochrane Database Syst Rev 2013: CD009098.

13. Bidani A, Tzouanakis AE, Cardenas VJ, Zwischenberger JB. Permissive hypercapnia in acute respiratory failure. JAMA 1994; 272:957–962.

14. Hickling KG, Walsh J, Henderson S, et al. Low mortality rate in adult respiratory distress syndrome using low-volume, pressure-limited ventilation with permissive hypercapnia: A prospective study. Crit Care Med 1994; 22:1568–1578.

15. The Acute Respiratory Distress Syndrome Network. Ventilation with lower tidal volumes as compared with traditional tidal volumes for acute lung injury and the acute respiratory distress syndrome. New Engl J Med 2000; 342:1301–1308.

16. Fan E, Needham DM, Stewart TE. Ventilator management of acute lung injury and acute respiratory distress syndrome. JAMA 2005; 294:2889–2896.

17. The Acute Respiratory Distress Syndrome Network. Comparison of two fluid management strategies in acute lung injury. N Engl J Med 2006; 354:2564–2575.

18. Murphy CV, Schramm GE, Doherty JA, et al. The importance of fluid management in acute lung injury secondary to septic shock. Chest 2009; 136:102–109.

19. Grissom CK, Hirshberg EL, Dickerson JB, et al. Fluid management with a simplified conservative protocol for the acute respiratory distress syndrome. Crit Care Med 2015; 43:288–295.

20. Marik PE, Meduri GU, Rocco PRM, Annane D. Glucocorticoid treatment in acute lung injury and acute respiratory distress syndrome. Crit Care Clin 2011; 27:589–607.

21. Meduri GU, Chinn A. Fibroproliferation in late adult respiratory distress syndrome. Chest 1994; 105(Suppl):127S–129S.

22. Guerin C, Baboi L, Richard JC. Mechanisms of the effects of prone positioning in acute respiratory distress syndrome. Intensive Care Med 2014; 40:16344–1642.

23. Bloomfield R, Noble DW, Sudlow A. Prone position for acute respiratory failure in adults. Cochrane Database Syst Rev 2015; 11:CD008095.

24. Berin T, Grasso S, Moerer O, et al. The standard of care of patients with ARDS: ventilatory settings and rescue therapies for refractory hypoxemia. Intensive Care Med 2016; 42:699–711.

25. Tonelli AR, Zein J, Adams J, Ioannidis JPA. Effects of interventions on survival in acute respiratory distress syndrome: an umbrella review of 159 published randomized trials and 29 meta-analyses. Intensive Care Med 2014; 40:769–787.

26. Pipeling MR, Fan E. Therapies for refractory hypoxemia in acute respiratory distress syndrome. JAMA 2010; 304:2521–2527.

27. Mercat A, Richard J-C, Vielle B, et al. Positive end-expiratory pressure setting in adults with acute lung injury and acute respiratory distress syndrome. JAMA 2008; 299:646–655.

28. Kallet RH. Patient-ventilator interaction during acute lung injury, and the role of spontaneous breathing: Part 2: airway pressure release ventilation. Respir Care 2011; 56:190–206.

29. Facchin F, Fan E. Airway pressure release ventilation and high-frequency oscillatory ventilation: potential strategies to treat severe hypoxemia and prevent ventilator-induced lung injury. Respir Care 2015; 60:1509–1521.

30. Ventetuolo CE, Muratore CS. Extracorporeal life support in critically ill adults. Am Rev Respir Crit Care Med 2014; 190:497–508.

31. Tramm R, Ilic D, Davies AR, et al. Extracorporeal membrane oxygenation for critically ill adults. Cochrane Database Syst Rev 2015; 1:CD010381.

Chapter 18

Asthma and COPD in the ICU

This chapter describes the management of acute exacerbations of asthma and chronic obstructive pulmonary disease (COPD), including the use of noninvasive and invasive ventilatory assistance. The recommendations in this chapter are drawn from clinical practice guidelines and pertinent reviews (1-3).

I. ACUTE ASTHMA

The flow diagram in Figure 18.1 shows the recommendations of the National Asthma Education Program for the initial management of adults with acute exacerbations of asthma (1). This protocol uses objective measures of airway obstruction (FEV_1 and peak expiratory flow rate) to determine disease severity, but these measures are difficult to obtain in acutely ill patients, so clinical assessment of disease severity is used to guide management (2,3). The drugs and dosing regimens used for acute asthma are shown in Table 18.1.

A. Short-Acting β_2 Agonists

Short-acting β_2-receptor agonists are the preferred bronchodilators for acute exacerbations of asthma, and are given as an inhaled aerosol, which is more effective than parenteral drug therapy, and has fewer side effects (4). Bronchodilator effects are usually apparent in 2–3 minutes, reach a peak at 30 minutes, and last for 2–5 hours (5).

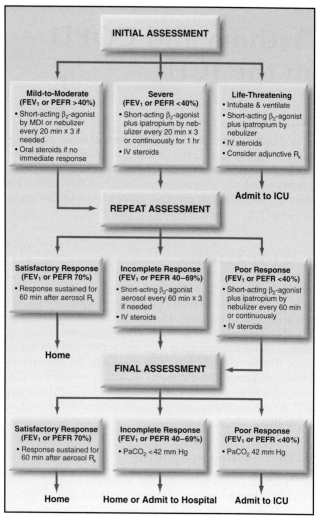

FIGURE 18.1 Flow diagram for the management of acute exacerbations of asthma. From the National Asthma Education Program (1). FEV$_1$ = forced expiratory volume in one second, PEFR = peak expiratory flow rate.

Table 18.1	Inhaled Bronchodilator Therapy in Acute Asthma
Drug	**Dosing Regimens**
Albuterol	Neb: 2.5–5 mg every 20 min for 3 doses, or 10–15 mg by continuous inhalation for 1 hr, then 2.5–10 mg every 1–4 hr as needed.
	MDI: 4–8 puffs (90 μg/puff) every 20 min up to 4 hr, then every 1–4 hr as needed. Use a holding chamber for inhalations.
Levalbuterol	Neb: Same regimen for intermittent dosing as albuterol, but at half the dose. Has not been evaluated for continuous inhalation.
	MDI: Same dosing regimen as albuterol (45 μg/puff).
Ipatropium	Neb: 0.5 mg every 20 min for 3 doses (can be added to albuterol or levalbuterol neb solution), then as needed.
	MDI: 8 puffs (18 μg/puff) every 20 min, as needed, for up to 3 hr. Use a holding chamber for inhalations.
Ipatropium with albuterol	Neb: 3 mL (0.5 mg ipatropium + 2.5 mg albuterol) every 20 min for 3 doses, then as needed.
	MDI: 8 puffs (18 μg ipatropium + 90 μg albuterol per puff) every 20 min, as needed, for up to 3 hr. Use holding chamber.

From Reference 1. Neb = nebulizer; MDI = metered dose inhaler.

1. The most widely used drug in this class is *albuterol,* which is a racemic mixture of two isomers, only one being active. *Levalbuterol* is the active isomer in albuterol, and was introduced as a more powerful bronchodilator than albuterol. However, clinical studies have shown no advantages with levalbuterol in acute asthma (6).

2. The dosing regimens for albuterol are shown in Table 18.1. Treatment usually begins with a series of 3 consecutive aerosol treatments at 20 minute intervals, and nebulizers are preferred to MDIs for moderate-to-severe airflow obstruction (1).

3. Albuterol can also be given as a continuous aerosol using a large-volume nebulizer and a dose of 10–15 mg for the first hour (1). This method has become popular, and is more effective than intermittent aerosol therapy for severe airflow obstruction (7).

4. When the acute episode begins to resolve, albuterol is given by intermittent aerosol treatments every 4–6 hours for the duration of the hospital stay.

5. Adverse effects of high-dose aerosol therapy with β_2-agonists include tachycardia, fine tremors, hyperglycemia, and electrolyte "hypos" (i.e., hypokalemia, hypomagnesemia, and hypophosphatemia) (8,9). Albuterol may also be responsible for the increase in serum lactate levels that are observed during acute exacerbations of asthma (10).

B. Anticholinergic Aerosols

1. Anticholinergic aerosols offer only marginal benefits in acute asthma, and their use is restricted to combination therapy with short-acting β_2-agonists for the first 3–4 hours of treatment in patients with moderate-to-severe airflow obstruction (1,11).

2. The only anticholinergic agent approved for use in asthma in the United States is *ipatropium bromide*, a derivative of atropine that blocks muscarinic receptors in the airways.

3. The dosing regimen for aerosolized ipatropium is shown in Table 18.1. Ipatropium can be mixed with albuterol for nebulizer treatments, and a premixed

preparation of albuterol and ipatropium is commercially available for nebulizers and MDIs (see Table 18.1).

4. Systemic absorption of ipatropium is minimal, and there is little risk of anticholinergic side effects (e.g., tachycardia, dry mouth, blurred vision, urinary retention).

5. Ipatropium has no proven benefit beyond the first few hours of treatment, and it *should not be used for daily maintenance therapy in asthma* (1).

C. Aerosol Intolerance

For the occasional patient that does not tolerate bronchodilator aerosols (usually because of excessive coughing), consider one of the following regimens (1):

1. *Epinephrine:* 0.3–0.5 mg subcutaneously every 20 minutes for 3 doses.

2. *Terbutaline:* 0.25 mg subcutaneously every 20 minutes for 3 doses.

3. Following the initial bronchodilator response, patients are more likely to tolerate aerosol treatments.

D. Corticosteroids

Systemic therapy with corticosteroids can accelerate the rate of improvement and reduce the risk of relapses (12), although *not all studies show a benefit from corticosteroids in acute asthma* (13,14).

1. **Relevant Observations**

   The following observations about steroid therapy in acute asthma deserve mention:

   a. There is no difference in efficacy between oral and intravenous steroids (12,15).

   b. The beneficial effects of steroids are often not apparent until 12 hours after therapy is started (19), and thus steroid therapy will not influence the clinical course of asthma in the emergency department.

c. There is no dose-response relationship for steroids in acute asthma (i.e., no evidence that larger steroid doses produce greater responses) (15).

d. A 10-day course of steroids can be stopped abruptly, without a tapering dose (12,16).

2. **Recommendations**

The recommendations for systemic steroid therapy in acute asthma are summarized in Table 18.2 (1). Inhaled corticosteroids can be added when the acute episode begins to resolve, and should continue for at least a few weeks after resolution to prevent relapses (3).

Table 18.2	Recommendations for Steroid Therapy

Acute Exacerbation of Asthma[1]

Indication:	Unsatisfactory bronchodilator response after 1 hr.
Route:	Oral route preferred.
Dose:	40–80 mg daily, in 1 or 2 divided doses, using prednisone (for PO) or methylprednisolone (for IV).
Duration:	Continue until resolution of signs and symptoms. No taper necessary if duration < 10 days.

Acute Exacerbation of COPD[2]

Indication:	Admission to hospital.
Route:	Oral route preferred.
Dose:	30–40 mg daily, in 1 or 2 divided doses, using prednisone (for PO) or methylprednisolone (for IV).
Duration:	Continue for 7–10 days. No taper necessary.

[1]From Reference 1. [2]From Reference 19.

E. Other Considerations

The following measures can be added to bronchodilator therapy, especially when the response to bronchodilators after one hour has not been satisfactory.

1. MAGNESIUM: Intravenous magnesium has mild bronchodilator effects (as "nature's calcium channel blocker"), and magnesium sulfate in a dose of 2 grams IV over 15–30 min has been shown to improve lung function and reduce hospital admissions in patients who respond poorly to initial bronchodilator therapy (17).

2. ANTIBIOTICS: Asthma exacerbations are often triggered by viral upper respiratory tract infections, and antibiotic therapy is *not advised unless there is evidence of a treatable infection* (1,3).

3. ABGs: Arterial blood gas analysis is advised for patients who show little or no clinical improvement after one hour of aggressive bronchodilator therapy. A normal PCO_2 in acute asthma is evidence of respiratory failure (because the minute ventilation is high, which should lower the arterial PCO_2), and hypercapnia is a sign that ventilatory assistance may be necessary.

F. Noninvasive Ventilation

1. For patients with hypercapnia after aggressive bronchodilator therapy, noninvasive ventilation (NIV) can be effective in correcting the hypercapnia and avoiding intubation and mechanical ventilation (18).

2. See Chapter 20, Section II for more information on NIV.

III. ACUTE EXACERBATION OF COPD

An acute exacerbation of COPD is described as "a change in the patient's baseline dyspnea, cough, or sputum production that is beyond the normal day-to-day variation" (23). Most cases are triggered by a lung infection (usually confined to the airways), and about 30% of cases have no apparent trigger (19).

A. Bronchodilator Therapy

1. Bronchodilator therapy for acute exacerbations of COPD involves the same aerosolized drugs used for acute asthma, but with different dosing regimens (see Table 18.3), and different expectations (i.e., unlike asthma, COPD is characterized by poor bronchodilator responsiveness, so bronchodilator therapy has much less influence on outcomes in COPD).

2. Ipatropium is used as combination therapy when the response to short-acting β_2-agonists is less than satisfactory (which is usually the case in COPD), although at least three clinical studies do not support this practice (20).

Table 18.3	Inhaled Bronchodilator Therapy for Exacerbation of COPD
Drug	**Dosing Regimens**
Albuterol	Neb: 2.5–5 mg every 4–6 hr.
	MDI: 2–8 puffs (90 μg/puff) every 4–6 hr.
Levalbuterol	Neb: 1.25–2.5 mg every 4–6 hr.
	MDI: 2–8 puffs (45 μg/puff) every 4–6 hr.
Ipatropium	Neb: 0.5 mg every 4–6 hr.
	MDI: 2–8 puffs (18 μg/puff) every 4–6 hr.
Ipatropium with albuterol	Neb: 3 mL (0.5 mg ipatropium + 3 mg albuterol) every 4–6 hr.
	MDI: 2–8 puffs (18 μg ipatropium + 90 μg albuterol per puff) every 4–6 hr.

From Reference 19. Neb = nebulizer; MDI = metered dose inhaler.

B. Corticosteroids

A brief course of corticosteroid therapy is recommended for all hospital admissions with acute exacerbation of COPD, and the recommended regimen is shown in Table 18.2 (19). Steroids have had limited success in exacerbations of COPD, and *at least 10 patients must be treated with steroids to produce one favorable response* (20).

C. Antibiotic Therapy

Bacterial pathogens are responsible for about half of the airway infections in acute exacerbations of COPD (2).

1. INDICATIONS: Clinical practice guidelines recommend antibiotics when either of the following conditions is satisfied (19):

   a. Increased volume and purulence of sputum.

   b. Noninvasive or mechanical ventilation.

2. ANTIBIOTICS: Gram-negative aerobic bacilli and *Strep pneumoniae* are the most frequent isolates in the sputum of hospitalized patients with COPD (21), and *Pseudomonas aeruginosa* can be prominent in ventilator-dependent patients (22). *Levofloxacin* should provide adequate coverage in non-ventilated patients, while *cefepime* or *piperacillin-tazobactam* are appropriate in ventilated patients. The duration of antibiotic therapy is typically 5–7 days.

D. Oxygen Therapy

1. In cases of severe COPD with chronic hypercapnia, high concentrations of inhaled O_2 can promote further increases in arterial PCO_2. This is not due to a decrease in ventilatory drive (23), as believed, but may be from CO_2 unloading by hemoglobin.

2. The best practice in this situation is to use the lowest FIO_2 (fractional concentration of inhaled O_2) that achieves an O_2 saturation by pulse oximetry (SpO_2) of 88–90%.

3. Monitor the mental status closely after initiating O_2 therapy, because a decrease in consciousness most likely signals progressive hypercapnia (CO_2 narcosis), and mandates immediate intubation and mechanical ventilation.

E. Noninvasive Ventilation

1. Noninvasive ventilation (NIV) has been successful in avoiding intubation in about 75% of patients with hypercapnic respiratory failure from COPD exacerbations (see Table 20.1) (24).

2. See Chapter 20, Section II for more information on NIV.

IV. MECHANICAL VENTILATION

Mechanical ventilation is required in fewer than 5% of hospitalized patients with acute asthma (25), but in more than 50% of patients with exacerbation of COPD (26). The following are some of the major considerations regarding positive pressure ventilation in these patients.

A. Dynamic Hyperinflation

1. In normal subjects, exhalation is completed before the end of expiration, and the end-expiratory pressure in the alveoli is equivalent to atmospheric (zero reference) pressure. This is illustrated in the lower pressure-volume loop in Figure 18.2.

2. In patients with severe airway obstruction from asthma or COPD, exhalation is prolonged, and is not completed before the next inhalation. This results in hyperinflation

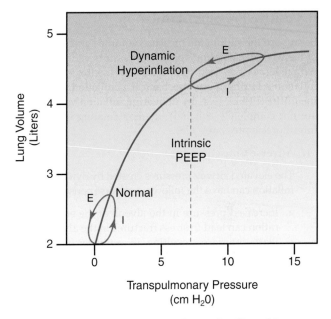

FIGURE 18.2 Pressure-volume curves showing the effects of dynamic hyperinflation. The hysteresis loops show the pressure and volume changes for a single breath. I = inspiration, E = expiration. See text for further explanation.

(called *dynamic hyperinflation*), and the trapped gas in the alveoli creates a positive end-expiratory pressure (PEEP), which is called *intrinsic PEEP* (27). This is illustrated by the upper pressure-volume loop in Figure 18.2

3. Note that, in the presence of intrinsic PEEP, the respiratory muscles must generate higher transpulmonary pressures to inflate the lungs (partly to overcome intrinsic PEEP, and partly because breathing occurs on a flat portion of the pressure-volume curve). This increases the work of breathing.

B. Positive Pressure Ventilation

Because of the shift in the pressure-volume curves caused by dynamic hyperinflation, positive-pressure ventilation will will generate increased intrathoracic pressures during lung inflation. Furthermore, mechanical ventilation can add to the intrinsic PEEP (e.g., by delivering inflation volumes that are not completely exhaled), thereby creating even higher intrathoracic pressures (28).

1. **Adverse Consequences**

   The elevated airway pressures created by dynamic hyper-inflation can have the following adverse consequences:

   a. Increased pressure in the alveoli at the end of inspiration can lead to stress fractures in the alveolar–capillary interface, resulting in *ventilator-induced lung injury* (described in Chapter 17, Section II-A).

   b. Increased alveolar pressure can also cause rupture of alveoli, with escape of air into the lung parenchyma or pleural space (i.e., *barotrauma*).

   c. Increased mean intrathoracic pressure can reduce cardiac output by increasing right ventricular afterload and decreasing right ventricular filling.

C. Monitoring

1. **Dynamic Hyperinflation**

   The presence of dynamic hyperinflation can be detected by monitoring the expiratory airflow during mechanical ventilation. This is illustrated in Figure 18.3. The normal flow waveforms in the upper panel show that the expiratory flow ceases before the next lung inflation, while the flow waveforms in the lower panel show that expiratory flow is continuing when the next lung inflation is delivered. *The presence of expiratory flow at the end of expiration is evidence of dynamic hyperinflation.*

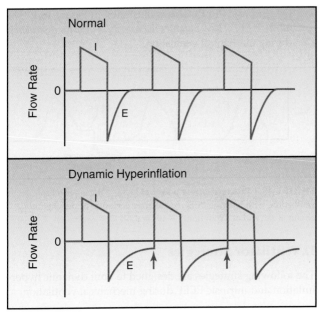

FIGURE 18.3 Flow waveforms during mechanical ventilation. The waveforms in the lower panel show that expiratory flow has not returned to zero at the end of expiration (indicated by the arrows), which indicates the presence of dynamic hyperinflation. I = inspiration, E = expiration.

2. **Intrinsic PEEP**

When there is evidence of dynamic hyperinflation on the flow waveforms, the severity of the problem can be evaluated by measuring the intrinsic PEEP level. Intrinsic PEEP is not evident in the proximal airway pressure (the pressure monitored by ventilators) because of the pressure drop along the airways at end-expiration. However, intrinsic PEEP can be revealed by occluding the expiratory tubing at the end of expiration. This creates a static column of air along the airways, and the proximal airway pressure is then equivalent to the alveolar pressure at end-expiration (i.e., intrinsic PEEP). This is illustrated in Figure 18.4. *The intrinsic PEEP level indicates the severity of airways obstruction* during mechanical ventilation.

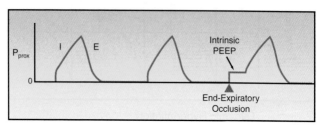

FIGURE 18.4 Proximal airway pressures (P_{prox}) during mechanical ventilation, with intrinsic PEEP revealed by occlusion of the expiratory circuit at the end of expiration. I = inspiration, E = expiration.

D. Ventilator Strategies

The following strategies are designed to limit dynamic hyperinflation and intrinsic PEEP during mechanical ventilation.

1. Ventilate with low tidal volumes (6 mL/kg predicted bogy weight) using the *lung protective ventilation* protocol described in Chapter 17, Section II-B (see Table 17.3).

2. Maximize the time for exhalation with the following measures:

   a. Avoid rapid respiratory rates (with sedation, if possible, or temporary neuromuscular paralysis, if absolutely necessary).

   b. Increase the inspiratory flow rate, if necessary, so that lung inflation accounts for only one-third of the respiratory cycle (i.e., I:E ratio of 1:2).

REFERENCES

1. National Asthma Education and Prevention Program Expert Panel Report 3: Guidelines for the diagnosis and management of

asthma. Full Report 2007. NIH Publication No. 07-4051; August, 2007. (Available at www.nhlbi.nih.gov/guidelines/asthma)

2. Suau SJ, DeBlieux PMC. Management of acute exacerbation of asthma and chronic obstructive pulmonary disease in the emergency department. Emerg Med Clin N Am 2016; 34:15–37.

3. Lazarus SC. Emergency treatment of asthma. N Engl J Med 2010; 363: 755–764.

4. Salmeron S, Brochard L. Mal H, et al. Nebulized versus intravenous albuterol in hypercapnic acute asthma. Am J Respir Crit Care Med 1994; 149:1466–1470.

5. Dutta EJ, Li JTC. β-agonists. Med Clin N Am 2002; 86:991–1008.

6. Jat KR, Khairwa A. Levalbuterol versus albuterol for acute asthma: A systematic review and meta-analysis. Pulm Pharmacol Ther 2013; 26:239–248.

7. Peters SG. Continuous bronchodilator therapy. Chest 2007; 131:286–289.

8. Truwit JD. Toxic effect of bronchodilators. Crit Care Clin 1991; 7:639–657.

9. Bodenhamer J, Bergstrom R, Brown D, et al. Frequently nebulized beta-agonists for asthma: effects on serum electrolytes. Ann Emerg Med 1992; 21:1337–1342.

10. Lewis LM, Ferguson I, House SL, et al. Albuterol administration is commonly associated with increases in serum lactate in patients with asthma treated for acute exacerbation of asthma. Chest 2014; 145:53–59.

11. Rodrigo G, Rodrigo C. The role of anticholinergics in acute asthma treatment. An evidence-based evaluation. Chest 2002; 121:1977–1987.

12. Krishnan JA, Davis SQ, Naureckas ET, et al. An umbrella review: corticosteroid therapy for adults with acute asthma. Am J Med 2009; 122:977–991.

13. Stein LM, Cole RP. Early administration of corticosteroids in emergency room treatment of asthma. Ann Intern Med 1990; 112:822–827.

14. Morrell F, Orriols R, de Gracia J, et al. Controlled trial of intravenous corticosteroids in severe acute asthma. Thorax 1992; 47:588–591.

15. Rodrigo G, Rodrigo C. Corticosteroids in the emergency department therapy of acute adult asthma. An evidence-based evaluation. Chest 1999; 116:285–295.

16. Cydulka RK, Emerman CL. A pilot study of steroid therapy after

emergency department treatment of acute asthma: Is a taper needed? J Emerg Med 1998; 16:15–19.

17. Kew KM, Kirtchik L, Mitchell CI. Intravenous magnesium sulfate for treating adults with acute asthma in the emergency department. Cochrane Database Syst Rev 2014; 5:CD010909.

18. Murase K, Tomii K, Chin K, et al. The use of non-invasive ventilation for life-threatening asthma attacks. Respirology 2010; 15:714–720.

19. Rabe KF, Hurd S, Anzueto A, et al. Global strategy for the diagnosis, management, and prevention of chronic obstructive pulmonary disease. The GOLD executive summary. Am J Respir Crit Care Med 2007; 176:532–555.

20. Walters JAE, Gibson PG, Wood-Baker R, et al. Systemic corticosteroids for acute exacerbations of chronic obstructive pulmonary disease. Cochrane Database of Systematic Reviews, 2009; 1:CD001288.

21. Stolz D, Christ-Crain M, Bingisser R, et al. Antibiotic treatment of exacerbations of COPD. A randomized-controlled trial comparing procalcitonin-guidance with standard therapy.

22. Murphy TF. *Pseudomonas aeruginosa* in adults with chronic obstructive pulmonary disease. Curr Opin Pulm Med 2009; 15:138–142.

23. Aubier M, Murciano D, Fournier M, et al. Central respiratory drive in acute respiratory failure of patients with chronic obstructive pulmonary disease. Am Rev Respir Dis 1980; 122:191–199.

24. Boldrini R, Fasano L, Nava S. Noninvasive mechanical ventilation. Curr Opin Crit Care 2012; 18:48–53.

25. Leatherman J. Mechanical ventilation for severe asthma. Chest 2015; 147:1671–1680.

26. Soo Hoo GW, Hakimian N, Santiago SM. Hypercapnic respiratory failure in COPD patients response to therapy. Chest 2000; 117:169–177.

27. Blanch L, Bernabe F, Lucangelo U. Measurement of air trapping, intrinsic positive end-expiratory pressure, and dynamic hyperinflation in mechanically ventilated patients. Respir Care 2005; 50:110–123.

28. Pepe P, Marini JJ. Occult positive end-expiratory pressure in mechanically ventilated patients with airflow obstruction. The auto-PEEP effect. Am Rev Respir Dis 1982; 126:166–170.

Chapter 19

Conventional Mechanical Ventilation

There are 174 methods of positive pressure ventilation (1), yet in the 50-plus years since positive pressure ventilation was introduced, the only method that has improved clinical outcomes is low-volume *lung protective ventilation* (see later), which uses less than traditional levels of ventilatory support (2). What this means is that positive pressure ventilation is much more complicated than it needs to be, and "less is better" (3).

This chapter describes six basic methods of positive pressure ventilation (volume control, pressure control, pressure-support, assist-control, intermittent mandatory ventilation, and positive end-expiratory pressure). These six methods should be sufficient for providing ventilatory support in a majority of patients.

I. METHODS OF LUNG INFLATION

A. Volume vs. Pressure Control

There are two basic modes of mechanical ventilation, based on the method used to inflate the lungs. These two methods are depicted in Figure 19.1.

1. With *volume control ventilation* (VCV), the inflation (tidal) volume is preselected, and the lungs are inflated at a constant flow rate until the desired volume is delivered. The inspiratory flow rate is adjusted so that the

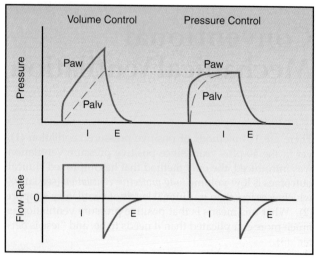

FIGURE 19.1 Pressure and flow changes during a single ventilator breath with volume control and pressure control methods of lung inflation, at equivalent inflation (tidal) volumes. Changes in airway pressure (Paw) indicated by the solid lines, and changes in alveolar pressure (Palv) indicated by the dashed lines. I = inspiration, E = expiration.

time for lung inflation is no more than one-third of the respiratory cycle (i.e., I:E ratio of 1:2).

2. With *pressure control ventilation* (PCV), the inflation pressure is preselected, and high flow rates are used at the onset of lung inflation to achieve the desired inflation pressure quickly. The flow rate decelerates during lung inflation, and the inspiratory time is adjusted to allow the flow rate to fall to zero at the end of inspiration.

B. Airway Pressures

Note in Figure 19.1 that the airway pressure (Paw) at the end of inspiration is higher with volume control, but the alveolar pressure (Palv) at end-inspiration is the same with both methods of lung inflation. This is explained below.

1. With VCV, the airway pressure at the end of inspiration (peak pressure) is the pressure needed to overcome both airway resistance, and the elastic recoil force of the lungs and chest wall. These two components can be separated by briefly holding the inflation volume in the lungs, as demonstrated in Figure 19.2.

   a. During the "inflation hold" maneuver (which typically lasts one second), the peak pressure drops to a steady "plateau" pressure. The difference between the peak and plateau pressure is the pressure needed to overcome airway resistance (Ppeak – Pplateau = Pres), and the plateau pressure is the elastic recoil pressure of the lungs and chest wall (Pplateau = Pel).

   b. Since there is no airflow during the inflation hold maneuver, the plateau pressure is equivalent to the alveolar pressure at the end of inspiration (Pplateau = Palv).

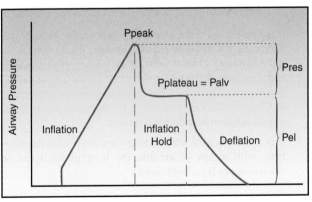

FIGURE 19.2 Airway pressure profile during volume control ventilation with an inspiratory hold maneuver. See text for explanation. Palv = alveolar pressure, Pres = pressure needed to overcome airway resistance, Pel = elastic recoil pressure (lungs and chest wall).

2. With PCV, there is no airflow at the end of the inspiration, so the airway pressure at end-inspiration is equivalent to the alveolar pressure (end-inspiratory Paw = Palv).

C. Alveolar Pressure

The alveolar pressure at the end of inspiration represents the following:

1. It is the elastic recoil pressure of the lungs and chest wall (Pel in Figure 19.2); as such, it can be used to compute the compliance (C) of the thorax (lungs and chest wall) at a particular tidal volume (V_T); i.e.,

$$C = V_T/Palv \quad \text{(mL/cm } H_2O) \quad (19.1)$$

a. The normal thoracic compliance is about 50 mL/cm H_2O.

b. Diffuse infiltrative lung diseases, like the acute respiratory distress syndrome (described in Chapter 17), cause a marked decrease in lung compliance (e.g., to <20 mL/cm H_2O), and monitoring compliance can be useful in following the clinical course of such diseases.

2. It is a reflection of the stress imposed on the walls of the alveoli by the inflation (tidal) volume. *An increase in the end-inspiratory alveolar pressure to >30 cm H_2O creates a risk for stress fractures in the alveolar-capillary interface, which results in ventilator-induced lung injury* (described in Chapter 17, Section II-A) (2,4). Alveolar injury from overdistension is called *volutrauma*.

3. It is a reflection of the tendency for overt alveolar rupture, with escape of air into the lung parenchyma or pleural space (i.e., *barotrauma*).

D. Which Method is Preferred?

Either method of lung inflation can be used effectively, but the following points deserve mention.

1. One advantage of VCV is the ability to maintain a constant level of alveolar ventilation, despite changes in the mechanical properties of the lungs. With PCV, alveolar ventilation will decrease if there is an increase in airways resistance (e.g., from secretions) or a decrease in lung compliance (e.g., from atelectasis or worsening of infiltrative lung disease).

2. Another advantage of VCV is the ability to use the *lung protective ventilation* protocol (see later).

3. A major advantage of PCV is patient comfort, which promotes synchronous breathing with the ventilator and reduces the work of breathing (5). This has been attributed to the high initial flow rates used during PCV (which are more likely to match the high flow demands of patients with respiratory failure), and the decelerating flow pattern (which promotes more even ventilation of the distal airspaces). A decelerating flow pattern is available for VCV, and has been shown to improve patient comfort (6).

4. Another stated advantage of PCV is the lower peak airway pressures. However, as shown in Figure 19.1, the end-inspiratory alveolar pressure is the same with PCV and VCV (at the same tidal volume), so *the lower peak airway pressures with PCV do not reduce the risk of alveolar overdistension and lung injury.* This only occurs when the tidal volume is reduced during PCV.

II. ASSIST-CONTROL VENTILATION

Assist-control ventilation (ACV) allows the patient to initiate a ventilator breath, but if this is not possible, ventilator breaths are delivered at a preselected rate. The ventilator breaths during ACV can be volume-controlled or pressure-controlled.

A. Triggers

Two examples of a ventilator breath during ACV are shown in the upper panel of Figure 19.3.

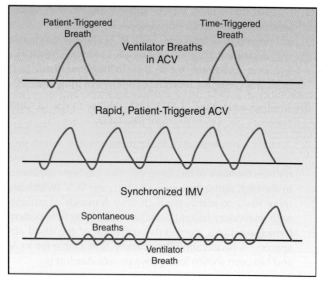

FIGURE 19.3 Airway pressure patterns in assist-control ventilation (ACV) and synchronized intermittent mandatory ventilation (SIMV). See text for explanation.

1. The ventilator breath on the left begins with a negative pressure deflection, which represents a spontaneous inspiratory effort by the patient. This is a *patient-triggered* ventilator breath.

2. The ventilator breath on the right does not begin with a negative pressure deflection, indicating the absence of a spontaneous inspiratory effort by the patient. This is a *time-triggered* ventilator breath, which is delivered at a preselected rate.

3. **Patient Triggers**

    a. NEGATIVE PRESSURE: The traditional trigger signal is a negative airway pressure (usually $2–3$ cm H_2O), which opens a pressure-sensitive valve in the ventilator.

b. INSPIRATORY FLOW RATE: Using inspiratory flow rate as a trigger requires less mechanical work by patients than negative pressure triggering (7). For this reason, flow has replaced pressure as the standard trigger signal. The flow rate that is required to trigger a ventilator breath differs (from 1–10 L/min) for each brand of ventilator. Auto-triggering from system leaks (which create flow changes) is the major problem associated with flow triggering (7).

B. Rapid Breathing

1. When each breath is a patient-triggered ventilator breath, rapid breathing like that shown in Figure 19.3 (middle panel) can have two adverse consequences:

   a. Severe respiratory alkalosis (pH >7.56).

   b. Incomplete alveolar emptying during exhalation, resulting in *dynamic hyperinflation* (described in Chapter 18, Section IV-A).

2. When uncontrolled rapid breathing has the above adverse effects, the appropriate mode of ventilation is *intermittent mandatory ventilation*, described next.

III. INTERMITTENT MANDATORY VENTILATION

A. The Method

1. Intermittent mandatory ventilation (IMV) allows patients to breathe spontaneously between ventilator breaths. This is accomplished by placing a spontaneous breathing circuit in parallel with the ventilator circuit, and using a unidirectional valve to open the spontaneous breathing circuit when a ventilator breath is not being delivered.

2. The ventilatory pattern for IMV is illustrated in the lower panel of Figure 19.3. Note that the ventilator breaths are delivered in synchrony with the patient's spontaneous breath; this is called *synchronized IMV* (SIMV).

3. The ventilator breaths during IMV can be volume-controlled or pressure-controlled. The rate of ventilator breaths can begin at 10 breaths/min, and then adjusted according to the severity of respiratory alkalosis, and/or the presence of dynamic hyperinflation (see Figure 18.3).

B. Adverse Effects

1. **Work of Breathing**

   There is an increased work of breathing during the spontaneous breathing periods in IMV, which can be reduced by *pressure-support ventilation* (described in the next section) during the spontaneous breathing periods (8).

2. **Cardiac Output**

   Positive pressure ventilation reduces left ventricular afterload and increases cardiac output in patients with left ventricular dysfunction (9). IMV has the opposite effect; i.e., it increases left ventricular afterload (attributed to the spontaneous breathing periods) and decreases cardiac output in patients with left ventricular dysfunction (10).

IV. PRESSURE SUPPORT VENTILATION

Pressure support ventilation (PSV) is pressure-augmented spontaneous breathing. PSV differs from pressure-control ventilation (PCV) in that the patient terminates the lung inflation in PSV, while the ventilator terminates the lung inflation in PCV.

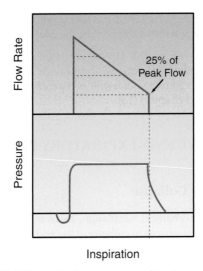

Inspiration

FIGURE 19.4 Changes in airway pressure and inspiratory flow during a single lung inflation with pressure support ventilation. The lung inflation is terminated when the flow rate falls to 25% of the peak flow, which allows the patient to determine the inspiratory time and tidal volume.

A. The Pressure-Supported Breath

The changes in pressure and flow during a lung inflation with PSV are shown in Figure 19.4. PSV monitors the patient's inspiratory flow rate, and the breath is terminated when the flow rate falls to 25% of the peak level. This *allows the patient to determine the duration of lung inflation, and the resulting tidal volume* (11).

B. Clinical Uses

1. Low levels of PSV (5–10 cm H_2O) can be used during weaning from mechanical ventilation, to overcome the resistance to flow in the artificial airways and ventilator

tubing. The goal of PSV in this setting is to reduce the work of breathing without augmenting the tidal volume (12).

2. Higher levels of PSV (15–30 cm H_2O) can be used to augment the tidal volume and provide full ventilatory support as a method of *noninvasive ventilation* (described in the next chapter) (13).

V. POSITIVE END-EXPIRATORY PRESSURE

A. Alveolar Collapse

1. During mechanical ventilation, there is a tendency for the distal airspaces to collapse at the end of expiration in dependent lung regions (14), and this tendency is magnified in patients with obstructive airway disease (e.g., COPD) and infiltrative diseases that reduce the distensibility of the lungs (e.g., acute respiratory distress syndrome). This has two adverse consequences:

   a. Alveoli that remain collapsed will impair gas exchange.

   b. Distal airspaces that repetitively close and open with each respiratory cycle can generate shear forces that damage the airway epithelium (15). This form of lung injury is called *atelectrauma* (16).

2. To prevent alveolar collapse at the end of expiration, a *positive end-expiratory pressure* (PEEP) (usually 5 cm H_2O) is routinely applied to the airways during mechanical ventilation, especially when low-volume ventilation is used (see later). This pressure is created by a pressure-relief valve in the expiratory limb of the ventilator circuit, which allows exhalation to proceed until a preselected pressure is reached, and this pressure (PEEP) is then maintained until the next inspiration.

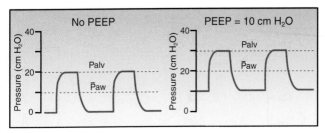

FIGURE 19.5 Airway pressure waveforms during pressure control ventilation showing the effects of positive end-expiratory pressure (PEEP) on end-inspiratory alveolar pressure (Palv) and mean airway pressure ($\overline{P}aw$).

B. Airway Pressures

The influence of PEEP on airway pressures are shown in Figure 19.5. Note that the addition of PEEP increases both the end-inspiratory alveolar pressure, and the mean airway pressure.

1. The increase in alveolar pressure determines the influence of PEEP on alveolar ventilation (and hence arterial oxygenation), and also determines the risk of ventilator-induced lung injury and barotrauma.

2. The increase in mean airway pressure determines the tendency for PEEP to decrease cardiac output (see later).

C. Alveolar Recruitment

In diffuse infiltrative lung diseases like the acute respiratory distress syndrome (ARDS), increases in PEEP to levels above those used to prevent alveolar collapse can be effective in opening collapsed alveoli (*alveolar recruitment*) to improve arterial oxygenation.

1. The use of increased PEEP levels is generally reserved for cases where the concentration of inhaled O_2 is at potentially toxic levels (>60%).

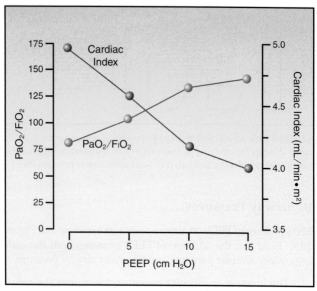

FIGURE 19.6 The opposing effects of positive end-expiratory pressure (PEEP) on arterial oxygenation (PaO_2/FiO_2) and cardiac output. Data from Reference 20.

2. If increased PEEP is used to improve arterial oxygenation, the end-inspiratory alveolar pressure should not exceed 30 cm H_2O, to limit the risk of ventilator-induced lung injury (17).

D. Hemodynamic Effects

1. PEEP can decrease cardiac output by several mechanisms, including impaired venous return, increased right ventricular afterload, and external constraint of the ventricles (18,19). These effects are exaggerated by hypovolemia, and can be mitigated by volume infusion (18).

2. PEEP-induced decreases in cardiac output can cancel the benefits of PEEP in improving arterial oxygenation, as demonstrated in Figure 19.6 (20).

3. Because of the tendency of PEEP to decrease cardiac output, some measure of cardiac output seems appropriate when using higher than usual levels of PEEP (e.g., >10 cm H_2O). The *central venous O_2 saturation* (which should decrease if there is a PEEP-induced decrease in cardiac output) might prove useful in this regard (see Chapter 6, Sections I-E and I-F).

VI. LUNG PROTECTIVE VENTILATION

When initiating mechanical ventilation for patients with acute respiratory failure, consider using the the *lung protective ventilation* protocol in Table 19.1. This protocol was developed to reduce the risk of ventilator-induced lung injury (described in Chapter 17, Section II-A) in patients with the acute respiratory distress syndrome (ARDS), and it has a proven survival benefit in these patients (2). However, it also improves outcomes in non-ARDS patients as well (21).

A. Design Features

Lung protective ventilation uses volume-controlled ventilation, and is designed to accomplish the following:

1. Reduce the risk of alveolar rupture from overdistension (volutrauma) by employing relatively low tidal volumes (6 mL/kg predicted body weight, instead of the standard 10–12 mL/kg ideal body weight), and by keeping the end-inspiratory alveolar pressure ≤30 cm H_2O.

2. Reduce the risk of epithelial injury from repetitive opening and closing of distal airspaces (atelectrauma) using low-level PEEP (5 cm H_2O) to prevent alveolar collapse.

Table 19.1	Protocol for Lung Protective Ventilation

I. FIRST STAGE:

1. Calculate patient's predicted body weight (PBW):

    Males: PBW = 50 + [2.3 x (height in inches − 60)]
    Females: PBW = 45.5 + [2.3 x (height in inches − 60)]

2. Set initial tidal volume (V_T) at 8 mL/kg PBW.

3. Add positive end-expiratory pressure (PEEP) at 5 cm H_2O.

4. Select the lowest FiO_2 that achieves an SpO_2 of 88−95%.

5. Reduce V_T by 1 mL/kg every 2 hrs until V_1 = 6 mL/kg.

II. SECOND STAGE:

1. When V_T = 6 mL/kg measure the end-inspiratory plateau pressure (Ppl).

2. If Ppl >30 cm H_2O, decrease V_T in 1 mL/kg increments until Ppl <30 cm H_2O or V_T = 4 mL/kg.

III. THIRD STAGE:

1. Monitor arterial blood gases for respiratory acidosis.

2. If pH = 7.15−7.30, increase respiratory rate (RR) until pH >7.30 or RR = 35 bpm.

3. If pH <7.15, increase RR to 35 bpm. If pH is still <7.15, increase V_T in 1 mL/kg increments until pH >7.15.

IV. OPTIMAL GOALS:

V_T = 6 mL/kg, Ppl ≤30 cm H_2O, SpO_2 = 88−95%, pH = 7.30−7.45

Adapted from the protocol developed by the ARDS Network, available at www.ardsnet.org.

REFERENCES

1. Cairo JM, Pilbean SP. Mosby's Respiratory Care Equipment. 8th ed. St. Louis: Mosby Elsevier; 2010.

2. The Acute Respiratory Distress Syndrome Network. Ventilation with lower tidal volumes as compared with traditional tidal volumes for acute lung injury and the acute respiratory distress syndrome. N Engl J Med 2000; 342(18): 1301–1308.

3. Mireles-Cabodevila E, Hatipoglu U, Chatburn RL. A rational framework for selecting modes of ventilation. Respir Care 2013; 58:348–366.

4. Petrucci N, Iacovelli W. Ventilation with lower tidal volumes versus traditional tidal volumes for acute lung injury and acute respiratory distress syndrome. Cochrane Database Syst Rev 2004; (2):CD003844.

5. Kallet RH, Campbell AR, Alonzo JA, et al. The effects of pressure control versus volume control on patient work of breathing in acute lung injury and acute respiratory distress syndrome. Respir Care 2000; 45:1085–1096.

6. Yang SC, Yang SP. Effects of inspiratory flow waveforms on lung mechanics, gas exchange, and respiratory metabolism in COPD patients during mechanical ventilation. Chest 2002; 122:2096–2104.

7. Laureen H, Pearl R. Flow triggering, pressure triggering, and autotriggering during mechanical ventilation. Crit Care Med 2000; 28:579–581.

8. Shelledy DC, Rau JL, Thomas-Goodfellow L. A comparison of the effects of assist-control, SIMV, and SIMV with pressure-support on ventilation, oxygen consumption, and ventilatory equivalent. Heart Lung 1995; 24:67–75.

9. Singh I, Pinsky MR. Heart-lung interactions. In Papadakos PJ, Lachmann B, eds. Mechanical ventilation: clinical applications and pathophysiology. Philadelphia: Saunders Elsevier, 2008:173–184.

10. Mathru M, et al. Hemodynamic responses to changes in ventilatory patterns in patients with normal and poor left ventricular reserve. Crit Care Med 1982; 10:423–426.

11. Hess DR. Ventilator waveforms and the physiology of pressure support ventilation. Respir Care 2005; 50:166–186.

12. Jubran A, Grant BJ, Duffner LA, et al. Effect of pressure support vs unassisted breathing through a tracheostomy collar on weaning duration in patients requiring prolonged mechanical ventilation: a randomized trial. JAMA 2013; 309:671–677.

13. Caples SM, Gay PC. Noninvasive positive pressure ventilation in the intensive care unit: a concise review. Crit Care Med 2005; 33:2651–2658.

14. Harris RS. Pressure-volume curves of the respiratory system. Respir Care 2005; 50:78–99.

15. Muscedere JG, Mullen JBM, Gan K, Slutsky AS. Tidal ventilation at low airway pressures can augment lung injury. Am J Respir Crit Care Med 1994; 149:1327–1334.

16. Gattinoni L, Protti A, Caironi P, Carlesso E. Ventilator-induced lung injury: the anatomical and physiological framework. Crit Care Med 2010; 38(Suppl):S539–S548.

17. Mercat A, Richard J-C, Vielle B, et al. Positive end-expiratory pressure setting in adults with acute lung injury and acute respiratory distress syndrome. JAMA 2008; 299:646–655.

18. Fougeres E, Teboul J-T, Richard C, et al. Hemodynamic impact of a positive end-expiratory pressure setting in acute respiratory distress syndrome: Importance of the volume status. Crit Care Med 2010; 38:802–807.

19. Takata M, Robotham JL. Ventricular external constraint by the lung and pericardium during positive end-expiratory pressure. Am Rev Respir Dis 1991; 43:872–875.

20. Gainnier M, Michelet P, Thirion X, et al. Prone position and positive end-expiratory pressure in acute respiratory distress syndrome. Crit Care Med 2003; 31:2719–2726.

21. Serpa Neto A, Cardoso SO, Manetta JA, et al. Association between the use of lung-protective ventilation with lower tidal volumes and clinical outcomes among patients without acute respiratory distress syndrome: a meta-analysis. JAMA 2012; 308:1651–1659.

Chapter 20

Alternative Modes of Ventilation

This chapter describes alternative methods of ventilatory support when conventional mechanical ventilation is not sufficient, or may not be necessary. Included are *rescue modes of ventilation* (i.e., high frequency oscillatory ventilation and airway pressure release ventilation) and *noninvasive modes of ventilation* (i.e., continuous positive airway pressure, bilevel positive airway pressure, and pressure support ventilation).

I. RESCUE MODES OF VENTILATION

A small percentage (10–15%) of patients with acute respiratory distress syndrome (ARDS) develop hypoxemia that is refractory to O_2 therapy and conventional mechanical ventilation (CMV) (1). The following methods of ventilation can be beneficial in these patients.

A. High Frequency Oscillation

High frequency oscillatory ventilation (HFOV) uses high-frequency, low volume oscillations like the ones shown in Figure 20.1. These oscillations create a high mean airway pressure, which improves gas exchange by opening collapsed alveoli (alveolar recruitment) and preventing further alveolar collapse. The small tidal volumes (typically 1–2 mL/kg) limit the risk of alveolar injury from overdistension (volutrauma) (2).

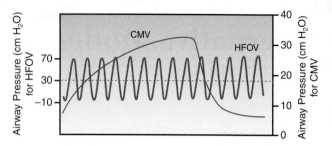

FIGURE 20.1 Airway pressure oscillations during high frequency oscillatory ventilation (HFOV) with a superimposed lung inflation during
conventional mechanical ventilation (CMV). Dotted line represents mean
airway pressure. From Reference 3.

1. **Ventilator Settings**

   HFOV requires a specialized ventilator (Sensormedics
   3100B, Viasys Healthcare, Yorba Linda, CA) that allows
   the following adjustments: (a) the frequency and amplitude of the oscillations, (b) the mean airway pressure, (c)
   the bias flow rate (similar to an inspiratory flow rate),
   and (d) the inspiratory time (time of the bias flow).

   a. The frequency range for oscillations is 4–7 Hz (oscilla-
      tions/sec). The frequency selected is determined by the
      arterial pH (which is a reflection of the CO_2 burden).
      Lower frequencies have higher pulse amplitudes, and
      are more effective for CO_2 removal, which reduces the
      risk of respiratory acidosis.

   b. The initial pulse amplitude is set at 70–90 cm H_2O.

   c. The mean airway pressure is usually set slightly
      above the end-inspiratory alveolar pressure during
      CMV (see Chapter 19, Figures 19.1 and 19.2) (3).

   d. The bias flow rate is usually set at 40 L/min.

2. **Advantages**

   Clinical trials comparing HFOV with CMV have shown 16–24% increase in the PaO_2/FiO_2 ratio associated with HFOV (2). However, there is no documented survival benefit with HFOV (3,4).

3. **Disadvantages**

   a. A special ventilator is needed, along with trained personnel to operate the device.

   b. Cardiac output is often decreased during HFOV because of the high mean airway (intrathoracic) pressures (3).

B. Airway Pressure Release Ventilation

Airway pressure release ventilation (APRV) is a modified form of *continuous positive airway pressure* (CPAP), and involves prolonged periods of spontaneous breathing with high-level CPAP, interrupted by brief periods of pressure release to atmospheric pressure. This is demonstrated in the middle panel of Figure 20.2. The high CPAP level improves arterial oxygenation by opening collapsed alveoli (alveolar recruitment), and the pressure release is designed to facilitate CO_2 removal (5). The increase in arterial oxygenation occurs gradually, over 24 hours (6).

1. **Ventilator Settings**

   APRV is available in most modern critical care ventilators. The variables that must be selected when initiating APRV include the high and low airway pressures, and the time spent at each pressure level. Suggested settings are as follows (3):

   a. The high airway pressure should be equivalent to the end-inspiratory alveolar pressure during CMV (see Chapter 19, Figures 19.1 and 19.2).

   b. The low airway pressure is set to zero.

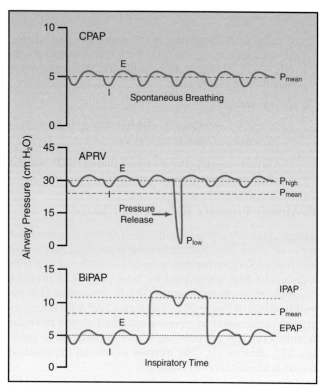

FIGURE 20.2 Related modes of pressure-regulated spontaneous ventilation. CPAP = continuous positive airway pressure, APRV = airway pressure release ventilation, BiPAP = bilevel positive airway pressure, IPAP = inspiratory positive airway pressure, EPAP = expiratory positive airway pressure, P_{mean} = mean airway pressure, I = inspiration, E = expiration. See text for explanation.

    c. The time spent at the high airway pressure is usually 85–90% of the total cycle time. Recommended times are 4–6 seconds for the high pressure level, and 0.6 to 0.8 seconds for the low pressure level.

2. **Advantages**

   a. APRV can achieve nearly complete recruitment of collapsed alveoli, more than can be achieved with HFOV or high-level PEEP (5). However, the improvement in arterial oxygenation occurs gradually, over 24 hours (6).

   b. APRV *can increase cardiac output* despite the high airway pressures that are used (5). This is attributed to the marked alveolar recruitment that occurs with APRV, which also reopens blood vessels and increases pulmonary blood flow.

3. **Disadvantages**

   a. The benefits of APRV are lost if the patient has no spontaneous breathing efforts.

   b. Severe asthma and COPD are relative contraindications to APRV because of the inability to empty the lungs rapidly during the pressure release phase (3).

II. NONINVASIVE VENTILATION

The term *noninvasive ventilation* (NIV) refers to pressure-augmented spontaneous breathing that is achieved with tight-fitting face masks instead of endotracheal intubation.

A. Modes of Noninvasive Ventilation

There are three types of NIV: (a) continuous positive airway pressure (CPAP), (b) bilevel positive airway pressure (BiPAP), and (c) pressure support ventilation (PSV).

1. **Continuous Positive Airway Pressure**

   Continuous positive airway pressure (CPAP) is spontaneous breathing at a positive end-expiratory pressure, as illustrated in the upper panel of Figure 20.2. CPAP is simple to use, and requires only a source of O_2 and a face mask with a pressure-relief valve (CPAP mask).

a. The principal effect of CPAP is an increase in functional residual capacity (the volume in the lungs at the end of expiration). CPAP does not augment the tidal volume, which limits its use in patients with acute respiratory failure.

b. SETTINGS: CPAP is usually set at 5–10 cm H_2O.

2. **Bilevel Positive Airway Pressure**

Bilevel positive airway pressure (BiPAP) is CPAP that alternates between two pressure levels, as illustrated in the lower panel of Figure 20.2. The high pressure level is called the *inspiratory positive airway pressure* (IPAP), and the low pressure level is called the *expiratory positive airway pressure* (EPAP).

a. BiPAP creates higher mean airway pressures than CPAP, and this helps to promote alveolar recruitment. BIPAP does not directly augment tidal volumes, but the alveolar recruitment will increase lung compliance (lung distensibility), which can result in higher tidal volumes.

b. SETTINGS: BiPAP requires a specialized ventilator, and can be started with the following settings: IPAP = 10 cm H_2O, EPAP = 5 cm H_2O, inspiratory time (the duration of IPAP) = 3 sec. Further adjustments in pressure are guided by blood gases, patient comfort, etc. Airway pressures above 20 cm H_2O are not advised because they are poorly tolerated by patients, and promote air leaks around the face masks.

3. **Pressure Support Ventilation**

Pressure support ventilation (PSV) is described in Chapter 19, Section IV.

a. PSV augments the tidal volume, and is usually combined with CPAP to increase the functional residual capacity. *PSV with CPAP is the preferred method of non-invasive ventilation* (with a few exceptions, described later).

b. SETTINGS: PSV is usually initiated with an inflation pressure of 10 cm H_2O and a CPAP level of 5 cm H_2O. Further adjustments are guided by blood gases, patient comfort, etc. Peak airway pressures above 20 cm H_2O are not advised because they are poorly tolerated by patients, and promote air leaks around the face masks.

B. Patient Selection

Patient selection is one of the most important determinants of the success or failure of NIV (7,8).

1. The first step is to identify patients who need ventilatory support; i.e., patients with persistent or progressive respiratory distress, severe hypoxemia ($PaO_2/FiO_2 < 200$ mm Hg), or severe or progressive hypercapnia.

2. The next step is to determine which of these patients are candidates for NIV. While some causes of acute respiratory failure are more successfully managed with NIV than others (see later), all patients with acute respiratory failure are candidates for NIV if all of the following conditions are satisfied:

    a. The respiratory failure is not an immediate threat to life.

    b. There is no life-threatening circulatory impairment (e.g., circulatory shock).

    c. The patient is alert or easily aroused, and is cooperative.

    d. The patient does not have an uncontrolled cough, or copious secretions.

   e. There is no facial trauma that will prevent the use of a tight-fitting face mask.

   f. The patient does not have hematemesis or recurrent vomiting.

   g. The patient does not have uncontrolled seizures.

3. Progression of the respiratory failure can limit the success of NIV (7,8), so there should be little delay in initiating NIV for appropriate candidates.

C. Success Rates

Table 20.1 shows the success rate of NIV in avoiding endotracheal intubation in relation to the cause of acute respiratory failure.

Table 20.1	Success Rates for Noninvasive Ventilation
Condition	**Success Rate**
Cardiogenic Pulmonary Edema	90%
Acute Exacerbation of COPD	76%
Community-Acquired Pneumonia	50%
Acute respiratory Distress Syndrome	40%

From References 9 and 10.

1. **Acute Exacerbations of COPD:**

   The greatest benefit with NIV in acute respiratory failure has generally been in patients with hypercapnic respiratory failure from acute exacerbations of COPD (9). As a result, *NIV is considered a first-line therapy for acute exacerbations of COPD* (7,8). The preferred mode of ventilation in this condition is PSV with CPAP.

2. **Hypoxemic Respiratory Failure**

   With the exception of cardiogenic pulmonary edema, NIV has been less successful in preventing endotracheal intubation in conditions that cause hypoxemic respiratory failure (e.g., acute respiratory distress syndrome) (10).

   a. CARDIOGENIC EDEMA: NIV can prevent endotracheal intubation in a large majority of patients with cardiogenic pulmonary edema (11,12). Most of the experience in this condition has been with CPAP (at 10 cm H_2O), but BiPAP produces equivalent results (13). This benefit may be related to improved cardiac performance because NIV increases cardiac output in patients with systolic heart failure (13), presumably as a result of the decrease in left-ventricular afterload caused by positive intrathoracic pressures (14).

   b. ARDS: NIV has had limited success in patients with acute respiratory distress syndrome (ARDS), and is more successful when ARDS has an extrapulmonary origin (10). The preferred method of NIV in patients with ARDS is PSV with CPAP, while CPAP alone should be avoided (8).

D. Monitoring

1. The success or failure of NIV in individual patients should be determined early (one hour) after initiating NIV (10,15).

2. *Failure to improve gas exchange significantly after one hour of NIV is evidence that NIV is failing as a support modality*, and should serve as an indication to proceed with immediate endotracheal intubation and mechanical ventilation.

3. Delays in recognizing progressive respiratory failure

during NIV can lead to impending respiratory arrest and a hazardous endotracheal intubation.

E. Adverse Events

Notable adverse events during NIV include gastric distension, pressure ulcers on the bridge of the nose (from tight-fitting masks), and nosocomial pneumonia.

1. **Gastric Distension**

    Gastric distension from insufflated gas is a common concern during NIV, but it should not be a common occurrence when inflation pressures are less than 30 cm H_2O (16). Gastric decompression with nasogastric tubes is not always necessary during NIV, but can be reserved for patients who develop abdominal distension during NIV (17).

2. **Nosocomial Pneumonia**

    Positive pressure ventilation can retard mucociliary clearance in the airways and predispose to nosocomial pneumonia. In studies comparing NIV to endotracheal intubation and mechanical ventilation, the incidence of nosocomial pneumonia was 8–10% during NIV, but was much higher (19–22%) after intubation and mechanical ventilation (18,19).

REFERENCES

1. Pipeling MR, Fan E. Therapies for refractory hypoxemia in acute respiratory distress syndrome. JAMA 2010; 304:2521–2527.

2. Ali S, Ferguson ND. High-frequency oscillatory ventilation in ALI/ARDS. Crit Care Clin 2011; 27:487–499.

3. Stawicki SP, Goyal M, Sarini B. High-frequency oscillatory ventilation (HFOV) and airway pressure release ventilation (APRV): a practical guide. J Intensive Care Med 2009; 24:215–229.

4. Sud S, Sud M, Freiedrich JO, et al. High-frequency oscillatory ventilation versus conventional ventilation for acute respiratory distress syndrome. Cochrane Database Syst Rev 2016; 4:CD004085.

5. Muang AA, Kaplan LJ. Airway pressure release ventilation in acute respiratory distress syndrome. Crit Care Clin 2011; 27:501–509.

6. Sydow M, Burchardi H, Ephraim E, et al. Long-term effects of two different ventilatory modes on oxygenation in acute lung injury. Comparison of airway pressure release ventilation and volume-controlled inverse ratio ventilation. Crit Care Med 1994; 149:1550–1556.

7. Hill NS, Brennan J, Garpestad E, Nava S. Noninvasive ventilation in acute respiratory failure. Crit Care Med 2007; 35:2402–2407.

8. Keenan SP, Sinuff T, Burns KEA, et al, as the Canadian Critical Care Trials Group/Canadian Critical Care Society Noninvasive Ventilation Guidelines Group. Clinical practice guidelines for the use of noninvasive positive-pressure ventilation and noninvasive continuous positive airway pressure in the acute care setting. Canad Med Assoc J 2011; 183:E195–E214.

9. Ram FSF, Picot J, Lightowler J, Wedzicha JA. Non-invasive positive pressure ventilation for treatment of respiratory failure due to exacerbations of COPD. Cochrane Database Syst Rev 2009; July 8:CD004104

10. Antonelli M, Conti G, Moro ML, et al. Predictors of failure of noninvasive positive pressure ventilation in patients with acute hypoxemic respiratory failure: a multi-center study. Intensive Care Med 2001; 27:1718–1728.

11. Masip J, Roque M, Sanchez B, et al. Noninvasive ventilation in cardiogenic pulmonary edema: systematic review and meta-analysis. JAMA 2005; 294:3124–3130.

12. Vital FM, Saconato H, Ladeira MT, et al. Non-invasive positive pressure ventilation (CPAP or bilevel NPPV) for cardiogenic pulmonary edema. Cochrane Database Syst Rev 2008; July 16:CD005351.

13. Acosta B, DiBenedetto R, Rahimi A, et al. Hemodynamic effects of noninvasive bilevel positive airway pressure on patients with chronic congestive heart failure with systolic dysfunction. Chest 2000; 118:1004–1009.

14. Singh I, Pinsky MR. Heart-lung interactions. In Papadakos PJ, Lachmann B, eds. Mechanical ventilation: clinical applications and pathophysiology. Philadelphia: Saunders Elsevier, 2008:173–184.

15. Anton A, Guell R, Gomez J, et al. Predicting the result of noninvasive ventilation in severe acute exacerbations of patients with chronic airflow limitation. Chest 2000; 117:828–833.

16. Wenans CS. The pharyngoesophageal closure mechanism: a manometric study. Gastroenterology 1972; 63:769–777.

17. Meduri GU, Fox RC, Abou-Shala N, et al. Noninvasive mechanical ventilation via face mask in patients with acute respiratory failure who refused endotracheal intubation. Crit Care Med 1994; 22:1584–1590.

18. Girou E, Schotgen F, Delclaux C, et al. Association of noninvasive ventilation with nosocomial infections and survival in critically ill patients. JAMA 2000; 284:2361–2367.

19. Carlucci A, Richard J-C, Wysocki M, et al. Noninvasive versus conventional mechanical ventilation: an epidemiological study. Am J Respir Crit Care Med 2001; 163:874–880.

Chapter 21

The Ventilator-Dependent Patient

This chapter describes the daily care and concerns for ventilator-dependent patients, with emphasis on the artificial airways (endotracheal and tracheostomy tubes) and mechanical complications of positive pressure ventilation. The infectious complications of mechanical ventilation are described in Chapter 16.

I. ARTIFICIAL AIRWAYS

A. Endotracheal Tubes

Endotracheal (ET) tubes vary in length from 25 to 35 cm, and are sized according to their internal diameter (ID), which varies from 5 to 10 mm (e.g., a "size 7" endotracheal tube indicates an ID of 7 mm). A size 8 ET tube (ID = 8 mm) is standard for adults (1).

1. **Subglottic Drainage Tube**

   The prominent role played by aspiration of mouth secretions in ventilator-associated pneumonias has led to the introduction of specially-designed ET tubes capable of draining mouth secretions that accumulate just above the inflated cuff (see Chapter 16, Figure 16.1). These tubes can reduce the incidence of ventilator-associated pneumonia (2), and should be considered when intubating patients who are likely to require more than 48 hours of ventilatory support.

2. **Tube Position**

Evaluation of tube position is mandatory after intubation, and Figure 21.1 shows the proper tube position. When the head is in a neutral position, *the tip of the ET tube should be 3 to 5 cm above the carina, or midway between the carina and vocal cords.* (If not visible, the main carina is usually over the T4–T5 interspace.)

a. ET tubes can migrate into the right mainstem bronchus (which runs a straight course down from the trachea). To reduce the risk of this complication, keep the tip of the endotracheal tube no further than 21 cm from the teeth in women, or 23 cm in men (3).

3. **Laryngeal Injury**

The risk for laryngeal injury from ET tubes is a major

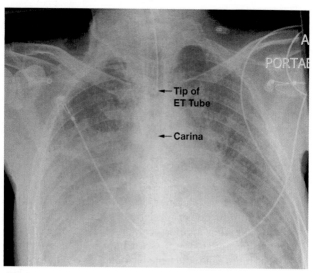

FIGURE 21.1 Portable chest x-ray showing proper position of an endotracheal tube, with the tip of the tube located midway between the thoracic inlet and the carina.

concern, and is one of the reasons for performing tracheostomies when prolonged intubation is anticipated. The spectrum of laryngeal damage includes ulceration, granulomas, vocal cord paresis, and laryngeal edema.

a. Laryngeal injuries are reported in three-quarters of patients who are intubated for longer than 24 hours (4), but most cases are not clinically significant, and do not result in permanent injury (5).

b. Airway obstruction from laryngeal edema is reported after 13% of extubations (4). (The management of this problem is described in Chapter 22.)

B. Tracheostomy

Tracheostomy is preferred in patients who require prolonged mechanical ventilation (>1–2 weeks). There are several advantages with tracheostomy, including greater patient comfort, easier access to airways for clearing secretions and bronchodilator administration, reduced resistance for breathing, and reduced risk of laryngeal injury.

1. **Timing**

   The optimal time for performing a tracheostomy has been debated for years. Recent studies comparing early tracheostomy (one week after intubation) with late tracheostomy (two weeks after intubation) have shown that early tracheostomy reduces sedative requirements and promotes early mobilization (6), but *does not reduce the incidence of ventilator-associated pneumonia, or the mortality rate* (6,7).

   a. Based on the pneumonia and mortality data, tracheostomy is recommended after 2 weeks of endotracheal intubation (8). However, if one considers patient comfort, it is reasonable to *consider tracheostomy after 7 days of intubation if there is little chance of extubation in the next few days.*

2. **Complications**

a. Percutaneous dilatational tracheostomy is associated with less blood loss and fewer local infections than surgically created tracheostomies (9).

b. Combining surgical and percutaneous tracheostomy, the mortality rate is <1%, and early complications (i.e., bleeding and infection) occur in <5% of cases (9,10).

c. TRACHEAL STENOSIS: Tracheal stenosis is a late complication that appears in the first 6 months after the tracheostomy tube is removed. Most cases of tracheal stenosis occur at the site of the tracheal incision, and are the result of tracheal narrowing after the stoma closes. The incidence of tracheal stenosis ranges from zero to 15% (10), but most cases are asymptomatic. The risk of tracheal stenosis is the same with surgical and percutaneous tracheostomies (8).

C. Cuff Management

Artificial airways are equipped with inflatable balloons (called cuffs) that are used to seal the trachea and prevent gas from escaping through the larynx during lung inflation. A tracheostomy tube with an inflated cuff is shown in Figure 21.2. Note the elongated design of the cuff, which allows for greater dispersion of pressure, and allows a tracheal seal at relatively low pressures.

1. **Cuff Inflation**

The cuff is attached to a pilot balloon that has a one-way valve. To inflate the cuff, a syringe is attached to the pilot balloon, and air is injected into the cuff through the pilot balloon (which will inflate as the cuff inflates).

a. The cuff is inflated until no audible leak is detected around the cuff.

b. The pressure in the cuff (measured with a pressure gauge attached to the pilot balloon) should be <25 mm

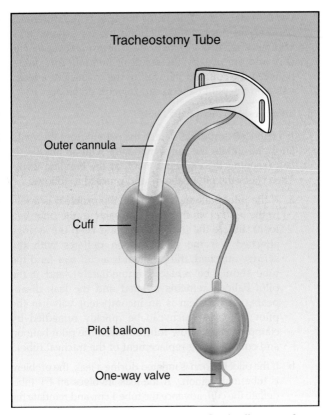

FIGURE 21.2 A tracheostomy tube with an inflated cuff. See text for further explanation.

Hg (11), which is the assumed hydrostatic pressure in capillaries within the wall of the trachea. (Cuff pressures >25 mm Hg could then compress adjacent capillaries and produce ischemic injury in the trachea.)

2. **Cuff Leaks**

Cuff leaks are usually detected by audible sounds during lung inflation (created by gas escaping through the vocal cords). The volume of the leak is the difference between the desired tidal volume and the exhaled tidal volume. *Cuff leaks are rarely caused by disruption of the cuff* (12), and are usually the result of nonuniform contact between the cuff and the wall of the trachea, or a leaky valve on the pilot balloon causing cuff deflation.

3. **Troubleshooting a Cuff Leak**

   If a cuff leak is audible, detach the patient from the ventilator and inflate the lungs manually with an anesthesia bag (keeping the end-tidal PCO_2 at the baseline level). Then check the pilot balloon, and proceed as follows:

   a. If the pilot balloon is deflated, the problem is a tear in the cuff, or an incompetent valve in the pilot balloon. Inflate the pilot balloon and keep the syringe attached. If the pilot balloon deflates with the syringe attached, the problem is a cuff tear (and the tube should be replaced immediately), and if the pilot balloon remains inflated and the leak disappears, the problem is an incompetent valve in the pilot balloon (which can be quickly remedied by clamping the narrow tube between the pilot balloon and cuff, pending replacement of the tracheal tube).

   b. If the pilot balloon is inflated during a leak, the problem is tube malposition. If the leak involves an ET tube, deflate the cuff, advance the tube 1 cm, and reinflate the cuff. If the leak persists, replace the ET tube with a larger size tube. If the leak involves a tracheostomy tube, replace the tube with a larger, or longer, tube.

II. AIRWAYS CARE

A. Suctioning

The inner surface of ET tubes and tracheostomy tubes becomes colonized with biofilms containing pathogenic organisms, and passing a suction catheter through the tubes can dislodge these biofilms and inoculate the lungs with pathogenic organisms (13). As a result, *endotracheal suctioning is no longer recommended as a routine procedure*, but should be performed only when it is necessary to clear respiratory secretions (14).

B. Pitfalls of Saline Instillation

Saline is often instilled into the trachea to facilitate the clearing of secretions, but this practice is *no longer advised as a routine procedure* (14) for two reasons: (a) saline will not liquefy or reduce the viscosity of respiratory secretions (explained next), and (b) saline injections can dislodge pathogenic organisms colonizing the inner surface of tracheal tubes (15).

1. Sputum Viscosity

   The respiratory secretions create a blanket that covers the mucosal surface of the airways. This blanket has a hydrophilic (water soluble) layer, and a hydrophobic (water insoluble) layer. The hydrophilic layer faces inward, and keeps the mucosal surface moist. The hydrophobic layer, which faces outward, is composed of a meshwork of mucoprotein strands that traps particles and debris in the airways, and the combination of the mucoprotein strands and the trapped debris determines the viscoelastic behavior of the respiratory secretions.

   a. Since the layer that contributes to the viscosity of respiratory secretions is not water soluble, *saline will not reduce the viscosity of respiratory secretions*. (Adding saline to respiratory secretions is like pouring water over grease.)

C. Mucolytic Therapy

1. The mucoprotein strands in respiratory secretions are held together by disulfide bridges, which can be dis-

rupted by *N-Acetylcysteine* (NAC) (19), a sulfhydryl-con-
taining tripeptide that is better known as the antidote
for acetaminophen overdose.

2. NAC is available in a liquid preparation (10 or 20% solution) that can be given as an aerosol spray, or injected
directly into the airways (see Table 21.1). Aerosolized
NAC can be irritating, and can provoke coughing and
bronchospasm (particularly in asthmatics). Direct instillation of NAC into the tracheal tube is preferred.

3. NAC instillation should not be continued for longer
than 48 hours because the drug solution is hypertonic,
and can provoke bronchorrhea with continued use.

Table 21.1	Mucolytic Therapy with N-Acetylcysteine (NAC)
Aerosol Therapy:	• Use 10% NAC solution.
	• Mix 2.5 mL NAC with 2.5 mL saline and place mixture (5 mL) in a small volume nebulizer for aerosol delivery.
	• *Warning:* this can provoke bronchospasm, and is not recommended in asthmatics
Tracheal Injection:	• Use 20% NAC solution.
	• Mix 2 mL NAC with 2 mL saline and inject 2 mL aliquots into the trachea.
	• *Warning:* Excessive volumes can produce bronchorrhea.

III. ALVEOLAR RUPTURE

One of the manifestations of ventilator-induced lung injury

is the overt rupture of alveoli, with escape of air into the lung parenchyma or pleural space. This form of injury is called *barotrauma*, even though it is a manifestation of *volutrauma* (i.e., alveolar overdistension).

A. Clinical Manifestations

Escape of air from the alveoli can result in the following:

1. The alveolar gas can dissect along tissue planes and produce *pulmonary interstitial emphysema*, and can move into the mediastinum and produce *pneumomediastinum*.

2. Mediastinal gas can move into the neck to produce *subcutaneous emphysema*, or can pass below the diaphragm to produce *pneumoperitoneum*.

3. If the rupture involves the visceral pleura, gas will collect in the pleural space and produce a *pneumothorax*.

4. Each of the above conditions can occur alone or in combination with the others (17,18).

B. Pneumothorax

Radiographic evidence of pneumothorax is reported in 5–15% of ventilator-dependent patients (20,21). (The incidence may be lower with low-volume, *lung protective ventilation*, described in Chapter 17, Section II-B.)

1. **Clinical Presentation**

   Clinical manifestations are either absent, minimal, or nonspecific. The *most valuable clinical sign is subcutaneous emphysema* in the neck and upper thorax, which is pathognomonic of alveolar rupture. Breath sounds are unreliable in ventilator-dependent patients because sounds transmitted from the ventilator tubing can be mistaken for airway sounds.

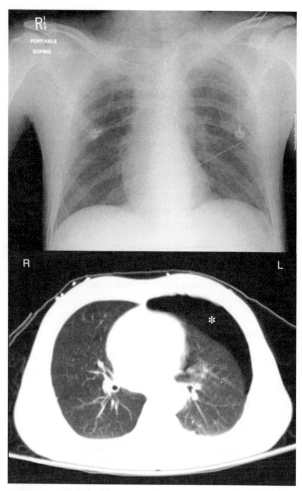

FIGURE 21.3 A portable chest x-ray and CT image of the thorax in a young male with blunt trauma to the chest. An anterior pneumothorax is evident on the CT image (indicated by the asterisk) but is not apparent on the portable chest x-ray. Images courtesy of Dr. Kenneth Sutin, MD.

2. Radiographic Detection

The radiographic detection of pleural air can be difficult in the supine position, because *pleural air does not collect at the lung apex when patients are supine* (19). Figure 21.3 illustrates this difficulty. In this case of a traumatic pneumothorax, the chest x-ray is unrevealing, but the CT scan reveals an anterior pneumothorax on the left. Pleural air will collect in the most superior region of the hemithorax; in the supine position, this region is just anterior to both lung bases. Therefore, *basilar and subpulmonic collections of air are characteristic of pneumothorax in the supine position* (19).

3. Evacuation of Pleural Air

Evacuation of pleural air is accomplished with a chest tube inserted through the fourth or fifth intercostal space along the mid-axillary line, and advanced in an anterior and superior direction (which is where pleural air collects in the supine position). The drainage system is a three-chamber arrangement like the one shown in Figure 21.4 (20).

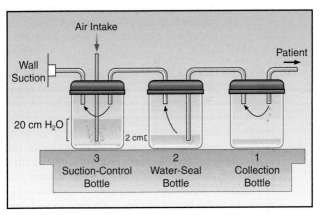

FIGURE 21.4 A standard pleural drainage system for evacuating air and fluid from the pleural space. See text for explanation.

a. COLLECTION CHAMBER: The first bottle in the system collects fluid from the pleural space and allows air to pass to the next bottle in the series. Because the inlet of this chamber is not in direct contact with the fluid, the pleural fluid that is collected does not impose a back pressure on the pleural space.

b. WATER-SEAL CHAMBER: The second bottle acts as a one-way valve that allows air to escape from the pleural space, but prevents air from entering the pleural space. This one-way valve is created by submerging the inlet tube under water, which imposes a back-pressure on the pleural space that is equal to the depth that the tube is submerged. The positive pressure in the pleural space then prevents atmospheric air (at zero pressure) from entering the pleural space. The water thus "seals" the pleural space from the surrounding atmosphere. This water-seal pressure is usually 2 cm H_2O.

c. DETECTING AIR LEAKS: Air that is evacuated from the pleural space passes through the water in the second bottle and creates bubbles. Thus, *the presence of bubbles in the water-seal chamber is evidence of a bronchopleural air leak.*

d. SUCTION-CONTROL CHAMBER: The third bottle in the system is used to set a maximum limit on the negative suction pressure that is imposed on the pleural space. This maximum pressure is determined by the height of the water column in the air inlet tube. Negative pressure (from wall suction) draws the water down the air inlet tube, and when the negative pressure exceeds the height of the water column, air is entrained from the atmosphere. Therefore, the pressure in the bottle can never become more negative than the height of the water column in the air inlet tube (which is usually set at 20 cm). The presence of bubbling in the suction control chamber means that the maximum suction pressure has been reached.

4. **The Dark Side of Suction**

   The use of suction to evacuate pleural air is often unnecessary, and potentially harmful, as explained below.

   a. The lungs will reinflate without the use of suction.

   b. Creating a negative pressure in the pleural space also creates a higher transpulmonary pressure (the pressure difference between alveoli and the pleural space), which is the driving pressure for air flow through a bronchopleural fistula. This means that *applying suction to the pleural space will increase the volume of air that leaks out from the lungs,* which is counterproductive.

   c. Although suction is used routinely to evacuate pleural air, the presence of a continuing air leak while pleural suction is applied should prompt you to discontinue the suction in an attempt to reduce or eliminate the air leak.

IV. INTRINSIC PEEP

As described in Chapter 18, Section IV, trapped gas in the alveoli from incomplete exhalation (called *dynamic hyperinflation*) creates a positive end-expiratory pressure (PEEP), which is called *intrinsic PEEP* (21).

A. Why Worry?

1. During conventional mechanical ventilation, intrinsic PEEP is universal in patients with severe asthma and COPD (22,23), and is common in patients with acute respiratory distress syndrome (ARDS) (24).

2. Intrinsic PEEP can have several adverse consequences

(see next), and it is not apparent during routine monitoring of airway pressures.

B. Adverse Effects

Intrinsic PEEP can have the following adverse effects (21).

1. Decreased cardiac output (caused by the increase in mean intrathoracic pressure).

2. Increased work of breathing (explained in Chapter 18, Section IV-A-3.)

3. Increased risk of alveolar overdistension and ventilator-induced lung injury (caused by the increase in end-inspiratory alveolar pressure).

4. Intrinsic PEEP can be transmitted into the superior vena cava, which increases the central venous pressure and gives the mistaken impression that the right ventricular end-diastolic pressure has increased.

5. The increase in end-inspiratory alveolar pressure caused by intrinsic PEEP can be misinterpreted as a decrease in the compliance of the lungs and chest wall (see Chapter 19, Section I-C). When thoracic compliance (C) is calculated at any given tidal volume (V_T), the PEEP level must be subtracted from the end-inspiratory alveolar pressure (Palv).

$$C = V_T/(Palv - PEEP) \quad \text{(mL/cm } H_2O) \quad (21.1)$$

C. Detection

Intrinsic PEEP is easy to detect but difficult to quantify.

1. The presence of dynamic inflation (and intrinsic PEEP) is detected by inspecting the expiratory flow waveform for the presence of airflow at the end of expiration (see Figure 18.3).

2. If intrinsic PEEP is evident on the expiratory flow wave-form, the level of intrinsic PEEP can be measured with the end-expiratory occlusion method (see Figure 18.4). However, accuracy requires that the occlusion occur at the very end of expiration, and this cannot be timed properly if patients are breathing spontaneously. Therefore, *the end-expiratory occlusion method performs best during controlled ventilation, when patients are not triggering ventilator breaths.*

D. Prevention

The maneuvers that prevent or limit dynamic hyperinflation and intrinsic PEEP are all aimed at promoting alveolar emptying during exhalation. These maneuvers are described in Chapter 18, Section IV-D.

E. Adding PEEP to Reduce PEEP (!)

1. The addition of external PEEP can reduce hyperinflation (and intrinsic PEEP) by holding the small airways open at end-expiration.

2. The level of applied PEEP must be enough to counterbalance the pressure causing small airways collapse, but should not exceed the level of intrinsic PEEP (so that it does not impair expiratory flow) (25).

3. The response to externally applied PEEP can be evaluated by monitoring the presence of airflow at the end of expiration; i.e., if the applied PEEP reduces or eliminates end-expiratory flow, then it is reducing or eliminating intrinsic PEEP.

4. Although the end result is still PEEP (applied PEEP instead of intrinsic PEEP), the applied PEEP will help to reduce the risk of lung injury (atelectrauma) from repetitive opening and closing of distal airspaces at end-expiration. (See Chapter 17, Section II-A-3.)

REFERENCES

1. Gray AW. Endotracheal tubes. Crit Care Clin 2003; 24:379–387.

2. Muscedere J, Rewa O, Mckechnie K, et al. Subglottic secretion drainage for the prevention of ventilator-associated pneumonia: a systematic review and meta-analysis. Crit Care Med 2011; 39:1985–1991.

3. Owen RL, Cheney FW. Endotracheal intubation: a preventable complication. Anesthesiology 1987; 67:255–257.

4. Tadie JM, Behm E, Lecuyer L, et al. Post-intubation laryngeal injuries and extubation failure: a fiberoptic endoscopic study. Intensive Care Med 2010; 36:991–998.

5. Colice GL. Resolution of laryngeal injury following translaryngeal intubation. Am Rev Respir Dis 1992; 145:361–364.

6. Trouillet JL, Luyt CE, Guiguet M, et al. Early percutaneous tracheotomy versus prolonged intubation of mechanically ventilated patients after cardiac surgery: A randomized trial. Ann Intern Med 2011; 154:373–383.

7. Terragni PP, Antonelli M, Fumagalli R, et al. Early vs late tracheotomy for prevention of pneumonia in mechanically ventilated adult ICU patients. JAMA 2010; 303:1483–1489.

8. Freeman BD, Morris PE. Tracheostomy practice in adults with acute respiratory failure. Crit Care Med 2012; 40:2890–2896.

9. Freeman BD, Isabella K, Lin N, Buchman TG. A meta-analysis of prospective trials comparing percutaneous and surgical tracheostomy in critically ill patients. Chest 2000; 118:1412–1418.

10. Tracheotomy: application and timing. Clin Chest Med 2003; 24:389–398.

11. Heffner JE, Hess D. Tracheostomy management in the chronically ventilated patient. Clin Chest Med 2001; 22:5; 10:561–568.

12. Kearl RA, Hooper RG. Massive airway leaks: an analysis of the role of endotracheal tubes. Crit Care Med 1993; 21:518–521.

13. Adair CC, Gorman SP, Feron BM, et al. Implications of endotracheal tube biofilm for ventilator-associated pneumonia. Intensive Care Med 1999; 25:1072–1076.

14. AARC Clinical Practice Guideline. Endotracheal suctioning of mechanically ventilated patients with artificial airways 2010. Respir Care 2010; 55:758–764.

15. Hagler DA, Traver GA. Endotracheal saline and suction catheters: sources of lower airways contamination. Am J Crit Care 1994; 3:444–447.

16. Holdiness MR. Clinical pharmacokinetics of N-acetylcysteine. Clin Pharmacokinet 1991; 20:123–134.

17. Gammon RB, Shin MS, Buchalter SE. Pulmonary barotrauma in mechanical ventilation. Chest 1992; 102:568–572.

18. Marcy TW. Barotrauma: detection, recognition, and management. Chest 1993; 104:578–584.

19. Tocino IM, Miller MH, Fairfax WR. Distribution of pneumothorax in the supine and semirecumbent critically ill adult. Am J Radiol 1985; 144:901–905.

20. Kam AC, O'Brien M, Kam PCA. Pleural drainage systems. Anesthesia 1993; 48:154–161.

21. Marini JJ. Dynamic hyperinflation and auto-positive end expiratory pressure. Am J Respir Crit Care Med 2011; 184:756–762.

22. Blanch L, Bernabe F, Lucangelo U. Measurement of air trapping, intrinsic positive end-expiratory pressure, and dynamic hyperinflation in mechanically ventilated patients. Respir Care 2005; 50:110–123.

23. Shapiro JM. Management of respiratory failure in status asthmaticus. Am J Respir Med 2002; 1:409–416.

24. Hough CL, Kallet RH, Ranieri M, et al. Intrinsic positive end-expiratory pressure in Acute Respiratory Distress Syndrome (ARDS) Network subjects. Crit Care Med 2005; 33:527–532.

25. Tobin MJ, Lodato RF. PEEP, auto-PEEP, and waterfalls. Chest 1989; 96:449–451

Chapter 22

Discontinuing Mechanical Ventilation

This chapter describes the process of removing patients from mechanical ventilation (also called *weaning* from mechanical ventilation), and the difficulties that can occur during the transition to unassisted breathing (1-4).

I. READINESS EVALUATION

The management of ventilator-dependent patients should include a daily evaluation for signs that ventilatory support may no longer be necessary. A checklist of the items in this evaluation is shown in Table 22.1.

A. Weaning Parameters

1. When the conditions in Table 22.1 are all present, the patient is removed from the ventilator briefly (for 1–2 minutes) to obtain the measurements listed in Table 22.2. These are called "weaning parameters", and they are used to predict the likelihood of success or failure in the transition to unassisted breathing.

2. Note the wide range of likelihood ratios in Table 22.1, which indicates that each of the weaning parameters can have a poor predictor value in individual patients. As a result, the emerging consensus is that weaning parameters are not necessary, and trials of spontaneous, unassisted breathing can begin when the readiness criteria in Table 22.1 are satisfied.

Table 22.1	Checklist for a Trial of Spontaneous Breathing

Respiratory Criteria:

☑ PaO_2/FiO_2 >150–200 mm Hg with FiO_2 ≤50% and PEEP ≤8 cm H_2O.

☑ $PaCO_2$ normal or at baseline levels.

☑ Patient is able to initiate an inspiratory effort.

Cardiovascular Criteria:

☑ No evidence of myocardial ischemia.

☑ Heart rate ≤140 beats/minute.

☑ Blood pressure adequate with minimal or no vasopressors.

Appropriate Mental Status:

☑ Patient is arousable, or Glasgow Coma Score ≥13.

Absence of Correctible Comorbid Conditions:

☑ No fever or uncontrolled sepsis.

☑ No troublesome electrolyte abnormalities.

From References 1 and 2.

Table 22.2	Measurements Used to Predict a Successful Trial of Spontaneous Breathing	
Measurement	**Threshold for Success**	**Likelihood Ratios[§]**
Tidal Volume (V_T)	4 – 6 mL/kg	0.7 – 3.8
Respiratory Rate (RR)	30 – 38 bpm	1.0 – 3.8
RR/V_T Ratio	60 – 105 bpm/L	0.8 – 4.7
Maximum Inspiratory Pressure (PI_{max})	-15 to -30 cm H_2O	0 – 3.2

[§]The likelihood ratio is the likelihood that the measurement will predict success, divided by the likelihood that the measurement will predict failure. From Reference 2.

II. SPONTANEOUS BREATHING TRIAL

The traditional approach to discontinuing mechanical ventilation emphasizes a gradual reduction in ventilatory support (over hours to days), and this creates unnecessary delays in removing ventilatory support for patients who are capable of unassisted breathing. (This delayed approach is evident in the practice of placing patients back on a ventilator at night to "rest them".) In contrast, spontaneous breathing trials (SBTs) are conducted with no ventilatory support, so that patients capable of unassisted breathing can be identified quickly. There are two methods for conducting an SBT, as described next.

A. Using the Ventilator Circuit

SBTs are often conducted while the patient breathes through the ventilator circuit.

1. The advantage of this method is the ability to monitor the patient's tidal volume (V_T) and respiratory rate (RR), which allows for the early detection of rapid, shallow breathing (indicated by an increase in the RR/V_T ratio), which is a sign of ventilatory failure (5).

2. The drawback of this method is the resistance to breathing through the ventilator tubing, and the work involved in opening a valve on the ventilator to receive inhaled O_2.

3. Low-level *pressure support ventilation* (5 cm H_2O) is used to counteract the resistance to breathing through the ventilator circuit, but does not augment the patient's tidal volume. (For a description of pressure support ventilation, see Chapter 19, Section IV.)

B. Disconnecting the Ventilator

SBTs can also be conducted when the patient is disconnected from the ventilator.

1. This method employs a simple circuit design, which is illustrated in Figure 22.1. A source of O_2 (usually from a wall outlet) is delivered to the patient at a high flow rate (higher than the patient's inspiratory flow rate).

2. The high flow rate in this circuit achieves 3 goals: (a) it promotes comfortable breathing in patients with increased ventilatory demands, (b) it prevents the patient from inhaling low O_2 gas from the expiratory limb of the circuit, and (c) it carries exhaled CO_2 away from the patient, and thereby prevents CO_2 rebreathing.

3. Because the breathing circuit employs a T-shaped adapter, this type of SBT is also known as a *T-piece weaning trial*.

4. The major disadvantage of the T-piece weaning trials is the inability to monitor the patient's tidal volume and respiratory rate.

C. Which Method is Preferred?

There is no evidence of superiority for either method of spontaneous breathing (3). However, T-piece weaning trials are favored because they more closely approximate the conditions after extubation (6).

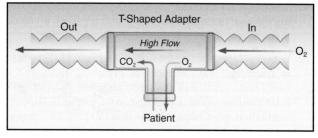

FIGURE 22.1 The design of the breathing circuit for spontaneous breathing trials while totally disconnected from the ventilator (also called *T-piece weaning* because of the T-shaped adapter in the circuit). See text for further explanation.

D. Success vs. Failure

A majority of patients (~ 80%) who tolerate SBTs for 2 hours can be permanently removed from the ventilator (1,2). Failure to tolerate spontaneous breathing is usually signaled by one or more of the following:

1. Signs of respiratory distress; e.g., agitation, rapid breathing, and use of accessory muscles of respiration.

2. Signs of respiratory muscle weakness; e.g., paradoxical inward movement of the abdominal wall during inspiration.

3. Progressive hypoxemia or hypercapnia.

E. Rapid Breathing

Rapid breathing during SBTs can be the result of anxiety rather than ventilatory failure (7). This is an important distinction because it is possible to manage anxiety without terminating the SBT trial (see later).

1. **Tidal Volumes**

   Monitoring the tidal volume can be useful in distinguishing anxiety from ventilatory failure; i.e., anxiety produces *hyperventilation*, which is characterized by an increase in the respiratory rate and an unchanged or increased tidal volume, whereas ventilatory failure is typically associated with rapid, shallow breathing (i.e., the respiratory rate is increased but the tidal volume is decreased) (5). Therefore, *rapid breathing without an associated decrease in tidal volume can represent anxiety, and not ventilatory failure.*

2. **Using Opiates**

   If anxiety is suspected as the cause of rapid breathing, administration of an anxiolytic agent should be considered, rather than terminating the SBT. Opiates can be useful in this setting because they are particularly effective in curbing the sensation of dyspnea (8). Contrary to the pervasive fear of opiate use in COPD, opiates have been used safely for the relief of dyspnea in patients with advanced COPD (8).

III. FAILURE OF SPONTANEOUS BREATHING

Factors other than intrinsic pulmonary disease can contribute to a failed trial of spontaneous breathing, and the principal ones are described next.

A. Acute Cardiac Dysfunction

1. Cardiac dysfunction can develop during a trial of spontaneous breathing (9), and can contribute to failed weaning trials by promoting pulmonary congestion, and decreasing the strength of diaphragmatic contractions (10). *Acute cardiac dysfunction has been identified in 40% of failed weaning trials* (11).

2. Potential sources of cardiac dysfunction in this situation include: (a) negative intrathoracic pressure, which increases left ventricular afterload (9), (b) hyperinflation and intrinsic PEEP from rapid breathing, which increases right ventricular afterload, and (c) silent myocardial ischemia (12).

3. Monitoring

   In addition to cardiac ultrasound, the following methods can be used to detect cardiac dysfunction in patients who fail spontaneous breathing trials.

   a. VENOUS O_2 SATURATION: Monitoring the mixed venous O_2 saturation (SvO_2) has been used to detect changes in cardiac output during trials of spontaneous breathing (13). The central venous O_2 saturation ($ScvO_2$) is a suitable alternative to SvO_2, and is more easily monitored. (The SvO_2 and $ScvO_2$ are described in Chapter 6, Sections I-E and I-F.)

b. β-TYPE NATRIURETIC PEPTIDE: Clinical studies have shown that plasma levels of β-type natriuretic peptide (BNP) are significantly increased when cardiac dysfunction develops during SBTs (11), and further, that increased BNP levels are associated with failure to sustain spontaneous breathing (14). Therefore, monitoring BNP levels can be useful in patients who are failing SBTs. (See Chapter 8, Section II-A for more information on plasma BNP levels in acute heart failure.)

4. **Management**

Weaning-induced cardiac dysfunction has been treated with *furosemide* (guided by plasma BNP levels in some studies), intravenous *nitroglycerin* (when systolic blood pressure is elevated), and a phosphodiesterase inhibitor (*enoximone*) (9). In most cases, this treatment improves the chances of discontinuing ventilatory support (9).

B. Respiratory Muscle Weakness

Respiratory muscle weakness is a common concern in patients who fail repeated attempts to wean from mechanical ventilation, but the prevalence of muscle weakness as a cause of failed wean attempts is unclear.

1. **Predisposing Conditions**

Potential sources of respiratory muscle weakness include controlled mechanical ventilation (especially during neuromuscular paralysis), electrolyte depletion (magnesium and phosphorous), prolonged steroid therapy, and *critical illness neuromyopathy*. This latter condition is an inflammatory-mediated polyneuropathy and/or myopathy that typically appears in patients with septic shock and multiorgan failure, and is recognized when patients fail to wean from mechanical ventilation (15). A more detailed description of this conditions is included in Chapter 41, Section II-C.

2. **Monitoring**

The standard measure of respiratory muscle strength in the ICU is the *maximum inspiratory pressure* (PI_{max}), which is the negative pressure generated by a maximum inspiratory effort against a closed airway (16,17).

a. The normal values of PI_{max} can vary widely, but mean values of -120 cm H_2O and -84 cm H_2O have been reported for adult men and women, respectively (17).

b. Spontaneous breathing is threatened, and acute CO_2 retention is a risk, when the PI_{max} drops below -30 cm H_2O (see Table 22.2).

IV. EXTUBATION

When there is evidence that mechanical ventilation is no longer necessary, the next step is to remove the artificial airway. This section focuses on the removal of endotracheal tubes (*extubation*), and the problem of postextubation laryngeal edema.

A. Airway Protection

Prior to extubation, the strength of the gag and cough reflexes should be checked to determine the patient's ability to protect the airways from aspirated secretions and food particles.

1. Cough strength can be assessed by holding a piece of paper 1–2 cm from the end of the endotracheal tube and asking the patient to cough. If wetness appears on the paper, the cough strength is considered adequate (18).

2. Diminished strength or even absence of cough or gag reflexes does not prevent extubation, but identifies patients who need special precautions to prevent aspiration.

B. Postextubation Laryngeal Edema

As many as 10% of extubations are followed by signs of respiratory insufficiency that mandates reintubation (19). Most reintubations are the result of traumatic laryngeal edema from the endotracheal tube, which has a reported incidence of 1.5% to 26.3% (19). Contributing factors include difficult or prolonged intubation, endotracheal tube size, and self-extubations.

1. Cuff-Leak Test

   The cuff leak test is performed prior to extubation, and is used to evaluate the risk of symptomatic laryngeal edema following extubation.

   a. To perform the test, the cuff on the endotracheal tube is deflated, and the volume of inhaled gas that leaks out through the larynx is determined (by comparing the inspiratory and expiratory tidal volumes). The lower the volume of the leak, the greater the risk of postextubation laryngeal edema.

   b. One problem with the cuff leak test is the lack of a standard cutoff value for the leak volume that identifies a high risk of postextubation laryngeal edema. Cutoff values have varied from 90 mL to 140 mL in individual studies (19).

   c. Another problem with this test is the positive predictive value, which is below 15% in several studies (19). This indicates that *the cuff leak test is unable to identify patients with a high risk of postextubation laryngeal edema.*

   d. Considering the above problems, avoiding the cuff leak test seems appropriate.

2. **Pretreatment with Steroids**

   At least four clinical studies have shown that pretreatment with steroids, starting 12–24 hours prior to extubation, can reduce the incidence of clinically significant laryngeal edema after extubation (19). The effective steroid regimens in two of these studies are listed below.

   a. *Methylprednisolone*: 20 mg IV every 4 hours, starting 12 hours before extubation (total of 4 doses) (20).

   b. *Dexamethasone:* 5 mg IV every 6 hours, starting 24 hours prior to extubation (total of 4 doses) (21).

3. **Clinical Detection**

   Laryngeal edema produces "noisy breathing" (called *stridor*) when the airway narrowing exceeds 50% (19). The sound is much more pronounced during inspiration (because the negative intrathoracic pressure during inspiration is transmitted to the larynx, and causes slight narrowing of the airway). When stridor develops, it's apparent within 30 minutes of extubation in a majority (80%) of cases (18).

4. **Management**

   If postextubation stridor is accompanied by signs of respiratory insufficiency, immediate reintubation is required. Otherwise, the following measures can be considered.

   a. AEROSOLIZED EPINEPHRINE: Inhalation of an epinephrine aerosol (2.5 mL of 1% epinephrine) is used to promote vasoconstriction and thereby reduce laryngeal edema (19). However, this is an unproven practice in adults.

   b. STEROIDS: Postextubation corticosteroids are recommended for laryngeal edema (19), even though this has not been studied. The preventive steroid regimens mentioned earlier (e.g., dexamethasone, 5 mg IV every 6 hrs for 24 hrs) have been suggested for this purpose (19).

5. **Noninvasive Ventilation**

Noninvasive ventilation (described in Chapter 20, Section II) does NOT reduce the reintubation rate in patients with postextubation respiratory failure (22), and thus is not advised (19).

REFERENCES

1. MacIntyre NR, Cook DJ, Ely EW Jr, et al. Evidence-based guidelines for weaning and discontinuing ventilatory support: a collective task force facilitated by the American College of Chest Physicians, the American Association for Respiratory Care, and the American College of Critical Care Medicine. Chest 2001; 120(Suppl):375S–395S.

2. MacIntyre NR. Evidence-based assessments in the ventilator discontinuation process. Respir Care 2012; 57:1611–1618.

3. McConville JF, Kress JP. Weaning patients from the ventilator. New Engl J Med 2012; 367:2233–2239.

4. Thille AW, Cortes-Puch I, Esteban A. Weaning from the ventilator and extubation in ICU. Curr Opin Crit Care 2013; 19:57–64.

5. Kreiger BP, Isber J, Breitenbucher A, et al. Serial measurements of the rapid-shallow breathing index as a predictor of weaning outcome in elderly medical patients. Chest 1997; 112:1029–1034.

6. Perren A, Brochard L. Managing the apparent and hidden difficulties in weaning from mechanical ventilation. Intensive Care Med 2013; 39:1885–1895.

7. Bouley GH, Froman R, Shah H. The experience of dyspnea during weaning. Heart Lung 1992; 21:471–476.

8. Raghavan N, Webb K, Amornputtisathaporn N, O'Donnell DE. Recent advances in pharmacotherapy for dyspnea in COPD. Curr Opin Pharmacol 2011; 11:204–210.

9. Teboul J-L. Weaning-induced cardiac dysfunction: where are we today. Intensive Care Med 2014; 40:1069–1079.

10. Nishimura Y, Maeda H, Tanaka K, et al. Respiratory muscle strength and hemodynamics in heart failure. Chest 1994; 105:355–359.

11. Grasso S, Leone A, De Michele M, et al. Use of N-terminal pro-brain natriuretic peptide to detect acute cardiac dysfunction during weaning failure in difficult-to-wean patients with chronic obstructive pulmonary disease. Crit Care Med 2007; 35:96–105.

12. Srivastava S, Chatila W, Amoateng-Adjepong Y, et al. Myocardial ischemia and weaning failure in patients with coronary artery disease: an update. Crit Care Med 1999; 27:2109–2112.

13. Jubran A, Mathru M, Dries D, Tobin MJ. Continuous recordings of mixed venous oxygen saturation during weaning from mechanical ventilation and the ramifications thereof. Am Rev Respir Crit Care Med 1998; 158:1763–1769.

14. Zapata L, Vera P, Roglan A, et al. β-type natriuretic peptides for prediction and diagnosis of weaning failure from cardiac origin. Intensive Care Med 2011; 37:477–485.

15. Hudson LD, Lee CM. Neuromuscular sequelae of critical illness. N Engl J Med 2003;348:745–747.

16. Mier-Jedrzejowicz A, Brophy C, Moxham J, Geen M. Assessment of diaphragm weakness. Am Rev Respir Dis 1988; 137:877–883.

17. Bruschi C, Cerveri I, Zoia MC, et al. Reference values for maximum respiratory mouth pressures: A population-based study. Am Rev Respir Dis 1992; 146:790–793.

18. Khamiees M, Raju P, DeGirolamo A, et al. Predictors of extubation outcome in patients who have successfully completed a spontaneous breathing trial. Chest 2001; 120:1262–1270.

19. Pluijms W, van Mook W, Wittekamp B, Bergmans D. Postextubation laryngeal edema and stridor resulting in respiratory failure in critically ill adult patients: updated review. Crit Care 2015; 19:295.

20. François B, Bellisant E, Gissot V, et al, for the Association des Réanimateurs du Centre-Quest (ARCO). 12-h pretreatment with methylprednisolone versus placebo for prevention of postextubation laryngeal oedema: a randomized double-blind trial. Lancet 2007; 369:1083–1089.

21. Lee CH, Peng MJ, Wu CL. Dexamethasone to prevent postextubation airway obstruction in adults: a prospective, randomized, double-blind, placebo-controlled study. Crit Care 2007; 11:R72.

22. Hess D. The role of noninvasive ventilation in the ventilator discontinuation process. Respir Care 2012; 57:1619–1625.

Chapter 23

Acid-Base Analysis

This chapter describes how to identify acid-base disorders using the pH, PCO_2 and bicarbonate (HCO_3) concentration in blood. Included are: (a) simple rules for the identification of primary, secondary, and mixed acid-base disorders, (b) formulas for determining the expected acid-base changes for each of the primary acid-base disorders, and (c) a description of the "anion gap" and how it is used.

I. ACID-BASE BALANCE

According to traditional concepts of acid-base physiology, the hydrogen ion (H^+) concentration in extracellular fluid is determined by the balance between the partial pressure of carbon dioxide (PCO_2) and the bicarbonate (HCO_3) concentration (1):

$$[H^+] = k \times (PCO_2/HCO_3) \qquad (23.1)$$

(k is a proportionality constant). This means that *all acid-base disorders are defined by two variables: PCO_2 and HCO_3.* This is shown in Table 23.1.

A. Types of Acid-Base Disorders

1. A *respiratory acid-base disorder* is a change in $[H^+]$ that is a direct result of a change in PCO_2. According to Equation 23.1, an increase in PCO_2 will increase the $[H^+]$ and produce a *respiratory acidosis*, while a decrease in PCO_2 will decrease the $[H^+]$ and produce a *respiratory alkalosis*.

2. A *metabolic acid-base disorder* is a change in $[H^+]$ that is a

direct result of a change in HCO_3. Equation 23.1 predicts that an increase in HCO_3 will decrease the $[H^+]$ and produce a *metabolic alkalosis*, while a decrease in HCO_3 will increase the $[H^+]$ and produce a *metabolic acidosis*.

3. Acid base disorders can be *primary* (the principal disturbance) or *secondary* (an additional disturbance).

Table 23.1	Acid-Base Disorders and Compensatory Responses	
$\Delta H^+ = \Delta PCO_2 / \Delta HCO_3$		
Acid-Base Disorder	Primary Change	Compensatory Response
Respiratory Acidosis	(↑ PCO_2)	(↑ HCO_3)
Respiratory Alkalosis	(↓ PCO_2)	(↓ HCO_3)
Metabolic Acidosis	(↓ HCO_3)	(↓ PCO_2)
Metabolic Alkalosis	(↑ HCO_3)	(↑ PCO_2)

B. Compensatory Responses

1. Compensatory responses are designed to limit the change in H^+ concentration produced by the primary acid-base disorder. This is accomplished by changing the secondary variable in the same direction as the primary variable (e.g., a primary increase in PCO_2 is accompanied by a compensatory increase in HCO_3), as shown in Table 23.1.

2. Compensatory responses do not completely correct the change in $[H^+]$ produced by the primary acid-base disorder (2).

3. The specific features of compensatory responses are described next. The equations that describe these responses are shown in Table 23.2.

C. Responses to Primary Metabolic Disorders

The response to a metabolic acid-base disorder involves a change in minute ventilation that is mediated by peripheral chemoreceptors in the carotid body, located at the carotid bifurcation in the neck.

1. **Response to Metabolic Acidosis**

   The compensatory response to metabolic acidosis is an increase in minute ventilation (tidal volume and respiratory rate) and a subsequent decrease in arterial PCO_2 ($PaCO_2$). This response appears in 30–120 minutes, and can take 12 to 24 hours to complete (2). The magnitude of the response is defined by the equation below (2).

$$\Delta\, PaCO_2 = 1.2 \times \Delta\, HCO_3 \qquad (23.2)$$

   Using a normal $PaCO_2$ of 40 mm Hg and a normal HCO_3 of 24 mEq/L, the above equation can be rewritten as follows:

$$\text{Expected } PaCO_2 = 40 - [1.2 \times (24 - HCO_3)] \qquad (23.3)$$

   a. EXAMPLE: For a primary metabolic acidosis with a plasma HCO_3 of 14 mEq/L, the ΔHCO_3 is 24 – 14 = 10 mEq/L, the $\Delta PaCO_2$ is 1.2 × 10 = 12 mm Hg, and the expected $PaCO_2$ is 40 – 12 = 28 mm Hg. If the measured $PaCO_2$ is >28 mm Hg, there is a secondary respiratory acidosis, and if the measured $PaCO_2$ is <28 mm Hg, there is a secondary respiratory alkalosis.

2. **Response to Metabolic Alkalosis**

   The compensatory response to metabolic alkalosis is a decrease in minute ventilation and a subsequent increase in $PaCO_2$. This response is not as vigorous as the response to metabolic acidosis (because the baseline activity of peripheral chemoreceptors is low, so they are easier to stimulate than inhibit). The magnitude of the response is defined by the equation below (2).

$$\Delta\, PaCO_2 \;=\; 0.7 \;\times\; \Delta\, HCO_3 \qquad (23.4)$$

Using a normal $PaCO_2$ of 40 mm Hg and a normal HCO_3 of 24 mEq/L, the above equation can be rewritten as follows:

$$\text{Expected } PaCO_2 = 40 + [0.7 \times (HCO_3 - 24)] \qquad (23.5)$$

a. EXAMPLE: For a metabolic alkalosis with a plasma HCO_3 of 40 mEq/L, the ΔHCO_3 is $40 - 24 = 16$ mEq/L, the $\Delta PaCO_2$ is $0.7 \times 16 = 11$ mm Hg, and the expected $PaCO_2$ is $40 + 11 = 51$ mm Hg.

Table 23.2	Equations for the Expected Response to Primary Acid-Base Disorders
Primary Disorder	**Compensatory Response**
Metabolic Acidosis	$\Delta PaCO_2 = 1.2 \times \Delta HCO_3$ Expected $PaCO_2 = 40 - [1.2 \times (24 - HCO_3)]$
Metabolic Alkalosis	$\Delta PaCO_2 = 0.7 \times \Delta HCO_3$ Expected $PaCO_2 = 40 + [0.7 \times (HCO_3 - 24)]$
Acute Respiratory Acidosis	$\Delta HCO_3 = 0.1 \times \Delta PaCO_2$ Expected $HCO_3 = 24 + [0.1 \times (PaCO_2 - 40)]$
Acute Respiratory Alkalosis	$\Delta HCO_3 = 0.2 \times \Delta PaCO_2$ Expected $HCO_3 = 24 - [0.2 \times (40 - PaCO_2)]$
Chronic Respiratory Acidosis	$\Delta HCO_3 = 0.4 \times \Delta PaCO_2$ Expected $HCO_3 = 24 + [0.4 \times (PaCO_2 - 40)]$
Chronic Respiratory Alkalosis	$\Delta HCO_3 = 0.4 \times \Delta PaCO_2$ Expected $HCO_3 = 24 - [0.4 \times (40 - PaCO_2)]$

From Reference 2.

D. Responses to Primary Respiratory Disorders

The compensatory response to changes in $PaCO_2$ occurs in the kidneys, where HCO_3 absorption in the proximal tubules is adjusted to produce the appropriate change in plasma HCO_3 (in the same direction as the change in $PaCO_2$). This renal response is relatively slow, and can take 2 or 3 days to reach completion. As a result, respiratory acid-base disorders are separated into acute and chronic disorders.

1. **Acute Respiratory Disorders**

   Acute changes in $PaCO_2$ are not accompanied by large changes in the plasma HCO_3, as demonstrated by the following equations (2).

   a. For acute respiratory acidosis:

   $$\Delta HCO_3 = 0.1 \times \Delta PaCO_2 \qquad (23.6)$$

   b. For acute respiratory alkalosis:

   $$\Delta HCO_3 = 0.2 \times \Delta PaCO_2 \qquad (23.7)$$

2. **Chronic Respiratory Disorders**

   The renal response to a chronic increase in $PaCO_2$ involves an increase in HCO_3 absorption in the proximal renal tubules, which increases the plasma HCO_3. The response to a chronic decrease in $PaCO_2$ is a decrease in renal HCO_3 absorption, which lowers the plasma HCO_3 concentration. The magnitude of this response is similar in chronic respiratory acidosis and chronic respiratory alkalosis, so the same formula can be used to describe the expected changes in both conditions.

   $$\Delta HCO_3 = 0.4 \times \Delta PaCO_2 \qquad (23.8)$$

Using a normal $PaCO_2$ of 40 mm Hg and a normal

HCO_3 of 24 mEq/L, the above equation can be rewritten as follows:

a. For chronic respiratory acidosis:

$$\text{Expected } HCO_3 = 24 + [0.4 \times (PaCO_2 - 40)] \quad (23.9)$$

b. For chronic respiratory alkalosis:

$$\text{Expected } HCO_3 = 24 - [0.4 \times (40 - PaCO_2)] \quad (23.10)$$

II. ACID-BASE EVALUATION

The following is a structured, rule-based approach to acid-base evaluations using the relationships between the $[H^+]$, PCO_2, and HCO_3 described in the previous section. The normal range of values for these variables are shown below.

$$pH = 7.36 - 7.44$$

$$PCO_2 = 36 - 44 \text{ mm Hg}$$

$$HCO_3 = 22 - 26 \text{ mEq/L}$$

Step 1: Identify Primary and Mixed Disorders

The first step in the evaluation focuses on the $PaCO_2$ and pH to identify primary and mixed acid-base disorders.

1. If the $PaCO_2$ and pH are both abnormal, compare the directional change.

   a. If the $PaCO_2$ and pH change in the same direction, there is a primary metabolic acid-base disorder (and the pH identifies whether it is an acidosis or alkalosis).

   b. If the $PaCO_2$ and pH change in opposite directions, there is a primary respiratory acid-base disorder.

c. EXAMPLE: Consider a case where the arterial pH is 7.23 and the $PaCO_2$ is 23 mm Hg. The pH and $PaCO_2$ are both decreased (indicating a primary metabolic disorder) and the pH is low (indicating an acidosis), so this represents a *primary metabolic acidosis*.

2. If only one variable (pH or $PaCO_2$) is abnormal, there is a mixed metabolic and respiratory disorder (of equivalent strength).

   a. If the $PaCO_2$ is abnormal, the directional change in $PaCO_2$ identifies the type of respiratory disorder, which then identifies the opposing metabolic disorder.

   b. If the pH is abnormal, the directional change in pH identifies the type of metabolic disorder (e.g., low pH indicates a metabolic acidosis) and the opposing respiratory disorder.

   c. EXAMPLE: Consider a case where the arterial pH is 7.38 and the $PaCO_2$ is 55 mm Hg. Only one variable (the $PaCO_2$) is abnormal, indicating a mixed metabolic and respiratory disorder. The $PaCO_2$ is elevated, indicating a respiratory acidosis, so the opposing metabolic disorder must be a metabolic alkalosis. Therefore, this condition is a *mixed respiratory acidosis and metabolic alkalosis*. Both disorders are equal in strength because the pH is normal.

Step 2: Identify Secondary Disorders

If the first step identified a primary disorder (instead of a mixed disorder), the next step is to calculate the expected acid-base changes using the equations in Table 23.2. The expected changes are then compared to the actual changes, and discrepancies between the two are used to identify secondary acid-base problems. This process is demonstrated in the following example.

1. EXAMPLE: Consider a case with the following arterial blood gas results: pH = 7.32, $PaCO_2$ = 23 mm Hg, HCO_3 = 16 mEq/L.

   a. This represents a primary metabolic acidosis because the pH and PCO_2 are both decreased.

   b. Equation 23.3 is then used to calculate the expected $PaCO_2$ from the compensatory response. The expected $PaCO_2$ is $40 - [1.2 \times (24 - 16)] = 30.4$ mm Hg.

   c. The expected and measured $PaCO_2$ are then compared. The measured $PaCO_2$ (23 mm Hg) is lower than the expected $PaCO_2$ (30.4 mm Hg), indicating a secondary respiratory alkalosis.

   d. Therefore, this case is a *primary metabolic acidosis with a secondary respiratory alkalosis.*

III. THE ANION GAP

The anion gap is a measure of the relative abundance of unmeasured anions in extracellular fluid, and can be useful in the evaluation of metabolic acidosis (6,7), as explained next.

A. Derivation

Electrochemical balance requires equal concentrations of negatively-charged anions and positively-charged cations in extracellular fluid. This balance is expressed in the equation below using the predominant anions and cations in plasma (sodium, chloride, and bicarbonate) as well as the unmeasured cations (UC) and unmeasured anions (UA).

$$Na + UC = CL + HCO_3 + UA \qquad (23.11)$$

Rearranging the terms in the above equation yields the following:

$$Na - (CL + HCO_3) = UA - UC \qquad (23.12)$$

1. The difference between unmeasured anions and unmeasured cations (UA – UC) is the anion gap (AG), so Equation 23.12 can be restated as:

$$AG = Na - (CL + HCO_3) \quad \text{(mEq/L)} \quad \quad (23.13)$$

The anion gap is thus a very simple calculation that involves routinely monitored electrolytes.

2. **Reference Range**

The reference range for the AG was originally 12±4 mEq/L (8–16 mEq/L) (7), but advances in automated electrolyte measurements led to a reduction in the reference range to *7±4 mEq/L* (3–11 mEq/L) (8). Unfortunately, this change is not universally recognized.

B. Using the Anion Gap

In the presence of a metabolic acidosis, an increase in the AG is evidence of an increase in strong (readily dissociated) acids in extracellular fluid, while a normal AG indicates that bicarbonate loss is the source of acidosis. The causes of metabolic acidosis can thus be separated into two groups, based on the AG, as shown in Table 23.3.

1. **High Anion Gap Acidosis**

Frequent sources of high AG metabolic acidosis include lactic acidosis, ketoacidosis, and end-stage renal failure (due to loss of H^+ secretion in the distal renal tubules). Other notable sources are toxic ingestions of methanol (which produces formic acid), ethylene glycol (which produces oxalic acid), and salicylates (which produce salicylic acid) (9).

2. **Normal Anion Gap Acidosis**

Common causes of metabolic acidosis with a normal AG include diarrhea (especially secretory diarrhea), isotonic saline infusion (see Chapter 10, Section I-B-3), and early renal failure (due to loss of HCO_3 reabsorption in the proximal tubules). The HCO_3 loss in these conditions is replaced by chloride for electrical neutrality, and the term *hyperchloremic metabolic acidosis* is also used for this type of metabolic acidosis. (In high AG metabolic acidoses, the acids dissociate and generate anions that balance the decrease in HCO_3, so there is no associated hyperchloremia.)

Table 23.3	Causes of Metabolic Acidosis, According to the Anion Gap (AG)
High AG	**Normal AG**
Lactic Acidosis	Diarrhea
Ketoacidosis	Isotonic saline infusion
End-stage renal failure	Early renal insufficiency
Methanol ingestion	Renal tubular acidosis
Ethylene glycol ingestion	Acetazolamide
Salicylate toxicity	Ureteroenterostomy

C. Reliability

The reliability of the anion gap for detecting strong acids has been inconsistent, and there are a number of reports showing a normal AG in patients with lactic acidosis (10,11) and ketoacidosis (see Reference 21 in Chapter 24).

1. **Correctable Factors**

   There are two correctable factors that limit the sensitivity of the AG.

   a. One factor is the continued use of the original, higher reference range for the AG, which substantially reduces the sensitivity of the AG for detecting lactic acidosis when compared to the lower, more current reference range (12).

b. The other factor is the ability of hypoalbuminemia to decrease the AG (13), which is described next.

Table 23.4	Determinants of the Anion Gap	
Unmeasured Anions	**Unmeasured Cations**	
Albumin (15 mEq/L)	Calcium (5 mEq/L)	
Organic Acids (5 mEq/L)	Potassium (4.5 mEq/L)	
Phosphate (2 mEq/L)		
Sulfate (1 mEq/L)	Magnesium (1.5 mEq/L)	
Total UA: (23 mEq/L)	Total UC: (11 mEq/L)	
Anion Gap = UA − UC = 12 mEq/L		

2. **Influence of Albumin**

The unmeasured anions and cations that normally contribute to the anion gap are shown in Table 23.4. Note that *albumin is the principal unmeasured anion, and the principal determinant of the anion gap.*

a. Albumin is a weak acid that contributes about 3 mEq/L to the AG for each 1 g/dL of albumin in plasma (at a normal pH) (3).

b. Hypoalbuminemia lowers the AG, and this could hinder or prevent an increase in AG in metabolic acidoses caused by the accumulation of strong acids. Considering that hypoalbuminemia is present in as many as 90% of ICU patients (13), the influence of albumin on the AG cannot be ignored.

c. The AG can be adjusted for low albumin levels by using the following formula for the corrected anion gap (AGc).

$$AGc = AG + [2.5 \times (4.5 - \text{Plasma Albumin in g/dL})] \quad (23.14)$$

(4.5 represents the normal concentration of albumin in plasma). The corrected AG has shown an improved diagnostic performance in critically ill patients (14).

REFERENCES

1. Adrogue HJ, Gennari J, Gala JH, Madias NE. Assessing acid-base disorders. Kidney Int 2009; 76:1239–1247.

2. Adrogue HJ, Madias NE. Secondary responses to altered acid-base status: The rules of engagement. J Am Soc Nephrol 2010; 21:920–923.

3. Kellum JA. Disorders of acid-base balance. Crit Care Med 2007; 35:2630–2636.

4. Whittier WL, Rutecki GW. Primer on clinical acid-base problem solving. Dis Mon 2004; 50:117–162.

5. Fencl V, Leith DE. Stewart's quantitative acid-base chemistry: applications in biology and medicine. Respir Physiol 1993; 91:1–16.

6. Narins RG, Emmett M. Simple and mixed acid-base disorders: a practical approach. Medicine 1980; 59:161–187.

7. Emmet M, Narins RG. Clinical use of the anion gap. Medicine 1977; 56:38–54.

8. Winter SD, Pearson JR, Gabow PA, et al. The fall of the serum anion gap. Arch Intern Med 1990;150:311–313.

9. Judge BS. Metabolic acidosis: differentiating the causes in the poisoned patient. Med Clin N Am 2005; 89:1107–1124.

10. Iberti TS, Liebowitz AB, Papadakos PJ, et al. Low sensitivity of the anion gap as a screen to detect hyperlactatemia in critically ill patients. Crit Care Med 1990; 18:275–277.

11. Schwartz-Goldstein B, Malik AR, Sarwar A, Brandtsetter RD. Lactic acidosis associated with a normal anion gap. Heart Lung 1996; 25:79–80.

12. Adams BD, Bonzani TA, Hunter CJ. The anion gap does not accurately screen for lactic acidosis in emergency department patients. Emerg Med J 2006; 23:179–182.

13. Figge J, Jabor A, Kazda A, Fencl V. Anion gap and hypoalbuminemia. Crit Care Med 1998; 26:1807–1810.

14. Mallat J, Barrailler S, Lemyze M, et al. Use of sodium chloride difference and corrected anion gap as surrogates of Stewart variables in critically ill patients. PLoS ONE 2013; 8:e56635.

Chapter 24

Organic Acidoses

This chapter describes two clinical disorders that involve excessive production of organic (carbon-based) acids by intermediary metabolism. Both of these disorders, lactic acidosis and ketoacidosis, can be adaptive processes in the right setting, but are pathological processes in the ICU setting.

I. LACTIC ACIDOSIS

Lactic acidosis is probably the most concerning of all metabolic acidoses, but the source of the concern is not the acidosis, but the condition that is responsible for the acidosis.

A. Responsible Conditions

(*Note*: Because the pertinent issues in lactic acidosis are often related to the lactate level rather than the acidosis, the term hyperlactatemia will be used interchangeably with lactic acidosis.) Several conditions can be responsible for hyperlactatemia, as shown in Table 24.1. The most prevalent of these conditions are sepsis and the clinical shock syndromes (i.e., hypovolemic, cardiogenic, and septic shock).

1. **Clinical Shock Syndromes**

    Hyperlactatemia is universal in the clinical shock syndromes (since it is required for the diagnosis) and the prognosis in these conditions is related to the severity of the lactate elevation, and the time required for the lactate levels to normalize (lactate clearance). These relationships are demonstrated in Figure 6.2 (Chapter 6).

Table 24.1	Sources of Hyperlactatemia in the ICU
Inflammatory:	sepsis
Shock syndrome:	hypovolemic, cardiogenic, septic
Drugs:	antiretroviral agents, β_2 agonists, epinephrine, linezolid, metformin, nitroprusside, propofol, salicylates
Toxins:	carbon monoxide, cyanide, propylene glycol
Nutritional:	thiamine deficiency
Others:	alkalosis (severe), fulminant hepatic failure, seizure

2. Sepsis

   Serum lactate levels have the same diagnostic and prognostic significance in sepsis as they do in in the shock syndromes. The lactic acidosis in sepsis is not the result of inadequate tissue oxygenation (see Chapter 6, Section III-F), which has important implications for the traditional emphasis on promoting tissue oxygenation in patients with lactic acidosis.

3. Thiamine Deficiency

   Thiamine deficiency is often overlooked as a cause of elevated blood lactate levels. Thiamine is a cofactor for pyruvate dehydrogenase (the enzyme that converts pyruvate to acetyl coenzyme A, and limits conversion to lactate), and thiamine deficiency can result in severe lactic acidosis (2). (See Chapter 36, Section III-A for more information on thiamine deficiency.)

4. Drugs

   A variety of drugs can produce hyperlactatemia, as indicated in Table 24.1. Most cases are due to an impaired oxidative metabolism, but epinephrine and high-dose β_2

agonists promote hyperlactatemia by increasing the production of pyruvate (1).

a. METFORMIN: Metformin is an oral hypoglycemic agent that produces lactic acidosis during therapeutic dosing. The mechanism is unclear, and it occurs primarily in patients with renal insufficiency (3). The lactic acidosis can be severe, with a mortality rate that exceeds 45% if untreated (3,4). Plasma metformin levels are not routinely available, and the diagnosis is based on excluding other causes of lactic acidosis. The preferred treatment is hemodialysis (3,4).

5. **Propylene Glycol**

   Propylene glycol is used as a solvent in intravenous preparations of lorazepam, diazepam, esmolol, nitroglycerin, and phenytoin. It is metabolized primarily in the liver, and the principal metabolites are lactate and pyruvate (5).

   a. Propylene glycol toxicity (i.e., agitation, coma, seizures, hypotension, and lactic acidosis) has been reported in 19–66% of patients receiving *high-dose IV lorazepam infusions for more than 48 hours* (5,6).

   b. The diagnosis can be elusive. There is an assay for propylene glycol in blood, but the acceptable range has not been determined.

   c. Prolonged infusions of lorazepam should be avoided. (In fact, prolonged infusions of any benzodiazepine should be avoided because these drugs accumulate in the brain and produce excessive and prolonged sedation.)

6. **Other Notable Conditions**

   a. Generalized seizures can produce marked increases in serum lactate levels, but this is a hypermetabolic effect, and it resolves quickly after the seizures subside (7).

b. The liver is responsible for 70% of lactate clearance. Hyperlactatemia is common in acute, fulminant liver failure (1), but is not a frequent finding in chronic liver failure unless there is a coexisting condition that increases lactate production (e.g., sepsis) (1).

B. Diagnostic Considerations

1. Serum lactate levels are readily available, and screening tests for lactic acidosis, such as the anion gap, are not necessary (and can be unreliable, as described in Chapter 23, Section III-C).

2. Lactate levels can be measured in venous or arterial blood, with equivalent results (1).

3. The upper limit of normal for serum lactate varies from 1.0 to 2.2 mmol/L in individual laboratories (1), but 2 mmol/L seems to be a common cutoff point. However, lactate levels must rise above 4 mmol/L to show an association with increased mortality (8), so a cutoff of 4 mmol/L may be more appropriate for clinically significant hyperlactatemia.

C. Alkali Therapy

Therapy aimed at correcting the acidosis does not have a major role in the management of patients with lactic acidosis. The following is a brief summary of the relevant issues in alkali therapy for lactic acidosis.

1. **The Bicarbonate Experience**

   Clinical studies have consistently shown that sodium bicarbonate infusions are without hemodynamic benefit or survival benefit in lactic acidosis (9-11). Furthermore, bicarbonate infusions are accompanied by several undesirable effects (see Table 24.2), including an increase in arterial PCO_2 and a paradoxical *decrease in intracellular pH* (attributed to transcellular movement of the generated CO_2) (9,12).

Table 24.2	Bicarbonate Replacement
7.5% NaHCO₃	**Undesirable Effects†**
Na: 0.9 mEq/L	↑ Arterial PCO_2
HCO₃: 0.9 mEq/L	↓ Intracellular pH
PCO₂: >200 mm Hg	↓ Ionized calcium
pH: 8.0	↑ Serum lactate
Osmolality: 1,461 mosm/kg	

†From References 9–12.

2. **Current Recommendations**

Given the lack of benefit, and the associated risk, bicarbonate therapy is not recommended as a treatment modality in lactic acidosis (9,13). Furthermore, bicarbonate therapy has been removed from the ACLS guidelines on cardiac arrest (14). Nevertheless, there continue to be recommendations for bicarbonate therapy in cases of severe acidosis, when the pH falls below 7.0 (15). The current use of bicarbonate is predominantly as a "desperation measure" to restore vasopressor responsiveness in patients who are rapidly deteriorating.

3. **Replacement Regimen**

The popular fluid for bicarbonate replacement is a 7.5% sodium bicarbonate solution, and Table 24.2 shows the composition of this fluid. Note the hyperosmolality (which mandates infusion through a large vein) and the extremely high PCO_2 (which explains the increase in arterial PCO_2 associated with bicarbonate infusions).

a. The bicarbonate dose is determined by estimating

the HCO$_3$ deficit with the following equation (15,16).

$$HCO_3 \text{ deficit } = 0.6 \times wt \text{ (kg)} \times (15 - \text{plasma HCO}_3) \quad (24.1)$$

where wt is ideal body weight, and 15 mEq/L is the desired plasma HCO$_3$. (For an adult with an ideal body weight of 70 kg and a plasma HCO$_3$ of 10 mEq/L, the HCO$_3$ deficit is $0.6 \times 70 \times (15 - 10) = 210$ mEq.)

b. The HCO$_3$ deficit can be replaced at a rate of 1 mEq/kg per hour (11). The PaCO$_2$ should be monitored during bicarbonate infusions, and increases in the PaCO$_2$ should be corrected by adjusting the ventilator settings to provide an increased minute ventilation.

c. If there is no hemodynamic or clinical improvement after a few hours, the bicarbonate infusion should be discontinued.

II. DIABETIC KETOACIDOSIS

When glucose movement into cells is impaired, adipose tissue releases free fatty acids that are taken up in the liver and metabolized to ketones that can be used as oxidative fuels. These ketones include acetone, acetoacetate (AcAc) and β-hydroxybutyrate (β-OHB).

A. Ketoacids

AcAc and β-OHB are strong acids (ketoacids), and plasma concentrations above 3 mmol/L produce a metabolic acidosis (17). β-OHB is the predominant ketoacid (see Figure 24.1), and is about three times more abundant than AcAc. Acetone is not a ketoacid, but is responsible for the characteristic "fruity" odor of the breath in patients with ketoacidosis.

1. The Nitroprusside Reaction

The nitroprusside reaction is a popular, colorimetric

method for detecting ketones in blood and urine. The test can be performed with tablets (Acetest) or reagent strips (Ketostix, Labstix, Multistix).

a. THE PROBLEM: The nitroprusside reaction has one major shortcoming; i.e., it detects only acetone and AcAc, and *does not detect β-OHB (17), the predominant ketoacid in blood.* This limitation is illustrated in Figure 24.1. Note that, in alcoholic ketoacidosis, the total concentration of ketoacids in blood is 13 mmol/L (about 4 times the concentration that produces an acidosis), but the ketoacids will not be detected because the AcAc level is below the threshold for detection (3 mmol/L).

2. β-hydroxybutyrate Monitoring

Portable "ketone meters" are now available that provide reliable measurements of β-OHB in fingerstick (capil-

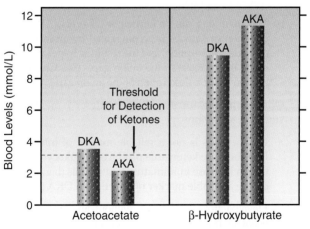

FIGURE 24.1 The concentrations of acetoacetate and β-hydroxybutyrate in the blood in diabetic ketoacidosis (DKA) and alcoholic ketoacidosis (AKA). The horizontal hatched line represents the threshold for a positive nitroprusside reaction.

lary) blood in about 10 seconds (18). The American Diabetes Association considers this the preferred method for monitoring ketoacidosis (19).

B. Clinical Features

1. According to the American Diabetes Association (ADA), diabetic ketoacidosis (DKA) has the following characteristics (19):

   a. Blood glucose >250 mg/dL.

   b. Plasma HCO_3 <18 mEq/L and plasma pH ≤7.3.

   c. Increased anion gap.

   d. Evidence of ketones in blood or urine.

2. The following are exceptions to the ADA criteria:

   a. The blood glucose is <250 mg/dL in about 20% of cases of DKA (20).

   b. The anion gap can be normal in DKA (21). The renal excretion of ketones is accompanied by an increase in chloride reabsorption, and the resulting hyperchloremia limits the increase in the anion gap. (See Chapter 23, Section III for a description of the anion gap.)

3. Other clinical features of DKA that deserve mention are summarized below.

   a. Leukocytosis is not a reliable marker of infection in DKA because ketonemia produces a leukocytosis (19), but an increase in immature neutrophils (band forms) can be a reliable marker of infection in DKA (22).

   b. Elevated troponin I levels without an acute coronary event has been reported in 27% of patients with DKA (23).

   c. Hyperamylasemia is common in DKA, but the amylase is extrapancreatic (19).

d. Dehydration is almost universal in DKA, but this may not be reflected in the plasma sodium concentration because hyperglycemia draws water from intracellular fluid, which causes a dilutional decrease in the serum sodium concentration, and this masks free-water loss (dehydration).

e. *The dilutional effect of hyperglycemia results in decrease in serum sodium of 1.6 to 2.4 mEq/L for every 100 mg/dL increase in the serum glucose concentration* (24,25).

C. Management

The management of DKA described here is based on the ADA guidelines (19).

1. **Intravenous Fluids**

   A protocol for intravenous fluid therapy in DKA is shown in Table 24.3. The following are some highlights of this protocol.

Table 24.3	Intravenous Fluid Protocol in Diabetic Ketoacidosis

1. Start with isotonic (0.9%) saline at 15–20 mL/kg/hr.
2. When BP stabilizes, reduce infusion rate to 4–14 mL/kg/hr and use 0.45% saline (if corrected serum Na^+ is normal or high) or 0.9% saline (if corrected serum Na^+ is low).
3. When the serum glucose falls to 250 mg/dL, change to 5% dextrose in 0.45% saline and infuse at 150–250 mL/hr.
4. Replace the volume deficit (50–100 mL/kg) in the first 24 hrs.

From the American Diabetes Association Guidelines (19).

a. Volume deficits in DKA average about 50 to 100 mL/kg, and fluid therapy begins with isotonic (0.9%)

saline at a rate of 15–20 mL/kg per hour (or 1–1.5 L/hr) until the patient is hemodynamically stable.

b. Note in Table 24.3 that the "corrected" serum sodium concentration is used to select the appropriate IV fluid after hemodynamic stability is achieved. This correction refers to the previously-described dilutional effect of hyperglycemia on the serum sodium concentration, which is 1.6 to 2.4 mEq/L for every 100 mg/dL increase in the serum glucose.

c. EXAMPLE: Using 2 mEq/L as the correction factor, if the sodium concentration is 140 mEq/L and the plasma glucose is 600 mg/dL, the dilutional effect is $2 \times 5 = 10$ mEq/L, so the corrected sodium concentration is $140 + 10 = 150$ mEq/L.

d. Note also in Table 24.3 that 5% dextrose is added to the IV fluids when the serum glucose falls to 250 mg/dL. This reduces the risk of hypoglycemia until food intake begins.

2. **Insulin**

A protocol for insulin therapy in DKA is shown in Table 24.4. The following are some highlights.

a. Note that insulin should not be started if the patient is hypokalemic (which is uncommon when DKA first presents).

b. Regular insulin is started with an IV bolus dose of 0.15 units/kg (some consider this unnecessary) followed by a continuous infusion at 0.1 units/kg/hr.

c. Insulin infusions are continued until the ketoacidosis has resolved (see later for how this is determined) and oral nutrient intake is possible. Thereafter, subcutaneous insulin is started as directed in Table 24.4.

d. Achieving euglycemia is never advised in the ICU setting because of the risk of hypoglycemia, and the goal of glycemic control is a serum glucose of 150–200 mg/dL (26).

Table 24.4	Insulin Protocol in Diabetic Ketoacidosis

1. Start insulin therapy if the serum K^+ is above 3.3 mEq/L.

2. Use regular insulin and give an IV bolus dose of 1–0.15 units/kg (if hypokalemia excluded), followed by a continuous infusion at 0.1 unit/kg/h.

3. Check serum glucose hourly. If serum glucose does not fall at least 50 mg/dL after 1 hour, double the infusion rate (0.2 units/kg/h).

4. Thereafter, adjust infusion rate, if necessary, so that serum glucose decreases by 50–75 mg/dL per hour.

5. When serum glucose falls to 250 mg/dL, decrease infusion rate to 0.05–0.1 units/kg/h, and add 5% dextrose to the infusate.

6. Maintain serum glucose at 150–200 mg/dL.

7. When ketoacidosis has resolved and oral fluids are tolerated, start subcutaneous insulin using the patient's prehospital regimen. For insulin-naive patients, start with 0.5–0.8 units/kg per day, in divided doses.

9. Continue insulin infusion for a few hours after the first subcutaneous dose.

From the American Diabetes Association Guidelines (19).

3. Potassium

   a. Potassium depletion is universal in DKA, with an average deficit of 3–5 mEq/kg (20), but the serum potassium is often normal (74% of patients) or elevated (22% of patients) when DKA presents (20).

   b. The serum potassium can fall precipitously during insulin therapy (transcellular shift), so potassium replacement should be started as soon as possible, and serum potassium levels should be monitored every 1–2 hours until levels stabilize. Adding potassium to the IV fluids, as indicated in Table 24.5, is usually effective in maintaining normokalemia (19).

Table 24.5	Potassium in Diabetic Ketoacidosis
Initial Serum K+	**Recommendations**
<3.3 mEq/L	Hold insulin infusion and give 40 mEq K+ per hour until serum K+ >3.3 mEq/L.
3.3–4.9 mEq/L	Add 20–30 mEq K+ to each liter of IV fluid to keep serum K+ at 4–5 mEq/L.
≥5 mEq/L	Check serum K+ every 2 hours.

From the American Diabetes Association Guidelines (19).

4. **Phosphate**

The situation with phosphate is very similar to potassium (i.e., depletion common but serum levels rarely low at presentation, and serum levels decline during insulin infusions) with one exception; i.e., routine phosphate replacement has no documented benefit in DKA, and is not recommended unless phosphate levels are <1 mg/dL (19,26).

5. **Alkali Therapy**

The recommendations for bicarbonate replacement in DKA are the same as those described earlier for lactic acidosis; i.e., bicarbonate therapy has no documented benefit in DKA, even when the acidosis is severe (pH 6.9–7.1) (27), and it is not recommended until the pH falls below 7.0 (19).

D. Acid-Base Monitoring

1. Resolution of DKA has been defined as a plasma

glucose <200 mg/dL, plasma HCO_3 ≥18 mEq/L, and venous pH >7.3 (19).

2. The HCO_3 and pH will be unreliable when isotonic (0.9%) saline is the predominant resuscitation fluid because the high chloride concentration in isotonic saline produces a hyperchloremic metabolic acidosis (see Chapter 10, Section I-B-3) that will counteract the increase in serum HCO_3 from the resolving ketoacidosis.

3. The *anion gap* should be a more reliable measure for monitoring the resolution of DKA.

III. ALCOHOLIC KETOACIDOSIS

Alcoholic ketoacidosis (AKA) is a sporadic disorder that occurs primarily in chronic alcoholics who binge drink (17,28).

A. Clinical Features

Clinical manifestations appear 1–3 days after a period of heavy, intense drinking.

1. Common manifestations include abdominal pain, vomiting, dehydration, and multiple electrolyte abnormalities (e.g., hypokalemia, hypomagnesemia, hypoglycemia, and hypophosphatemia).

2. The electrolyte abnormalities might explain why *as many as 10% of patients with AKA experience an unexpected cardiac arrest* (17).

B. Diagnosis

1. The diagnosis of AKA can be elusive because the *nitroprusside reaction for detecting ketones can be negative in AKA.* This is illustrated in Figure 24.1.

2. Figure 24.1 also shows that betahydroxybutyrate (β-OHB) is present in high concentrations in AKA (higher than DKA), so measuring the β-OHB level in blood should be a sensitive method for the detection of ketones in AKA.

C. Management

1. The management of AKA is notable for its simplicity; i.e., infusion of dextrose-containing saline solutions is usually all that is required. The glucose infusion slows hepatic ketone production, while the infused volume promotes the renal clearance of ketones.

2. Thiamine supplementation is recommended because glucose infusions can deplete marginal thiamine reserves.

3. The ketoacidosis usually resolves within 24 hours.

REFERENCES

1. Kraut JA, Madias NE. Lactic acidosis. N Engl J Med 2014; 371:2309–2319.

2. Campbell CH. The severe lactic acidosis of thiamine deficiency: acute, pernicious or fulminating beriberi. Lancet 1984; 1:446–449.

3. Seidowsky A, Nseir S, Houdret N, Fourrier F. Metformin-associated lactic acidosis: a prognostic and therapeutic study. Crit Care Med 2009; 37:2191–2196.

4. Perrone J, Phillips C, Gaieski D. Occult metformin toxicity in three patients with profound lactic acidosis. J Emerg Med 2011; 40:271–275.

5. Wilson KC, Reardon C, Theodore AC, Farber HW. Propylene glycol toxicity: a severe iatrogenic illness in ICU patients receiving IV benzodiazepines. Chest 2005; 128:1674–1681.

6. Arroglia A, Shehab N, McCarthy K, Gonzales JP. Relationship of continuous infusion lorazepam to serum propylene glycol con-

centration in critically ill adults. Crit Care Med 2004; 32:1709–1714.

7. Orringer CE, Eusace JC, Wunsch CD, Gardner LB. Natural history of lactic acidosis after grand-mal seizures. A model for the study of anion-gap acidoses not associated with hyperkalemia. N Engl J Med 1977; 297:796–781.

8. Okorie ON, Dellinger P. Lactate: biomarker and potential therapeutic target. Crit Care Clin 2011; 27:299–326.

9. Forsythe SM, Schmidt GA. Sodium bicarbonate for the treatment of lactic acidosis. Chest 2000; 117:260–267

10. Cooper DJ, Walley KR, Wiggs RR, et al. Bicarbonate does not improve hemodynamics in critically ill patients who have lactic acidosis: a prospective, controlled clinical study. Ann Intern Med 1990; 112:492–498.

11. Mathieu D, Neviere R, Billard V, et al. Effects of bicarbonate therapy on hemodynamics and tissue oxygenation in patients with lactic acidosis: A prospective, controlled clinical study. Crit Care Med 1991; 19:1352–1356.

12. Kimmoun A, Novy E, Auchet T, et al. Hemodynamic consequences of severe lactic acidosis in shock states: from bench to bedside. Crit Care 2015; 19:175.

13. Dellinger RP, Levy MM, Rhodes A, et al. Surviving Sepsis Campaign: International guidelines for management of severe sepsis and septic shock, 2012. Intensive Care Med 2013; 39:165–228.

14. Link MS, Berkow LC, Kudenchuk PJ, et al. Part 7: Adult advanced cardiovascular life support: 2015 American Heart Association Guidelines Update for Cardiopulmonary Resuscitation and Emergency Cardiovascular Care. Circulation. 2015; 132(Suppl 2):S444–S464.

15. Sabatini S, Kurtzman NA. Bicarbonate therapy in severe metabolic acidosis. J Am Soc Nephrol 2009; 20:692–695.

16. Rose BD, Post TW. Clinical physiology of acid-base and electrolyte disorders. 5th ed. New York: McGraw-Hill, 2001:630–632.

17. Cartwright MM, Hajja W, Al-Khatib S, et al. Toxigenic and metabolic causes of ketosis and ketoacidotic syndromes. Crit Care Clin 2012; 601–631.

18. Plüdderman A, Hemeghan C, Price C, et al. Point-of-care blood test for ketones in patients with diabetes: primary care diagnostic technology update. Br J Clin Pract 2011; 61:530–531.

19. American Diabetes Association. Hyperglycemic crisis in diabetes. Diabetes Care 2004; 27(Suppl):S94–S102.

20. Charfen MA, Fernandez-Frackelton M. Diabetic ketoacidosis. Emerg Med Clin N Am 2005; 23:609–628.

21. Gamblin GT, Ashburn RW, Kemp DG, Beuttel SC. Diabetic ketoacidosis presenting with a normal anion gap. Am J Med 1986; 80:758–760.

22. Slovis CM, Mork VG, Slovis RJ, Brain RP. Diabetic ketoacidosis and infection: leukocyte count and differential as early predictors of serious infection. Am J Emerg Med 1987; 5:1–5.

23. AlMallah M, Zuberi O, Arida M, Kim HE. Positive troponin in diabetic ketoacidosis without evident acute coronary syndrome predicts adverse cardiac events. Clin Cardiol 2008; 31:67–71.

24. Rose BD, Post TW. Hyperosmolal states: hyperglycemia. In: Clinical physiology of acid-base and electrolyte disorders. 5th ed. New York, NY: McGraw-Hill, 2001; 794–821.

25. Moran SM, Jamison RL. The variable hyponatremic response to hyperglycemia. West J Med 1985; 142:49–53.

26. Westerberg DP. Diabetic ketoacidosis: evaluation and treatment. Am Fam Physician 2013; 87:337–346.

27. Morris LR, Murphy MB, Kitabchi AE. Bicarbonate therapy in severe diabetic ketoacidosis. Ann Intern Med 1986; 105:836–840.

28. McGuire LC, Cruickshank AM, Munro PT. Alcoholic ketoacidosis. Emerg Med J 2006; 23:417–420.

Chapter 25

Metabolic Alkalosis

Metabolic acidosis gets all the headlines, but metabolic alkalosis is the most common acid-base disorder in hospitalized patients (1-3). The prevalence of metabolic alkalosis can be attributed to three factors: (a) common etiologies (e.g., diuretic therapy), (b) a tendency for the alkalosis to be sustained (thanks to chloride), and (c) failure to identify and correct the factors that maintain the alkalosis.

I. ORIGINS

Metabolic alkalosis is defined as an increase in the bicarbonate (HCO_3) concentration in extracellular fluid (plasma) that is not an adaptive response to hypercapnia. The normal range for the plasma HCO_3 is 22–26 mEq/L.

A. Pathogenesis

1. Metabolic alkalosis is usually the result of one of the following conditions (3):

   a. Loss of gastric acid from vomiting or nasogastric suction.

   b. Enhanced secretion of hydrogen ions (H^+) in the distal renal tubules (e.g., from diuretics or mineralocorticoid excess).

   c. Transcellular shift of H^+ as a result of hypokalemia.

   d. Loss of fluids that contain little or no HCO_3 (contraction alkalosis).

2. The normal response to metabolic alkalosis is an increase in the renal excretion of HCO_3. This response is reversed by chloride depletion and hypokalemia (3,4), and this helps to maintain a metabolic alkalosis.

   a. Chloride depletion promotes the renal retention of HCO_3 by increasing HCO_3 reabsorption, and inhibiting HCO_3 secretion, in the distal renal tubules. Both effects are mediated by a decrease in the luminal chloride concentration. The renal actions of *chloride depletion* are considered *the principal cause of sustained cases of metabolic alkalosis* (3,4).

   b. Hypokalemia has the same effects as chloride depletion (though the mechanisms differ).

B. Etiologies

The common conditions that precipitate and/or maintain a metabolic alkalosis are shown in Table 25.1, along with the mechanisms involved in each condition.

1. **Volume Loss**

   Loss of fluids that contain little or no HCO_3 is a well-known cause of metabolic alkalosis, and has been called *contraction alkalosis* because the assumed mechanism was a simple concentrating effect on the plasma HCO_3. However, *the real culprit is chloride depletion*, because the alkalosis is not corrected by replacing the fluid deficit unless the chloride deficit is also replaced (4).

2. **Loss of Gastric Secretions**

   Gastric secretions are rich in H^+ (50–100 mEq/L), CL^- (120–160 mEq/L), and, to a lesser extent, K^+ (10–15 mEq/L) (5). As a result, loss of gastric secretions (e.g., from nasogastric suction) creates multiple risks for metabolic alkalosis (i.e., loss of H^+, CL^-, K^+, and volume loss).

Table 25.1	Potential Sources of Metabolic Alkalosis in the ICU
Condition	**Mechanisms**
Volume Loss	• Chloride loss
Loss of Gastric Secretions	• Loss of H^+, CL^-, and K^+ • Volume loss
Diuretics†	• Loss of H^+, CL^-, and K^+ • Volume loss
Hypokalemia	• Transcellular H^+ flux • Increased H^+ loss in urine • Renal retention of HCO_3
Chloride Depletion	• Renal retention of HCO_3
Posthypercapnic Alkalosis	• $PaCO_2$ lower than expected
Massive Transfusion	• Administration of citrate (metabolized to HCO_3)

†Thiazides and "loop" diuretics (e.g., furosemide).

3. **Diuretics**

   Thiazide diuretics and "loop" diuretics like furosemide promote metabolic alkalosis via urinary losses of H^+, CL^-, K^+, and volume (1-3). Urinary chloride losses (chloruresis) match the sodium losses (natriuresis), and must be replaced to correct the alkalosis.

4. **Hypokalemia**

   Hypokalemia can precipitate a metabolic alkalosis (via transcellular shift of H^+) and also helps to maintain the alkalosis (by decreasing the renal excretion of HCO_3) (1-3).

5. **Chloride Depletion**

   As mentioned, chloride depletion helps to maintain the metabolic alkalosis by promoting renal HCO_3 retention.

6. **Posthypercapnic Alkalosis**

   Chronic CO_2 retention is associated with an increase in plasma HCO_3 (from enhanced HCO_3 reabsorption in the kidneys), and patients with chronic CO_2 retention who are placed on mechanical ventilation can experience an abrupt decrease in arterial PCO_2 from overventilation. In this situation, the plasma HCO_3 remains elevated and resembles a metabolic alkalosis. This condition is often sustained because of coexisting chloride depletion (3).

7. **Massive Transfusion**

   Each unit of packed red blood cells (PRBCs) contains about 17 mEq of citrate (used as an anticoagulant), which generates HCO_3 when metabolized. Transfusion of more than 8 units of PRBCs can produce a metabolic alkalosis (3).

8. **Others**

   Other causes of metabolic alkalosis include mineralocorticoid excess (primary hyperaldosteronism), hypercalcemia and milk-alkali syndrome (chronic ingestion of calcium carbonate-containing antacids that promote hypercalcemia), and laxative abuse.

II. CLINICAL MANIFESTATIONS

Metabolic alkalosis has remarkably few adverse effects.

A. Hypoventilation

1. Metabolic alkalosis produces respiratory depression and a subsequent increase in the arterial PCO_2 ($PaCO_2$). However, *this is not a vigorous response* (unlike the respi-

ratory stimulation produced by a metabolic acidosis) (6). The magnitude of the response is defined by the following equation (7):

$$\Delta PaCO_2 = 0.7 \times \Delta HCO_3 \qquad (25.1)$$

2. Using a normal $PaCO_2$ of 40 mm Hg, and a normal plasma HCO_3 of 24 mEq/L, the expected $PaCO_2$ can be calculated as follows:

$$\text{Expected } PaCO_2 = 40 + [0.7 \times (\text{plasma } HCO_3 - 24)] \qquad (25.2)$$

3. EXAMPLE: For a patient with a metabolic alkalosis and a plasma HCO_3 of 40 mEq/L, the ΔHCO_3 is 40 − 24 = 16 mEq/L, the $\Delta PaCO_2$ is 0.7 × 16 = 11.2 mm Hg, and the expected $PaCO_2$ is 40 + 11.2 = 51.2 mm Hg. This example demonstrates that a *considerable rise in plasma HCO_3 (to 40 mEq/L) is needed to produce significant hypercapnia* (i.e., $PaCO_2$ >50 mm Hg).

B. Oxyhemoglobin Dissociation Curve

Alkalosis shifts the oxyhemoglobin dissociation curve to the left (Bohr effect), which results in a decreased tendency for hemoglobin to release oxygen into the tissues.

1. When the O_2 extraction from capillary blood is constant, a leftward shift of the oxyhemoglobin dissociation curve results in a decrease in venous PO_2 (8), which typically indicates a decrease in tissue PO_2. However, there is no evidence of inadequate tissue oxygenation from this effect.

III. EVALUATION

The likely source(s) of metabolic alkalosis is usually apparent. In the rare case of uncertainty, the urinary chloride concentration can be informative, as described next.

A. Urinary Chloride

The urinary chloride concentration can be used to classify metabolic alkalosis as *chloride-responsive* or *chloride-resistant*; the conditions associated with each category are listed in Table 25.2.

Table 25.2	Classification of Metabolic Alkalosis	
Category	**Urine [CL⁻]**	**Conditions**
Chloride-Responsive	<15 mEq/L	Volume loss
		Vomiting, NG suction
		Loop diuretics
		Hypokalemia
		Chloride depletion
Chloride-Resistant	>25 mEq/L	Mineralocorticoid excess

1. **Chloride-Responsive Alkalosis**

   A chloride-responsive metabolic alkalosis is characterized by a low urinary chloride concentration (<15 mEq/L), indicating chloride depletion.

   a. This category includes all of the common causes of metabolic alkalosis in the ICU.

   b. During therapy with *chloruretic* diuretics, the urinary chloride may be inappropriately high.

2. **Chloride-Resistant Alkalosis**

   A chloride-resistant metabolic alkalosis is characterized by an elevated urinary chloride concentration (>25 mEq/L).

   a. Most cases of chloride-resistant alkalosis are caused by primary mineralocorticoid excess (e.g., primary aldosteronism).

b. Whereas hypovolemia is common in chloride-responsive alkalosis, hypervolemia is typical in chloride-resistant alkalosis.

IV. MANAGEMENT

A. Saline Infusion

Saline infusion is used to correct chloride-responsive metabolic alkalosis.

1. As mentioned earlier, volume infusion will not correct metabolic alkaloses unless the chloride deficit is replaced, so isotonic saline is used for volume infusion, as directed by the estimated chloride (CL^-) deficit (2,9):

$$CL^- \text{ deficit (mEq)} = 0.2 \times wt \text{ (kg)} \times (100 - plasma\ CL^-) \quad (25.3)$$

(wt is lean body weight in kg, and 100 is the desired plasma chloride in mEq/L). The corresponding volume of isotonic saline (0.9% NaCL) is determined as follows:

$$\text{Volume (L)} = CL^- \text{ deficit} / 154 \quad (25.4)$$

(154 is the chloride concentration in mEq/L in isotonic saline). This method is summarized in Table 25.3. If the patient is hemodynamically stable, the infusion rate of saline should be 125–150 mL/hr above the hourly fluid losses.

2. EXAMPLE. A 70 kg adult with protracted vomiting has a metabolic alkalosis with a plasma chloride of 80 mEq/L. The chloride deficit in this case is $0.2 \times 70 \times (100 - 80) = 280$ mEq. The volume of isotonic saline needed to correct this deficit is $280/154 = 1.8$ liters.

Table 25.3	Isotonic Saline Infusions for Metabolic Alkalosis

1. Estimate the chloride deficit:

$$CL^- \text{ deficit (mEq)} = 0.2 \times \text{wt (kg)} \times (100 - \text{plasma } CL^-)$$

2. Determine the corresponding volume of isotonic saline:

$$\text{Volume (liters)} = \frac{CL^- \text{ deficit}}{154}$$

From References 2 and 9.

B. Edematous States

The following measures are available for treating metabolic alkalosis in edematous patients.

1. **Correct Hypokalemia**

   If hypokalemia is present, potassium replacement can proceed as described in Chapter 28, Section II-D.

2. **Acetazolamide**

   Acetazolamide (Diamox) is well suited for treating metabolic alkalosis in edematous patients because it can promote diuresis while correcting the alkalosis.

   a. Acetazolamide increases urinary HCO_3 excretion by inhibiting carbonic anhydrase (the enzyme involved in HCO_3 reabsorption).

   b. The increased HCO_3 excretion is accompanied by increased sodium excretion; hence the dual benefit of diuresis and correction of the metabolic alkalosis.

c. The recommended dose is 5–10 mg/kg (PO or IV), and the peak effect occurs about 15 hours later (10).

C. Hydrochloric Acid

Intravenous infusions of hydrochloric acid (HCL) are reserved for the rarest cases of metabolic alkalosis that are: (a) severe (pH >7.6), (b) uncorrected by other means, and (c) appear to be harmful.

1. The dose of HCL is determined by estimating the hydrogen ion (H^+) deficit with the following equation (2,9):

$$H^+ \text{ deficit (mEq)} = 0.5 \times wt \text{ (kg)} \times (\text{plasma } HCO_3 - 30) \quad (25.5)$$

(wt is the lean body weight in kg, and 30 is the desired plasma HCO_3).

2. The preferred HCL solution for intravenous use is 0.1N HCL, which contains 100 mEq H^+ per liter. The volume of 0.1N HCL (in liters) needed to replace the H^+ deficit is calculated as follows:

$$\text{Volume (L)} = H^+ \text{ Deficit } / 100 \quad (25.6)$$

This method is summarized in Table 25.4.

3. HCL solutions are extremely corrosive, and extravasation can result in life-threatening tissue necrosis (11). Infusion through a large, central vein is advised, and the *infusion rate should not exceed 0.2 mEq/kg/hr* (9).

4. EXAMPLE. A 70 kg adult has a refractory metabolic alkalosis with a plasma HCO_3 of 50 mEq/L and an arterial pH of 7.61. The H^+ deficit is $0.5 \times 70 \times (50 - 30) = 700$ mEq. The corresponding volume of 0.1N HCL is $700/100 = 7$ liters, and the maximum infusion rate is $(0.2 \times 70)/100 = 0.14$ L/hour (140 mL/hr).

Table 25.4	Hydrochloric Acid Infusions

1. Estimate the hydrogen ion deficit:

$$H^+ \text{ deficit (mEq)} = 0.5 \times wt \text{ (kg)} \times (\text{plasma } HCO_3 - 30)$$

2. Determine the corresponding volume of 0.1N HCL:

$$\text{Volume (liters)} = \frac{H^+ \text{ deficit}}{100}$$

3. Maximum rate = 0.2 mEq/kg/hr.

From References 2 and 9.

5. The entire H^+ deficit does not have to be replaced, and the HCL infusion can be stopped when the plasma pH falls below 7.6.

REFERENCES

1. Laski ME, Sabitini S. Metabolic alkalosis, bedside and bench. Semin Nephrol 2006; 26:404–421.

2. Khanna A, Kurtzman NA. Metabolic alkalosis. Respir Care 2001; 46:354–365.

3. Rose BD, Post TW. Metabolic alkalosis. In: Clinical Physiology of Acid-Base and Electrolyte Disorders. 5th ed. New York: McGraw-Hill, 2001:551–577.

4. Luke RG, Galla JH. It is chloride depletion alkalosis, not contraction alkalosis. J Am Soc Nephrol 2012; 23:204–207.

5. Gennari FJ, Weise WJ. Acid-base disturbances in gastrointestinal disease. Clin J Am Soc Nephrol 2008; 3:1861–1868.

6. Javaheri S, Kazemi H. Metabolic alkalosis and hypoventilation in humans. Am Rev Respir Dis 1987; 136:1011–1016.

7. Adrogue HJ, Madias NE. Secondary responses to altered acid-base status: The rules of engagement. J Am Soc Nephrol 2010; 21:920–923.

8. Nunn JF. Nunn's Applied Respiratory Physiology. 4th ed. Oxford: Butterworth-Heinemann Ltd, 1993:275–276.

9. Androgue HJ, Madias N. Management of life-threatening acid-base disorders. Part 2. N Engl J Med 1998; 338:107–111.

10. Marik PE, Kussman BD, Lipman J, Kraus P. Acetazolamide in the treatment of metabolic alkalosis in critically ill patients. Heart Lung 1991; 20:455–458.

11. Buchanan IB, Campbell BT, Peck MD, Cairns BA. Chest wall necrosis and death secondary to hydrochloric acid infusion for metabolic alkalosis. South Med J 2005; 98:822.

Chapter 26

Acute Kidney Injury

As many as 70% of ICU patients have some degree of acute renal dysfunction, and about 5% require renal replacement therapy (1). The acute renal dysfunction that occurs in critically ill patients is called *acute kidney injury,* and this chapter describes the diagnostic and therapeutic considerations related to this entity.

I. DIAGNOSTIC CONSIDERATIONS

Acute kidney injury (AKI) is defined as an abrupt (within 48 hrs) decrease in renal function that is clinically significant (i.e., can have adverse consequences) (2).

A. Diagnostic Criteria

The Acute Kidney Injury Network has proposed the following criteria for the diagnosis of AKI (2):

1. An increase in serum creatinine of ≥0.3 mg/dL within 48 hours, or

2. An increase in serum creatinine of ≥50% within 48 hours, or

3. A decrease in hourly urine output to <0.5 mL/kg (oliguria) for more than 6 hours.

   a. Ideal body weight is recommended for weight-based urine output measurements (3).

B. Etiologies

The common predisposing conditions for AKI are listed in Table 26.1 (1). These conditions can be categorized by their location in relation to the kidneys; i.e., prerenal, renal, or postrenal.

Table 26.1	Common Causes of Acute Kidney Injury
Most Common	**Others**
Sepsis (#1)	Trauma
Major Surgery	Rhabdomyolysis
Hypovolemia	Abdominal Compartment Syndrome
Low Cardiac Output	Cardiopulmonary Bypass
Nephrotoxic Agents	Hepatorenal Syndrome

From Reference 1.

1. **Prerenal Disorders**

   Prerenal disorders are extrarenal, and promote AKI by decreasing renal blood flow (e.g., hypovolemia). Correcting these disorders may, or may not, improve renal function, depending on the severity and duration of the flow impairment in the kidneys.

2. **Renal Disorders**

   The principal renal disorders that produce AKI are *acute tubular necrosis* (ATN) and *acute interstitial nephritis* (AIN).

   a. *ATN is responsible for over 50% of cases of AKI* (4), and is the result of injury involving the epithelial cell lining of the renal tubules. Common inciting conditions include septic shock, trauma, major surgery, radiocontrast dye, nephrotoxic drugs, and rhabdomyolysis.

b. AIN involves inflammatory injury in the renal parenchyma, and is described later in the chapter.

3. **Postrenal Obstruction**

Postrenal obstruction is responsible for 10% of cases of AKI (4). The obstruction can involve the most distal portion of the renal collecting ducts (papillary necrosis), the ureters (from a retroperitoneal mass), or the urethra (strictures or prostatic enlargement). Obstructing renal calculi do not cause AKI unless there is a solitary functional kidney.

C. Diagnostic Evaluation

The evaluation of AKI begins with a bedside ultrasound evaluation of the kidneys for evidence of postrenal obstruction (hydronephrosis). If there is no obstruction, the measurements in Table 26.2 can help to distinguish prerenal from intrinsic renal disorders, but *only in the setting of oliguria*.

Table 26.2	Urinary Measurements for the Evaluation of Oliguria	
Measurement	**Prerenal Disorder**	**Renal Disorder**
Spot Urine Sodium	<20 mEq/L	>40 mEq/L
Fractional Excretion of Na	<1%	>2%
Fractional Excretion of Urea	<35%	>50%
Urine Osmolality	>500 mosm/kg	300–400 mosm/kg
U/P Osmolality	>1.5	1–1.3

1. **Spot Urine Sodium**

a. In prerenal disorders (e.g., hypovolemia), there is an

increase in sodium reabsorption in the renal tubules, which results in a low urine sodium concentration (<20 mEq/L).

b. The renal tubular dysfunction in ATN impairs sodium reabsorption, resulting in a high urine sodium concentration (>40 mEq/L).

c. EXCEPTIONS: A prerenal disorder can be associated with a high urine sodium if there is ongoing diuretic therapy, or the patient has chronic renal disease with an obligatory sodium loss in urine (5).

2. **Fractional Excretion of Sodium**

The fractional excretion of sodium (FENa) is the fraction of filtered sodium that is excreted in the urine, and is equivalent to the fractional sodium (Na) clearance divided by the fractional creatinine (Cr) clearance, as expressed by the following equation:

$$\text{FENa (\%)} = \frac{U/P\,[\text{Na}]}{U/P\,[\text{Cr}]} \qquad (26.1)$$

(U/P is the urine-to-plasma ratio.)

a. In prerenal disorders, the FENa is <1%, reflecting sodium conservation.

b. In renal disorders like ATN, the FENa is typically >2%, indicating inappropriate sodium loss in the urine (6).

c. EXCEPTIONS: Like the spot urine sodium, the FENa can be increased (>1%) by diuretic therapy and chronic renal insufficiency (6). In addition, the FENa can be inappropriately low (<1%) in patients with AKI from sepsis (7), radiocontrast dyes (8), and myoglobinuria (9).

3. **Fractional Excretion of Urea**

The fractional excretion of urea (FEU) is conceptually

similar to the FENa, but it *is not influenced by diuretics* (10), which is a major advantage over the FENa. The FEU is equivalent to the fractional urea clearance divided by the fractional creatinine clearance, as expressed by the following equation:

$$\text{FEU (\%)} \;=\; \frac{\text{U/P [Urea]}}{\text{U/P [Cr]}} \qquad (26.2)$$

(U/P is the urine-to-plasma ratio.) The FEU is low (<35%) in prerenal disorders, and high (>50%) in intrinsic renal disorders.

4. **Uncertainty**

   Distinguishing between prerenal and intrarenal causes of AKI can be difficult, especially when there is both a prerenal and renal component that coexist (e.g., in trauma, where hypovolemia and rhabdomyolysis can both contribute to AKI). Uncertainty in the setting of oliguria should prompt a fluid challenge (see next section).

II. INITIAL MANAGEMENT

The following are recommendations for the initial encounter with a patient who develops AKI, especially when associated with oliguria.

A. What to Do

1. As just mentioned, it is often difficult to rule out a prerenal component in oliguric AKI, and uncertainty should prompt a fluid challenge. (See Chapter 7, Section III-A, for recommendations on fluid challenges.)

2. If volume infusion is not indicated, or does not correct the problem, then proceed as follows:

    a. Reduce fluid intake as much as possible.

    b. Discontinue potentially nephrotoxic drugs. Common offenders are listed in Table 26.3.

    c. Adjust the dose of drugs that are excreted in the urine.

Table 26.3	Drugs Most Often Implicated in Acute Kidney Injury

Intrarenal Hemodynamics

    Most Frequent: Nonsteroidal anti-inflammatory agents (NSAIDs)

           Others: ACE inhibitors, angiotensin receptor-blocking drugs, cyclosporine, tacrolimus

Renal Tubular Injury

    Most Frequent: Aminoglycosides

           Others: Amphotericin B, antiretrovirals, cisplatin

Interstitial Nephritis

    Most Frequent: Antimicrobials (penicillins, cephalosporins, sulfonamides, vancomycin, macrolides, tetracyclines, rifampin)

           Others: Anticonvulsants (phenytoin, valproic acid), H_2 blockers, NSAIDs, proton pump inhibitors

Adapted from Reference 11.

B. What Not to Do

1. Do not give furosemide to correct oliguria (3). Intravenous furosemide does not improve renal function in AKI, and does not convert oliguric to non-oliguric renal failure (1,3,12). Furosemide can increase urine output during the recovery phase of AKI (13), and can be used at that time if volume overload is a problem.

2. Do not use low-dose dopamine to increase renal blood flow in AKI (3,14,15). Low-dose dopamine does not improve renal function in patients with AKI (14,15), and it can have deleterious effects (e.g., decreased splanchnic blood flow, inhibition of T-cell lymphocyte function) (15).

III. SPECIFIC CONDITIONS

A. Contrast-Induced Nephropathy

Iodinated contrast agents can damage the kidneys in several ways, including direct renal tubular toxicity, renal vasoconstriction, and the generation of toxic oxygen metabolites (16). The incidence of contrast-induced nephropathy (CIN) is 8–9% (17). CIN appears within 72 hours after the contrast study, and most cases resolve within two weeks without renal replacement therapy (24).

1. **Predisposing Conditions**

   The risk of CIN is increased by diabetes, dehydration, renal dysfunction (serum creatinine >1.3 mg/dL in males, and >1.0 mg/dL in females), and the use of nephrotoxic drugs (3).

2. **Prevention**

   a. INTRAVENOUS HYDRATION: The most effective preventive measure in high-risk patients is *intravenous hydration* (if permitted) *with isotonic saline at 100–150 mL/hr started 3 to 12 hours before the procedure and continued for 6–24 hours after the procedure* (18). For emergency procedures, at least 300–500 mL isotonic saline should be infused just prior to the procedure.

   b. N-ACETYLCYSTEINE: N-acetylcysteine (NAC) is a glutathione surrogate with antioxidant actions that has had mixed results as a protective agent for CIN (1). However, the pooled results of 16 studies using high-dose NAC show a 50% risk-reduction for CIN (18). *The high-dose NAC regimen is 1,200 mg orally twice daily for 48 hours, beginning the night before the contrast procedure.* For emergency procedures, the first 1,200 mg dose should be given just prior to the procedure.

B. Acute Interstitial Nephritis (AIN)

1. AIN is an inflammatory condition involving the renal parenchyma that presents as AKI, often without oliguria (20).

2. Most cases of AIN are the result of a hypersensitivity drug reaction, but infections (usually viral or atypical pathogens) can also be involved. The drugs most often implicated in AIN are listed in Table 26.3 (11). Antibiotics are the leading offenders, particularly the penicillins.

3. Drug-induced AIN is often (but not always) accompanied by signs of a hypersensitivity reaction; i.e., fever, rash, and eosinophilia.

4. The onset of renal injury is usually several weeks after the first exposure (11), but can appear within a few days after a second exposure. Sterile pyuria and eosinophiluria are common (11). A renal biopsy can secure the diagnosis, but is rarely performed.

5. AIN usually resolves after the offending agent is discontinued, but recovery can take months.

C. Myoglobinuric Renal Injury

AKI develops in one-third of patients with diffuse muscle injury (*rhabdomyolysis*) (21,22). The culprit is myoglobin, which is released by the injured muscle, and can damage the renal tubular epithelial cells.

1. Diagnosis

The widespread myocyte injury in rhabdomyolysis produces marked elevations in the creatine kinase (CK) levels in blood (CK levels of 20,000–30,000 U/L are not uncommon). However, the diagnosis of AKI can be difficult in this setting because the injured myocytes release creatine, which elevates the serum creatinine, and oliguria can be the result of hypovolemia, which occurs with rhabdomyolysis (23). The distinguishing feature in this setting is the presence or absence of myoglobin in the urine.

2. **Myoglobin in Urine**

Myoglobin can be detected in urine with the orthotoluidine dipstick reaction (Hemastix) for heme-bound iron, which is used to detect occult blood in urine. If the test is positive, the urine is centrifuged (to separate erythrocytes) and the supernatant is passed through a micropore filter (to remove hemoglobin). A positive test after these measures is evidence of myoglobin in urine. A positive dipstick test with no red blood cells in the urine sediment also provides supportive evidence of myoglobinuria.

a. The presence of myoglobin in urine does not ensure the diagnosis, but *the absence of myoglobin in urine excludes the diagnosis of myoglobinuric renal injury* (22).

3. **Management**

Aggressive *volume resuscitation* to promote renal blood flow is the most effective measure for preventing or limiting myoglobinuric renal injury. Alkalinizing the urine can also limit the renal injury, but is difficult to accomplish. About 30% of patients with myoglobinuric renal injury require dialysis (22).

D. Abdominal Compartment Syndrome

An increase in intraabdominal pressure (IAP) can adversely affect renal function by decreasing both renal perfusion pressure and the net filtration pressure across the glomerulus

454 section x Renal and Electrolyte Disorders

(24). As a result, oliguria is one of the first signs of intraabdominal hypertension (IAH) (24). When IAH is associated with organ dysfunction, the condition in called *abdominal compartment syndrome* (ACS).

1. **Predisposing Conditions**

   ACS is traditionally associated with abdominal trauma, but several conditions can raise the IAP and predispose to ACS, including gastric distension, bowel obstruction, ileus, ascites, bowel wall edema, hepatomegaly, positive-pressure breathing, upright body position, and obesity (25). Several of these factors can co-exist in critically ill patients, which explains why *IAH is discovered in as many as 60% of patients in medical and surgical ICUs* (26).

   a. LARGE VOLUME RESUSCITATION: Large-volume resuscitation can raise IAP by promoting edema in the abdominal organs (particularly the bowel). One report of ICU patients with a positive fluid balance >5 liters over 24 hours found that 85% of the patients had ICH, and 25% had ACS (27).

2. **Measuring Intraabdominal Pressure**

   IAP is measured as the pressure in a decompressed urinary bladder (intravesicular method), using specialized bladder drainage catheters (Bard Medical, Covington, GA). Patients must be in the supine position, with no abdominal muscle contractions, and the pressure transducer should be zeroed in the mid-axillary line. The IAP is then measured (in mm Hg) at the end of expiration (24).

3. **Diagnostic Criteria**

   a. The normal IAP is 5–7 mm Hg in the supine position.

   b. IAH is defined as a sustained IAP ≥12 mm Hg (24).

   c. ACS is defined as an IAP >20 mm Hg plus acute organ dysfunction (24).

4. **Management**

   a. General measures for reducing IAP include sedation (to reduce abdominal muscle contractions), avoiding elevation of the head more than 20° above the horizontal plane (28), and avoiding a positive fluid balance.

   b. Specific measures are dictated by the responsible condition, and can include decompression of the stomach, or bowel, percutaneous drainage of ascites, or surgery (e.g., for abdominal injuries or bowel obstruction).

   c. ABDOMINAL PERFUSION PRESSURE: The abdominal perfusion pressure (APP) is the pressure gradient across the abdominal organs and kidneys, and is equivalent to the difference between the mean arterial pressure (MAP) and the IAP;

$$APP = MAP - IAP \qquad (26.3)$$

   Maintaining an APP >60 mm Hg is associated with improved outcomes in ACS, so this should be one of the goals of management.

IV. RENAL REPLACEMENT THERAPY

Renal replacement therapy (RRT) refers to artificial methods of solute clearance. Several methods are available, including hemodialysis, hemofiltration, hemodiafiltration, high-flux dialysis, and plasmafiltration. The first two methods (used most often) are described here, and these methods are illustrated in Figure 26.1.

A. Indications

1. The usual indications for RRT include:

   a. Volume overload

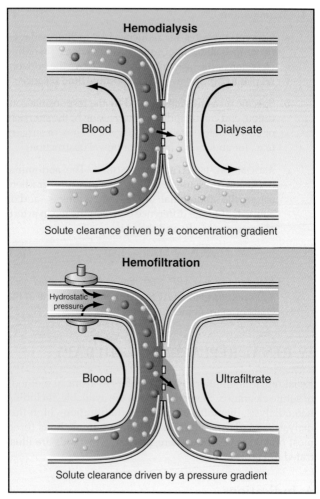

FIGURE 26.1 Mechanisms of solute clearance by hemodialysis and hemofiltration. The smaller yellow particles represent small solutes (e.g., urea), and the larger red particles represent larger molecules (e.g., toxins). See text for explanation.

b. Life-threatening hyperkalemia or metabolic acidosis

c. Manifestations of uremia (e.g., encephalopathy)

d. Removal of toxins (e.g., ethylene glycol)

2. Otherwise, the optimal timing for RRT in acute renal failure is unclear (29).

B. Hemodialysis

Hemodialysis removes solutes by *diffusion*, which is driven by the concentration gradient of the solutes across a semipermeable membrane. To maintain this concentration gradient, the blood and dialysis fluid are driven in opposite directions across the dialysis membrane (see Figure 26.1). This is known as *countercurrent exchange*.

1. **Method**

    To perform acute hemodialysis, a large-bore double-lumen catheter is inserted percutaneously into the internal jugular or femoral veins, and advanced into the superior or inferior vena cava. (See Appendix 3 for the size and flow characteristics of hemodialysis catheters.) Venous blood is withdrawn through one lumen of the catheter by a pump in the dialysis machine, which propels the blood at a rate of 200–300 mL/min as it passes the dialysis membrane and returns through the other lumen of the catheter (29).

2. **Advantages**

    The principal benefit of hemodialysis is rapid clearance of small solutes. Only a few hours of hemodialysis is needed to remove a day's worth of nitrogenous waste.

3. **Disadvantages**

    The need to maintain a blood flow of 200–300 mL/min through the dialysis chamber creates a risk for hypotension, especially in hemodynamically compromised patients. Hypotension occurs in about one of every three hemodialysis treatments (30).

C. Hemofiltration

Hemofiltration removes solutes by *convection*, where a hydrostatic pressure gradient is used to move a solute-containing fluid across a semipermeable membrane. Since the bulk movement of fluid "drags" the solute across the membrane, this method of solute removal is also known as *solvent drag* (30).

1. **Fluid vs. Solute Removal**

   a. Hemofiltration can remove large volumes of fluid (up to 3 liters per hour), but the rate of solute clearance is slow, requiring continuous hemofiltration for effective solute clearance.

   b. Because solutes are cleared with water, the plasma concentration of cleared solutes does not decrease during hemofiltration unless a solute-free intravenous fluid is infused to replace some of the ultrafiltrate that is lost.

2. **Method**

   The popular method at present is *continuous venovenous hemofiltration* (CVVH), which has a circuit design similar to hemodialysis (i.e., a large-bore, double-lumen catheter is used to cannulate one of the vena cavae, and a pump is used to circulate blood through the hemofiltration chamber).

3. **Advantages**

   There are two advantages with hemofiltration.

   a. It allows more gradual fluid removal than hemodialysis, and is less likely to produce hemodynamic instability.

b. It removes larger molecules than hemodialysis, and is more effective for removing toxins like ethylene glycol.

4. **Disadvantages**

The disadvantages of hemofiltration include slow solute removal, and the need to infuse solute-free fluid to decrease the solute concentration in blood. As a result, it is not as efficient as hemodialysis as a surrogate kidney, and is not recommended for rapid correction of life-threatening hyperkalemia or metabolic acidosis.

REFERENCES

1. Dennen P, Douglas IS, Anderson R. Acute kidney injury in the intensive care unit: an update and primer for the intensivist. Crit Care Med 2010; 38:261–275.

2. Mehta RL, Kellum JA, Shaw SV, et al. Acute Kidney Injury Network: Report of an initiative to improve outcomes in acute kidney injury. Crit Care 2007; 11:R31.

3. Fliser D, Laville M, Covic A, et al. A European Renal Best Practice (ERBP) Position Statement on Kidney Disease Improving Global Outcomes (KDIGO) clinical practice guidelines on acute kidney injury. Nephrol Dial Transplant 2012, 27:4263–4272.

4. Abernathy VE, Lieberthal W. Acute renal failure in the critically ill patient. Crit Care Clin 2002; 18:203–222.

5. Subramanian S, Ziedalski TM. Oliguria, volume overload, Na^+ balance, and diuretics. Crit Care Clin 2005; 21:291–303.

6. Steiner RW. Interpreting the fractional excretion of sodium. Am J Med 1984; 77:699–702.

7. Vaz AJ. Low fractional excretion of urine sodium in acute renal failure due to sepsis. Arch Intern Med 1983; 143:738–739.

8. Fang LST, Sirota RA, Ebert TH, Lichtenstein NS. Low fractional excretion of sodium with contrast media-induced acute renal failure. Arch Intern Med 1980; 140:531–533.

9. Corwin HL, Schreiber MJ, Fang LST. Low fractional excretion of sodium. Occurrence with hemoglobinuric- and myoglobinuric-induced acute renal failure. Arch Intern Med 1984; 144:981–982.

10. Gottfried J, Wiesen J, Raina R, Nally JV Jr. Finding the cause of acute kidney injury: which index of fractional excretion is better? Clev Clin J Med 2012; 79:121–126.

11. Bentley ML, Corwin HL, Dasta J. Drug-induced acute kidney injury in the critically ill adult: Recognition and prevention strategies. Crit Care Med 2010; 38(Suppl):S169–S174.

12. Venkataram R, Kellum JA. The role of diuretic agents in the management of acute renal failure. Contrib Nephrol 2001; 132:158–170.

13. van der Voort PH, Boerma EC, Koopmans M, et al. Furosemide does not improve renal recovery after hemofiltration for acute renal failure in critically ill patients. A double blind randomized controlled trial. Crit Care Med 2009; 37:533–538.

14. Kellum JA, Decker JM. Use of dopamine in acute renal failure: a meta-analysis. Crit Care Med 2001; 29:1526–1531.

15 Holmes CL, Walley KR. Bad medicine. Low-dose dopamine in the ICU. Chest 2003; 123:1266–1275.

16. Pierson PB, Hansell P, Lias P. Pathophysiology of contrast medium-induced nephropathy. Kidney Int 2005; 68:14–22.

17. Ehrmann S, Badin J, Savath L, et al. Acute kidney injury in the critically ill: Is iodinated contrast medium really harmful? Crit Care Med 2013; 41:1017–1025.

18. McCullough PA, Soman S. Acute kidney injury with iodinated contrast. Crit Care Med 2008; 36(Suppl):S204–S211.

19. Triverdi H, Daram S, Szabo A, et al. High-dose N-acetylcysteine for the prevention of contrast-induced nephropathy. Am J Med 2009; 122:874.e9–15.

20. Ten RM, Torres VE, Millner DS, et al. Acute interstitial nephritis. Mayo Clin Proc 1988; 3:921–930.

21. Beetham R. Biochemical investigation of suspected rhabdomyolysis. Ann Clin Biochem 2000; 37:581–587.

22. Sharp LS, Rozycki GS, Feliciano DV. Rhabdomyolysis and secondary renal failure in critically ill surgical patients. Am J Surg 2004; 188:801–806.

23. Visweswaran P, Guntupalli J. Rhabdomyolysis. Crit Care Clin 1999; 15:415–428.

24. Malbrain MLNG, Cheatham ML, Kirkpatrick A, et al. Results from the International Conference of Experts on Intra-abdominal Hypertension and Abdominal Compartment Syndrome. I. Definitions. Intensive Care Med 2006; 32:1722–1723.

25. Al-Mufarrej F, Abell LM, Chawla LS. Understanding intra-abdominal hypertension: from bench to bedside. J Intensive Care Med 2012; 27:145–160.

26. Malbrain ML, Chiumello D, Pelosi P, et al. Prevalence of intra-abdominal hypertension in critically ill patients: A multicenter epidemiological study. Intensive Care Med 2004; 30:822–829.

27. Daugherty EL, Hongyan L, Taichman D, et al. Abdominal compartment syndrome is common in medical ICU patients receiving large-volume resuscitation. J Intensive Care Med 2007; 22:294–299.

28. Cheatham ML, Malbrain MLNG, Kirkpatrick A, et al. Results from the International Conference of Experts on Intra-abdominal Hypertension and Abdominal Compartment Syndrome. II. Recommendations. Intensive Care Med 2007; 33:951–962.

29. Pannu N, Klarenbach S, Wiebe N, et al. Renal replacement therapy in patients with acute renal failure. A systematic review. JAMA 2008; 299:793–805.

30. O'Reilly P, Tolwani A. Renal replacement therapy III. IHD, CRRT, SLED. Crit Care Clin 2005; 21:367–378.

Chapter 27

Osmotic Disorders

As many as 40% of ICU patients have a problem with the osmotic balance between intracellular and extracellular fluid (1). The signal for this problem is a change in the plasma sodium concentration, but the real problem is a change in cell volume, which is most apparent in the central nervous system. This chapter presents a simple approach to osmotic disorders based on a single variable: the extracellular volume.

I. OSMOTIC ACTIVITY

The concentration of solutes in a solution can be expressed in terms of *osmotic activity*, which is a reflection of the number of solute particles in a solution. The unit of measurement is the osmole (osm), which is 6×10^{23} particles (Avogadro's Number) for a non-dissociable substance (2). The osmotic activity in a fluid compartment determines its water content.

A. Relative Osmotic Activity

1. When two fluid compartments are separated by a semipermeable membrane (not freely permeable to solutes), the solutes will not distribute evenly in the fluid compartments, and the osmotic activity will be higher in one fluid compartment. Water then moves from the fluid with the lower osmotic activity into the fluid with the higher osmotic activity.

2. The difference in osmotic activity between the fluid compartments is called the *effective osmotic activity*, and it is the force that drives the movement of water between fluid compartments. This force is also called the *osmotic pressure*.

3. The fluid with the higher osmotic activity is described as *hypertonic*, and the fluid with the lower osmotic activity is described as *hypotonic*.

4. If the two fluid compartments are the intracellular and extracellular volumes, then:

   a. When the extracellular fluid is hypertonic, water will move out of cells.

   b. When the extracellular fluid is hypotonic, water will move into cells.

B. Units of Osmotic Activity

Osmotic activity can be expressed in relation to the volume of the solution, or the volume of water in the solution (3,4).

1. Osmotic activity per volume of solution is called *osmolarity*, and is expressed as milliosmoles per liter (mosm/L).

2. Osmotic activity per volume of water is called *osmolality*, and is expressed as milliosmoles per kilogram of H_2O (mosm/kg H_2O, or mosm/kg).

3. Plasma is mostly (95%) water, so osmolality is typically used to described the osmotic activity of plasma. However, there is little difference between the osmolality and osmolarity of plasma, and the two terms are often used interchangeably (4).

C. Plasma Osmolality

The osmotic activity of plasma can be measured or calculated.

1. **Measured Plasma Osmolality**

   Plasma osmolality is measured with the *freezing point depression* method. The freezing point of water (0° C) decreases 1.86° C for each osmole of solute that is added to one kilogram (liter) of water. Therefore, the freezing point of an aqueous solution (relative to water) can be used to determine the osmotic activity of the solution. This is the "gold-standard" method for measuring plasma osmolality.

2. **Calculated Plasma Osmolality**

   Plasma osmolality can be calculated using the concentrations of the principal solutes in plasma (sodium, chloride, glucose, and urea) (3); i.e.,

   $$\text{Posm} = 2 \times \text{Plasma Na} + \frac{\text{glucose}}{18} + \frac{\text{BUN}}{2.8} \quad (27.1)$$

   a. Posm is the plasma osmolality in mosm/kg H_2O (or mosm/kg).

   b. Plasma Na is the sodium concentration in mEq/L, and is doubled to include the osmotic activity of chloride.

   c. Glucose and BUN are the plasma concentrations of each in mg/dL.

   d. 18 and 2.8 are the molecular weights of glucose and urea divided by 10 (to express their concentrations in mosm/kg).

   e. EXAMPLE: Using normal plasma concentrations of Na (140 mEq/L), glucose (90 mg/dL), and BUN (14 mg/dL), the plasma osmolality is: $(2 \times 140) + 90/18 + 14/2.8 = 290$ mosm/kg.

3. **Effective Plasma Osmolality**

   Urea readily crosses cell membranes, so an increase in

BUN will not increase the effective osmotic activity of plasma (i.e., *azotemia is a hyperosmotic, but not a hypertonic, condition*). Therefore, the calculation of effective plasma osmolality does not include the BUN; i.e.,

$$\text{Posm} = 2 \times \text{Plasma Na} + \frac{\text{glucose}}{18} \qquad (27.2)$$

a. EXAMPLE: Using normal plasma concentrations of Na (140 mEq/L) and glucose (90 mg/dL), the effective plasma osmolality is: $(2 \times 140) + 90/18 = 285$ mosm/kg.

b. Note that the plasma sodium accounts for 98% (280 of 285 mosm/kg) of the effective osmotic activity of the extracellular fluid. In other words, *the plasma sodium concentration is the principal determinant of the distribution of total body water in the intracellular and extracellular fluid compartments.*

D. Osmolal Gap

1. Because solutes other than sodium, chloride, glucose, and urea are present in the extracellular fluid, the measured plasma osmolality will be greater than the calculated osmolality. This *osmolal gap* is normally ≤10 mosm/kg (3,5).

2. The presence of a toxin or drug will increase the osmolal gap, and this makes the osmolal gap a useful measurement in cases of suspected toxin exposure or drug overdose (6).

II. HYPERNATREMIA

The normal plasma sodium is 135–145 mEq/L, so hypernatremia is defined as a plasma sodium >145 mEq/L.

A. Extracellular Volume

Three conditions can produce hypernatremia (7):

1. Loss of sodium and water, with water loss > sodium loss (i.e., hypotonic fluid loss). This results in a decreased extracellular volume (ECV).

2. Loss of water only (free water loss), which results in an unchanged ECV.

3. Gain of sodium and water, with sodium gain > water gain (i.e., gain of hypertonic fluid), which results in an increased ECV.

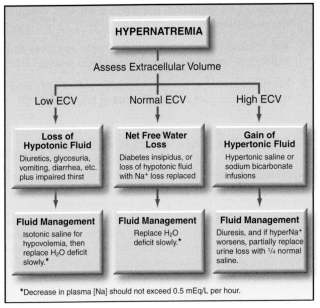

FIGURE 27.1 Flow diagram for the approach to hypernatremia based on the extracellular volume (ECV).

Since each of these conditions is associated with a different ECV, assessment of the ECV can be used to identify the condition responsible for hypernatremia. This is shown in Figure 27.1. (Assessment of the ECV is not presented here. See Chapter 7 for the evaluation of hypovolemia.)

B. Encephalopathy

The clinical consequences of hypernatremia (i.e., hypertonicity) include insulin resistance, cardiac dysfunction, and encephalopathy (1), with the latter condition being the most significant.

1. Encephalopathy is more likely to occur with a rapid rise in plasma sodium (8). Possible mechanisms include shrinkage of neuronal cell bodies (8) and osmotic demyelination (9).

2. The clinical manifestations range from agitation and lethargy to coma and generalized or focal seizures (1).

3. Encephalopathy is a poor prognostic sign in hypernatremia, and carries a mortality rate as high as 50% (9).

III. HYPOVOLEMIC HYPERNATREMIA

Hypernatremia associated with a low ECV is the result of loss of hypotonic fluids (i.e., fluids with a sodium concentration <135 mEq/L). Common sources of hypotonic fluid loss include: (a) diuretic-induced urine loss, (b) osmotic diuresis from glycosuria, (c) vomiting and diarrhea, (d) excessive sweat loss in heat-related illnesses, and (e) normal fluid losses without sodium or water intake (e.g., in elderly, debilitated patients).

A. Management

Management is aimed at correcting the two consequences of hypotonic fluid loss: (a) loss of sodium, which reduces the

ECV, and (b) loss of water in excess of sodium (the *free water deficit*), which creates a hypertonic plasma.

1. **Sodium Replacement**

   The most immediate concern with sodium loss is a decrease in plasma volume, which can decrease cardiac output and impair tissue perfusion. Therefore, the management of hypovolemic hyponatremia begins with sodium replacement using isotonic saline.

2. **Free Water Replacement**

   When hypovolemia has been corrected, the next step is to replace the free water deficit. The free water deficit can be estimated, based on the assumption that the product of total body water (TBW) and plasma sodium concentration (PNa) is always constant (7).

   $$\text{Current (TBW} \times \text{PNa)} = \text{Normal (TBW} \times \text{PNa)} \qquad (27.3)$$

   Substituting 140 mEq/L for a normal PNa and rearranging terms yields the following relationship:

   $$\text{Current TBW} = \text{Normal TBW} \times (140/\text{Current PNa}) \qquad (27.4)$$

   a. The normal TBW (in liters) is usually 60% of lean body weight (in kg) in men and 50% of lean body weight in women, but a 10% reduction in the normal TBW has been suggested for hypernatremic patients who are water depleted (10).

   b. For patients who are hyperglycemic, *the plasma sodium should be corrected for the dilutional effect of hyperglycemia*. This effect averages 2 mEq/L for every 100 mg/dL increase in plasma glucose (see Section V-A-2).

   c. Once the current TBW is calculated, the free water deficit is calculated as:

   $$\text{Free Water Deficit (L)} = \text{Normal TBW} - \text{Current TBW} \qquad (27.5)$$

d. EXAMPLE: For an adult male with a lean body weight of 70 kg and a plasma Na of 160 mEq/L, the normal TBW is 0.6 × 70 = 42 L, the current TBW is 42 × (140/160) = 36.8 L, and the free water deficit is (42 − 36.8 = 5.2 liters.

e. Free water deficits are corrected with sodium-containing fluids such as 0.45% NaCL to replace ongoing sodium losses. The volume needed to correct the free water deficit can be estimated as follows (11):

Liters of 0.45% NaCL = Free Water Deficit × (140/77) (27.6)

where 140 is the desired plasma Na concentration, and 77 is the Na concentration in 0.45% NaCL.

3. **Rate of Change in Plasma Sodium**

Neuronal cells initially shrink in response to hypertonic extracellular fluid, but cell volume is restored within hours; an effect attributed to the generation of osmotically active substances within brain cells, called *idiogenic osmoles* (7). Once the cell volume is restored to normal, aggressive replacement of free water deficits can produce cell swelling and cerebral edema.

a. To limit the risk of cerebral edema, *the decrease in plasma sodium should not exceed 0.5 mEq/L per hour* (1,7,8).

IV. HYPERNATREMIA WITHOUT HYPO-VOLEMIA

Hypernatremia with a normal ECV is the result of free water loss with no net sodium loss. This condition is common in ICU patients with hypernatremia (1), and *usually occurs when sodium losses are replaced, leaving a net free water deficit.* The condition described next is probably the best example of a pure water deficit.

A. Diabetes Insipidus

Diabetes insipidus (DI) is a disorder of renal water conservation, and is characterized by loss of urine that is largely devoid of solute (12). The underlying problem in DI is a defect related to antidiuretic hormone (ADH), which promotes water reabsorption in the distal renal tubules. DI can involve two distinct defects related to ADH:

1. *Central DI* is characterized by failure of ADH release from the posterior pituitary (13). Common causes include traumatic brain injury, anoxic encephalopathy, meningitis, and brain death. The onset is heralded by polyuria that usually is evident within 24 hours of the inciting event.

2. *Nephrogenic DI* is characterized by impaired end-organ responsiveness to ADH (14). Potential causes include amphotericin, aminoglycosides, radiocontrast dye, dopamine, lithium, hypokalemia, and the recovery (polyuric) phase of ATN. The defect in renal concentrating ability is less severe in nephrogenic DI than in central DI.

3. **Diagnosis**

   The hallmark of DI is a dilute urine in the face of hypertonic plasma.

   a. In central DI, the urine osmolarity is often below 200 mosm/L, whereas in nephrogenic DI, the urine osmolarity is usually between 200 and 500 mosm/L (15).

   b. The diagnosis of DI is confirmed by noting the urinary response to fluid restriction. Failure of the urine osmolarity to increase more than 30 mosm/L in the first few hours of complete fluid restriction is diagnostic of DI.

   c. Once the diagnosis of DI is confirmed, the response to vasopressin (5 units IV) will differentiate central from nephrogenic DI. In central DI, the urine osmolarity increases by at least 50% almost immediately after vasopressin administration, whereas in nephrogenic DI, the urine osmolarity is unchanged after vasopressin.

4. **Management**

The fluid loss in DI is almost pure water, so the replacement strategy is aimed at replacing free water deficits using Equations 27.4–27.6 and limiting the rate of sodium correction to ≤0.5 mEq/L per hour.

VASOPRESSIN: In central DI, vasopressin administration is also required. The usual dose is *2–5 Units of aqueous vasopressin given subcutaneously every 4 to 6 hours* (16). The serum sodium must be monitored carefully during vasopressin therapy because of the risk of water intoxication.

B. Hypervolemic Hypernatremia

Hypernatremia with a high ECV is uncommon, and is usually the result of sodium bicarbonate infusions for metabolic acidosis, or aggressive use of hypertonic saline for intracranial hypertension. Excessive ingestion of table salt (often in females with a psychiatric disorder) should be considered in outpatients who present with hypervolemic hypernatremia (17).

1. **Management**

If renal function is normal, excess sodium and water are excreted rapidly. If renal sodium excretion is impaired, it can be increased by a diuretic (e.g., furosemide), but the urinary sodium during diuresis (~80 mEq/L) is less than the plasma sodium, which will aggravate the hypernatremia, so urine losses should be partially replaced with a fluid that is hypotonic to urine.

V. HYPERTONIC HYPERGLYCEMIA

Severe hyperglycemia has a considerable influence on plasma osmolality; e.g., a plasma glucose of 600 mg/dL will increase plasma osmolality by 600/18 = 40 mosm/kg.

A. Non-Ketotic Hyperglycemia

The syndrome of *non-ketotic hyperglycemia* (NKH) is characterized by severe hyperglycemia without ketoacidosis. This condition typically occurs in elderly patients with type 2 diabetes, and is precipitated by a physiological stress (e.g., infection, trauma). Blood glucose levels are typically >600 mg/dL, and can reach levels in excess of 1,000 mg/dL. Glycosuria is marked, and the resulting osmotic diuresis results in hypovolemia. The combination of hyperglycemia and hypotonic fluid loss produces a considerable increase in plasma osmolality. The mortality rate in NKH (5–20%) is higher than in diabetic ketoacidosis (1–5%) (18).

1. **Clinical Manifestations**

   The manifestations of NKH include (18):

   a. Severe hyperglycemia (glucose levels typically >600 mg/dL)

   b. Absent (or mild) ketosis

   c. Evidence of hypovolemia

   d. ENCEPHALOPATHY: Mental status changes begin when the plasma osmolality rises to 320 mosm/kg, and coma can develop at 340 mosm/kg (18). Generalized and focal seizures can appear, as well as involuntary movements such as chorea and hemiballismus (19).

2. **Hyperglycemia and Plasma Sodium**

   Hyperglycemia draws water from the intracellular space, and creates a dilutional effect on the plasma sodium. *For every 100 mg/dL increment in plasma glucose, the plasma sodium is decreased by 1.6 to 2.4 mEq/L (average of 2 mEq/L)* (20,21).

a. EXAMPLE: Using a correction factor of 2 mEq/L per 100 mg/dL increment in plasma glucose, if the measured plasma sodium is 140 mEq/L and the plasma glucose is 800 mg/dL, the corrected plasma sodium is 140 + (7 × 2) = 154 mEq/L.

3. **Fluid Management**

Volume deficits can be profound in NKH, and aggressive volume infusion with isotonic fluids (1–2 liters in the first hour) is often necessary. Thereafter, volume infusion should be guided by signs of hypovolemia and by the corrected plasma sodium concentration.

4. **Insulin Therapy**

a. Because insulin drives both glucose and water into cells, insulin therapy can aggravate hypovolemia, so *insulin should be withheld until the vascular volume is restored*. This is a safe practice because patients with NKH usually have some endogenous insulin, and volume infusion will reduce insulin resistance as it corrects the hypertonicity.

b. When hypovolemia is corrected, *insulin therapy can begin with an infusion of regular insulin at 0.1 units/kg/hr*, using the protocol for diabetic ketoacidosis outlined in Chapter 24, Table 24.4. The insulin requirement will diminish as the hypertonic condition is corrected, so monitoring plasma glucose levels hourly is especially important.

VI. HYPONATREMIA

Hyponatremia (plasma sodium <135 mEq/L) is reported in 40–50% of ICU patients (22,23), and is particularly prevalent in neurosurgical patients (27).

A. Pseudohyponatremia

1. Automated plasma electrolyte measurements include both aqueous and nonaqueous phases of plasma, while only the aqueous phase is osmotically important. Plasma is mostly (95%) water, so the difference between measured and aqueous-phase sodium concentrations is usually negligible.

2. Extreme elevations of plasma lipid or protein levels add to the nonaqueous phase of plasma, and this can significantly lower the measured plasma sodium relative to the aqueous-phase sodium level. This condition is called *pseudohyponatremia*, and it is not usually seen until the plasma lipid levels rise above 1,500 mg/dL, or the plasma protein levels are above 12–15 g/dL (24).

3. If this condition is suspected, clinical laboratories have ion-specific electrodes that can measure the aqueous-phase sodium concentration. Alternately, measuring the plasma osmolality will distinguish pseudohyponatremia (which has a normal osmolality) from "true" hyponatremia (which has a reduced osmolality).

B. Hypotonic Hyponatremia

Hypotonic hyponatremia is the result of excess free water relative to sodium in the extracellular fluid. Most cases involve loss of the normal control mechanisms for antidiuretic hormone (ADH) release.

1. **Nonosmotic ADH Release**

   Antidiuretic hormone (ADH) is released by the posterior pituitary in response to an increase in the osmolality of extracellular fluid, and it helps to curb hypertonicity by promoting water reabsorption in the distal renal tubules.

a. ADH is also released by nonosmotic factors like a decrease in blood pressure (via baroreceptors) or "physiological stress" (i.e., the same stress that stimulated ACTH release from the anterior pituitary).

b. ADH release is usually suppressed when the plasma sodium falls below 135 mEq/L (1). However, when nonosmotic stimuli for ADH release are active, ADH release persists despite hyponatremia, and the resulting water reabsorption in the kidneys aggravates the hyponatremia.

c. *Nonosmotic or "inappropriate" release of ADH is an important cause of sustained hyponatremia in hospitalized patients* (25).

2. **Encephalopathy**

The principal consequence of hypotonic hyponatremia is a life-threatening encephalopathy characterized by cerebral edema, increased intracranial pressure, and the risk of brain herniation (25,26). Symptoms range from headache, nausea and vomiting to seizures, coma, and brain death. The risk and severity of encephalopathy are greater with acute (<48 hrs) hyponatremia (25,26).

3. **Extracellular Volume:**

Like hypernatremia, the extracellular volume can be low, normal, and high in hyponatremia, and the approach can be organized according to the extracellular volume (ECV), as shown in Figure 27.2.

C. Hypovolemic Hyponatremia

Hyponatremia with a low ECV is the result of sodium loss with excess free water retention. The free water retention in hospitalized patients is often the result of nonosmotic ADH release (25), combined with unrestricted water intake.

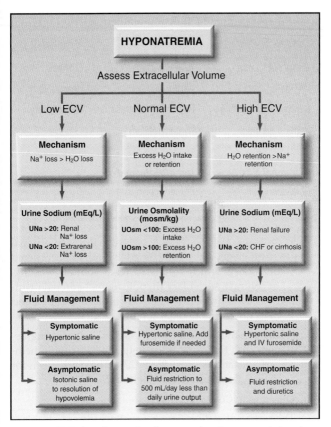

FIGURE 27.2 Flow diagram for the approach to hyponatremia based on the extracellular volume (ECV).

1. **Etiologies**

   The principal conditions associated with hypovolemic hyponatremia are shown in Table 27.1. Thiazide diuretics are common offenders, probably because they impair renal diluting ability.

Table 27.1	Predisposing Conditions for Hyponatremia	
Low ECV†	**Normal ECV**	**High ECV**
Renal NA+ Loss	***ADH-Related***	Cirrhosis
Diuretics	SIADH	Heart failure
Cerebral salt wasting	Physiological stress	Renal failure
Primary adrenal insufficiency	Hypothyroidism	
Extrarenal NA+ Loss	***Not ADH-Related***	
GI losses	Primary polydipsia	

†Must be combined with water retention to produce hyponatremia.

a. PRIMARY ADRENAL INSUFFICIENCY: Primary adrenal insufficiency is accompanied by mineralocorticoid deficiency, which results in renal sodium wasting. In contrast, secondary (hypothalamic) adrenal insufficiency is primarily a glucocorticoid deficiency, and does not promote renal sodium loss.

b. CEREBRAL SALT WASTING: Cerebral salt wasting occurs with traumatic brain injury, subarachnoid hemorrhage, and neurosurgery (23). The mechanism for the renal sodium loss is unclear (23).

2. **Diagnostic Considerations**

The source of sodium loss is usually apparent. If this is unclear, the spot urine sodium can help to distinguish renal from extrarenal losses; i.e., a high urine sodium (>20 mEq/L) suggests renal sodium loss, while a low urine sodium (<20 mEq/L) suggests an extrarenal source.

D. Euvolemic Hyponatremia

1. **Etiologies**

The principal causes of euvolemic hyponatremia include:

a. Nonosmotic ADH release from physiologic stress, which is typically seen in hospitalized patients (25).

b. The *syndrome of inappropriate ADH* (SIADH), which is a condition of nonosmotic ADH release associated with numerous malignancies, infections, and drugs (25).

c. Excessive water intake (primary or psychogenic polydipsia).

2. **Diagnostic Considerations**

Nonosmotic ADH release is characterized by an inappropriately concentrated urine (urine osmolality >100 mosm/kg), while excessive water intake is characterized by a dilute urine (urine osmolality <100 mosm/kg) (25).

E. Hypervolemic Hyponatremia

1. Hypervolemic hyponatremia is the result of both sodium and water retention, and occurs in advanced cases of heart failure, cirrhosis, and renal failure.

2. Renal failure is associated with a high urine sodium (>20 mEq/L), while the urine sodium is low (<20 mEq/L) in heart failure and cirrhosis, except when diuretics are given.

F. Fluid Management

The management of hyponatremia is determined by the ECV, and the presence or absence of neurological symptoms. Symptomatic hyponatremia requires a more rapid increase in the plasma sodium level (with hypertonic saline), but an increase that is too rapid can be deleterious, as described next.

1. **Osmotic Demyelination**

Rapid correction of the plasma sodium (i.e., >10–12 mEq/L in 24 hrs) can produce an osmotic demyelination syndrome (sometimes called *central pontine myelinolysis*) characterized by dysarthria, quadriparesis, and loss of consciousness (23,25). Chronic hyponatremia poses a greater risk than acute (within 48 hrs) hyponatremia. The following measures are recommended for avoiding osmotic demyelination:

a. For chronic hyponatremia, the plasma sodium should not rise faster than 0.5 mEq/L per hour (or 10–12 mEq/L in 24 hours), and the rapid correction phase should stop when the plasma sodium reaches 120 mEq/L (25).

b. For acute hyponatremia, the plasma sodium can be increased by 4–6 mEq/L in the first 1–2 hrs (23), but the final plasma sodium should not exceed 120 mEq/L.

2. **Infusion Rate for Hypertonic Saline**

   The infusion rate of hypertonic saline (3% NaCL) can be estimated by multiplying the patient's body weight (in kg) by the desired rate of increase in plasma sodium (25).

   a. EXAMPLE: If the patient weighs 70 kg and the desired rate of rise in plasma sodium is 0.5 mEq/L per hour, the infusion rate of hypertonic (3%) saline is $70 \times 0.5 = 35$ mL/hr. The plasma sodium is then monitored periodically to determine when the target plasma sodium (120 mEq/L) is achieved.

3. **Strategies**

   The following are some general strategies for fluid management based on the ECV. (These are summarized in Figure 27.2.)

   a. LOW ECV: For symptomatic patients, infuse hypertonic saline (3% NaCL) using the rapid correction guidelines in the prior section. For asymptomatic patients, infuse isotonic saline until the hypovolemia is corrected.

b. NORMAL ECV: For symptomatic patients, infuse hypertonic saline (3% NaCL) using the rapid correction guidelines in the prior section. If volume overload is a concern, give furosemide (20–40 mg IV) (25). For asymptomatic patients, restrict fluid intake to 500 mL below the daily urine output (25). If fluid restriction is ineffective or intolerable, consider the drug therapies described later.

c. HIGH ECV: There are no guidelines for treating hypervolemic hyponatremia. Hypertonic saline could be used for severely symptomatic patients, but should be combined with furosemide diuresis (25). For asymptomatic patients, fluid restriction and furosemide diuresis are the standard measures.

G. Pharmacotherapy

The following drugs are used primarily for chronic hyponatremia associated with SIADH, especially when fluid restriction is ineffective or is not tolerated.

1. **Demeclocycline**

   Demeclocycline is a tetracycline derivative that blocks the effects of ADH in the renal tubules. The drug is *given orally, and the dose is 600–1,200 mg daily in divided doses* (25). Maximum effect takes several days, and success is variable. Demeclocycline can be nephrotoxic, so monitoring renal function is advised.

2. **Vasopressin Antagonists**

   Two drugs (*conivaptan* and *tolvaptan*) are available that block receptors for arginine vasopressin (the other term for ADH) (27,28).

   a. CONIVAPTAN: Conivaptan blocks vasopressin effects in the kidneys and elsewhere. The drug is *given intravenously, with a loading dose of 20 mg, followed by a con-*

tinuous infusion of 40 mg/day for 96 hours (28). The increment in plasma sodium is about 6–7 mEq/L (28).

b. TOLVAPTAN: Tolvaptan selectively blocks vasopressin effects in the kidneys. The drug is *given orally, starting at a dose of 15 mg once daily, which can be
increased to 60 mg daily, if needed.* The peak effect is an
increase in plasma sodium of 6–7 mEq/L, which
occurs in the first 4 days of treatment (27).

c. These "vaptans" provide little or no advantage for
the acute management of hyponatremia in the ICU.

REFERENCES

1. Pokaharel M, Block CA. Dysnatremia in the ICU. Curr Opin Crit
Care 2011; 17:581–593.

2. Rose BD, Post TW. The total body water and the plasma sodium
concentration. In: Clinical physiology of acid-base and electrolyte
disorders. 5th ed. New York, NY: McGraw-Hill, 2001; 241–257.

3. Gennari FJ. Current concepts. Serum osmolality. Uses and limitations. N Engl J Med 1984; 310:102–105.

4. Erstad BL. Osmolality and osmolarity: narrowing the terminology gap. Pharmacother 2003; 23:1085–1086.

5. Turchin A, Seifter JL, Seely EW. Clinical problem-solving. Mind
the gap. N Engl J Med 2003; 349:1465–1469.

6. Purssell RA, Lynd LD, Koga Y. The use of the osmole gap as a
screening test for the presence of exogenous substances. Toxicol
Rev 2004; 23:189–202.

7. Adrogue HJ, Madias NE. Hypernatremia. N Engl J Med 2000;
342:1493–1499.

8. Arieff AI, Ayus JC. Strategies for diagnosing and managing
hypernatremic encephalopathy. J Crit Illness 1996; 11:720–727.

9. Naik KR, Saroja AO. Seasonal postpartum hypernatremic
encephalopathy with osmotic extrapontine myelinolysis and
rhabdomyolysis. J Neurol Sci 2010; 291:5–11.

10. Rose BD, Post TW. Hyperosmolal states: hypernatremia. In: Clinical physiology of acid-base and electrolyte disorders. 5th ed. New York, NY: McGraw-Hill, 2001; 746–792.

11. Marino PL, Krasner J, O'Moore P. Fluid and electrolyte expert, Philadelphia, PA: WB Saunders, 1987.

12. Makaryus AN, McFarlane SI. Diabetes insipidus: diagnosis and treatment of a complex disease. Cleve Clin J Med 2006; 73:65–71.

13. Ghirardello S, Malattia C, Scagnelli P, et al. Current perspective on the pathogenesis of central diabetes insipidus. J Pediatr Endocrinol Metab 2005; 18:631–645.

14. Garofeanu CG, Weir M, Rosas-Arellano MP, et al. Causes of reversible nephrogenic diabetes insipidus: a systematic review. Am J Kidney Dis 2005; 45:626–637.

15. Geheb MA. Clinical approach to the hyperosmolar patient. Crit Care Clin 1987; 3: 797–815.

16. Blevins LS, Jr., Wand GS. Diabetes insipidus. Crit Care Med 1992; 20:69–79.

17. Ofran Y, Lavi D, Opher D, et al. Fatal voluntary salt intake resulting in the highest ever documented sodium plasma level in adults (255 mmol/L): a disorder linked to female gender and psychiatric disorders. J Intern Med 2004; 256:525–528.

18. Chaithongdi N, Subauste JS, Koch CA, Geraci SA. Diagnosis and management of hyperglycemic emergencies. Hormones 2011; 10:250–260.

19. Awasthi D, Tiwari AK, Upadhyaya A, et al. Ketotic hyperglycemia with movement disorder. J Emerg Trauma Shock 2012; 5:90–91.

20. Moran SM, Jamison RL. The variable hyponatremic response to hyperglycemia. West J Med 1985; 142:49–53.

21. Hiller TA, Abbott RD, Barrett EJ. Hyponatremia: evaluating the correction factor for hyperglycemia. Am J Med 1999; 106:399–403.

22 Hoorn EJ, Lindemans J, Zietse R. Development of severe hyponatremia in hospitalized patients: treatment-related risk factors and inadequate management. Nephrol Dial Transplant 2006; 21:70–76.

23. Upadhyay UM, Gormley WB. Etiology and management of hyponatremia in neurosurgical patients. J Intensive Care Med 2012; 27:139–144.

24. Weisberg LS. Pseudohyponatremia: A reappraisal. Am J Med 1989; 86:315–318.

25. Verbalis JG, Goldsmith SR, Greenberg A, et al. Hyponatremia treatment guidelines 2007: Expert panel recommendations. Am J Med 2007; 120(Suppl): S1–S21.

26. Arieff AI, Ayus JC. Pathogenesis of hyponatremic encephalopathy. Current concepts. Chest 1993; 103:607–610.

27. Lehrich RW, Greenberg A. Hyponatremia and the use of vasopressin receptor antagonists in critically ill patients. J Intensive Care Med 2012; 27:207–218.

28. Zeltser D, Rosansky S, van Rensburg H, et al. Assessment of efficacy and safety of intravenous conivaptan in euvolemic and hypervolemic hyponatremia. Am J Nephrol 2007; 27:447–457.

Chapter 28

Potassium

Monitoring the plasma potassium (K^+) level as an index of total body K^+ is like evaluating the size of an iceberg by its visible tip, because less than 1% of the total body K^+ is located in plasma (1). With this limitation in mind, this chapter describes the causes and consequences of abnormalities in the plasma K^+ concentration (1-3).

I. BASICS

A. Potassium Distribution

1. The intracellular preponderance of K^+ is the result of a sodium-potassium (Na^+-K^+) exchange pump on cell membranes that moves Na^+ out of cells and moves K^+ into cells (1).

2. The total body K^+ in healthy adults is about 50 mEq/kg, and only 2% is in the extracellular fluid (1). Since the plasma accounts for about 20% of the extracellular fluid, *the K^+ content of plasma is only 0.4% of the total body K^+.*

   a. EXAMPLE: A 70 kg adult is expected to have a total body K^+ of 3,500 mEq, with only 70 mEq K^+ in the extracellular fluid, and a miniscule 14 mEq of K^+ in plasma.

B. Plasma Potassium

1. The influence of changes in total body K^+ on plasma K^+ is described by the curve in Figure 28.1 (4). Note the

shape of the curve, with the flat portion in the region of K⁺ deficiency.

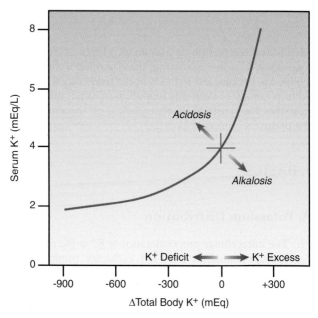

FIGURE 28.1 Relationship between changes in total body K⁺ and the serum K⁺ concentration. Redrawn from Reference 4.

2. In an average-sized adult with a normal plasma K⁺, a total body K⁺ deficit of 200–400 mEq is required to produce a 1 mEq/L decrease in plasma K⁺, while a total body K⁺ excess of 100–200 mEq is required to produce a 1 mEq/L increase in plasma K⁺ (5). Therefore, *for a given change in serum K⁺, the change in total body K⁺ is twofold greater with K⁺ depletion (hypokalemia) than with K⁺ excess (hyperkalemia).*

C. Potassium Excretion

1. Small amounts of K^+ are lost in stool (5–10 mEq/day) and sweat (0–10 mEq/day), but the majority of K^+ loss is in urine (40–120 mEq/day, depending on K^+ intake) (1).

2. **Renal Excretion**

   Most of the filtered K^+ is reabsorbed in the proximal tubules, and K^+ is then secreted in the distal tubules and collecting ducts (1).

   a. Potassium loss in urine is primarily a function of K^+ secretion in the distal nephron, which is controlled by plasma K^+ and aldosterone (which stimulates K^+ secretion as it promotes sodium retention).

   b. When renal function is normal, the capacity for K^+ excretion is great enough to prevent a sustained rise in plasma K^+ in response to an increased K^+ load (1).

II. HYPOKALEMIA

Hypokalemia (plasma K^+ <3.5 mEq/L) can be the result of K^+ movement into cells (transcellular shift), or a decrease in total body K^+ (K^+ depletion) (6).

A. Transcellular Shift

The following conditions can result in hypokalemia from K^+ movement into cells.

1. Inhaled *β_2-agonist bronchodilators* (e.g., albuterol) can produce a mild decrease in plasma K^+ (≤ 0.5 mEq/L) in therapeutic doses (7). The mechanism is stimulation of β_2 receptors on cell membranes of myocytes in skeletal muscle. The effect on plasma K^+ is magnified when inhaled β_2 agonists are used in combination with insulin (7) or diuretics (8).

2. *Alkalosis* can promote the intracellular movement of K^+ in exchange for intracellular H^+ via a membrane H^+-K^+ exchange pump. However, alkalosis has a variable and unpredictable effect on plasma K^+ (9).

3. *Hypothermia* causes a transient drop in plasma K^+ that resolves on rewarming (10).

4. *Insulin* drives K^+ into cells via the glucose transporter, and the effect lasts 1–2 hours (7).

B. Potassium Depletion

Potassium depletion can be the result of K^+ loss via the kidneys or GI tract.

1. **Renal Potassium Loss**

   a. *Diuretics* (thiazides and loop diuretics) promote K^+ secretion in the distal nephron via two mechanisms: (a) increased sodium delivery to the distal nephron, and (b) enhanced aldosterone secretion (from volume loss) (6).

   b. *Magnesium depletion* is a well-known cause of enhanced urinary K^+ loss, but the exact mechanism is unclear (6). Hypomagnesemia is found in about 40% of patients with hypokalemia (6), and is considered an important factor in promoting K^+ depletion in critically ill patients (11).

   c. *Loss of gastric secretions* is often accompanied by hypokalemia (11). Gastric secretions have a relatively low concentration of K^+ (10–15 mEq/L), but the resulting volume loss and alkalosis promote K^+ loss in the urine (12).

   d. *Amphotericin B* promotes K^+ secretion in the distal nephron, and hypokalemia occurs in up to half of patients treated with this antifungal agent (6).

2. **GI Potassium Loss**

The major cause of extrarenal K^+ loss is *secretory diarrhea*, where the concentration of K^+ is 15–40 mEq/L (12). The daily stool volume can reach 10 liters in severe cases of secretory diarrhea, resulting in daily K^+ losses up to 400 mEq (12).

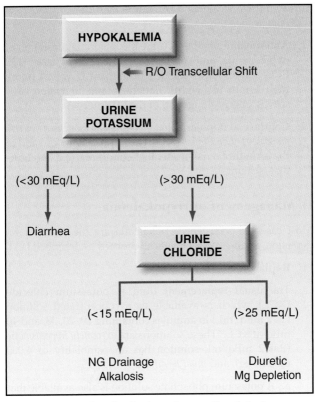

FIGURE 28.2 An algorithm for the evaluation of hypokalemia.

3. **Diagnostic Evaluation**

   If the source of the K^+ loss is not evident, the urinary K^+ and chloride concentrations can be useful, as shown in Figure 28.2.

C. Clinical Manifestations

Severe hypokalemia (serum K^+ <2.5 mEq/L) can produce diffuse muscle weakness (3,6), but *in most cases, hypokalemia is asymptomatic.*

1. Abnormalities in the ECG are the major manifestation of hypokalemia, and can be present in 50% of cases (13). ECG abnormalities include prominent U waves (more than 1 mm in height), flattening and inversion of T waves, and prolongation of the QT interval.

2. Contrary to popular belief, *hypokalemia alone is not a risk for serious arrhythmias* (3,13), but hypokalemia can add to the arrhythmia risk from other conditions (e.g., myocardial ischemia).

D. Management of Hypokalemia

Most cases of persistent hypokalemia are the result of K^+ depletion, and K^+ replacement can proceed as described next.

1. **Replacement Fluids**

   The usual replacement fluid is potassium chloride (KCL), which is available as a concentrated solution (1–2 mEq/mL) in ampules containing 10, 20, 30, and 40 mEq of KCL. These solutions are *extremely hyperosmotic* (the 2 mEq/mL solution has an osmolality of 4,000 mosm/kg), and *must be diluted* (14).

   a. A potassium phosphate solution is also available that contains 4.5 mEq of K^+ and 3 mmol of PO_4 per mL.

This solution is preferred by some for K^+ replacement in diabetic ketoacidosis (because PO_4 depletion is also common in ketoacidosis).

2. **Rate of Replacement**

The standard method of intravenous K^+ replacement is to add 20 mEq of KCL to 100 mL of isotonic saline and infuse this mixture over 1 hour (15).

a. The *standard rate of intravenous K^+ replacement is 20 mEq/hr* (15) but replacement of 40 mEq/hr may be necessary for severe hypokalemia (<1.5 mEq/L) or troublesome arrhythmias, and *replacement rates as high as 100 mEq/hr have been used safely* (16).

b. Infusion through a large, central vein is preferred because of the irritating properties of the hyperosmotic KCL solutions. However, *delivery into the superior vena cava is not advised if the replacement rate exceeds 20 mEq/hr* because of the (poorly documented) risk of asystole from an an abrupt rise in plasma K^+ in the right heart chambers.

3. **Response**

The plasma K^+ may be slow to rise initially, as predicted by the flat portion of the curve in Figure 28.1. If the hypokalemia is refractory to K^+ replacement, magnesium depletion should be considered, because, *in the presence of magnesium depletion, hypokalemia is often refractory to K^+ replacement until the magnesium deficit is replaced* (17).

III. HYPERKALEMIA

While hypokalemia is often well tolerated, hyperkalemia (serum K^+ >5.5 mEq/L) can be a life-threatening condition.

A. Pseudohyperkalemia

1. Hyperkalemia that is present *ex vivo* (in the blood sample) but not *in vivo*, is known as *pseudohyperkalemia*, and has been reported in 20% of blood samples that show hyperkalemia (18).

2. Causes of pseudohyperkalemia include (19):

   a. Traumatic hemolysis during collection of the blood sample (most common cause).

   b. Fist clenching (K^+ release from muscles) or tourniquet stasis.

   c. K^+ release from WBCs in severe leukocytosis ($>50,000/mm^3$), or from platelets in severe thrombocytosis (>1 million/mm^3).

   d. K^+ release during clot formation (serum $K^+ >$ plasma K^+).

3. Conditions a, b, or d should be suspected if hyperkalemia is abrupt and unexpected, and a repeat blood sample should be collected using special precautions (e.g., minimum suction during blood collection).

B. Transcellular Shift

Hyperkalemia can be the result of K^+ release from cells (transcellular shift) in the following conditions:

1. **Tumor Lysis Syndrome**

   Tumor lysis syndrome is an acute, life-threatening condition that appears within 7 days after the initiation of cytotoxic therapy for selected malignancies (e.g., acute leukemia, non-Hodgkin's lymphoma). Clinical features include hyperkalemia, hyperphosphatemia, hypocalcemia, and hyperuricemia, often accompanied by acute kidney injury (20). Hyperkalemia is the most immediate threat to life.

2. **Drugs**

The drugs that promote K^+ movement out of cells are listed in Table 28.1.

a. Digitalis inhibits the membrane Na^+-K^+ exchange pump, but hyperkalemia occurs only with acute *digitalis toxicity* (21).

b. *Succinylcholine* (depolarizing neuromuscular blocker) also inhibits the membrane Na^+-K^+ exchange pump (depolarizing effect), causing a minor increase in serum K^+ (<1 mEq/L) that lasts 5–10 minutes in most cases (22). However, life-threatening hyperkalemia can occur in patients with malignant hyperthermia, skeletal muscle myopathies, or a variety of neurologic conditions associated with skeletal muscle denervation (e.g., spinal cord injury).

Table 28.1	Drugs That Promote Hyperkalemia
Transcellular Shift	**Impaired Renal Excretion**
β-blockers	ACE Inhibitors
Digitalis	Angiotensin-receptor blockers
Succinylcholine	K^+- sparing diuretics
	NSAIDs
	Heparin
	Trimethoprim-sulfamethoxazole

3. **Acidosis:**

The traditional teaching that acidosis promotes hyperkalemia via K^+ release from cells is being questioned because the organic acidoses (lactic acidosis and ketoacidosis) do not promote hyperkalemia (9).

C. Impaired Renal Excretion

1. Hyperkalemia from impaired renal K^+ excretion is usually the result of renal failure, or drugs that inhibit the renin-angiotensin-aldosterone system (which are listed in Table 28.1) (22,23).

2. Adrenal insufficiency impairs renal potassium excretion, but *hyperkalemia is seen only in chronic adrenal insufficiency*.

3. **Massive Transfusion**

   A steady leakage of K^+ from stored RBCs results, after 18 days of storage (the average time that blood is stored), in a K^+ load of 2–3 mEq per unit of packed RBCs (24). The significance of this K^+ load is demonstrated by the fact that the average-sized adult has only 14–15 mEq of K^+ in the plasma (see Section I-A).

   a. The K^+ load in transfused blood is normally cleared by the kidneys, but when systemic blood flow is compromised (e.g., from hemorrhage), renal K^+ excretion is impaired, and the K^+ in packed RBC transfusions will accumulate.

   b. One study has shown that hyperkalemia appears after transfusion of 7 units of packed RBCs (25).

D. ECG Abnormalities

1. The principal threat of hyperkalemia is slowed impulse transmission in the heart.

2. The ECG changes in progressive hyperkalemia are shown in Figure 28.3. The earliest change is the appearance of a tall, tapering (tented) T wave that is most evident in precordial leads V_2 and V_3. As the hyperkalemia progresses, the P wave amplitude decreases and the PR

interval lengthens. The P waves eventually disappear and the QRS complex widens. The final event is ventricular fibrillation or asystole.

3. ECG changes usually begin to appear when the serum K⁺ reaches 6–7 mEq/L (26), but the threshold for ECG changes can vary widely.

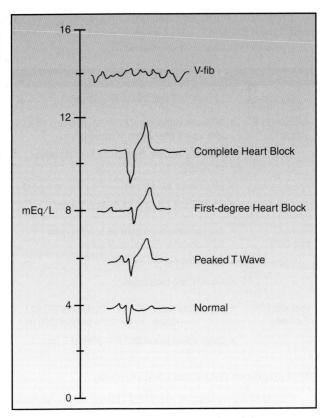

FIGURE 28.3 ECG abnormalities in progressive hyperkalemia.

E. Management of Severe Hyperkalemia

Severe hyperkalemia is defined as a serum K^+ >6.5 mEq/L, or any serum K^+ associated with ECG changes (26).

1. **Goals**

   The management of severe hyperkalemia has 3 goals: (a) antagonize the cardiac effects of hyperkalemia, (b) promote K^+ movement into cells, and (c) remove excess K^+ from the body. The methods used to achieve these goals are summarized in Table 28.2.

Table 28.2	Management of Severe Hyperkalemia
Goal	**Treatment Regimen**
Antagonize K^+ Effects	• 10% calcium gluconate; 10 mL IV over 3 min, and repeat after 5 min, if necessary
	• Use 10% calcium chloride for hemodynamic instability
	• Effect lasts 30–60 min
	• Do NOT use calcium for digitalis toxicity
Move K^+ into Cells	• Regular insulin (10 units as IV bolus) plus 50% dextrose (50 mL as IV bolus)
	• Peak effect at 30–60 min
	• Do NOT use bicarbonate
Promote K^+ Excretion	• Kayexalate (oral): 30 g in 20% sorbitol (50 mL) (rectal): 50 g in 20% sorbitol (200 mL)
	• Slow-acting (onset at 2 hrs, peak at 6 hrs)

2. **Antagonize Potassium Cardiotoxicity**

   Calcium increases the electrical charge across myocardial cell membranes and opposes the depolarization produced by hyperkalemia. Calcium antagonism is recommended for a serum K^+ >6.5 mEq/L (with or without

ECG changes), and for any serum K^+ associated with ECG changes (26). *Calcium is contraindicated in hyper-kalemia from digitalis toxicity.*

a. CALCIUM GLUCONATE: The preferred calcium preparation is *calcium gluconate*, which is given in the dosing regimen shown in Table 28.2. The response is short-lived (30–60 minutes), so efforts to move K^+ into cells should be started as well.

b. CALCIUM CHLORIDE: For hyperkalemia associated with hemodynamic instability, calcium chloride is preferred because the calcium in one ampule (10 mL) of 10% calcium chloride is three times greater than one ampule of 10% calcium gluconate (see Chapter 30, Table 30.3), and the extra calcium is a potential advantage by promoting cardiac output and preserving peripheral vascular tone.

3. **Move Potassium into Cells**

The preferred method for the transcellular movement of K^+ is the combination of insulin and dextrose.

a. INSULIN-DEXTROSE: Insulin drives K^+ into skeletal muscle cells by activating the membrane Na^+-K^+ exchange pump (27), and the insulin-dextrose regimen in Table 28.2 will decrease the serum K^+ by at least 0.6 mEq/L (26). Insulin can be used without dextrose in hyperglycemic patients (26). The insulin effect is temporary (peak effect between 30–60 min), so measures that promote potassium excretion should be started as well.

b. β_2 AGONISTS: Inhaled β_2 agonists produce a small decrease in plasma K^+ (<0.5 mEq/L) in therapeutic doses (7), but a much (4-fold) larger dose is needed to produce a significant (0.5–1 mEq/L) drop in serum K^+ (26), and this larger dose can produce unwanted side effects (e.g., tachycardia). Therefore, this approach is not advised (at least as a sole measure).

    c. SODIUM BICARBONATE: There are two reasons to *avoid bicarbonate* in this setting: (a) short-term infusions of sodium bicarbonate (up to 4 hrs) have no effect on serum K^+ levels (26), and (b) bicarbonate can form complexes with calcium, which is counterproductive.

4. **Promote Potassium Excretion**

    a. CATION EXCHANGE RESIN: *Sodium polystyrene sulfonate* (Kayexalate) is a cation exchange resin that promotes K^+ excretion via the bowel (each gram of resin binds 0.65 mEq of K^+). It is given orally (preferred) or by retention enema, using the dosing regimens in Table 28.2, and is mixed with sorbitol to prevent concretions. At least 6 hours is required for peak effect (26), so treatment should be started as soon as possible. There are several case reports of life-threatening, necrotic lesions in the bowel linked to Kayexalate (28).

    b. HEMODIALYSIS: The most effective method of K^+ removal is hemodialysis, which can produce a 1 mEq/L drop in serum K^+ after one hour, and a 2 mEq/L drop after 3 hrs (26).

REFERENCES

1. Rose BD, Post TW. Potassium homeostasis. In: Clinical physiology of acid-base and electrolyte disorders. 5th ed. New York, NY: McGraw-Hill, 2001; 372–402.

2. Alfonzo AVM, Isles C, Geddes C, Deighan C. Potassium disorders—clinical spectrum and emergency management. Resusc 2006; 70:10–25.

3. Schaefer TJ, Wolford RW. Disorders of potassium. Emerg Med Clin North Am 2005; 23:723–747.

4. Brown RS. Extrarenal potassium homeostasis. Kidney Int 1986; 30:116–127.

5. Sterns RH, Cox M, Feig PU, et al. Internal potassium balance and the control of the plasma potassium concentration. Medicine 1981; 60:339–354.

6. Rose BD, Post TW. Hypokalemia. In: Clinical Physiology of Acid-Base and Electrolyte Disorders. 5th ed. New York, NY: McGraw-Hill, 2001:836–887.

7. Allon M, Copkney C. Albuterol and insulin for treatment of hyperkalemia in hemodialysis patients. Kidney Int 1990; 38:869–872.

8. Lipworth BJ, McDevitt DG, Struthers AD. Prior treatment with diuretic augments the hypokalemic and electrocardiographic effects of inhaled albuterol. Am J Med 1989; 86:653–657.

9. Adrogue HJ, Madias NE. Changes in plasma potassium concentration during acute acid-base disturbances. Am J Med 1981; 71:456–467.

10. Bernard SA, Buist M. Induced hypothermia in critical care medicine: a review. Crit Care Med 2003; 31:2041–2051.

11. Salem M, Munoz R, Chernow B. Hypomagnesemia in critical illness. A common and clinically important problem. Crit Care Clin 1991; 7:225–252.

12. Gennari FJ, Weise WJ. Acid-base disturbances in gastrointestinal disease. Clin J Am Soc Nephrol 2008; 3:1861–1868.

13. Flakeb G, Villarread D, Chapman D. Is hypokalemia a cause of ventricular arrhythmias? J Crit Illness 1986; 1:66–74.

14. Trissel LA. Handbook on Injectable Drugs. 13th ed. Bethesda, MD: Amer Soc Health System Pharmcists, 2005; 1230.

15. Kruse JA, Carlson RW. Rapid correction of hypokalemia using concentrated intravenous potassium chloride infusions. Arch Intern Med 1990;150:613–617.

16. Kim GH, Han JS. Therapeutic approach to hypokalemia. Nephron 2002;92 Suppl 1:28–32.

17. Whang R, Flink EB, Dyckner T, et al. Magnesium depletion as a cause of refractory potassium repletion. Arch Intern Med 1985;145:1686–1689.

18. Rimmer JM, Horn JF, Gennari FJ. Hyperkalemia as a complication of drug therapy. Arch Intern Med 1987;147:867–869.

19. Wiederkehr MR, Moe OW. Factitious hyperkalemia. Am J Kidney Dis 2000; 36:1049–1053.

20. Howard SC, Jones DP, Pui C-H. The tumor lysis syndrome. N Engl J Med 2012; 364:1844–1854.

21. Krisanda TJ. Digitalis toxicity. Postgrad Med 1992; 91:273–284.

22. Ponce SP, Jennings AE, Madias N, Harington JT. Drug-induced hyperkalemia. Medicine 1985; 64:357–370.

23. Perazella MA. Drug-induced hyperkalemia: old culprits and new offenders. Am J Med 2000; 109:307–314.

24. Vraets A, Lin Y, Callum JL. Transfusion-associated hyperkalemia. Transfus Med Rev 2011; 25:184–196.

25. Aboudara MC, Hurst FP, Abbott KC, et al. Hyperkalemia after packed red blood cell transfusion in trauma patients. J Trauma 2008; 64:S86–S91.

26. Weisberg L. Management of severe hyperkalemia. Crit Care Med 2008; 36:3246–3251.

27. Clausen T, Everts ME. Regulation of the Na, K-pump in skeletal muscle. Kidney Int 1989; 35:1–13.

28. Harel Z, Harel S, Shah PS, et al. Gastrointestinal adverse events with sodium polystyrene sulfonate (Kayexalate) use: a systematic review. Am J Med 2013; 126:264.e9–264.e24.

Chapter 29

Magnesium

Magnesium is the second most abundant intracellular cation, and is an essential element for the utilization of energy in the organic world. Unfortunately, the "tip of the iceberg" analogy used for potassium also applies to magnesium; i.e., only a minor fraction (0.3%) of total body magnesium is located in plasma (1-3), so monitoring the plasma magnesium provides little information about total body magnesium.

I. BASICS

A. Distribution

1. The average-sized adult contains approximately 24 g (1 mole, or 2,000 mEq) of magnesium (Mg); a little over half is located in bone, whereas less than 1% is located in plasma (2).

2. The lack of representation in the plasma limits the value of the plasma Mg as an index of total body magnesium; e.g., *plasma Mg levels can be normal in the face of total body Mg depletion* (2-3).

B. Serum Magnesium

1. Serum is favored over plasma for Mg assays because the anticoagulant used for plasma samples can be contaminated with citrate or other anions that bind Mg (2).

2. The normal reference range for serum Mg (in healthy adults in the United States) is shown in Table 29.1 (4).

Table 29.1	Reference Ranges for Magnesium	
Fluid	**Traditional Units**	**SI Units**
Serum Magnesium:		
Total	1.7–2.4 mg/dL	0.7–1.0 mmol/L
	1.4–2.0 mEq/L	
Ionized	0.8–1.1 mEq/L	0.4–0.6 mmol/L
Urinary Magnesium:	5–15 mEq/24 hr	2.5–7.5 mmol/24 hr

From Reference 4. Conversions: mEq/L = [(mg/dL x 10)/24] x 2; mEq/L = mmol/L x 2.

C. Ionized Magnesium

1. Only 67% of the Mg in plasma is in the ionized (active) form, and the remaining 33% is either bound to plasma proteins or chelated with divalent anions such as phosphate and sulfate (2).

2. The standard assay for Mg includes all plasma fractions. Therefore, when the serum Mg is abnormally low, it is not possible to determine whether the problem is a decrease in the ionized (active) fraction or a decrease in the bound fractions (e.g., hypoproteinemia).

3. Since the total amount of Mg in plasma is small, the difference between the ionized and bound Mg may not be large enough to be clinically relevant.

D. Urinary Magnesium

1. The normal range for urinary Mg excretion is shown in Table 29.1. Urinary Mg excretion is dependent on the Mg intake.

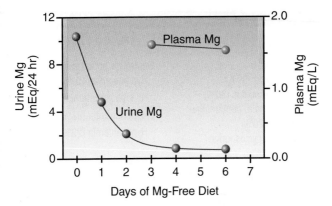

FIGURE 29.1 Urinary Mg excretion and plasma Mg levels in a healthy volunteer placed on a Mg-free diet. Solid bars on the vertical axes indicate the normal range for each variable. (Adapted from Shils ME. Medicine 1969; 48:61–82.)

2. When Mg intake is deficient, the kidneys conserve Mg, and urinary Mg excretion falls to negligible levels. This is shown in Figure 29.1. Note that after one week of a Mg-free diet, the plasma Mg remains in the normal range, while the urinary Mg excretion has decreased to negligible levels. This illustrates the relative value of urinary Mg excretion for monitoring Mg balance.

II. MAGNESIUM DEFICIENCY

Hypomagnesemia is reported in as many as 65% of ICU patients (1,6), and the incidence of Mg depletion is even higher (because the serum Mg level can be normal in patients with Mg deficiency) (2,3).

A. Predisposing Conditions

Several conditions promote Mg depletion, and these are listed in Table 29.2.

Table 29.2	Causes & Consequences of Mg Depletion	
Predisposing Conditions	**Clinical Findings**	
Drug Therapy:	Electrolyte abnormalities:	
Furosemide (50%)	Hypokalemia (40%)	
Aminoglycosides (30%)	Hypophosphatemia (30%)	
Amphotericin, pentamidine	Hyponatremia (27%)	
Digitalis (20%)	Hypocalcemia (22%)	
Cisplatin, cyclosporine		
Diarrhea (secretory)	Cardiac manifestations:	
Alcohol abuse (chronic)	Arrhythmias	
	Digitalis toxicity	
Diabetes mellitus		
Acute MI	Reactive CNS Syndrome	

Numbers in parentheses indicate incidence of associated hypomagnesemia.

1. **Diuretic Therapy**

   Diuretics are the leading cause of Mg deficiency. Diuretic-induced inhibition of sodium reabsorption also interferes with Mg reabsorption, and the urinary Mg losses can parallel urinary sodium losses.

   a. Urinary Mg excretion is most pronounced with loop diuretics like furosemide. *Mg deficiency has been reported in 50% of patients receiving chronic therapy with furosemide* (7).

   b. The thiazide diuretics also promote Mg depletion, primarily in elderly patients (8).

   c. Mg depletion is not a complication of "potassium-sparing" diuretics (9).

2. **Antibiotic Therapy**

   The antibiotics that promote Mg depletion are the aminoglycosides, amphotericin and pentamidine (10,11). The aminoglycosides block Mg reabsorption in the ascending loop of Henle, and hypomagnesemia has been reported in 30% of patients receiving aminoglycoside therapy (11).

3. **Other Drugs**

Prolonged use of proton pump inhibitors can be associated with severe hypomagnesemia (12). Other drugs associated with Mg depletion include digitalis and epinephrine (shift Mg into cells), and the chemotherapeutic agents cisplatin and cyclosporine (promote renal Mg excretion) (10,13).

4. **Alcohol-Related Illness**

Hypomagnesemia is reported in 30% of hospital admissions for alcohol abuse, and in 85% of admissions for delirium tremens (14). Malnutrition and chronic diarrhea may play a role in the Mg depletion in these conditions.

5. **Secretory Diarrhea**

Secretions from the lower GI tract are rich in Mg (10 to 14 mEq/L) (15), and secretory diarrhea can lead to profound Mg depletion. Upper GI tract secretions are not rich in Mg (1–2 mEq/L), so vomiting is not a risk for Mg depletion.

6. **Diabetes Mellitus**

Mg depletion is common in insulin-dependent diabetics, probably as a result of glycosuria-induced urinary Mg loss (16). Hypomagnesemia is reported in only 7% of admissions for diabetic ketoacidosis, but the incidence increases to 50% over the first 12 hours after admission (17), probably as a result of insulin-induced movement of Mg into cells.

7. **Acute Myocardial Infarction**

Hypomagnesemia is reported in as many as 80% of patients with acute myocardial infarction (18). The mechanism is unclear, but may be due to an intracellular shift of Mg from excess catecholamines.

B. Clinical Manifestations

There are no specific clinical manifestations of Mg depletion, but the following clinical findings can suggest an underlying Mg deficiency.

1. **Other Electrolyte Abnormalities**

   Mg depletion is often accompanied by other electrolyte abnormalities (see Table 29.2) (19):

   a. HYPOKALEMIA: Mg depletion enhances renal K^+ excretion, and hypokalemia develops in almost half of patients with Mg depletion (19). The *hypokalemia that accompanies Mg depletion is often refractory to K^+ replacement therapy, and Mg repletion is necessary before the hypokalemia can be corrected* (20).

   b. HYPOCALCEMIA: Mg depletion can cause hypocalcemia as a result of impaired parathyroid hormone release, and impaired end-organ response to parathyroid hormone (21,22). The hypocalcemia resolves when Mg deficits are corrected.

   c. HYPOPHOSPHATEMIA: Phosphate depletion is a cause rather than an effect of Mg depletion. The mechanism is enhanced renal excretion of Mg (23).

2. **Arrhythmias**

   a. Mg depletion prolongs the QT interval on the ECG and can provoke a polymorphic ventricular tachycardia known as *torsade de pointes* (see Chapter 13, Section V-C).

   b. Mg deficiency promotes digitalis cardiotoxicity (because both digitalis and Mg deficiency inhibit the Na-K exchange pump on cell membranes). Intravenous Mg can suppress digitalis-toxic arrhythmias, even when serum Mg levels are normal (24-25).

3. **Neurologic Findings**

   a. The neurologic manifestations of Mg deficiency include altered mentation, tremors, and generalized seizures.

   b. *Reactive central nervous system Mg deficiency* is a syndrome that is characterized by ataxia, slurred speech, metabolic acidosis, excessive salivation, diffuse muscle spasms, generalized seizures, and progressive obtundation (26). The clinical features are often triggered by loud noises or bodily contact. The treatment is Mg replacement.

C. Diagnosis

As emphasized throughout this chapter, the serum Mg level is an insensitive marker of Mg depletion. The urinary Mg excretion is more reliable (see Figure 29.1), and the urinary Mg excretion in response to a Mg load is even better (see next).

1. **Magnesium Retention Test**

   Mg reabsorption in the renal tubules is close to the maximum rate, so most of an infused Mg load will be excreted in the urine when total body Mg stores are normal. However, when Mg stores are deficient, Mg is reabsorbed in the renal tubules, and a smaller fraction of an infused Mg load is excreted in the urine.

   a. The Mg retention test, which is outlined in Table 29.3, measures the fraction of an intravenous Mg load that is excreted in the urine (27).

   b. When less than 50% of the infused Mg is recovered in the urine, Mg deficiency is likely, and when more than 80% of the infused Mg is excreted in the urine, Mg deficiency is unlikely.

c. This test is reliable only when renal function is normal, and when there is no condition that promotes renal Mg wasting.

Table 29.3	Renal Magnesium Retention Test

Indications:

1. For suspected Mg deficiency when serum Mg is normal
2. For identifying the end-point of Mg replacement therapy

Contraindications:

1. Renal failure or ongoing renal Mg wasting

Protocol:

1. Add 24 mmol of Mg (6g of $MgSO_4$) to 250 mL of isotonic saline and infuse over 1 hour.
2. Collect urine for 24 hrs, beginning at the onset of the Mg infusion.

Results:

1. Urinary Mg excretion <12 mmol (24 mEq) in 24 hrs (i.e., less than 50% of the infused Mg) is evidence of Mg depletion.
2. Urinary Mg excretion >19 mmol (38 mEq) in 24 hrs (i.e., more than 80% of the infused Mg) is evidence against Mg depletion.

From Reference 27.

D. Magnesium Preparations

1. The Mg preparations available for oral and parenteral use are listed in Table 29.4. Oral preparations can be used for daily maintenance (5 mg/kg in normal subjects), but IV Mg is preferred for replacement therapy because intestinal absorption of Mg is erratic.

2. The standard IV preparation is magnesium sulfate ($MgSO_4$). Each gram of $MgSO_4$ has 8 mEq (4 mmol) of elemental Mg.

3. The 50% $MgSO_4$ solution (500 mg/mL) has an osmolarity of 4,000 mosm/L, so it must be diluted to a 10% (100 mg/mL) or 20% (200 mg/mL) solution for IV use. Saline solutions should be used as the diluent. Ringer's solutions are not advised because the calcium in Ringer's solutions will counteract the actions of Mg.

Table 29.4	Oral and Parenteral Magnesium Preparations
Preparation	**Elemental Mg**
Oral Preparations:	
Magnesium chloride tablets	64 mg (5.3 mEq)
Magnesium oxide tablets (400 mg)	241 mg (19.8 mEq)
Magnesium oxide tablets (140 mg)	85 mg (6.9 mEq)
Magnesium gluconate tablets (500 mg)	27 mg (2.3 mEq)
Parenteral solutions	
Magnesium sulfate (50%)*	500 mg/dL (4 mEq/L)
Magnesium sulfate (12.5%)	120 mg/dL (1 mEq/L)

*Should be diluted to a 20% solution for intravenous injection.

E. Replacement Protocols

The following Mg replacement protocols are recommended for patients with normal renal function (28).

1. **Mild, Asymptomatic Hypomagnesemia**

   a. Assume a total Mg deficit of 1 to 2 mEq/kg.

   b. Because 50% of the infused Mg can be lost in the urine, assume that the total Mg requirement is twice the Mg deficit.

   c. Replace 1 mEq/kg for the first 24 hours, and 0.5 mEq/kg daily for the next 3 to 5 days.

2. **Moderate Hypomagnesemia**

   The following therapy is intended for patients with a serum Mg <1 mEq/L, or when hypomagnesemia is accompanied by other electrolyte abnormalities:

   a. Add 6 grams $MgSO_4$ (48 mEq Mg) to 250 or 500 mL isotonic saline and infuse over 3 hours.

   b. Follow with 5 grams $MgSO_4$ (40 mEq Mg) in 250 or 500 mL isotonic saline infused over the next 6 hours.

   c. Continue with 5 grams $MgSO_4$ every 12 hours (by continuous infusion) for the next 5 days.

3. **Life-Threatening Hypomagnesemia**

   The following protocol is recommended when hypomagnesemia is accompanied by serious cardiac arrhythmias (e.g., torsade de pointes) or generalized seizures.

   a. Infuse 2 grams $MgSO_4$ (16 mEq Mg) intravenously over 2–5 minutes.

   b. Follow with 5 grams $MgSO_4$ (40 mEq Mg) in 250 or 500 mL isotonic saline infused over the next 6 hours.

   c. Continue with 5 grams $MgSO_4$ every 12 hours (by continuous infusion) for the next 5 days.

4. **Renal Insufficiency**

   For patients with renal insufficiency, no more than 50% of the Mg in the standard replacement protocols should be administered (28) and the serum Mg should be monitored carefully.

III. HYPERMAGNESEMIA

Hypermagnesemia (>2 mEq/L) is reported in 5% of hospitalized patients (29), and is found almost exclusively in patients with renal insufficiency.

A. Etiologies

1. **Hemolysis**

   The Mg concentration in erythrocytes is approximately three times greater than that in serum, and hemolysis can increase the serum Mg by 0.1 mEq/L for every 250 mL of lysed RBCs (30).

2. **Renal Insufficiency**

   The renal excretion of Mg becomes impaired when the creatinine clearance falls below 30 mL/minute (31). However, hypermagnesemia is not a prominent feature of renal insufficiency unless magnesium intake is increased.

3. **Other Conditions**

   Other conditions that can be associated with hypermagnesemia include diabetic ketoacidosis (transient), adrenal insufficiency, hyperparathyroidism, and lithium intoxication (30). The hypermagnesemia in these conditions is usually mild.

B. Clinical Manifestations

1. The clinical consequences of progressive hypermagnesemia are listed below (30).

Serum Mg	Manifestation
>4 mEq/L	Hyporeflexia
>5 mEq/L	1st° AV Block
>10 mEq/L	Complete Heart Block
>13 mEq/L	Cardiac Arrest

2. The serious consequences of hypermagnesemia are due to calcium antagonism in the cardiovascular system. The predominant effect is delayed cardiac conduction, while contractility and vascular tone are relatively unaffected.

C. Management

1. Hemodialysis is the treatment of choice for severe hypermagnesemia.

2. Intravenous calcium gluconate (1 g IV over 2 to 3 minutes) can be used to antagonize the cardiovascular effects of hypermagnesemia, but the effects are transient, and should not delay hemodialysis (32).

3. If fluids are permissible and some renal function is preserved, aggressive volume infusion combined with furosemide may be effective in reducing the serum magnesium levels in less advanced cases of hypermagnesemia.

REFERENCES

1. Noronha JL, Matuschak GM. Magnesium in critical illness: metabolism, assessment, and treatment. Intensive Care Med 2002; 28:667–679.

2. Elin RJ. Assessment of magnesium status. Clin Chem 1987; 33:1965–1970.

3. Reinhart RA. Magnesium metabolism. A review with special reference to the relationship between intracellular content and serum levels. Arch Intern Med 1988; 148:2415–2420.

4. Lowenstein FW, Stanton MF. Serum magnesium levels in the United States, 1971–1974. J Am Coll Nutr 1986; 5:399–414.

5. Altura BT, Altura BM. A method for distinguishing ionized, complexed and protein-bound Mg in normal and diseased subjects. Scand J Clin Lab Invest 1994; 217:83–87.

6. Tong GM, Rude RK. Magnesium deficiency in critical illness. J Intensive Care Med 2005;20:3–17.

7. Dyckner T, Wester PO. Potassium/magnesium depletion in patients with cardiovascular disease. Am J Med 1987; 82:11–17.

8. Hollifield JW. Thiazide treatment of systemic hypertension: effects on serum magnesium and ventricular ectopic activity. Am J Cardiol 1989; 63:22G–25G.

9. Ryan MP. Diuretics and potassium/magnesium depletion. Directions for treatment. Am J Med 1987; 82:38–47.

10. Atsmon J, Dolev E. Drug-induced hypomagnesaemia : scope and management. Drug Safety 2005; 28:763–788.

11. Zaloga GP, Chernow B, Pock A, et al. Hypomagnesemia is a common complication of aminoglycoside therapy. Surg Gynecol Obstet 1984; 158:561–565.

12. Hess MW, Hoenderop JG, Bindeis RJ, Drenth JP. Systematic review: hypomagnesemia induced by proton pump inhibition. Ailement Pharmacol Ther 2012; 36:405–413.

13. Whang R, Oei TO, Watanabe A. Frequency of hypomagnesemia in hospitalized patients receiving digitalis. Arch Intern Med 1985; 145:655–656.

14. Balesteri FJ. Magnesium metabolism in the critically ill. Crit Care Clin 1985; 5:217–226.

15. Kassirer J, Hricik D, Cohen J. Repairing Body Fluids: Principles and Practice. 1st ed. Philadelphia, PA: WB Saunders, 1989; 118–129.

16. Sjogren A, Floren CH, Nilsson A. Magnesium deficiency in IDDM related to level of glycosylated hemoglobin. Diabetes 1986; 35:459–463.

17. Lau K. Magnesium metabolism: normal and abnormal. In: Arieff AI DeFronzo RA, eds. Fluids, electrolytes, and acid base disorders. New York, NY: Churchill Livingstone, 1985; 575–623.

18. Abraham AS, Rosenmann D, Kramer M, et al. Magnesium in the prevention of lethal arrhythmias in acute myocardial infarction. Arch Intern Med 1987; 147:753–755.

19. Whang R, Oei TO, Aikawa JK, et al. Predictors of clinical hypomagnesemia. Hypokalemia, hypophosphatemia, hyponatremia, and hypocalcemia. Arch Intern Med 1984; 144:1794–1796.

20. Whang R, Flink EB, Dyckner T, et al. Magnesium depletion as a cause of refractory potassium repletion. Arch Intern Med 1985; 145:1686–1689.

21. Anast CS, Winnacker JL, Forte LR, et al. Impaired release of parathyroid hormone in magnesium deficiency. J Clin Endocrinol Metab 1976; 42:707–717.

22. Rude RK, Oldham SB, Singer FR. Functional hypoparathyroidism and parathyroid hormone end-organ resistance in human magnesium deficiency. Clin Endocrinol 1976; 5:209–224.

23. Dominguez JH, Gray RW, Lemann J, Jr. Dietary phosphate deprivation in women and men: effects on mineral and acid balances, parathyroid hormone and the metabolism of 25-OH-vitamin D. J Clin Endocrinol Metab 1976; 43:1056–1068.

24. Cohen L, Kitzes R. Magnesium sulfate and digitalis-toxic arrhythmias. JAMA 1983; 249:2808–2810.

25. French JH, Thomas RG, Siskind AP, et al. Magnesium therapy in massive digoxin intoxication. Ann Emerg Med 1984; 13:562–566.

26. Langley WF, Mann D. Central nervous system magnesium deficiency. Arch Intern Med 1991; 151:593–596.

27. Clague JE, Edwards RH, Jackson MJ. Intravenous magnesium loading in chronic fatigue syndrome. Lancet 1992; 340:124–125.

28. Oster JR, Epstein M. Management of magnesium depletion. Am J Nephrol 1988; 8:349–354.

29. Whang R, Ryder KW. Frequency of hypomagnesemia and hypermagnesemia. Requested vs routine. JAMA 1990; 263:3063–3064.

30. Elin RJ. Magnesium metabolism in health and disease. Dis Mon 1988; 34:161–218.

31. Van Hook JW. Hypermagnesemia. Crit Care Clin 1991; 7:215–223.

32. Mordes JP, Wacker WE. Excess magnesium. Pharmacol Rev 1977; 29:273–300

Chapter 30

Calcium and Phosphorus

Calcium and phosphorus are responsible for much of the structural integrity of the bony skeleton. Although neither is found in abundance in the soft tissues, both have an important role in vital cell functions. Phosphorus participates in energy storage and utilization, while calcium participates in blood coagulation, neuromuscular transmission, and smooth muscle contraction.

I. CALCIUM IN PLASMA

Calcium is the most abundant electrolyte in the human body (the average adult has more than half a kilogram of calcium), but 99% is in bone (1,2).

A. Plasma Fractions

1. About half of the calcium in plasma is ionized (biologically active), and the other half is either bound to albumin (80%) or complexed to phosphates and sulfates (20%) (1).

2. The concentration of total and ionized calcium in plasma is shown in Table 30.1.

3. Hypoalbuminemia decreases the total plasma calcium without changing the ionized calcium. A variety of correction factors have been proposed for adjusting the total plasma calcium in patients with hypoalbuminemia, but none are reliable (3,4). However, this adjust-

ment is not necessary, since the ionized calcium fraction is not altered by hypoalbuminemia.

4. Ionized calcium can be measured in whole blood, plasma, or serum with ion-specific electrodes that are now available in most clinical laboratories.

Table 30.1	Normal Ranges for Calcium and Phosphate in Blood		
Serum Electrolyte	**Traditional Units (mg/dL)**	**Conversion Factor***	**SI Units (mmol/L)**
Total calcium	9.0–10.0	0.25	2.25–2.50
Ionized calcium	4.6–5.0	0.25	1.15–1.25
Phosphorus	2.5–5.0	0.32	0.8–1.6

*Multiply traditional units by conversion factor to obtain SI units or divide SI units by conversion factor to obtain traditional units.

II. IONIZED HYPOCALCEMIA

Ionized hypocalcemia is extremely common in ICU patients (with an incidence of 88% in one study) (5), and there are several predisposing conditions.

A. Etiologies

The common disorders associated with hypocalcemia in ICU patients are listed in Table 30.2. Hypoparathyroidism is a leading cause of hypocalcemia in outpatients, but is not a consideration in the ICU unless neck surgery has been performed recently.

Table 30.2	Causes of Ionized Hypocalcemia in the ICU

Alkalosis
Blood Transfusions (15%)
Drugs:
    Aminoglycosides (40%)
    Heparin (10%)
	Fat embolism
	Magnesium depletion (70%)
	Pancreatitis
	Renal insufficiency (50%)
	Sepsis (30%)

Numbers in parentheses show the frequency of ionized hypocalcemia reported in each condition.

1. *Magnesium depletion* promotes hypocalcemia by inhibiting parathormone secretion, and reducing end-organ responsiveness to parathormone (see References 21 and 22 in Chapter 29). The hypocalcemia in these cases is refractory to calcium replacement, and correction requires magnesium replacement.

2. *Sepsis* is a common cause of hypocalcemia in the ICU (6,7), but the mechanism is unclear.

3. *Alkalosis* promotes the binding of calcium to albumin, and thereby reduces the fraction of ionized calcium in blood.

4. Ionized hypocalcemia has been reported in 20% of patients receiving *blood transfusions* (6). The culprit is citrate anticoagulant in banked blood, which binds calcium.

5. A number of *drugs* can bind calcium and reduce ionized calcium levels (6). These include aminoglycosides, cimetidine, heparin, and theophylline.

6. Ionized hypocalcemia can accompany *renal failure* as a

result of phosphate retention and impaired conversion of vitamin D to its active form in the kidneys. Treatment is aimed at lowering phosphate levels in blood.

   a. The acidosis in renal failure can decrease the binding of calcium to albumin, so a decrease in total serum calcium in renal failure does not always indicate the presence of ionized hypocalcemia.

7. *Necrotizing pancreatitis* can produce hypocalcemia via several mechanisms. The appearance of hypocalcemia in pancreatitis carries a poor prognosis (8).

B. Clinical Manifestations

The potential consequences of hypocalcemia include increased neuromuscular excitability, and reduced contractile force in cardiac muscle and vascular smooth muscle. However, *most cases of ionized hypocalcemia have no adverse consequences* (5,9).

1. **Neuromuscular**

   Hypocalcemia is reported to cause tetany (of peripheral or laryngeal muscles), hyperreflexia, paresthesias, and seizures (10).

   a. Chvostek's and Trousseau's signs are often listed as manifestations of hypocalcemia, but *Chvostek's sign is nonspecific* (and present in 25% of normal adults), and *Trousseau's sign is insensitive* (absent in ≥30% of cases of hypocalcemia) (11).

2. **Cardiovascular**

   The cardiovascular complications of hypocalcemia, which include hypotension, decreased cardiac output, and ventricular ectopic activity, are reported only in cases of severe ionized hypocalcemia (<0.65 mmol/L) (6).

C. Calcium Replacement Therapy

1. The treatment of ionized hypocalcemia should be directed at the underlying cause of the problem. *Calcium replacement should be reserved only for symptomatic hypocalcemia, which is uncommon.*

2. The available calcium solutions and a recommended replacement regimen are shown in Table 30.3 (6).

   a. Note that the calcium chloride solution contains three times more elemental calcium than calcium gluconate.

   b. Calcium gluconate is usually preferred because it has a lower osmolarity, and is less irritating when injected. However, both calcium solutions are hyperosmolar, and should be given via a large central vein, if possible.

Table 30.3	Intravenous Calcium Replacement Therapy		
Intravenous Solution	**Elemental Calcium**	**Unit Volume**	**Osmolarity (mosm/L)**
10% calcium chloride	27 mg/mL	10 mL	2,000
10% calcium gluconate	9 mg/mL	10 mL	680

For symptomatic hypocalcemia:
1. Give a bolus dose of 200 mg elemental calcium in 100 mL isotonic saline over 10 minutes.
2. Follow with a continuous infusion of 1–2 mg/kg/hr for 6–12 hrs.
3. Monitor ionized calcium levels hourly for the first few hours.

3. CAUTION: Intravenous calcium can be risky; i.e., calcium infusions can promote vasoconstriction and ischemia in

vital organs (12), and intracellular calcium accumulation can produce lethal cell injury (13). These risks emphasize the importance of avoiding calcium replacement therapy unless there is evidence of an adverse effect of hypocalcemia.

III. IONIZED HYPERCALCEMIA

In one large survey, 23% of ICU patients had at least one episode of ionized hypercalcemia (5). The source of hypercalcemia in ICU patients has not been adequately studied, but common causes of hypercalcemia outside the ICU are hyperparathyroidism and malignancy (14-16).

A. Clinical Manifestations

1. The manifestations of hypercalcemia are nonspecific, and include the following (15):

   a. *Gastrointestinal:* nausea, vomiting, constipation, ileus, and pancreatitis.

   b. *Cardiovascular:* hypovolemia, hypotension, and shortened QT interval.

   c. *Renal:* polyuria and nephrocalcinosis.

   d. *Neurologic:* confusion and depressed consciousness, including coma.

2. These manifestations can be evident when the total serum calcium is >12 mg/dL (or the ionized calcium is >3.0 mmol/L), and they are almost always present when the total serum calcium is >14 mg/dL (or the ionized calcium is >3.5 mmol/L) (16).

B. Management

Treatment is indicated when the hypercalcemia is associated

with adverse effects, or when the serum calcium is greater than 14 mg/dL (or ionized calcium >3.5 mmol/L). Most cases of severe, symptomatic hypercalcemia (*hypercalcemic crisis*) are cancer-related, and the treatment is summarized in Table 30.4 (1,14-16).

1. **Saline Infusion**

   Hypercalcemia is accompanied by hypercalciuria, which produces an osmotic diuresis. This leads to hypovolemia, which reduces calcium excretion in the urine and precipitates a rapid rise in the serum calcium.

   a. *Volume infusion to correct hypovolemia and promote renal calcium excretion is the first goal of management for hypercalcemia.*

   b. Isotonic saline (200–500 mL/hr) is recommended for the volume infusion (15) because natriuresis promotes *calciuresis*.

   c. The goal is a urine output of 100–150 mL/hr (14-16).

   d. Saline infusion does not completely correct hypercalcemia in >70% of cases (14).

2. **Furosemide**

   Furosemide (40 to 80 mg IV every 2 hours) promotes urinary calcium excretion, but it also promotes hypovolemia (which is counterproductive), so *furosemide is advised only in cases of volume overload* (14,16).

3. **Calcitonin**

   a. Calcitonin (a naturally occurring hormone) inhibits bone resorption, and is available as salmon calcitonin, which is given subcutaneously or intramuscularly in a dose of 4 U/kg every 12 hours.

   b. Although the response is rapid (within 2 hours), the effect is modest (maximum drop in serum calcium is

0.5 mmol/L) and tachyphylaxis is common (14), so *calcitonin is no longer favored* for the treatment of severe hypercalcemia (14).

Table 30.4	Management of Severe Hypercalcemia	
Agent	**Dosing Regimens and Comments**	
Isotonic saline	Dosing:	200–500 ml/hr, to maintain a urine output of 100–150 mL/hr.
	Comment:	Reduces, but does not usually normalize, the serum calcium.
Furosemide	Dosing:	40–80 mg IV every 2 hrs to maintain urine output of 100–150 mL/hr.
	Comment:	Promotes calciuria, but also promotes hypovolemia (which is counterproductive), so only advised for cases of volume overload.
Calcitonin	Dosing:	4 units/kg by subcutaneous or intramuscular injection every 12 hrs.
	Comment:	No longer favored because of modest effect, and tachyphylaxis.
Glucocorticoids	Dosing:	Oral prednisone (20–100 mg daily) or IV hydrocortisone (200–400 mg daily) for 3–5 days.
	Comment:	Useful in lymphoma and myeloma. Effects may not be evident for 4 days.
Bisphosphonates	Dosing:	Zoledronate (4–8 mg IV over 15 min) or pamidronate (90 mg IV over 2 hrs). Can be repeated in 10 days.
	Comment:	First line drugs, but effect is not apparent for 2 days. Zoledronate is more effective than pamidronate, but the higher dose can be nephrotoxic.

From References 1,14–16.

4. **Glucocorticoids**

   Glucocorticoids increase the renal excretion of calcium, decrease osteoclast activity in bone, and decrease extrarenal production of calcitriol in lymphoma and myeloma (14). (See Table 30.4 for the glucocorticoid dosing regimens.) On the negative side, effects may not be evident for 4 days, and tumor lysis syndrome is a risk (14).

5. **Bisphosphonates**

   a. Bisphosphonates are potent inhibitors of osteoclast activity, and are considered *first line agents* in the treatment of severe hypercalcemia (14).

   b. Two drugs are available: *zoledronate* (4 or 8 mg IV over 15 min) and *pamidronate* (90 mg IV over 2 hours). Zoledronate is the more effective agent, but the higher dose carries a risk of renal injury.

   c. Both drugs have a delayed onset of action (2–4 days). The peak effect is at 4–7 days, and the effect lasts 1–4 weeks (14).

6. **Dialysis**

   Hemodialysis and peritoneal dialysis are effective in removing calcium in patients with renal failure.

IV. HYPOPHOSPHATEMIA

The normal concentration of inorganic phosphate (PO_4) in plasma is shown in Table 30.1 (17). Hypophosphatemia (serum PO_4 <2.5 mg/dL or <0.8 mmol/L) is reported in 17 to 28% of critically ill patients (18,19). Most cases are the result of an intracellular shift of PO_4. Less common causes are an increase in the renal excretion of PO_4, and a decrease in PO_4 absorption from the GI tract.

A. Predisposing Conditions

1. **Glucose Loading**

   The movement of glucose into cells is accompanied by a similar movement of PO_4 into cells. *Glucose loading is the most common cause of hypophosphatemia in hospitalized patients* (18,20,21), and typically occurs during refeeding in malnourished or debilitated patients (21). The influence of total parenteral nutrition (TPN) on serum PO_4 levels is shown in Figure 30.1.

   a. A similar effect occurs in patients with prolonged or severe hyperglycemia who receive insulin. An example of this is the hypophosphatemia that appears during the treatment of diabetic ketoacidosis (see Chapter 24, Section II-C-4).

2. **Respiratory Alkalosis**

   Respiratory alkalosis can increase intracellular pH, and this accelerates glycolysis. The increase in glucose utilization is accompanied by an increase in glucose and phosphorus movement into cells (22).

3. **β-Receptor Agonists**

   Stimulation of β-adrenergic receptors can move PO_4 into cells and promote hypophosphatemia. This effect is evident in patients with acute asthma who are treated with high-dose β-agonist bronchodilators (23).

4. **Systemic Inflammation**

   There is an inverse relationship between serum PO_4 and circulating levels of inflammatory cytokines (24). This may be the result of increased PO_4 utilization by activated neutrophils.

5. **Phosphate-Binding Agents**

   Aluminum forms insoluble complexes with inorganic

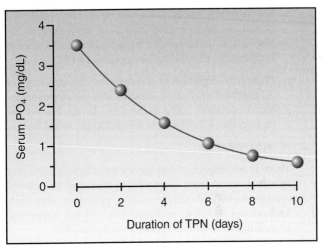

FIGURE 30.1 The cumulative effect of total parenteral nutrition (TPN) on the serum phosphate level. Data from Reference 20.

phosphates, and aluminum-containing compounds like sucralfate can impede the absorption of phosphate in the upper GI tract and promote hypophosphatemia (25).

B. Clinical Manifestations

Hypophosphatemia is often clinically silent; e.g., in one study of patients with severe hypophosphatemia (i.e., serum PO_4 <1 mg/dL), none of the patients showed evidence of harm (26). However, the following adverse effects create the potential for harm.

1. **Adverse Effects**

   a. Phosphate depletion can impair myocardial contractility, and hypophosphatemic patients with heart failure have shown improved cardiac performance after PO_4 supplementation (27).

b. Severe hypophosphatemia can be accompanied by a hemolytic anemia (25), which is attributed to reduced RBC deformability from limited availability of high-energy phosphate compounds (ATP).

c. Phosphate depletion is accompanied by depletion of 2,3-diphosphoglycerate, which shifts the oxyhemoglobin dissociation curve to the left. When this occurs, hemoglobin is less likely to release oxygen to the tissues.

2. **Muscle Weakness**

There is one report of respiratory muscle weakness and failure to wean from mechanical ventilation in patients with severe hypophosphatemia (28). However, other studies have not shown a significant link between hypophosphatemia and respiratory muscle weakness (29).

C. Phosphate Replacement

Table 30.5	Phosphate Replacement Therapy	
Solution	**PO₄ Content**	**Other Content**
Sodium Phosphate	93 mg (3 mmol)/mL	Na⁺: 4.0 mEq
Potassium Phosphate	93 mg (3 mmol)/mL	K⁺: 4.3 mEq

PO$_4$ Replacement IV by Body Weight†			
Serum PO$_4$ (mg/dL)	40–60 kg	61–80 kg	81–120 kg
<1	30 mmol	40 mmol	50 mmol
1–1.7	20 mmol	30 mmol	40 mmol
1.8–2.5	10 mmol	15 mmol	20 mmol

†If the plasma K⁺ is ≥4 mEq/L, use sodium phosphate, and if the plasma K⁺ is <4 mEq/L, use potassium phosphate. From Reference 30.

1. Intravenous phosphate replacement is recommended for all patients with severe hypophosphatemia (i.e.,

serum PO_4 <1.0 mg/dL or <0.3 mmol/L), and for select-ed patients with hypophosphatemia (e.g., those with systolic heart failure). The phosphate solutions and dosing regimen are shown in Table 30.5 (30).

2. The daily maintenance dose of PO_4 is 1,200 mg PO, or 800 mg IV (31).

V. HYPERPHOSPHATEMIA

Most cases of hyperphosphatemia are the result of either impaired renal PO_4 excretion, or PO_4 release from disrupted cells (e.g., rhabdomyolysis, tumor lysis syndrome).

A. Clinical Manifestations

The clinical manifestations of hyperphosphatemia include: (a) the formation of insoluble calcium–phosphate complexes (with deposition into soft tissues), and (b) acute hypocal-cemia (with tetany) (10). Neither of these is a documented risk in ICU patients.

B. Management

1. Enhanced binding of PO_4 in the upper GI tract lowers the serum PO_4, even in the absence of oral PO_4 intake (i.e., GI dialysis) (32,33).

    a. Sucralfate or aluminum-containing antacids can be used for this purpose.

    b. In patients with hypocalcemia, calcium acetate tablets can raise the serum calcium while lowering the serum PO_4. Each calcium acetate tablet (667 mg) contains 8.45 mEq elemental calcium. The recom-mended dose is 2 tablets three times a day.

2. Hemodialysis can increase PO_4 clearance in patients with renal failure, but this is rarely necessary.

REFERENCES

1. Bushinsky DA, Monk RD. Electrolyte quintet: Calcium. Lancet 1998; 352:306–311.

2. Baker SB, Worthley LI. The essentials of calcium, magnesium and phosphate metabolism: part I. Physiology. Crit Care Resusc 2002; 4:301–306.

3. Slomp J, van der Voort PH, Gerritsen RT, et al. Albumin-adjusted calcium is not suitable for diagnosis of hyper- and hypocalcemia in the critically ill. Crit Care Med 2003; 31:1389–1393.

4. Byrnes MC, Huynh K, Helmer SD, et al. A comparison of corrected serum calcium levels to ionized calcium levels among critically ill surgical patients. Am J Surg 2005; 189:310–314.

5. Moritoki E, Kim I, Nichol A, et al. Ionized calcium concentration and outcome in critical illness. Crit Care Med 2011; 39:314–321.

6. Zaloga GP. Hypocalcemia in critically ill patients. Crit Care Med 1992; 20:251–262.

7. Burchard KW, Simms HH, Robinson A, et al. Hypocalcemia during sepsis. Relationship to resuscitation and hemodynamics. Arch Surg 1992; 127:265–272.

8. Steinberg W, Tenner S. Acute pancreatitis. N Engl J Med 1994; 330:1198–1210.

9. Aberegg SK. Ionized calcium in the ICU: should it be measured and corrected. Chest 2016; 149:846–855.

10. Baker SB, Worthley LI. The essentials of calcium, magnesium and phosphate metabolism: part II. Disorders. Crit Care Resusc 2002; 4:307–315.

11. Zaloga G. Divalent cations: calcium, magnesium, and phosphorus. In Chernow B, ed. The Pharmacologic approach to the critically ill patient. 3rd ed. Baltimore: Williams & Williams, 1994.

12. Shapiro MJ, Mistry B. Calcium regulation and nonprotective properties of calcium in surgical ischemia. New Horiz 1996; 4:134–138.

13. Trump BF, Berezesky IK. Calcium-mediated cell injury and cell death. Faseb J 1995; 9:219–228.

14. McCurdy MT, Shanholtz CB. Oncologic emergencies. Crit Care Med 2012; 40:2212–2222.

15. Stewart AF. Clinical practice. Hypercalcemia associated with cancer. N Engl J Med 2005; 352:373–379.

16. Body JJ. Hypercalcemia of malignancy. Semin Nephrol 2004; 24:48–54.

17. Geerse DA, Bindels AJ, Kuiper MA, et al. Treatment of hypophosphatemia in the intensive care unit: a review. Crit Care 2010; 14:R147.

18. French C, Bellomo R. A rapid intravenous phosphate replacement protocol for critically ill patients. Critical Care Resusc 2004; 6:175–179.

19. Fiaccadori E, Coffrini E, Fracchia C, et al. Hypophosphatemia and phosphorus depletion in respiratory and peripheral muscles of patients with respiratory failure due to COPD. Chest 1994; 105:1392–1398.

20. Knochel JP. The pathophysiology and clinical characteristics of severe hypophosphatemia. Arch Intern Med 1977; 137:203–220.

21. Marinella MA. Refeeding syndrome and hypophosphatemia. J Intensive Care Med 2005; 20:155–159.

22. Paleologos M, Stone E, Braude S. Persistent, progressive hypophosphataemia after voluntary hyperventilation. Clin Sci 2000; 98:619–625.

23. Bodenhamer J, Bergstrom R, Brown D, et al. Frequently nebulized beta-agonists for asthma: effects on serum electrolytes. Ann Emerg Med 1992; 21:1337–1342.

24. Barak V, Schwartz A, Kalickman I, et al. Prevalence of hypophosphatemia in sepsis and infection: the role of cytokines. Am J Med 1998; 104:40–47.

25. Brown GR, Greenwood JK. Drug- and nutrition-induced hypophosphatemia: mechanisms and relevance in the critically ill. Ann Pharmacother 1994; 28:626–632.

26. King AL, Sica DA, Miller G, et al. Severe hypophosphatemia in a general hospital population. South Med J 1987; 80:831–835.

27. Davis SV, Olichwier KK, Chakko SC. Reversible depression of myocardial performance in hypophosphatemia. Am J Med Sci 1988; 295:183–187.

28. Agusti AG, Torres A, Estopa R, et al. Hypophosphatemia as a cause of failed weaning: the importance of metabolic factors. Crit Care Med 1984; 12:142–143.

29. Gravelyn TR, Brophy N, Siegert C, et al. Hypophosphatemia-associated respiratory muscle weakness in a general inpatient population. Am J Med 1988; 84:870–876.

30. Taylor BE, Huey WY, Buchman TG, et al. Treatment of hypophosphatemia using a protocol based on patient weight and serum phosphorus level in a surgical intensive care unit. J Am Coll Surg 2004; 198:198–204.

31. Knochel JP. Phosphorous. In: Shils ME, et al., eds. Modern nutrition in health and disease. 10th ed. Philadelphia, PA: Lippincott, Williams & Wilkins, 2006; 211–222.

32. Kraft MD, Btaiche IF, Sacks GS, et al. Treatment of electrolyte disorders in adult patients in the intensive care unit. Am J Health Syst Pharm 2005; 62:1663–1682.

33. Lorenzo Sellares V, Torres Ramirez A. Management of hyperphosphataemia in dialysis patients: role of phosphate binders in the elderly. Drugs Aging 2004; 21:153–165.

Chapter 31

Pancreatitis and Liver Failure

The conditions described in this chapter (i.e., necrotizing pancreatitis and liver failure) share the following features: (a) both are associated with injury in multiple organs, (b) both are plagued by infections from pathogens that reside in the bowel, (c) the management of both conditions is mostly supportive care, and (d) mortality rates remain high.

I. ACUTE PANCREATITIS

A. Classification

Two types of acute pancreatitis are identified (1):

1. *Edematous pancreatitis* is the most common form of pancreatitis, and is characterized by inflammatory infiltration of the pancreas without involvement of other organs. The clinical presentation is usually a self-limited period of abdominal pain, nausea, and vomiting. The mortality rate is low (<2%) (2), and management rarely requires ICU-level care.

2. *Necrotizing pancreatitis* occurs in 10–15% of cases (1), and is characterized by areas of necrotic destruction in the pancreas, usually accompanied by progressive systemic inflammation and inflammatory injury in one or more extrapancreatic sites (e.g., lungs, kidneys, and circulatory system) (3). The mortality rate can be as high as 40% (2), and management requires ICU-level care.

B. Etiology and Diagnosis

1. The conditions that produce pancreatitis are shown in Table 31.1. About 90% of cases are the result of gallstones (40%), alcohol abuse (30%), or are idiopathic (20%) (2,4,5).

2. The diagnosis of acute pancreatitis requires the following (1):

   a. An increase in the serum levels of pancreatic enzymes (amylase and lipase) to at least 3 times the upper limit of normal.

   b. Evidence of pancreatitis on contrast-enhanced computed tomography.

Table 31.1	Etiology of Acute Pancreatitis
Leading Causes	
• Gallstones (40%)	
• Alcohol (30%)	
• Idiopathic (20%)	
Other Causes	
• Abdominal trauma	
• Vasculitis	
• Hypertriglyceridemia	
• Infection (HIV, CMV, *Mycoplasma, Legionella*)	
• Drugs (acetaminophen, omeprazole, pentamidine, metronidazole, trimethoprim-sulfamethoxazole, furosemide, valproic acid)	

From References 2, 4, and 5.

C. Pancreatic Enzymes

1. **Amylase**
   Amylase is an enzyme that cleaves starch into smaller

polysaccharides. The principal sources of amylase are the pancreas, salivary glands, and fallopian tubes.

a. Serum amylase levels begin to rise 6–12 hours after the onset of acute pancreatitis, and they return to normal in 3–5 days.

b. An increase in serum amylase levels to 3 times the upper limit of normal (the threshold for the diagnosis of acute pancreatitis) has a high sensitivity (>90%) but a low specificity (as low as 70%) for the diagnosis of acute pancreatitis (6).

c. The low specificity of serum amylase is a reflection of the numerous conditions that can elevate serum amylase levels, which are listed in Table 31.2 (7).

d. *Note:* The reference range for serum amylase is not mentioned because it often varies in different clinical laboratories.

2. **Lipase**

Lipase is an enzyme that hydrolyses triglycerides to form glycerol and free fatty acids. The principal sources of lipase are the tongue, pancreas, liver, intestine, and circulating lipoproteins.

a. Serum lipase levels begin to rise 4–8 hours after the onset of acute pancreatitis (earlier than the rise in serum amylase), and the serum levels remain elevated for 8–14 days (longer than the rise in serum amylase).

b. Like amylase, there are several conditions that can elevate serum lipase levels, as shown in Table 31.2. However, unlike amylase, nonpancreatic conditions rarely raise serum lipase levels high enough to overlap with the levels seen in acute pancreatitis (8).

c. An increase in serum lipase to three times the upper limit of normal has a sensitivity and specificity of 80–100% for acute pancreatitis (6). Therefore, serum lipase is more specific than serum amylase for the diagnosis of acute pancreatitis.

d. RECOMMENDATION: *The serum lipase can be used alone for the diagnostic evaluation of pancreatitis.* Adding the serum amylase does not increase diagnostic accuracy (6).

Table 31.2	Sources of Elevated Serum Amylase and Lipase	
Conditions	**Drugs and Other Agents†**
Pancreatitis	**Amylase:**
Cholecystitis	Ethanol intoxication
Renal Failure	Hydroxyethyl starch
Parotitis (amylase)	Histamine H_2 blockers
Peptic Ulcer Disease	Metoclopramide
Bowel Obstruction or Infarction	Opiates
Liver Disease	**Lipase:**
Ruptured Ectopic Pregnancy (amylase)	Lipid infusions
	Methylprednisolone
Diabetic Ketoacidosis	Opiates

†Includes only substances that are likely to be encountered in ICU patients. For a more complete list, see Reference 7.

D. Computed Tomography

Contrast-enhanced computed tomography (CT) is the most reliable diagnostic test for acute pancreatitis, and can identify the type of pancreatitis (edematous vs. necrotizing) and localized complications (e.g., infection).

1. A contrast-enhanced CT image of edematous pancreatitis is shown in Figure 31.1. The pancreas is thickened and enhances completely, and the border of the pan-

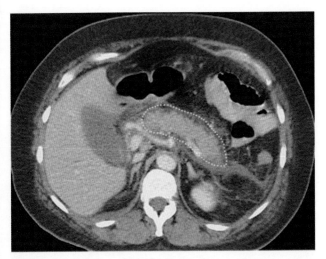

FIGURE 31.1 Contrast-enhanced CT image showing edematous pancreatitis. The pancreas (outlined by the dotted line) is enlarged and enhances completely. There is also blurring of the pancreatic border, which is characteristic of edema formation.

creas is blurred, which is characteristic of pancreatic edema.

2. A contrast-enhanced CT image of necrotizing pancreatitis is shown in Figure 31.2. Note the large area that is not contrast-enhanced in the region of the neck and body of the pancreas. This represents pancreatic necrosis. The full extent of pancreatic necrosis may not be evident on CT imaging for the first week after the onset of symptoms (1).

3. Without IV contrast, CT imaging is less likely to distinguish between edematous and necrotizing pancreatitis.

E. Biliary Evaluation

Since gallstones are the leading cause of acute pancreatitis in the United States (4), an evaluation of the gall bladder and biliary tree is advised in all cases of acute pancreatitis. Contrast-enhanced CT images may suffice for this evaluation; otherwise, ultrasonography is recommended.

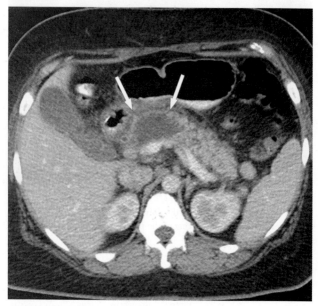

FIGURE 31.2 Contrast-enhanced CT image showing necrotizing pancreatitis, which is shown by the spotty enhancement of the pancreas. A large area of necrosis is indicated by the arrows. Image from Reference 1.

II. SEVERE PANCREATITIS

1. Severe pancreatitis is defined as acute (usually necrotizing) pancreatitis that is associated with persistent (>48 hrs) injury in at least one other organ system (1).

2. The extrapancreatic organ injury is inflammatory in origin, and typically involves the lungs (acute respiratory

distress syndrome), kidneys (acute kidney injury), and circulatory system (hypotension and circulatory shock).

3. The management of severe pancreatitis in the ICU includes: (a) circulatory support, (b) nutritional support, and (c) treating intraabdominal complications (e.g., infection).

A. Circulatory Support

Circulatory support includes volume resuscitation and vasopressor drugs, if necessary.

1. **Volume Resuscitation**

   Severe pancreatitis is accompanied by loss of intravascular fluid through leaky systemic capillaries, and the resulting hypovolemia can produce additional pancreatic necrosis. As a result, aggressive volume resuscitation is advised early in the course of severe pancreatitis (9). The typical regimen for volume resuscitation is summarized as follows:

   a. Using an isotonic crystalloid fluid, begin by infusing 20 mL/kg (about 1.5 liters) over 60 to 90 minutes.

   b. Follow with an infusion rate up to 250 mL/hr for the next 24–48 hours, to maintain a mean arterial pressure ≥65 mm Hg, and a urine output ≥0.5 mL/kg/hr.

   c. CAUTION: Aggressive volume infusion has not been shown to improve outcomes in severe pancreatitis (10), and this practice promotes edema formation, which can aggravate conditions like ARDS (see Chapter 17, Section III-A), and increases the risk of abdominal compartment syndrome (see Chapter 26, Section III-D-1). Therefore, after the initial 24–48 hours of aggressive volume infusion, the infusion rate of IV fluids should be reduced to match the urine output.

2. **Vasopressor Therapy**

   There are no official recommendations regarding vaso-pressor therapy in severe pancreatitis, but *norepinephrine* (2–20 µg/min) is an appropriate choice. All vasocon-strictor drugs can reduce splanchnic blood flow (especially epinephrine), and could aggravate pancreatic necrosis, so careful titration of infusion rates (and avoiding epinephrine) is advised.

B. Nutrition Support

1. Nutrition support should be started early (within 48 hours after the onset of illness) using enteral tube feedings, if possible (11).

2. The preference for enteral nutrition is based on the ability of tube feedings to exert a trophic effect on the bowel mucosa (see Chapter 37). *Enteral nutrition is associated with fewer infections, less multiorgan failure, and a lower mortality rate than total parenteral nutrition* in patients with severe pancreatitis (12).

3. Tube feedings should be infused into the jejunum using long feeding tubes that can be placed with fluoroscopic or endoscopic guidance. Although intragastric feedings are not currently advised, one small study has shown no apparent harm from nasogastric feedings in severe pancreatitis (13).

C. Pancreatic Infections

1. About one-third of patients with necrotizing pancreatitis develop infections in the necrotic areas of the pancreas (14). These infections typically appear 7–10 days after the onset of illness, and gram-negative enteric organisms are the responsible pathogens.

2. The diagnosis is confirmed by either of the following:

   a. A contrast-enhanced CT scan showing gas bubbles in the necrotic areas of the pancreas.

   b. A positive culture from necrotic areas of the pancreas (using CT-guided needle aspiration).

3. These infections are refractory to antibiotic therapy, and the treatment of choice is surgical debridement (necrosectomy) (14).

4. Antibiotic prophylaxis does not reduce the incidence of pancreatic infections (15); as a result, *prophylactic antibiotics are not recommended in necrotizing pancreatitis* (14).

D. Abdominal Compartment Syndrome

Abdominal compartment syndrome (ACS) is reported in about half of patients with severe pancreatitis (16). Since ACS can cause acute oliguric renal failure, abdominal pressure should be measured in any patient with acute pancreatitis who develops oliguric renal failure. (See Chapter 26, Section III-D for more information on ACS.)

III. LIVER FAILURE

A. Classification

There are two types of liver failure: (a) acute (fulminant) liver failure, and (b) acute-on-chronic liver failure.

1. **Acute Liver Failure**

   Acute liver failure occurs without prior liver disease, and is an uncommon disorder (annual incidence is <10 per million). Acetaminophen is the leading cause of acute liver failure in the United States, and is responsible for 40% of cases (17). (Acetaminophen hepatotoxicity is described in Chapter 46, Section I.) Other causes include viral hepatitis, ischemic hepatitis, other drugs (e.g., cocaine), and heat stroke. About 20% of cases are idiopathic (17).

2. **Acute-on-Chronic Liver Failure**

Most cases of acute-on-chronic liver failure are exacerbations of chronic liver disease in patients with cirrhosis, often precipitated by infection or variceal hemorrhage (18).

B. Clinical Features

Both types of liver failure share similar features (e.g., increased risk of infection, renal dysfunction, hypoalbuminemia), but there are some differences.

1. Acute liver failure has the following characteristics (17):

    a. It is often associated with systemic inflammation, which leads to multiorgan failure.

    b. The dominant feature is hepatic encephalopathy, which appears within 8 weeks of symptom onset, and can raise intracranial pressure.

    c. Portal hypertension is not prominent, and overt bleeding is uncommon.

    d. There is a chance for improvement with N-acetylcysteine (even in cases of acute liver failure unrelated to acetaminophen) (17).

2. Acute-on-chronic liver failure (cirrhosis) differs in the following ways:

    a. Portal hypertension is prominent, and variceal hemorrhage is common.

    b. Ascites is prominent, and there is a risk of spontaneous bacterial peritonitis and hepatorenal syndrome (see next sections).

C. Spontaneous Bacterial Peritonitis

Evidence of infection in the peritoneal fluid is found in 10–27% of patients with acute-on-chronic liver failure and ascites (19). This condition is called *spontaneous bacterial peritonitis* (SBP), and the presumed mechanism is peritoneal seeding from translocation of enteric pathogens across the bowel mucosa. The responsible pathogens are gram-negative aerobic bacilli in 75% of cases, and gram-positive aerobic cocci (especially streptococci) in 25% of cases (19).

1. Clinical features include fever, abdominal pain, and rebound tenderness in at least 50% of patients, but the condition can be asymptomatic in one-third of patients (19).

2. Culture of the peritoneal fluid is required for the diagnostic evaluation of SBP. An absolute neutrophil count of ≥ 250 cells/mm^3 in the peritoneal fluid is presumptive evidence of infection, and is an indication to begin empiric antimicrobial therapy. The preferred antibiotic is *cefotaxime* (2 grams IV every 8 hours), or another third-generation cephalosporin (19-21).

3. The mortality rate in SBP is 30–40% despite adequate antibiotic coverage (20). About one-third of patients with SBP develop the hepatorenal syndrome (21), and this might explain the high mortality rate (see next).

D. Hepatorenal Syndrome

Hepatorenal syndrome (HRS) is a functional renal failure (i.e., occurs without intrinsic renal disease) that occurs in patients with cirrhosis and ascites, especially those with spontaneous bacterial peritonitis or sepsis from another source (22). HRS is considered a fatal illness without liver transplantation (22,23).

1. Pathogenesis

   HRS is caused by hemodynamic alterations in the

splanchnic and renal circulations. Cirrhosis is associated with splanchnic vasodilation, and the neurohumoral (renin system) response to this vasodilation results in vasoconstriction in the kidneys (22). The renal vasoconstriction makes the glomerular filtration rate vulnerable to small decrements in cardiac output.

2. **Diagnosis**

The diagnostic criteria for HRS are shown in Table 31.3. These criteria include evidence of acute kidney injury (an increase in serum creatinine ≥0.3 mg/dL within 48 hrs) that does not respond to albumin infusions (volume resuscitation), and no other likely source of acute kidney injury (i.e., circulatory shock or nephrotoxic drugs) (22,24).

Table 31.3	Clinical Approach to Hepatorenal Syndrome
Diagnostic Criteria	**Management**
1. Cirrhosis with ascites	1. Terlipressin: 1–2 mg IV q 4–6 hr
2. Increase in serum creatinine of 0.3 mg/dL or more within 48 hr	Albumin: 1 g/kg (to 100 mg) on day 1, then 20–40 g daily†
3. No improvement in renal function after 2 days of albumin infusions (1g/kg/day to max of 100 g/day) and no diuretics	2. Evaluate for liver transplant
4. No other source of acute injury (e.g., shock, nephrotoxic drugs)	

†Stop if serum albumin >4.5. From References 22-24.

3. **Management**

The acute management of HRS includes a splanchnic

vasoconstrictor (*terlipressin*, a vasopressin analogue) to redirect blood flow to the kidneys, combined with a volume expander (albumin). The dosing regimens are shown in Table 31.3. Over 50% of patients with HRS will show improvement in renal function with the regimens in Table 31.3 (22,23), but the response is short-lived, and long term survival requires liver transplantation (23).

IV. HEPATIC ENCEPHALOPATHY

The hallmark of the advanced stages of liver failure is an encephalopathy that is characterized by cerebral edema and increased intracranial pressure. Ammonia has been identified as a key factor in the pathogenesis of hepatic encephalopathy (HE) (25-28).

A. Pathogenesis

The normal clearance of ammonia (NH_3) by conversion to urea in the liver is impaired in liver failure, and the resulting increase in plasma NH_3 eventually leads to accumulation of NH_3 in the brain, where it is taken up by astrocytes and used to convert glutamate to glutamine; i.e.,

$$\text{glutamate} + NH_3 + ATP \rightarrow \text{glutamine} + ADP \quad (31.1)$$

The intracellular accumulation of glutamine creates an osmotic force that draws water into the astrocytes, thereby promoting cerebral edema (25).

B. Clinical Features

The principal features of progressive HE are shown in Table 31.4 (27).

1. The earliest signs of encephalopathy include personality changes, altered cognition, and *asterixis* (irregular move-

ments produced by sustained dorsiflexion of the wrist), while disorientation and depressed consciousness become prominent as the encephalopathy progresses.

2. Extrapyramidal signs (e.g., rigidity, Parkinsonian tremor) are common in HE, and a positive Babinski sign can be observed (27).

3. Focal neurological deficits and seizures are uncommon in HE (27).

Table 31.4	Progressive Stages of Hepatic Encephalopathy
Stage	**Features**
Stage 0	• No encephalopathy
Stage 1	• Short attention span • Euphoria or depression • Asterixis may be present
Stage 2	• Lethargy or apathy • Disorientation • Asterixis usually present
Stage 3	• Somnolent, but responsive to verbal commands • Severe disorientation • Asterixis absent
Stage 4	• Coma

The "West Haven Criteria", from Reference 27.

C. Diagnostic Evaluation

The clinical features of HE are nonspecific (including asterixis, which can be observed with metabolic encephalopathies and drug overdoses), and the diagnosis is made by excluding other causes of altered mentation.

1. **Serum Ammonia**

   Despite the importance of NH_3 in the pathogenesis of HE, monitoring serum NH_3 levels has a limited role in HE.

   a. The major role for serum NH_3 levels is in acute liver failure, where there is a good correlation between NH_3 levels and both the presence and severity of HE (26-28).

   b. *In patients with cirrhosis, serum NH_3 levels are unreliable* for both detecting HE and determining the severity of illness (27,28). This is demonstrated by the results of one study (28), which showed that serum NH_3 levels were normal in over 50% of cirrhotic patients with HE.

D. Reducing the Ammonia Burden

The principal site of NH_3 production is the lower GI tract, where NH_3 is a byproduct of protein degradation, and urease-producing gut microbes promote the breakdown of urea to generate additional NH_3. The following measures are used to reduce the NH_3 burden from the bowel.

1. **Lactulose**

   Lactulose is a nonabsorbable disaccharide that is metabolized by gut microbes to form short-chain fatty acids, and the resulting acidification of the bowel lumen has two advantages: (a) it promotes the conversion of NH_3 to NH_4 (ammonium), which is not readily absorbed from the bowel, and (b) it eradicates urease-producing microbes (27,29). (The bactericidal actions of an acidic pH are shown in Figure 3.1.) The dosing recommendations for lactulose are shown in Table 31.5. Lactulose is considered a first-line agent for the treatment of HE (27,29).

Table 31.5	Reducing the Ammonia Burden in Hepatic Encephalopathy
Lactulose	
Oral Regimen:	Start with 20–30 g (30–45 mL) every hour until defecation occurs, then reduce to 20 g (30 mL) every 6 hrs.
Retention Enema:	Add 200 g (300 mL) to 700 mL tap water. Administer by high rectal enema and retain for 1 hr. Can be repeated every 4–6 hrs.
Neomycin	1–2 grams PO every 8 hours for 1–2 weeks
Rifaximin	400 mg PO every 8 hours for 10–21 days

From References 27 and 29.

2. **Nonabsorbable Antibiotics**

Nonabsorbable antibiotics are used to eradicate urease-producing bacteria in the gut. Two antibiotics have been used for this purpose: *neomycin* (an aminoglycoside) and *rifaximin* (a rifampin analogue). The dosing regimens for each are shown in Table 31.5.

a. Neomycin has shown no benefit in HE, while creating a (small) risk of ototoxicity and nephrotoxicity (29); as a result *rifaximin is the preferred antibiotic for HE* (27,29,30).

b. Rifaximin is used as an adjunct to lactulose, and is not used alone.

E. Reducing Intracranial Pressure

1. Increased intracranial pressure is predominantly seen in acute liver failure, and is an ominous sign (17).

2. A sustained increase in serum NH_3 levels to $\geq 150 \ \mu mol/L$ ($\geq 255 \ \mu g/dL$) is associated with a high risk of intracranial hypertension (17), and can be used as an indication to monitor intracranial pressure (ICP). Either of the following regimens is recommended for lowering the ICP (17).

   a. HYPERTONIC SALINE: Administer 20 mL of 30% NaCL or 200 mL of 3% NaCL, as an IV bolus, and keep the serum sodium below 150 mEq/L.

   b. MANNITOL: Using a 20% solution, give 2 mL/kg body weight, and keep the serum osmolality below 320 mosm/kg H_2O.

F. Maintaining Protein Intake

Restricting protein intake can reduce the NH_3 burden in the gut, but protein restriction does not hasten the resolution of HE, and it promotes muscle breakdown (31). Therefore, patients with HE should receive the standard protein intake (1.2–2 g/kg/day) recommended for all critically ill patients.

G. The Future?

Although liver transplantation is an option for selected cases of advanced liver failure, only 10% of liver transplant procedures are performed on patients with fulminant liver failure (17). Other therapies are emerging as a bridge or replacement for liver transplantation, and the most promising of these is *high-volume plasma exchange*, which removes NH_3 and other toxins from the bloodstream. Preliminary studies have shown improved transplant-free survival with this strategy (32).

REFERENCES

1. Banks PA, Bollen TL, Dervenis C, et al. Classification of acute pancreatitis—2012: revision of the Atlanta classification and definitions by international consensus. Gut 2012; 62:102–111.

2. Cavallini G, Frulloni L, Bassi C, et al. Prospective multicentre survey on acute pancreatitis in Italy (Proinf-AISP). Dig Liver Dis 2004; 36:205–211.

3. Greer SE, Burchard KW. Acute pancreatitis and critical illness. A pancreatic tale of hypoperfusion and inflammation. Chest 2009; 136:1413–1419.

4. Forsmark CE, Baille J. AGA Institute technical review on acute pancreatitis. Gastroenterol 2007; 132:2022–2044.

5. Yang AL, Vadhavkar S, Singh G, Omary MB. Epidemiology of alcohol-related liver and pancreatic disease in the United States. Arch Intern Med 2008; 168:649–656.

6. Yadav D, Agarwal N, Pitchumoni CS. A critical evaluation of laboratory tests in acute pancreatitis. Am J Gastroenterol 2002; 97:1309–1318.

7. Gelrud D, Gress FG. Elevated serum amylase and lipase. UpToDate (accessed on July 26, 2016).

8. Gumaste VV, Roditis N, Mehta D, Dave PB. Serum lipase levels in nonpancreatic abdominal pain versus acute pancreatitis. Am J Gastroenterol 1993; 88:2051–2055.

9. Tenner S. Initial management of acute pancreatitis: critical issues in the first 72 hours. Am J Gastroenterol 2004; 99:2489–2494.

10. Haydock MD, Mittal A, Wilms HR, et al. Fluid therapy in acute pancreatitis: anybody's guess. Ann Surg 2013; 257:182–188.

11. Parrish CR, Krenitsky J, McClave SA. Pancreatitis. 2012 A.S.P.E.N. Nutrition Support Core Curriculum. Silver Spring, MD: American Society of Parenteral and Enteral Nutrition, 2012:472–490.

12. Al-Omran M, AlBalawi ZH, Tashkandi MF, Al-Ansary LA. Enteral versus parenteral nutrition for acute pancreatitis. Cochrane Database Syst Rev 2010:CD002837.

13. Eatock FC, Chong P, Menezes N, et al. A randomized study of early nasogastric versus nasojejunal feeding in severe acute pancreatitis. Am J Gastroenterol 2005; 100:432–439.

14. Banks PA, Freeman ML, Practice Parameters Committee of the American College of Gastroenterology. Practice guidelines in acute pancreatitis. Am J Gastroenterol 2006; 101:2379–2400.

15. Hart PA, Bechtold ML, Marshall JB, et al. Prophylactic antibiotics in necrotizing pancreatitis: a meta-analysis. South Med J 2008; 101:1126–1131.

16. Al-Bahrani AZ, Abid GH, Holt A, et al. Clinical relevance of intra-abdominal hypertension in patients with severe acute pancreatitis. Pancreas 2008; 36:39–43.

17. Bernal W, Wendon J. Acute liver failure. N Engl J Med 2013; 369:2525–2534.

18. Olson JC, Kamath PS. Acute-on-chronic liver failure: concept, natural history, and prognosis. Curr Opin Crit Care 2011; 17:165–169.

19. Gilbert JA, Kamath PS. Spontaneous bacterial peritonitis: an update. Mayo Clin Proc 1995; 70:365–370.

20. Runyon BA. Management of adult patients with ascites caused by cirrhosis. Hepatology 1998; 27:264–272.

21. Moore CM, van Thiel DH. Cirrhotic ascites review: pathophysiology, diagnosis, and management. World J Hepatol 2013; 5:251–263.

22. Dalerno F, Gerbes A, Gines P, et al. Diagnosis, prevention and treatment of hepatorenal syndrome in cirrhosis. Gut 2007; 56:131–1318.

23. Rajekar H, Chawla Y. Terlipressin in hepatorenal syndrome: evidence for present indications. J Gastroenterol Hepatol 2011; 26(Suppl):109–114.

24. Wong F. The evolving concept of acute kidney injury in patients with cirrhosis. Nat Rev Gastroenterol Hepatol 2015; 12:711–719.

25. Clay AS, Hainline BE. Hyperammonemia in the ICU. Chest 2007; 132:1368–1378.

26. Ferenci P, Lockwood A, Mullen K, et al. Hepatic encephalopathy—definition, nomenclature, diagnosis and quantification: Final report of the Working Party at the 11th World Congress of Gastroenterology, Vienna, 1998. Hepatol 2002; 55:716–721.

27. Vilstrup H, Amodio P, Bajaj J, et al. Hepatic encephalopathy in chronic liver disease: 2014 practice guideline by the American Association for the Study of Liver Diseases and the European Association for the Study of the Liver. Hepatology 2014; 60:715–735.

28. Kundra A, Jain A, Banga A, et al. Evaluation of plasma ammonia levels in patients with acute liver failure and chronic liver disease and its correlation with the severity of hepatic encephalopathy and clinical features of raised intracranial pressure. Clin Biochem 2006; 38:696–699.

29. Leise MD, Poterucha JJ, Kamath PS, Kim WR. Management of hepatic encephalopathy in the hospital. Mayo Clin Proc 2014; 89:241–253.

30. Lawrence KR, Klee JA. Rifaximin for the treatment of hepatic encephalopathy. Pharmacotherapy 2008; 28:1019–1032.

31. Cordoba J, Lopez-Hellin J, Planas M, et al. Normal protein diet for episodic hepatic encephalopathy: results of a randomized trial. J Hepatol 2004; 41:38–43.

32. Karvellas CJ, Subramanian RM. Current evidence for extracorporeal liver support systems in acute liver failure and acute-on-chronic liver failure. Crit Care Clin 2016; 32:439–451.

Chapter 32

Abdominal Infections

This chapter describes abdominal infections that you are likely to encounter in the ICU, including infections of the biliary tree (acalculous cholecystitis), bowel (*Clostridium difficile* infections), and peritoneal cavity (postoperative infections).

I. ACALCULOUS CHOLECYSTITIS

Acalculous cholecystitis accounts for less than 15% of cases of acute cholecystitis (1), but it is more common in critically ill patients, and it has a mortality rate (about 45%) that rivals septic shock (1,2).

A. Predisposing Conditions

1. Common conditions associated with acalculous cholecystitis include the postoperative period, trauma, circulatory shock, and prolonged bowel rest (4 weeks or longer) (1,2).

2. Bowel rest during total parenteral nutrition (TPN) is usually less than 4 weeks in duration, so TPN should not be a risk factor for acalculous cholecystitis (3).

3. Possible mechanisms include hypoperfusion, gallbladder distension from diminished contractions, and a change in the composition of bile.

B. Clinical Features

1. Right upper quadrant pain and tenderness are com-

mon, but can be *absent in one-third of patients with acalculous cholecystitis* (4).

2. Other common findings include fever (100%), elevated bilirubin (90%), hypotension (90%) and multiorgan failure (65–80%) (1,2).

3. Blood cultures are positive in 90% of cases (4) and gram-negative aerobic bacilli are isolated in almost all cases.

C. Diagnosis

1. Ultrasound is the favored diagnostic test for acalculous cholecystitis.

2. Sonographic features include distension of the gallbladder (diameter >40 mm in the short-axis view), wall thickening (>3 mm), and the presence of sludge (a mixture of particulate matter that has precipitated from bile) (5). These features are shown in Figure 32.1. The presence of sludge is nonspecific, and is seen in critically ill patients without cholecystitis.

3. The diagnostic yield from ultrasound is as high as 95% when performed by ultrasound technicians (5). Nuclear medicine imaging is an option when ultrasound is not helpful, but the diagnostic yield may be lower in critically ill patients (5).

D. Management

1. Empiric antibiotic therapy should be started as soon as the diagnosis is confirmed. The recommended antibiotics are *piperacillin-tazobactam*, or a carbapenem (e.g., *meropenem*) (2). (See Chapter 44, Sections III and VI for dosing recommendations.)

2. Laparoscopic cholecystectomy is favored in clinically stable (non-ICU) patients, but percutaneous cholecys-

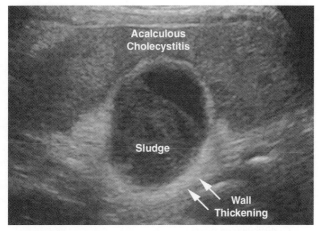

FIGURE 32.1 Sonogram showing a short-axis view of the gallbladder in a patient with acalculous cholecystitis. See text for explanation.

tostomy is the safest and most successful intervention in critically ill patients (7).

II. CLOSTRIDIUM DIFFICILE INFECTION

Clostridium difficile infection (CDI) is the most common health-care-associated infection in the United States, and is also the leading cause of nosocomial diarrhea worldwide (8). The incidence of CDI almost doubled during the past decade (9).

A. Pathogenesis

1. *C. difficile* is a spore-forming, toxin-producing, gram-positive, anaerobic bacillus. It does not inhabit the bowel in healthy subjects, but colonizes the bowel when the normal microflora has been altered (e.g., by antibiotic therapy).

2. CDI is transmitted via the fecal-oral route, and patient-to-patient transmission occurs on the hands of hospital personnel. The use of disposable gloves for patient contact reduces the transmission of CDI (10).

3. *C. difficile* is not an invasive organism, but releases cytotoxins that damage the bowel mucosa. This leads to inflammatory infiltration of the bowel wall and a secretory diarrhea. Severe inflammation produces raised, plaque-like lesions on the mucosal surface of the bowel. These are called "pseudomembranes," and the condition is called *pseudomembranous colitis*.

4. Antibiotic use is the most noted risk factor for CDI, but gastric acid suppression is emerging as a significant risk factor because it promotes the fecal-oral transmission of *C. difficile* (see next).

5. **Gastric Acid Suppression**

Gastric acidity plays a major role in eradicating organisms that invade the upper GI tract (see Chapter 3, Section I-C-3, and Figure 3.1), and there are several reports showing an increased incidence of CDI associated with the use of acid-suppressing drugs, particularly proton pump inhibitors (11-13). In fact, the marked increase in the incidence of CDI mentioned earlier coincides with the marked increase in the use of proton pump inhibitors for prophylaxis of stress ulcer bleeding, and *it is possible that the recent surge in frequency and severity of CDI is a reflection of the escalating use of proton pump inhibitors* in hospitalized patients (14).

B. Clinical Features

The clinical features of CDI are shown in Table 32.1. The information in this table is taken directly from the most recent clinical practice guidelines on CDI (15). The following points deserve mention:

1. The diarrhea in CDI is watery (not grossly bloody), and is often foul-smelling.

2. *Toxic megacolon* is a life-threatening complication of CDI. Clinical features include the abrupt onset of ileus and marked abdominal distension, with rapid progression to circulatory shock. Emergent surgical intervention is mandatory, and the preferred surgical procedure is subtotal colectomy (8).

Table 32.1	Clinical Features of *Clostridium difficile* Infection (CDI)

Mild to Moderate CDI

Diarrhea alone, or combined with features not present in other categories (e.g., fever to 101.2° F)

Severe CDI

Diarrhea PLUS serum albumin <3 g/dL AND one of the following: WBC's ≥15,000/mm^3 or abdominal tenderness

Severe CDI with Complications

Diarrhea PLUS any of the following attributed to CDI:

- admission to an ICU
- WBC's ≥35,000/mm^3 or <2,000/mm^3
- hypotension
- significant abdominal distension or ileus

- temp. >101.3° F
- serum lactate >2.2 mmol/L
- mental status changes
- failure of one major organ (e.g., lungs, kidneys)

Recurrent CDI

Recurrence within 8 weeks of completion of treatment.

From the Clinical Practice Guidelines in Reference 15.

C. Diagnostic Evaluation

The diagnosis of CDI requires evidence of *C. difficile* cytotoxins in stool, or the presence of toxigenic strains of *C. difficile* in stool. Growth of *C. difficile* in stool cultures is unreliable because it does not distinguish toxigenic from nontoxigenic strains of the organism.

1. **Toxin Assay**

   The diagnosis of CDI has been based on the detection of *C. difficile* toxins A and B in stool (both toxins must be detected to produce a positive result). The toxin assays have a sensitivity of 75–95%, and a specificity of 83–98%, for the diagnosis of CDI (15). The sensitivity of the toxin assay is considered substandard (15), and the toxin assay is being replaced by gene-targeted testing, described next.

2. **Gene-Targeted Testing**

   The newer diagnostic tests for CDI use nuclear amplification techniques like the polymerase chain reaction (PCR) to detect toxin-producing genes in *C. difficile*. The PCR-based tests are highly-sensitive tools for identifying toxigenic strains of *C. difficile*, and they are now *the preferred diagnostic tests for CDI* (15).

   CAVEAT: A recent study of PCR-based testing has revealed a high rate of false-positive results (16), so abandoning the toxin assays may be premature.

3. **Colonoscopy**

   Direct visualization of pseudomembranes on the mucosal surface of the large bowel can provide confirmatory evidence of CDI, but this is rarely necessary.

D. Antibiotic Treatment

The recommended antibiotic regimens for CDI are shown in

Table 32.2, using the same severity-of-illness classification in Table 32.1. Some additional points deserve mention.

Table 32.2	Antibiotic Therapy for *Clostridium difficile* Infection (CDI)

Mild to Moderate CDI

Preferred: metronidazole, 500 mg PO every 8 hrs for 10 days

Alternate: vancomycin, 125 mg PO every 6 hrs for 10 days

Severe CDI

Preferred: vancomycin, 125 mg PO every 6 hrs for 10 days

Severe CDI with Complications

Preferred: vancomycin, 500 mg PO or per rectum every 6 hrs, plus metronidazole, 500 mg IV every 8 hrs for 10 days

For ileus: Give vancomycin both orally and rectally (500 mg for each) every 6 hrs, plus IV metronidazole (same as above).

Recurrent CDI

1st Recurrence: same regimen as initial episode

2nd Recurrence: vancomycin, 125 mg PO every 6 hrs for 10–14 days

3rd Recurrence: fecal microbiota transplantation plus vancomycin

From the Clinical Practice Guidelines in Reference 15.

1. A favorable antibiotic response is characterized by resolution of fever (if present) in 24–48 hrs, and resolution of the diarrhea in 4–5 days (17).

2. The use of anti-peristalsis agents to control diarrhea should be limited or avoided because of the potential for aggravating the mucosal inflammation (15).

3. Although *metronidazole* is typically the preferred antibi-

otic for mild-to-moderate CDI, *vancomycin* is preferred in the following situations (15):

a. The patient is intolerant, or allergic, to metronidazole.

b. The patient is pregnant or breastfeeding.

c. The response to metronidazole is inadequate after 5–7 days.

4. *Fidaxomicin* (200 mg PO BID for 10 days) is equivalent to vancomycin for eradicating CDI, and may have fewer recurrences (15). It is currently approved for use as an additional alternative to metronidazole in mild-to-moderate CDI, but it is not favored in the current guidelines for CDI because it is costly (15).

5. There is no proven alternative to vancomycin in patients with severe CDI. For patients who are responding poorly to vancomycin, two alternatives can be considered (18):

a. Increase the vancomycin dose to 500 mg PO every 6 hours.

b. Switch to fidaxomicin (200 mg PO BID for 10 days).

6. The relapse rate for CDI is 10–20% after the initial episode, and 40–65% after a second episode (15). Relapses occur within 8 weeks after treatment is completed, and are probably the result of persistent alterations in the bowel microflora rather than resistant organisms. This is the basis for the recolonization efforts described next.

E. Recolonization

Recolonization of the bowel with normal microflora is used primarily to prevent recurrent episodes of CDI. There are two methods of recolonization: ingestion of probiotics, and fecal transplantation.

1. **Probiotics**

   Probiotics are nonpathogenic organisms that bind to epithelial cells in the bowel and impede colonization with *C. difficile*. These organisms are ingested in pill form or capsules, starting at the onset of antibiotic therapy for CDI, and continuing for 3–4 weeks. There are occasional reports of a decrease in recurrences with probiotic therapy, but a meta-analysis of the accumulated experience with probiotics found no convincing evidence of a treatment effect (19). As a result, the use of probiotics is not supported in the current guidelines for CDI (15).

2. **Fecal Microbiota Transplantation**

   Instillation of liquid preparations of stool from healthy donors (via nasogastric tubes, retention enemas, or colonoscopy) can prevent recurrent episodes of CDI in 90% of cases (15). *Fecal microbiota transplantation* is currently recommended for patients with 3 or more recurrences of CDI (see Table 32.2).

   a. Fecal transplantation has also had remarkable success in cases of life-threatening CDI. (See Reference 20 for more on this promising therapy.)

III. POSTOPERATIVE INFECTIONS

Postoperative abdominal infections are located in the peritoneal cavity, and are the result of peritoneal seeding during the procedure, or leakage of bowel contents from an anastomotic site or undetected injury to the bowel. These infections can present as diffuse peritonitis, or an abdominal abscess.

A. Peritonitis

Generalized peritonitis is not a common presentation for

postoperative infections, and is usually the result of an anastomotic leak or an accidental tear in the bowel.

1. **Clinical Features**

   Small leaks often present with non-specific abdominal pain, and the first sign of a leak may be the presence of air under the diaphragm. (This is not a useful finding after a laparoscopic procedure, because the instillation of CO_2 during laparoscopy can produce residual air under the diaphragm for days.) Persistent leakage will eventually produce signs of peritoneal irritation (e.g., rebound tenderness) and a systemic inflammatory response (fever, leukocytosis, etc). Progression to circulatory shock can be rapid.

2. **Management**

   Signs of diffuse peritonitis warrants immediate surgical exploration. The initial management should include the following measures.

   a. FLUIDS: Peritonitis can result in considerable fluid loss into the peritoneal cavity, and the hemodynamic consequences of hypovolemia will be aggravated by ongoing sepsis, and by general anesthesia for surgical exploration. Therefore, attention to fluid needs is essential.

   b. ANTIBIOTICS: Empiric antibiotic therapy should begin as soon as possible using antibiotics that are active against the frequent isolates in Table 32.3. Single-agent coverage using *piperacillin-tazobactam*, or a carbapenem (e.g., *meropenem*) is recommended (4). (See Chapter 44, Sections III and VI, for dosing recommendations for these antibiotics.)

   c. CANDIDIASIS: Empiric coverage for candidiasis is recommended for all postoperative intra-abdominal infections (21). The echinocandins (e.g., *caspofungin*) are the favored antifungal agents in this setting (21). (See Chapter 44, Section II-C, for the dosing regimens of these agents.)

Table 32.3	Organisms Involved in Complicated Abdominal Infections	
Organism	**Patients (%)**	
Gram-negative Bacilli		
Escherichia coli	71%	
Klebsiella spp	14%	
Pseudomonas aeruginosa	14%	
Gram-positive Cocci		
Streptococci	38%	
Enterococci	23%	
Staphylococcus aureus	4%	
Anaerobes		
Bacteroides fragilis	35%	
Other anaerobes	55%	

From Reference 4.

B. Abdominal Abscess

Abdominal abscesses are difficult to detect on routine physical examination, and they often serve as an occult source of sepsis.

1. Clinical Features

Fever is almost always present (22), but localized abdominal tenderness can be absent in 60% of cases, and a palpable abdominal mass is evident in less than 10% of cases (22,23).

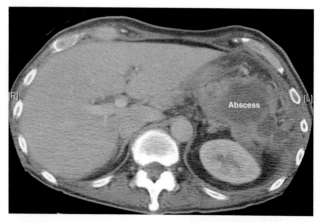

FIGURE 32.2 Abdominal CT scan showing a multiloculated abscess in the left upper quadrant of a post-splenectomy patient.

2. **Computed Tomography**

Computed tomography (CT) is the most reliable method for the detection for abdominal abscesses, with a sensitivity and specificity ≥90% (23). However, CT imaging in the first postoperative week can be misleading because collections of blood or irrigant solutions in the peritoneal cavity can be misread as an abscess (23). The CT appearance of an abdominal abscess is shown in Figure 32.2.

3. **Management**

Immediate drainage is required, and this is often achieved with CT-guided drainage catheters (22). Empiric antibacterial and antifungal coverage is required, using the same agents described for peritonitis.

REFERENCES

1. McChesney JA, Northrup PG, Bickston SJ. Acute acalculous cholecystitis associated with systemic sepsis and visceral arterial

hypoperfusion. A case series and review of pathophysiology. Dig Dis Sci 2003; 48:1960–1967.

2. Laurila J, Syrjälä H, Laurila PA, et al. Acute acalculous cholecystitis in critically ill patients. Acta Anesthesiol Scand 2004; 48:986–991.

3. Messing B, Bories C, Kuntslinger C. Does parenteral nutrition induce gallbladder sludge formation and lithiasis? Gastroenterology 1983; 84:1012–1019.

4. Solomkin JS, Mazuski JE, Bradley JS, et al. Diagnosis and management of complicated intra-abdominal infection in adults and children: guidelines by the Surgical Infection Society and the Infectious Disease Society of America. Clin Infect Dis 2010; 50:133–164.

5. Frankel HL, Kirkpatrick AW, Elbarbary M, et al. Guidelines for the appropriate use of bedside general and cardiac ultrasonography in the evaluation of critically ill patients—Part I: General ultrasonography. Crit Care Med 2015; 43:2479–2502.

6. Puc MM, Tran HS, Wry PW, Ross SE. Ultrasound is not a useful screening tool for acalculous cholecystitis in critically ill trauma patients. Am Surg 2002; 68:65–69.

7. Treinen C, Lomelin D, Krause C, et al. Acute acalculous cholecystitis in the critically ill: risk factors and surgical strategies. Langenbacks Arch Surg 2015; 400:421–427.

8. Ofosu A. *Clostridium difficile* infection: a review of current and emerging therapies. Ann Gastroenterol 2016; 29:147–154.

9. Reveles KR, Lee GC, Boyd NK, Frei CR. The rise in *Clostridium difficile* infection incidence among hospitalized adults in the United States: 2001–2010. Am J Infect Control 2014; 42:1028–1032.

10. Johnson S, Gerding DN, Olson MM, et al. Prospective, controlled study of vinyl glove use to interrupt *Clostridium difficile* nosocomial transmission. Am J Med 1990; 88:137–140.

11. Dial S, Alrasadi K, Manoukian C, et. al. Risk of *Clostridium-difficile* diarrhea among hospitalized patients prescribed proton pump inhibitors: cohort and case-control studies. Canad Med Assoc J 2004; 171:33–38.

12. Dial S, Delaney JA, Barkun AN, Suissa S. Use of gastric acid-suppressing agents and the risk of community-acquired *Clostridium difficile*-associated disease. JAMA 2005; 294:2989–2995.

13. Aseri M, Schroeder T, Kramer J, Kackula R. Gastric acid suppression by proton pump inhibitors as a risk factor for *Clostridium difficile*-associated diarrhea in hospitalized patients. Am J Gastroenterol 2008; 103:2308–2313.

14. Cunningham R, Dial S. Is over-use of proton pump inhibitors fueling the current epidemic of *Clostridium-difficile*-associated diarrhea? J Hosp Infect 2008; 70:1–6.

15. Surawicz CM, Brandt LJ, Binion DG, et al. Guidelines for diagnosis, treatment, and prevention of *Clostridium difficile* infections. Am J Gastroenterol 2013; 108:478–498.

16. Polage CR, Gyorke CE, Kennedy MA, et al. Overdiagnosis of *Clostridium difficile* infection in the molecular test era. JAMA Intern Med 2015; 175:1792–1801.

17. Bartlett JG. Antibiotic-associated diarrhea. N Engl J Med 2002; 346:334–339.

18. Ofosu A. *Clostridium difficile* infection: a review of current and emerging therapies. Ann Gastroenterol 2016; 29:147–154.

19. Pillai A, Nelson RL. Probiotics for treatment of *Clostridium difficile*-associated colitis in adults. Cochrane Database Syst Rev 2008; 1:CD004611.

20. Bakken JS, Borody T, Brandt LJ, et al. Fecal Microbiota Transplantation (FMT) Workgroup. Treating *Clostridium difficile* infection with fecal microbiota transplantation. Clin Gastroenterol Hepatol 2011; 9:1044–1049.

21. Pappas PG, Kauffman CA, Andes DR, et al. Clinical practice guideline for the management of candidiasis: 2016 update by the Infectious Disease Society of America. Clin Infect Dis 2016; 62:e1–e50.

22. Khurrum Baig M, Hua Zao R, Batista O, et al. Percutaneous postoperative intra-abdominal abscess drainage after elective colorectal surgery. Tech Coloproctol 2002; 6:159–164.

23. Fry DE. Noninvasive imaging tests in the diagnosis and treatment of intra-abdominal abscesses in the postoperative patient. Surg Clin North Am 1994; 74:693–709.

Chapter 33

Urinary Tract Infections

Urinary tract infections (UTIs) associated with bladder drainage catheters account for 40% of all hospital-acquired infections in the United States (1), but a majority of these infections represent asymptomatic bacteriuria, and do not require antimicrobial therapy. This chapter describes the diagnosis and treatment of *symptomatic* catheter-associated UTIs.

I. BACTERIAL INFECTIONS

A. Pathogenesis

1. The presence of a urethral catheter is associated with a 3–8% incidence of significant bacteriuria ($\geq 10^5$ colony forming units/mL) *per day* (1). This is assumed to be the result of bacterial migration along the outer surface of the catheter and into the bladder.

2. Bacteria also form *biofilms* on the inner and outer surface of urethral catheters (2), and these biofilms can serve as a source of continued microbial colonization in the bladder.

3. Bacterial migration and biofilm formation are not the whole story, because direct injection of pathogens into the bladder of healthy subjects does not result in a UTI (3). Epithelial cells of the bladder are coated with non-pathogenic organisms (4), which prevent the attach-

ment of pathogens (5), and it is possible that a change in bacterial adherence serves as a prelude to UTI.

B. Microbiology

1. The pathogens isolated in catheter-associated bacteriuria are shown in Table 33.1 (6).

Table 33.1	Pathogens Isolated in Catheter-Associated Bacteriuria	
Pathogen	**% of Infections**	
	Hospital	**ICU**
Escherichia coli	21.4	22.3
Enterococci	15.5	15.8
Candida albicans	14.5	15.3
Other *Candida* species	6.5	9.5
Pseudomonas aeruginosa	10.0	13.3
Klebsiella pneumoniae	7.7	7.5
Enterobacter species	4.1	5.5
Coag-neg staphylococci	2.5	4.6
Staphylococcus aureus	2.2	2.5
Acinetobacter baumannii	1.2	1.5

Adapted from Reference 6. Some of the percentages represent median values.

2. The predominant organisms are gram-negative aerobic bacilli (especially *Escherichia coli*), enterococci, and *Candida* species, while staphylococci are infrequent isolates.

3. A single organism predominates in bacteriuria associated with short-term catheterization (<30 days), whereas bacteriuria is often polymicrobial in long-term catheterization ($\geq$30 days).

C. Prevention

1. The risk of catheter-associated infection is determined primarily by the duration of catheterization (1), so *removing catheters when they are no longer necessary is the single most effective prophylactic measure* for catheter-associated infections.

2. Urinary catheters impregnated with antimicrobial agents (silver alloy or nitrofurazone) can reduce the incidence of asymptomatic bacteriuria in short-term catheterization (<1 week) (7), but the benefit in preventing symptomatic urinary tract infections is not clear (1).

3. The following practices are NOT recommended (1):

   a. Daily cleansing of catheter insertion sites (with antiseptic solutions, antibiotic creams, or soap and water), which can increase the risk of bacteriuria.

   b. Prophylaxis with systemic antibiotics.

D. Diagnosis

The criteria for the diagnosis of catheter-associated urinary tract infection (CAUTI) are shown in Table 33.2 (8).

1. Significant bacteriuria in catheterized patients is defined as a urine culture that grows $\geq 10^5$ colony forming units (cfu) per mL (1). However, over 90% of patients with significant bacteriuria have no other evidence of infection (asymptomatic bacteriuria) (9).

2. The diagnosis of CAUTI requires significant bacteriuria plus evidence of infection (e.g., new-onset fever).

Common symptoms of UTI such as dysuria and frequency are not relevant in catheterized patients.

3. The presence of white blood cells in urine (pyuria) is not predictive of CAUTI, but the absence of pyuria can be used as evidence against the diagnosis of CAUTI (1).

Table 33.2	Diagnostic Criteria for Catheter-Associated Urinary Tract Infection (CAUTI)

All three conditions must be satisfied for the diagnosis of CAUTI:

1. Urine culture growing no more than 2 organisms, one with growth of $\geq 10^5$ cfu/mL

2. Urethral catheter has been in place for more than 2 days prior to the event

3. Any of the following conditions is present:
   a. Fever (>38°C or >100.4°F)
   b. Suprapubic pain or tenderness
   c. Costovertebral pain or tenderness

From Reference 8.

E. Treatment

1. Antibiotic therapy is *not* advised for asymptomatic bacteriuria unless the patient is scheduled for a urologic procedure (10).

2. Empiric antibiotics are recommended for patients with suspected CAUTI. Single agent therapy with *piperacillin-tazobactam* (see Chapter 44, Section VI-A for dosing information) or a *carbapenem* (see Table 44.3 for drugs and dosing information) is recommended (11).

3. If the diagnosis of CAUTI is confirmed by urine culture, antibiotic therapy should be adjusted accordingly, and catheters that have been in place for longer than 2 weeks should be replaced.

4. The duration of antibiotic therapy for CAUTI should be 7 days for patients who respond promptly, and 10–14 days for patients with a delayed response.

II. CANDIDURIA

The presence of *Candida* species in urine usually represents colonization in patients with indwelling urethral catheters, but candiduria can also be a sign of disseminated candidiasis (i.e., the candiduria being the result, not the cause, of the disseminated candidiasis).

A. Microbiology

1. The most frequent isolate is *Candida albicans* (about 50% of cases), followed by *Candida glabrata* (about 15% of cases) (12). The latter organism is resistant to the antifungal agent fluconazole.

2. In cases of candiduria, the colony count has no predictive value for identifying renal or disseminated candidiasis (12).

B. Asymptomatic Candiduria

1. Asymptomatic candiduria does not require treatment unless the patient is neutropenic, or will undergo urologic manipulation (13).

   a. Neutropenic patients should receive an *echinocandin* (see Chapter 44, Section II-C-2 for drugs and dosing recommendations) (13).

b. Patients undergoing urologic procedures should receive oral *fluconazole*, 400 mg daily, or *amphotericin B*, 0.3–0.6 mg/kg IV daily, for several days before and after the procedure (13).

2. Removal of the catheter is advised, when possible (13).

3. Repeat urine cultures are recommended, and persistent candiduria in neutropenic patients should be investigated with blood cultures and imaging studies of the kidneys.

C. Symptomatic Candiduria

Symptomatic candiduria (i.e., associated with fever, suprapubic tenderness, etc.) requires blood cultures and imaging studies of the kidneys (ultrasound or computed tomography) to search for renal abscesses or urinary tract obstruction. The following recommendations for antifungal therapy are from the 2016 guidelines on treating candidiasis (13):

1. **Cystitis**

   a. For fluconazole-susceptible organisms, give oral fluconazole, 200 mg daily, for 2 weeks.

   b. For fluconazole-resistant *C. glabrata*, give oral *flucytosine*, 25 mg/kg, 4 times daily, for 7–10 days.

   c. For *C. krusei*, give amphotericin B, 0.3–0.6 mg/kg daily, for up to 7 days.

2. **Pyelonephritis**

   a. For fluconazole-susceptible organisms, give oral fluconazole, 200–400 mg daily, for 2 weeks.

   b. For fluconazole-resistant *C. glabrata*, give amphotericin B, 0.3–0.6 mg/kg daily, for up to 7 days, with or without oral flucytosine, 25 mg/kg, 4 times daily.

   c. For *C. krusei*, give amphotericin B, 0.3–0.6 mg/kg daily, for up to 7 days.

3. **Fluconazole**

Fluconazole is concentrated in the urine, and is well suited for treating *Candida* UTIs caused by susceptible organisms. Decreasing the dose of fluconazole for a creatinine clearance <50 mL/min (which is normally recommended) is not advised for *Candida* UTIs because this decreases the urinary concentration of fluconazole to subtherapeutic levels (14). (For more information on fluconazole, see Chapter 44, Section II-B.)

REFERENCES

1. Hooton TM, Bradley SF, Cardenas DD, et al. Diagnosis, prevention, and treatment of catheter-associated urinary tract infections in adults: 2009 international clinical practice guidelines from the Infectious Disease Society of America. Clin Infect Dis 2010; 50:625–663.

2. Ganderton L, Chawla J, Winters C, et al. Scanning electron microscopy of bacterial biofilms on indwelling bladder catheters. Eur J Clin Microbiol Infect Dis 1992; 11:789–796.

3. Howard RJ. Host defense against infection—Part 1. Curr Probl Surg 1980;27:267–316.

4. Sobel JD. Pathogenesis of urinary tract infections: host defenses. Infect Dis Clin North Am 1987; 1:751–772.

5. Daifuku R, Stamm WE. Bacterial adherence to bladder uroepithelial cells in catheter-associated urinary tract infection. N Engl J Med 1986; 314:1208–1213.

6. Shuman EK, Chenoweth CE. Recognition and prevention of healthcare-associated urinary tract infections in the intensive care unit. Crit Care Med 2010; 38(Suppl):S373–S379.

7. Schumm K, Lam TB. Types of urethral catheters for management of short-term voiding problems in hospitalized adults. Cochrane Database Syst Rev 2008:CD004013.

8. Centers for Disease Control and Prevention. Urinary tract infection (catheter-associated urinary tract infection [CAUTI] and non-

catheter-associated urinary tract infection [UTI]) and other urinary system infection events. January 2016. Accessed August, 2016 at http://www.cdc.gov/nhsn/pdfs/pscmanual/7psccauti-current.pdf

9. Tambyah PA, Maki DG. Catheter-associated urinary tract infection is rarely symptomatic. Arch Intern Med 2000; 160:678–682.

10. Nicolle LE, Bradley S, Colgan R, et al. Infectious Disease Society of America guidelines for the diagnosis and treatment of asymptomatic bacteriuria in adults. Clin Infect Dis 2005; 40:643–654.

11. Gilbert DN, Moellering RC, Eliopoulis, et al, eds. The Sanford guide to antimicrobial therapy, 2009. 39th ed. Sperryville, VA: Antimicrobial Therapy, Inc, 2009:31.

12. Hollenbach E. To treat or not to treat—critically ill patients with candiduria. Mycoses 2008; 51(Suppl 2):12–24.

13. Pappas PG, Kauffman CA, Andes DR, et al. Clinical practice guidelines for the management of candidiasis: 2016 update by the Infectious Disease Society of America. Clin Infect Dis 2016; 62:e1–50.

14. Fisher JF, Sobel JD, Kauffman CA, Newman CA. *Candida* urinary tract infections—treatment. Clin Infect Dis 2011; 52(Suppl 6):S457–S466.

Chapter 34

Thermoregulatory Disorders

The human thermoregulatory system limits the daily variation in body temperature to $\pm 0.6°C$ (1). This chapter describes what happens when this system fails, and allows the body temperature to rise or fall to dangerous levels.

I. HEAT STROKE

A. Clinical Features

Heat stroke is a life-threatening condition that can be precipitated by environmental temperatures (classic heart stroke) or strenuous exercise (exertional heat stroke). The clinical features include the following (2-4):

1. Body temperature $>40°C$ ($104°F$)

2. Altered mentation (e.g., delirium, coma) and seizures

3. Severe volume depletion with hypotension

4. Multiorgan involvement, including rhabdomyolysis, acute kidney injury, acute liver failure, and disseminated intravascular coagulopathy (DIC).

5. The inability to produce sweat (anhidrosis) is typical, but not universal.

B. Management

Management includes volume resuscitation (to replace volume losses, and reduce the risk of myoglobinuric renal injury from rhabdomyolysis), and cooling measures to *reduce the core temperature to 38°C (100.4°F)* (4). Thermistor-equipped bladder catheters can be used to monitor core body temperature.

1. *External cooling* is the easiest and quickest way to reduce the body temperature. This involves placing ice packs in the groin and axilla and covering the upper thorax and neck with ice, then placing cooling blankets over the entire length of the body.

2. *Evaporative cooling* is the most effective method of external cooling (3,4), and is typically used in the field. The skin is sprayed with cool water and then fanned to promote evaporation of the water. The evaporation of water from the skin requires body heat, called the *heat of vaporization*. (This is how sweating reduces body temperature.) This method can reduce the body temperature at a rate of 0.31°C (0.56°F) per minute (3).

3. The major drawback of external cooling is the risk of shivering, which raises the body temperature.

4. *Internal cooling* is easily implemented by infusing cooled (or even room temperature) intravenous fluids. Measures such as cold water lavage of the stomach or bladder are usually not necessary, and heroic measures like cold peritoneal lavage are rarely necessary.

C. Rhabdomyolysis

1. Skeletal muscle injury (rhabdomyolysis) is a common complication of hyperthermia syndromes, including heat stroke and drug-induced hyperthermia (described in the next sections).

2. Disruption of myocytes in skeletal muscle releases creatine kinase (CK) into the bloodstream. There is no stan-

dard plasma CK level for the diagnosis of rhabdomyolysis, but CK levels that are five times higher than normal (about 1,000 units/L) have been used in clinical studies of rhabdomyolysis (5).

3. Skeletal muscle injury also releases myoglobin into the bloodstream, and the myoglobin can damage the renal tubules and produce acute kidney injury (5). This condition is described in Chapter 26, Section III-C.

II. MALIGNANT HYPERTHERMIA

Malignant hyperthermia (MH) is an inherited disorder characterized by excessive calcium release from the sarcoplasmic reticulum in skeletal muscle in response to halogenated inhalational anesthetic agents (e.g., isoflurane) and succinylcholine. The genetic prevalence is about 1 in 2,000 (males >females), and the incidence of MH varies from 1 in 5,000 to 1 in 100,000 exposures to inhalational anesthesia (6).

A. Clinical Features

The clinical manifestations of MH are listed in Table 34.1 (6).

1. The first sign of MH may be a sudden, unexpected rise in end-tidal PCO_2 (from hypermetabolism). This is followed (within minutes to a few hours) by generalized muscle rigidity and rhabdomyolysis.

2. Trismus is often the first sign of MH from succinylcholine.

3. The heat generated by the muscle rigidity is responsible for the rise in body temperature (often >40°C or 104°F), which is a late occurrence in MH.

4. Autonomic instability can lead to cardiac arrhythmias and hypotension.

5. The mortality rate in untreated MH is 70–80% (6).

Table 34.1	Clinical Features of Malignant Hyperthermia
Early	**Late**
Masseter spasm	Hyperthermia
Muscle rigidity	Rhabdomyolysis
Hypercapnia	Acute Kidney Injury
Lactic acidosis	Hypotension
Tachycardia	Cardiac arrhythmias

From Reference 6.

B. Management

The first suspicion of MH should prompt immediate discontinuation of the inhalational anesthetic, and administration of the following drug.

1. **Dantrolene**

   Dantrolene sodium is a muscle relaxant that blocks the release of calcium from the sarcoplasmic reticulum. When given early in the course of MH, the mortality rate is as low as 5% (6).

   a. The dosing regimen is 2 mg/kg as an IV bolus, repeated every 5 minutes, if needed, to a total dose of 20 mg/kg (6). Some recommend a maintenance dose of 1 mg/kg IV or 2 mg/kg PO, four times daily for 3 days, to prevent recurrences (7).

   b. Dantrolene is not advised in patients with advanced liver disease (because it can be hepatotoxic), but this applies more to long-term use of the drug.

   c. Side effects of dantrolene, which are uncommon with short-term use, include tissue necrosis from extravasation, muscle weakness, headache, and vomiting (6).

2. **Other Measures**

   a. Minute ventilation should be increased (by adjustments on the ventilator) to keep the end-tidal PCO_2 within normal limits.

   b. Volume resuscitation is often necessary to combat hypotension and reduce the risk of myoglobinuric renal damage. Vasopressor support may also be necessary.

   c. Plasma levels of the following should be monitored: lactate, potassium, creatinine, and creatine kinase.

   d. Cooling measures may not be needed once the muscle rigidity is controlled.

C. Follow-up

All patients who survive an episode of MH should be given a medical bracelet that identifies their susceptibility to MH. Immediate family members should also be tested to identify the gene responsible for MH (6).

III. NEUROLEPTIC MALIGNANT SYNDROME

The neuroleptic malignant syndrome (NMS) is similar to malignant hyperthermia in that it is a drug-induced disorder characterized by hyperthermia, muscle rigidity, altered mental status, and autonomic instability (8).

A. Pathogenesis

1. NMS is typically associated with drugs that influence dopamine-mediated synaptic transmission in the brain.

2. As indicated in Table 34.2, NMS can be caused by drugs that inhibit dopaminergic transmission (most cases), or

it can be triggered by discontinuing drugs that facilitate dopaminergic transmission.

3. The incidence of NMS during therapy with neuroleptic agents is 0.2% to 1.9% (9), and the drugs most frequently implicated are *haloperidol* and *fluphenazine* (8).

4. There is no relationship between the intensity or duration of drug therapy and the risk of NMS (8).

Table 34.2	Drugs Implicated in the Neuroleptic Malignant Syndrome

Drugs that Inhibit Dopaminergic Transmission

Neuroleptics:	Butyrophenones (e.g., haloperidol), phenothiazines, clozapine, olanzapine, respiradone
Antimimetics:	Metaclopramide, droperidol, prochlorperazine
CNS stimulants:	Amphetamines, cocaine
Others:	Lithium, tricyclic antidepressants (overdose)

Discontinuing Drugs that Facilitate Dopaminergic Transmission

Dopaminergics:	Amantidine, bromocriptine, levodopa

B. Clinical Features

1. Most cases of NMS begin to appear 24–72 hours after the onset of drug therapy, and almost all cases are apparent in the first 2 weeks of drug therapy. The onset is usually gradual, and can take days to fully develop.

2. In 80% of cases, the initial manifestation is muscle rigidity or altered mental status (8). The muscle rigidity has been described as *lead-pipe rigidity*, to distinguish it

from the rigidity associated with tremulousness (cog-wheel rigidity).

3. A body temperature $\geq 40°C$ ($104°F$) is required for the diagnosis of NMS (8), but it can be delayed for 8–10 hours after the onset of muscle rigidity (10).

4. Autonomic instability can produce hypotension and cardiac arrhythmias.

C. Laboratory Studies

1. Dystonic reactions to neuroleptic agents may be difficult to distinguish from the muscle rigidity in NMS. The creatine kinase (CK) level in plasma can help in this regard because serum CK levels are only mildly elevated in dystonic reactions, but are higher than 1,000 units/L in NMS (9).

2. The blood leukocyte count in NMS can increase to $40,000/\mu L$, with increased immature neutrophils (8), so the clinical presentation of NMS (fever, leukocytosis, altered mental status) can be mistaken as sepsis.

D. Management

Discontinuing (or restarting) the offending drug is mandatory. The remainder of the management involves general support measures (e.g., volume resuscitation for hypotension, cooling measures) and the following drugs.

1. **Dantrolene**

   Dantrolene sodium (the same muscle relaxant used in the treatment of MH) can be given intravenously for severe cases of muscle rigidity. The optimal dose is not clearly defined, but one suggestion is shown below.

   a. DOSING REGIMEN: 2 mg/kg as IV bolus, and repeat

as needed to a total dose of 10 mg/kg, then follow with oral doses of 50–200 mg daily in 3–4 divided doses (8,11).

2. **Bromocriptine**

Bromocriptine mesylate is a dopamine agonist that has been successful in treating NMS in oral doses of 2.5–10 mg three times daily (11). Some improvement in muscle rigidity can be seen within hours, but the full response often takes days to develop. *Bromocriptine offers no advantage over dantrolene*, except possibly in patients with advanced liver disease (because dantrolene can be hepatotoxic, usually with prolonged use).

3. **Duration of Treatment**

Treatment of NMS should continue for about 10 days after clinical resolution, because of delayed clearance of many neuroleptics. When depot preparations are implicated, therapy should continue for 2 to 3 weeks after clinical resolution (8).

IV. SEROTONIN SYNDROME

Overstimulation of serotonin receptors in the central nervous system produces a combination of mental status changes, autonomic hyperactivity, and neuromuscular abnormalities, known as the *serotonin syndrome* (SS) (12).

A. Pathogenesis

Serotonin is a neurotransmitter that participates in sleep-wakefulness cycles, mood, and thermoregulation. A variety of drugs can enhance serotonin neurotransmission and produce SS, and a list of these drugs is shown in Table 34.3 (12,13). More than one drug is often involved.

Table 34.3	Drugs that can Produce the Serotonin Syndrome
Effect on Serotonin	**Drugs**
Increased Synthesis	L-tryptophan
Increased Release	Amphetamines, MDMA (ecstasy), cocaine, fenfluramine
Decreased Breakdown	MAO inhibitors (including linezolid), ritonavir
Decreased Reuptake	SSRIs, TCAs, dextromethorphan, meperidine, fentanyl, tramadol
Stimulates Receptors	Lithium, sumitriptan, buspirone, LSD

MDMA = methylenedioxy-methamphetamine; MAO = monoamine oxidase; SSRIs = selective serotonin reuptake inhibitors; TCAs = tricyclic antidepressants.

B. Clinical Features

1. The onset of SS is usually abrupt (in contrast to NMS), and over half of the cases are evident within 6 hours after ingestion of the responsible drug(s) (12).

2. The clinical findings include mental status changes (e.g., confusion, delirium, coma), hyperthermia, autonomic hyperactivity (e.g., mydriasis, tachycardia, hypertension), and neuromuscular abnormalities (e.g., hyperkinesis, clonus, and muscle rigidity).

3. Life-threatening cases are marked by rhabdomyolysis, renal failure, metabolic acidosis, and hypotension (12).

4. The clinical presentation can vary markedly. Hyperthermia and muscle rigidity can be absent in mild cases

of the illness. *The features that most distinguish SS from other drug-induced hyperthermia syndromes are hyperkinesis and clonus (inducible, spontaneous, or horizontal ocular clonus)* (12). Inducible clonus is most obvious in the patellar deep-tendon reflexes.

C. Management

Discontinuing the responsible drug(s) is mandatory.

1. Sedation with *benzodiazepines* is recommended for controlling agitation in SS (8). (For information on benzodiazepine dosing, see Chapter 43, Section II-B, and Table 43.5.)

2. The serotonin antagonist *cyproheptadine* can be given in severe cases of SS (14). This drug is available for oral administration only, but tablets can be broken up and administered through a nasogastric tube. The initial dose is 12 mg, followed by 2 mg every 2 hours for persistent symptoms (14). The maintenance dose is 8 mg every 6 hours.

3. Other measures may include volume resuscitation to combat hypotension and reduce the risk of myoglobinuric renal damage, and cooling measures for persistent hyperpyrexia ($\geq 40°C$), as described for heat stroke.

4. Neuromuscular paralysis may be required in severe cases of SS to control muscle rigidity and extreme temperature elevations ($>41°C$). Nondepolarizing agents (e.g., *vecuronium*) should be used for muscle paralysis (12).

5. Many cases of SS will resolve within 24 hours after initiation of therapy, but seritonergic drugs with long elimination half-lives can produce a more prolonged toxidrome.

V. HYPOTHERMIA

Hypothermia (body temperature $<35°C$ or $<95°F$) can be the result of environmental exposure, a metabolic disorder, or a therapeutic intervention. This section will focus on environmental (accidental) hypothermia.

A. Predisposing Conditions

Environmental hypothermia is most likely to occur in the following situations (15):

1. Prolonged submersion in cold water (the transfer of heat to cold water occurs much more readily than the transfer of heat to cold air) or prolonged exposure to cold wind (which promotes heat loss by convection).

2. When the physiological response to cold is impaired (e.g., the vasoconstrictive response to cold is impaired by alcohol consumption), or behavioral responses to cold are impaired (e.g., a confused or intoxicated person may fail to seek shelter from the cold).

B. Clinical Features

The consequences of progressive hypothermia are summarized in Table 34.4.

1. *Mild Hypothermia* ($32-35°C$ or $90-95°F$): Patients are often confused, and show signs of adaptation to cold, such as brisk shivering, and cold, pale skin from cutaneous vasoconstriction. The heart rate is usually rapid.

2. *Moderate Hypothermia* ($28-31.9°C$ or $82-89.9°F$): Patients are lethargic, and shivering may be absent. Bradycardia and a decreased respiratory rate (bradypnea) become evident, and pupillary light reflexes can be absent.

3. *Severe Hypothermia* ($<28°C$ or $<82°F$): Patients are usually obtunded or comatose, with dilated, fixed pupils (not a sign of brain death in this situation). Additional findings include hypotension, severe bradycardia, oliguria, and generalized edema. Apnea and asystole are expected at body temperatures below $25°C$ ($77°F$).

Table 34.4	Manifestations of Progressive Hypothermia	
Severity	**Body Temp**	**Clinical Manifestations**
Mild	32–35°C 90–95°F	Confusion, cold and pale skin, shivering, tachycardia
Moderate	28–31.9°C 82–89.9°F	Lethargy, reduced or absent shivering, bradycardia, bradypnea
Severe	<28°C <82°F	Obtundation or coma, no shivering, edema, dilated and fixed pupils, bradycardia, hypotension, oliguria
Fatal	<25°C <77°F	Apnea, asystole

C. Electrocardiogram

1. About 80% of patients with hypothermia have prominent J waves at the QRS-ST junction on the electrocardiogram (see Figure 34.1). These waves, called *Osborn waves*, are not specific for hypothermia, and can occur with hypercalcemia, subarachnoid hemorrhage, cerebral injuries, and myocardial ischemia (16). Despite their notoriety, these waves have no diagnostic value in hypothermia (which is diagnosed by body temperature).

2. A variety of arrhythmias can occur in hypothermia, including first, second, and third-degree heart block, sinus and junctional bradycardia, idioventricular rhythm, premature atrial and ventricular beats, and atrial and ventricular fibrillation (16).

D. Laboratory Tests

1. A generalized coagulopathy (with elevation of the INR and prolonged partial thromboplastin times) is common in hypothermia (15), but may not be evident if the coagulation profile is run at normal body temperatures.

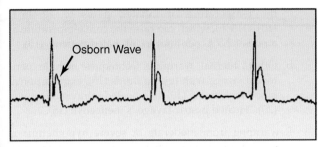

FIGURE 34.1 The (overhyped) Osborn wave.

2. Arterial blood gases (which should be run at normal body temperatures) can reveal a respiratory acidosis or a metabolic acidosis (15).

3. Serum electrolytes can reveal hyperkalemia from potassium release by skeletal muscle due to shivering or rhabdomyolysis.

4. Serum creatinine levels can be elevated as a result of rhabdomyolysis, acute renal failure, or *cold diuresis* (caused by diminished renal tubular responsiveness to antidiuretic hormone).

E. Rewarming

1. *External rewarming* is adequate for most cases of hypothermia (17). There can be a further decrease in body temperature during external rewarming (called afterdrop) from central displacement of cold blood in cutaneous blood vessels, and this is considered a risk for ventricular fibrillation (18). However, serious cardiac arrhythmias are uncommon during external rewarming (17,18).

2. *Internal rewarming* is generally reserved for the most severe cases of hypothermia.

   a. The easiest method of internal warming is to increase

the temperature of inhaled gases to 40–45°C (104–113°F), which can raise the core temperature at a rate of 2.5°C per hour in intubated patients (15).

b. Other internal warming techniques include peritoneal lavage with heated fluids (15), extracorporeal blood rewarming (19), and heated intravenous fluids (20). Heated gastric lavage is ineffective (15).

3. Rewarming from moderate or severe hypothermia is often accompanied by hypotension (rewarming shock), which is attributed to a combination of factors, including hypovolemia (from cold diuresis), myocardial depression, and vasodilation (17,18).

a. Volume infusion will help to alleviate this problem, but infusing fluids at room temperature (21°C or 70°F) can aggravate the hypothermia, so the infused fluids should be heated.

b. Vasopressors are required in about half of patients with severe hypothermia, and indicates a poor prognosis (18).

REFERENCES

1. Guyton AC, Hall JE. Body temperature, temperature regulation, and fever. In: Medical Physiology, 10th ed. Philadelphia, WB Saunders, 2000: 822–833.

2. Lugo-Amador NM, Rothenhaus T, Moyer P. Heat-related illness. Emerg Med Clin N Am 2004; 22:315–327.

3. Hadad E, Rav-Acha M, Heled Y, et al. Heat stroke: a review of cooling methods. Sports Med 2004; 34:501–511.

4. Glazer JL. Management of heat stroke and heat exhaustion. Am Fam Physician 2005; 71:2133–2142.

5. Ward MM. Factors predictive of acute renal failure in rhabdomyolysis. Arch Intern Med 1988; 148:1553–1557.

6. Schneiderbanger D, Johannsen S, Roewer N, Schuster F.

Management of malignant hyperthermia: diagnosis and treatment. Ther Clin Risk Manag 2014; 10:355–362.

7. McEvoy GK, ed. AHFS Drug Information, 2014. Bethesda, MD: American Society of Health-System Pharmacists, 2014:1439–1442.

8. Bhanushali NJ, Tuite PJ. The evaluation and management of patients with neuroleptic malignant syndrome. Neurol Clin N Am 2004; 22:389–411.

9. Khaldarov V. Benzodiazepines for treatment of neuroleptic malignant syndrome. Hosp Physician, 2003 (Sept): 51–55.

10. Lev R, Clark RF. Neuroleptic malignant syndrome presenting without fever: case report and review of the literature. J Emerg Med 1996; 12:49–55.

11. Guze BH, Baxter LR. Neuroleptic malignant syndrome. N Engl J Med 1985; 13:163–166.

12. Boyer EH, Shannon M. The serotonin syndrome. N Engl J Med 2005; 352:1112–1120.

13. Demirkiran M, Jankivic J, Dean JM. Ecstacy intoxication: an overlap between serotonin syndrome and neuroleptic malignant syndrome. Clin Neuropharmacol 1996; 19:157–164.

14. Graudins A, Stearman A, Chan B. Treatment of serotonin syndrome with cyproheptadine. J Emerg Med 1998; 16:615–619.

15. Hanania NA, Zimmerman NA. Accidental hypothermia. Crit Care Clin 1999; 15: 235–249.

16. Aslam AF, Aslam AK, Vasavada BC, Khan IA. Hypothermia: evaluation, electrocardiographic manifestations, and management. Am J Med 2006; 119:297–301.

17. Cornell HM. Hot topics in cold medicine: controversies in accidental hypothermia. Clin Ped Emerg Med 2001; 2:179–191.

18. Vassal T, Bernoit-Gonin B, Carrat F, et al. Severe accidental hypothermia treated in an ICU. Chest 2001; 120:1998–2003.

19. Ireland AJ, Pathi VL, Crawford R, et al. Back from the dead: Extracorporeal rewarming of severe accidental hypothermia victims in accidental emergency. J Accid Emerg Med 1997; 14:255–303.

20. Handrigen MT, Wright RO, Becker BM, et al. Factors and methodology in achieving ideal delivery temperatures for intravenous and lavage fluid in hypothermia. Am J Emerg Med 1997; 15:350–359.

Chapter 35

Fever in the ICU

The appearance of a new fever is always a source of concern in a hospitalized patient. This chapter presents the general considerations for a new-onset fever in ICU patients (1), including the potential sources of fever, empiric antibiotic coverage, and the benefits vs. harm of antipyretic therapy.

I. FEVER

A. Fever in the ICU

The current guidelines on fever in ICU patients (1) has the following recommendations:

1. A body temperature $\geq 38.3°C$ ($101°F$) represents a fever, while a lower threshold of $38.0°C$ ($100.4°F$) can be used for immunocompromised patients, particularly those with neutropenia.

2. The most accurate measurements of core body temperature are obtained with thermistor-equipped catheters placed in the pulmonary artery, esophagus, or urinary bladder. Less accurate measurements are obtained with rectal, oral, and tympanic temperature recordings, in that order. The axillary and temporal artery sites are not recommended for temperature measurements.

3. *Comment:* Thermistor-equipped urinary bladder catheters seem ideal for temperature monitoring in patients who require a bladder catheter (which includes most ICU patients). These devices not only provide reliable

measurements of core body temperature, they also permit continuous temperature monitoring, which has obvious advantages over periodic measurements.

B. Inflammation vs. Infection

Fever is the result of inflammatory cytokines (called *endogenous pyrogens*) that act on the hypothalamus to elevate the body temperature. Any condition that triggers a systemic inflammatory response will produce a fever.

1. Fever is thus a sign of inflammation, not infection, and about 50% of ICU patients who develop a fever have no apparent infection (2,3).

2. The severity of a fever does not correlate with the presence or severity of infection. High fevers can be the result of a noninfectious condition such as a drug fever (see later), while fever can be minimal or absent in life-threatening infections (1).

3. The distinction between inflammation and infection is an important one, not only for the evaluation of fever, but also for curtailing the "knee jerk" response of using antibiotics to treat fever.

II. NONINFECTIOUS SOURCES

Noninfectious sources of fever in the ICU include major surgery, venous thromboembolism, blood transfusions, and drugs.

A. Early Postop Fever

The incidence of fever in the first postoperative day following major surgery is 15–40%, and in most cases, there is no apparent infection (3-5). These fevers usually resolve within 24 to 48 hours, and most likely represent an inflammatory response to tissue injury sustained during the surgical procedure.

1. Atelectasis Does Not Cause Fever

There is a longstanding misconception that atelectasis is a common cause of fever in the early postoperative period. One possible source of this misconception is the high incidence of atelectasis in patients who develop a postoperative fever. This is demonstrated in the graph on the left in Figure 35.1 (5), which shows that close to 90% of the patients with fever on the first postoperative day had radiographic evidence of atelectasis. This, however, is not evidence that the atelectasis is the source of fever, as verified by the graph on the right (from the same study), which shows that most (75%) of the patients with atelectasis did not have a fever.

a. The lack of a causal relationship between atelectasis and fever was demonstrated over 65 years ago in an

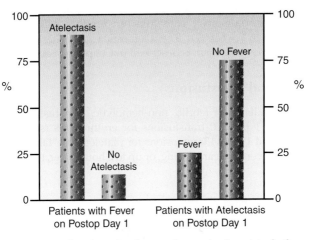

FIGURE 35.1 The relationships between fever and atelectasis in the first postoperative day in 100 consecutive patients who had open heart surgery. The graph on the left shows that most patients with fever had atelectasis, but the graph on the right shows that most patients with atelectasis did not have a fever. Data from Reference 5.

animal study that showed the absence of fever after lobar atelectasis was produced by ligation of a mainstem bronchus (6).

2. **Malignant Hyperthermia**

An uncommon but treatable cause of elevated body temperatures in the immediate postoperative period is *malignant hyperthermia*, an inherited disorder that produces muscle rigidity, hyperpyrexia ($>40°C$ or $>104°F$), and rhabdomyolysis in response to halogenated inhalational anesthetics. This disorder is described in Chapter 34, Section II.

B. Venous Thromboembolism

Several groups of patients are at risk for venous thromboembolism, as described in Chapter 4, Section I. Most cases of hospital-acquired deep vein thrombosis are asymptomatic, but acute pulmonary embolism can produce a fever that lasts up to 1 week (7). The diagnostic evaluation for acute pulmonary embolism is described in Chapter 4, Section III.

C. Blood Transfusions

The incidence of febrile, non-hemolytic, transfusion reactions is 1 per 200 transfusions for erythrocytes (see Table 11.3), and 1 per 14 transfusions for platelets (see Table 12.4). These fevers appears during, or up to 6 hours after, the transfusion.

D. Drug Fever

Any drug can trigger a fever (as a hypersensitivity reaction), but ones that are typically implicated in drug fever are listed in Table 35.1.

1. Drug fever is poorly understood. Over 75% of drug fevers

show no evidence of a hypersensitivity reaction (8).

2. The onset of the fever varies from a few hours to more than three weeks after the onset of drug therapy (1).

3. Drug fever can appear as an isolated finding, or it can be accompanied by the other manifestations listed in Table 35.1 (8). These manifestations indicate that *drug fever can present as a serious, life-threatening illness.*

4. Suspicion of drug fever usually occurs when there are no other likely sources of fever. When suspected, possible offending drugs should be discontinued. The fever should disappear in 2 to 3 days, but it can persist for up to 7 days (9).

Table 35.1	Drug-Associated Fever in the ICU	
Common Offenders	**Occasional Offenders**	**Clinical Findings**
Amphotericin	Cimetidine	Rigors (53%)
Cephalosporins	Carbamazepine	Myalgias (25%)
Penicillins	Hydralazine	Leukocytosis (22%)
Phenytoin	Rifampin	Eosinophilia (22%)
Procainamide	Streptokinase	Rash (18%)
Quinidine	Vancomycin	Hypotension (18%)

From Reference 8.

E. Iatrogenic Fever

Faulty thermal regulators in water mattresses and aerosol humidifiers can cause fever by transference (10). It takes only a few minutes to check the temperature settings on heated mattresses and ventilators, but it can take far longer to explain why such a simple cause of fever was overlooked.

III. NOSOCOMIAL INFECTIONS

The incidence of ICU-acquired infections in medical and surgical ICU patients is shown in Table 35.2 (11). Four infections account for about three-quarters of the infections: pneumonia (mostly ventilator-associated pneumonia), urinary tract infection, bloodstream infection (mostly catheter-related infection), and surgical site infection. Three of these infections are described elsewhere in the book.

1. Ventilator-associated pneumonias are described in Chapter 16.

2. Urinary tract infections are described in Chapter 33.

3. Catheter-related infections are described in Chapter 2, Section III.

   The following are the remaining nosocomial infections that deserve mention.

Table 35.2	Nosocomial Infections in Medical and Surgical ICU Patients	
Infection	**% Total Infections**	
	Medical ICU	**Surgical ICU**
Pneumonia	30%	33%
Urinary Tract Infection	30%	18%
Bloodstream Infection	16%	13%
Surgical Site Infection	—	14%
Others	24%	22%

From Reference 11.

A. Surgical Site Infections

1. Surgical site infections (SSIs) typically appear after 5–7 days, and can be superficial (involves skin and subcutaneous tissue) or deep (extends to fascia, muscle, etc); only the latter are associated with fever (12).

2. The management of deep SSIs includes a combination of drainage, debridement, and antibiotics. The pathogens involved in SSIs can differ; e.g., *Staph epidermidis* is the leading pathogen in SSIs following open heart surgery (13), while SSIs following bowel surgery typically involve gram-negative aerobic bacilli and anaerobes (1).

3. *Necrotizing wound infections* appear in the first few postoperative days, and are produced by *Clostridium* species or β-hemolytic streptococci (1). There is often marked edema and fluid-filled bullae around the incision, and crepitance may be present. Spread to deeper structures is rapid, leading to rhabdomyolysis and myoglobinuric renal failure. Treatment involves extensive debridement and intravenous penicillin. The mortality is high (>60%) when treatment is delayed.

B. Paranasal Sinusitis

Sinusitis is an underappreciated cause of fever in ICU patients with nasogastric tubes or endotracheal tubes (which can block the ostia draining the paranasal sinuses). In one study of unexplained fever in intubated patients (with orotracheal tubes), 42% had culture-proven evidence of sinusitis (14).

1. The diagnosis is suggested by radiographic evidence of sinusitis (i.e., opacification or air–fluid levels in the involved sinuses), and is then confirmed by a positive culture of an aspirate obtained from the involved sinus (14,15).

2. CT scans are optimal for the detection of sinusitis, but portable sinus films (obtained at the bedside) can suffice (14). The maxillary sinuses (which are almost always involved) can be viewed with a single occipitomental view, called a "Waters view" (15), as shown in Figure 35.2.

3. The most common isolates in ICU-acquired sinusitis are gram-negative aerobic bacilli (60% of cases), followed

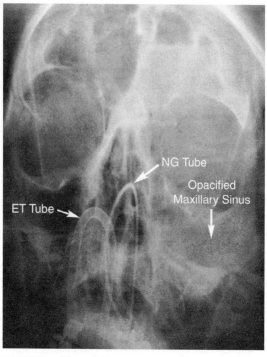

FIGURE 35.2 Portable sinus film (Waters view) showing opacification of the left maxillary and frontal sinuses in a patient with indwelling endotracheal (ET) and nasogastric tubes (NG).

by gram-positive aerobic cocci (particularly *Staph aureus* and *Staph epidermidis*) in 30% of cases, and yeasts (mostly *Candida albicans*) in 5–10% of cases (1).

4. Empiric antibiotic therapy should be guided by a Gram stain of the sinus aspirate. Aspiration of the involved sinus is necessary to document infection, because about 30% of patients with radiographic evidence of sinusitis have sterile sinus aspirates (15).

C. *Clostridium difficile* Infection

ICU-acquired fever that is associated with new-onset diarrhea should always prompt suspicion of *Clostridium difficile* enterocolitis. The diagnosis and management of this condition is described in Chapter 32, Section II.

D. Invasive Candidiasis

1. About 15% of infections in ICU patients are attributed to *Candida* species (17). Risk factors include indwelling central venous catheters, abdominal surgery, and recent exposure to broad spectrum antibiotics (18).

2. Invasive candidiasis often goes undetected because blood cultures are sterile in 30% to 80% of cases (18). More sensitive methods of detection (e.g., polymerase chain reaction) have been developed, but are still investigational.

3. Candidiasis should be suspected in high-risk patients who have persistent fever after 3 days of broad-spectrum antibiotic therapy.

E. Patient-Specific Infections

Nosocomial infections that should be considered in specific patient populations include: (a) abdominal abscesses in patients who have had major abdominal surgery (described in Chapter 32, Section III-B), (b) meningitis in neurosurgery patients, and (c) endocarditis in patients with damaged or prosthetic heart valves.

IV. CONSIDERATIONS

A. Blood Cultures

Blood cultures are recommended for all cases of ICU-related fever where a noninfectious source is unlikely (1). The yield from blood cultures is dependent on the volume of blood cultured, and the number of venipuncture sites.

1. The yield from blood cultures is optimal when 20–30 mL of blood is withdrawn from each venipuncture site (1). The standard practice is to withdraw 20 mL of blood from a venipuncture site, and inject 10 mL into each bottle of broth (one aerobic and one anaerobic) in the blood culture set. Increasing from 20 ml to 30 mL of blood increases the yield from blood cultures by about 10% (19).

2. Over 90% of bacteremias are detected with 3 blood cultures obtained over a 24-hour period, and for endocarditis, 2 blood cultures obtained over a 24-hour period will detect over 90% of the bacteremias (20). (One blood culture refers to a single venipuncture site.)

B. Procalcitonin?

Procalcitonin (PCT) has been proposed as a marker of sepsis in critically ill patients, and Table 35.3 shows the predictive value of serum PCT levels for detecting infection in febrile ICU patients (21). PCT levels above normal (>0.5 ng/mL) had the same predictive value as leukocytosis (and were more predictive than C-reactive protein), but when a higher cutoff value was used (1 ng/mL), elevated PCT levels were highly predictive of infection. These results suggest a potential role for PCT in guiding decisions about empiric antibiotic therapy in ICU patients with fever.

Table 35.3	Markers of Infection in Febrile ICU Patients		
Marker	**PPV**	**NPV**	**PLR**
WBC >12,000/mm^3	76%	62%	2.7
CRP >100 mg/dL	62%	54%	1.4
PCT >0.5 ng/dL	75%	68%	2.6
PCT >1.0 ng/dL	90%	72%	8.1

CRP = C-reactive protein; PCT = procalcitonin; PPV = positive predictive ratio; NPV = negative predictive ratio; PLR = positive likelihood ratio.
From Reference 21

C. Empiric Antimicrobial Therapy

Empiric antibiotic therapy is recommended for all ICU patients with fever, unless there is a high likelihood of a non-infectious source. Prompt initiation of therapy is considered essential, *particularly in patients with neutropenia* (absolute neutrophil count <500), where delays of only a few hours can have a negative impact on outcomes (22). However, appropriate cultures should be obtained prior to antibiotic administration, whenever possible.

1. The most frequently isolated pathogens in ICU infections in North America are shown in Table 35.4. Empiric antibiotic coverage should include the bacterial pathogens in this table.

2. Recommended antibiotics for empiric coverage include *cefepime*, a carbapenem (*meropenem* or *imipenem-cilastatin*), or *piperacillin/tazobactam*, plus *vancomycin* if methicillin-resistant *Staph aureus* (MRSA) is a potential pathogen (22).

a. For dosing recommendations, see Table 44.3 for the carbapenems, Table 44.4 for cefepime, Chapter 44, Section VI-A for piperacillin/tazobactam, and Chapter 44, Section VII-B for vancomycin.

Table 35.4	Common Isolates in ICU Infections	
Gram-Positive (55%)	**Gram-Negative (50%)**	
Staph aureus (27%)	*Escherichia coli* (14%)	
MRSA (18%)	*Pseudomonas* spp (13%)	
Staph epidermidis (9%)	*Klebsiella* spp (9%)	

Data from 607 ICUs in North America (17).

3. An *antifungal agent* should be considered when unexplained fever persists for longer than 3 days after the start of antibiotics, particularly in patients with risk factors for invasive candidiasis mentioned previously. The preferred agents are the echinocandins (*caspofungin, micafungin,* or *anidulafungin*) because of their broad spectrum of activity against *Candida* species (22). Dosing recommendations for these drugs are presented in Chapter 44, Section II-C-2.

V. ANTIPYRETIC THERAPY

The popular perception of fever as a malady that must be suppressed is rooted in parental misconceptions about fever, known as *fever phobia* (23). In fact, *fever is a normal adaptive response that enhances the ability to eradicate infection* (24). A review of the ongoing debate about the benefits vs. harm of fever is beyond the scope of this book, but the following information deserves mention.

A. Fever as a Host Defense Mechanism

1. Fever is not the result of abnormal temperature regulation (like the disorders in Chapter 34) but involves an intact thermoregulatory system operating at a higher set point (25).

2. Fever enhances immune function by increasing the production of antibodies and cytokines, activating T-lymphocytes, and enhancing phagocytosis by neutrophils and macrophages (26).

3. Increased body temperatures also suppress bacterial growth and viral replication, as demonstrated in Figure 35.3 (27).

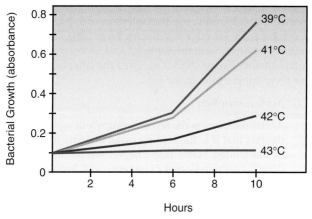

FIGURE 35.3 The influence of body temperature on the growth of *Pasteurella multocida* in blood cultures from infected laboratory animals. The range of temperatures in the figure corresponds to the range of febrile temperatures for the study animal (rabbits). Data from Reference 27.

B. Is Fever Harmful?

1. One of the presumed adverse effects of fever is the associated tachycardia, which is undesirable in patients with heart disease. However, the association between fever and tachycardia was established in animal models of sepsis, and tachycardia can be viewed as part of the inflammatory response to sepsis, rather than a specific effect of fever.

2. There is convincing evidence that increased body temperatures aggravate ischemic brain injury following cardiac arrest (see Chapter 15, Section III-B) and ischemic stroke (see Chapter 42, Section IV-B). However, there is no evidence that fever damages the non-ischemic brain.

C. Antipyretic Drugs

Prostaglandin E mediates the febrile response to endogenous pyrogens, and drugs that interfere with prostaglandin E synthesis are effective in reducing fever (28). These drugs include aspirin, acetaminophen, and nonsteroidal anti-inflammatory agents (NSAIDs). Only the latter two are used for fever suppression in the ICU.

1. **Acetaminophen**

   Acetaminophen is the favored antipyretic agent, despite the fact that it is the leading cause of acute liver failure in the United States (see Chapter 46, Section I). This drug is contraindicated in patients with hepatic insufficiency.

   a. DOSING REGIMENS: Acetaminophen is usually given PO or by rectal suppository in a dose of 650 mg every 4–6 hrs, with a maximum daily dose of 4 grams. An intravenous preparation is now available (OFIRMEV), and the recommended dose for adults (50 kg or heavier) is 650 mg every 4 hrs, or 1,000 mg every 6 hrs, with a maximum dose of 4 grams daily (29).

b. Intravenous acetaminophen is costly, and is not more effective than oral acetaminophen (30).

2. **NSAIDs**

a. *Ibuprofen* is a popular over-the-counter NSAID that has been given intravenously (10 mg/kg, up to 800 mg, every 6 hrs, for 48 hrs) to septic ICU patients, with satisfactory results (31).

b. *Ketorolac* is an intravenous NSAID that is normally used as an opioid-sparing analgesic (see Chapter 43, Section I-E), but has been shown to suppress fever in a single dose of 0.5 mg/kg (32). Use of this drug is usually restricted to a few days, to limit the risk of renal toxicity and GI hemorrhage.

D. External Cooling

Although the febrile response mimics the physiological response to a cold environment, external cooling has been used effectively for short-term (48 hours) fever suppression in patients with septic shock (33). External cooling (to maintain a body temp around 37°C or 98.6°F) may be preferred to antipyretic drugs because it provides more continuous temperature control, and it avoids the risk of adverse effects from antipyretic drugs.

REFERENCES

1. O'Grady NP, Barie PS, Bartlett J, et al. Guidelines for the evaluation of new fever in critically ill adult patients: 2008 update from the American College of Critical Care Medicine and the Infectious Disease Society of America. Crit Care Med 2008; 36:1330–1349.

2. Commichau C, Scarmeas N, Mayer SA. Risk factors for fever in the intensive care unit. Neurology 2003; 60:837–841.

3. Peres Bota D, Lopes Ferriera F, Melot C, et al. Body temperature alterations in the critically ill. Intensive Care Med 2004; 30:811–816.

4. Freischlag J, Busuttil RW. The value of postoperative fever evaluation. Surgery 1983; 94:358–363.

5. Engoren M. Lack of association between atelectasis and fever. Chest 1995; 107:81–84.

6. Shelds RT. Pathogenesis of postoperative pulmonary atelectasis: an experimental study. Arch Surg 1949; 48:489–503.

7. Murray HW, Ellis GC, Blumenthal DS, et al. Fever and pulmonary thrombo-embolism. Am J Med 1979; 67:232–235.

8. Mackowiak PA, LeMaistre CF. Drug fever: a critical appraisal of conventional concepts. Ann Intern Med 1987; 106:728–733.

9. Cunha B. Drug fever: The importance of recognition. Postgrad Med 1986; 80:123–129.

10. Gonzalez EB, Suarez L, Magee S. Nosocomial (water bed) fever. Arch Intern Med 1990; 150:687 (letter).

11. Richards MJ, Edwards JR, Culver DH, Gaynes RP. The National Nosocomial Infections Surveillance System. Nosocomial infections in combined medical-surgical intensive care units in the United States. Infect Control Hosp Epidemiol 2000; 21:510–515.

12. Horan TC, Andrus M, Dudeck MA. CDC/NHSN surveillance definition of healthcare-associated infection and criteria for specific types of infections in the acute care setting. Am J Infect Control 2008; 36:309–332.

13. Gudbjartsson T, Jeppson A, Sjogren J, et al. Sternal wound infections following open heart surgery—a review. Scand Cardiovasc J 2016; May 20:1–8.

14. van Zanten ARH, Dixon JM, Nipshagen MD, et al. Hospital-acquired sinusitis as a common cause of fever of unknown origin in orotracheally intubated critically ill patients. Crit Care 2005 9:R583–R590.

15. Holzapfel L, Chevret S, Madinier G, et al. Influence of long-term oro- or nasotracheal intubation on nosocomial maxillary sinusitis and pneumonia: results of a prospective, randomized, clinical trial. Crit Care Med 1993; 21:1132–1138.

16. Diagnosing sinusitis by x-ray: is a single Waters view adequate? J Gen Intern Med 1992; 7:481–485.

17. Vincent J-L, Rello J, Marshall J, et al. International study of the prevalence and outcomes of infection in intensive care units. JAMA 2009; 302:2323–2329.

18. Kullberg BJ, Arendrup MC. Invasive candidiasis. N Engl J Med 2015; 373:1445–1456.

29. Patel R, Vetter EA, Harmsen WS, et al. Optimized pathogen detection with 30- compared to 20-milliliter blood culture draws. J Clin Microbiol 2011; 49:4047–4051.

20. Cockerill FR, Wilson JW, Vetter EA, et al. Optimal testing parameters for blood cultures. Clin Infect Dis 2004; 38:1724–1730.

21. Tsangaris I, Plachouras D, Kavatha D, et al. Diagnostic and prognostic value of procalcitonin among febrile critically ill patients with prolonged ICU stay. BMC Infect Dis 2009; 9:213.

22. Freifeld AG, Bow EJ, Sepkowitz KA, et al. Clinical practice guidelines for the use of antimicrobial agents in neutropenic patients with cancer. 2010 update by the Infectious Diseases Society of America. Clin Infect Dis 2011; 52:e56–e93.

23. Schmitt BD. Fever phobia: misconceptions of parents about fevers. Am J Dis Child 1980; 134:176–181.

24. Kluger MJ, Kozak W, Conn CA, et al. The adaptive value of fever. Infect Dis Clin North Am 1996; 10:1–20.

25. Saper CB, Breder CB. The neurologic basis of fever. N Engl J Med 1994; 330:1880–1886.

26. van Oss CJ, Absolom DR, Moore LL, et al. Effect of temperature on the chemotaxis, phagocytic engulfment, digestion, and O_2 consumption of human polymorphonuclear leukocytes. J Reticuloendothel Soc 1980; 27:5610565.

27. Small PM, Tauber MG, Hackbarth CJ, Sande MA. Influence of body temperature on bacterial growth rates in experimental pneumococcal meningitis in rabbits. Infect Immun 1986; 52:484–487.

28. Plaisance KI, Mackowiak PA. Antipyretic therapy. Physiologic rationale, diagnostic implications, and clinical consequences. Arch Intern Med 2000; 160:449–456.

29. OFIRMEV package insert, Cadence Pharmaceuticals, 2010.

30. Peacock WF, Breitmeyer JB, Pan C, et al. A randomized study of the efficacy and safety of intravenous acetaminophen compared

to oral acetaminophen for the treatment of fever. Acad Emerg Med 2011; 18:360–366.

31. Bernard GR, Wheeler AP, Russell JA, et al. The effects of ibuprofen on the physiology and survival of patients with sepsis. N Engl J Med 1997; 336:912–918.

32. Gerhardt RT, Gerharst DM. Intravenous ketorolac in the treatment of fever. Am J Emerg Med 2000; 18:500–501 (Letter).

33. Schortgen F, Clabault K, Katashian S, et al. Fever control using external cooling in septic shock. Am J Respir Crit Care Med 2012; 185:1088–1095.

Chapter 36

Nutritional Requirements

The fundamental goal of nutritional support is to provide the daily nutrient and energy needs of each patient. This chapter will describe how to determine those needs in critically ill patients (1).

I. CALORIE REQUIREMENTS

A. Oxidation of Nutrient Fuels

Oxidative metabolism captures the energy stored in nutrient fuels (carbohydrates, lipids, and proteins), and uses this energy to sustain life. This process consumes O_2, and generates CO_2, H_2O, and heat. The quantities involved in the oxidation of each nutrient fuel are shown in Table 36.1.

1. The heat generated by the complete oxidation of a nutrient fuel is the energy yield (in kcal/g) of that fuel. Lipids have the highest energy yield (9.1 kcal/g), while glucose has the lowest energy yield (3.7 kcal/g).

2. The summed oxidation of all three nutrient fuels determines the whole-body O_2 consumption (VO_2), CO_2 production (VCO_2), and heat production for any given time period. *The 24-hour heat production (daily energy expenditure) in kcal, determines how many calories to provide each day in nutritional support.* The daily energy expenditure can be measured (indirectly) or estimated, as described next.

Table 36.1	Oxidation of Nutrient Fuels		
Fuel	O_2 Consumption	CO_2 Production	Heat Production[†]
Glucose	0.74 L/g	0.74 L/g	3.7 kcal/g
Lipid	2.00 L/g	1.40 L/g	9.1 kcal/g
Protein	0.96 L/g	0.78 L/g	4.0 kcal/g

[†]The energy yield from each nutrient fuel.

B. Indirect Calorimetry

1. **The Principle**

   It is not possible to measure metabolic heat production in hospitalized patients, so the daily energy expenditure is determined indirectly using the whole-body O_2 consumption (VO_2) and CO_2 production (VCO_2), and the relationships in Table 36.1. This is the principle of *indirect calorimetry*, which measures the resting energy expenditure (REE) in kcal/min, using the following relationships (2):

   $$REE = (3.6 \times VO_2) + (1.1 \times VCO_2) - 61 \quad \text{(kcal/min)} \quad (36.1)$$

2. **The Method**

   Indirect calorimetry is performed with "metabolic carts" that measure whole-body VO_2 and VCO_2 at the bedside by measuring the concentrations of O_2 and CO_2 in inhaled and exhaled gas (usually in intubated patients). Steady-state measurements are obtained for 15–30 minutes to determine the REE (kcal/min), which is then multiplied by 1,440 (the number of minutes in 24 hours) to derive the daily energy expenditure (kcal/24 hr) (3).

3. Indirect calorimetry is not readily available in many ICUs, and daily energy requirements are usually estimated, as described next.

C. The Simple Way

1. More than 200 cumbersome equations are available for estimating daily energy requirements (1), but none is more accurate than the following simple relationship (1,4):

$$REE \ (kcal/day) = 25 \times body \ weight \ (kg) \qquad (36.2)$$

2. Body weight adjustments have been proposed for obese patients (5), but such adjustments are not recommended in the current guidelines on nutrition support (1).

Table 36.2	Calorie-Restricted, High-Protein Feeding Regimen for Obese ICU Patients

1. If indirect calorimetry is available, measure the REE, and provide 70% of the daily calorie requirement.

2. If indirect calorimetry is not available, use the patient's body mass index (BMI), in kg/m^2, to determine the daily calorie and protein intake.

3. The daily calorie intake should be 11–14 kcal/kg (*actual* body weight) for a BMI of 30–50, and 22–25 kcal/kg (*ideal* body weight) for a BMI >50.

4. The daily protein intake should be 2 g/kg (*ideal* body weight) for a BMI of 30–40, and 2.5 g/kg (*ideal* body weight) for a BMI >40.

From the Clinical Practice Guidelines in Reference 1.

D. Calorie Restriction

1. Calorie restriction has several potential advantages, including a decrease in O_2 consumption (which creates less demand on the cardiac output), a decrease in CO_2

production (which is advantageous in ventilator-dependent patients), and improved glycemic control.

2. At least six clinical trials have shown no apparent harm when the daily caloric intake is reduced by about 50% (while protein intake is maintained) (6).

3. The current guidelines for nutrition support in the ICU includes a recommendation for *calorie restriction in obese patients* (1). This recommendation is summarized in Table 36.2.

II. SUBSTRATE REQUIREMENTS

The daily energy requirement is provided by nonprotein calories (from carbohydrates and lipids), while protein intake is used to maintain lean body mass (among other things).

Table 36.3	Endogenous Fuel Stores in Healthy Adults	
Fuel Source	**Amount (kg)**	**Energy Yield (kcal)**
Adipose Tissue Fat	15.0	141,000
Muscle Protein	6.0	24,000
Total Glycogen	0.09	900
		Total: 165,900

Data from Cahill GF, Jr. N Eng J Med 1970; 282:668–675.

A. Carbohydrates

Standard nutrition regimens use carbohydrates (dextrose) to provide about *70% of the nonprotein calories*. The human body has limited carbohydrate stores (see glycogen stores in Table 36.3), and daily intake of carbohydrates is essential for proper functioning of the brain, which relies heavily on glucose as a nutritive fuel.

B. Lipids

Lipids are used to provide about *30% of the nonprotein calories*. As mentioned, lipids have the highest energy yield of the three nutrient fuels (see Table 36.1), and lipid stores in adipose tissues represent the major endogenous fuel source in healthy adults (see Table 36.3).

1. **Linoleic Acid**

   Dietary lipids are triglycerides, which are composed of a glycerol molecule linked to three fatty acids. The only dietary fatty acid that is essential (i.e., must be provided in the diet) is *linoleic acid*, a long chain, polyunsaturated fatty acid.

   a. A deficient intake of linoleic acid produces a clinical disorder characterized by a scaly dermopathy, cardiac dysfunction, and increased susceptibility to infections (7). This disorder is prevented by providing 0.5% of the dietary fatty acids as linoleic acid.

   b. Safflower oil is the source of linoleic acid in most nutritional regimens.

2. **Propofol**

   Propofol (a popular agent for short-term sedation in the ICU) is mixed in a 10% lipid emulsion that provides 1.1 kcal/mL. As a result, *the calories provided by propofol infusions must be considered when determining the nonprotein calories in a nutrition support regimen* (1).

C. Protein

1. Protein is the most important nutrient substrate for healing wounds, supporting immune function, and maintaining lean body mass (1).

2. The normal daily protein intake is 0.8–1 grams per kg

(actual body weight), but in ICU patients, the daily protein intake is higher at 1.2–2 g/kg (1), to compensate for the hypercatabolism in critically ill patients.

3. Monitoring the adequacy of protein intake with the nitrogen balance (the difference between intake and excretion of protein-derived nitrogen), or plasma protein levels (e.g., albumin, prealbumin) is unreliable in critically ill patients, and is not recommended (1).

III. VITAMIN REQUIREMENTS

Fourteen vitamins are considered an essential part of the daily diet, and the daily requirement for these vitamins *in healthy adults* is shown in Table 36.4. The vitamin requirements in critically ill patients are not defined, and probably cannot be defined (because the clinical condition of these patients is constantly changing). Vitamin deficiencies are likely to occur in critically ill patients, and the following deficiencies deserve mention.

A. Thiamine Deficiency

Thiamine (vitamin B_1) plays an essential role in carbohydrate metabolism, where it serves as a coenzyme (thiamine pyrophosphate) for pyruvate dehydrogenase, the enzyme that draws pyruvate into the mitochondria to participate in the production of high-energy ATP molecules. Thiamine deficiency can adversely affect cellular energy metabolism, particularly in the central nervous system, which relies heavily on glucose metabolism.

1. **Predisposing Factors**

   Several conditions promote thiamine deficiency that are also prevalent in ICU patients. These include alcoholism, hypermetabolic states like trauma (8), increased urinary excretion of thiamine by furosemide (9), and magnesium depletion (10). Thiamine is also degraded by sulfites, which are used as preservatives in parenteral nutrition solutions (11).

Table 36.4	Dietary Allowances for Vitamins	
Vitamin	**Recommended Daily Intake**	**Maximum Daily Intake**
Vitamin A	900 μg	3,000 μg
Vitamin B_{12}	2 μg	5 μg
Vitamin C	90 mg	2,000 mg
Vitamin D	15 μg	100 μg
Vitamin E	15 mg	1,000 mg
Vitamin K	120 μg	ND
Thiamine (B_1)	1 mg	ND
Riboflavin (B_2)	1 mg	ND
Niacin (B_3)	16 mg	35 mg
Pyridoxine (B_6)	2 mg	100 mg
Pantothenic acid (B_1)	5 mg	ND
Biotin	30 μg	ND
Folate	400 μg	1,000 μg
Choline	500 mg	ND

Intakes for adult males, age 51–70 yrs. From the Food & Nutrition Board, Institute of Medicine. Available at the Food and Nutrition Information Center (http://fnic.nal.usda.gov). Accessed Aug., 2016. Doses rounded off to the nearest whole number. ND = not determined.

2. Clinical Features

There are 4 manifestations of thiamine deficiency (12): cardiomyopathy (wet beriberi), Wernicke's encephalopathy (nystagmus, lateral gaze palsy, ataxia, and confusion), lactic acidosis, and peripheral neuropathy (dry beriberi).

3. **Diagnosis**

   a. The plasma thiamine level can be measured: the reference range is 5.3–7.9 µg/dL (13). Plasma levels can correct within 24 hours after starting thiamine replacement (13).

   b. The most reliable measure of thiamine stores is the *erythrocyte transketolase assay* (14), which measures the activity of a thiamine pyrophosphate (TPP)–dependent transketolase enzyme in the patient's red blood cells in response to the addition of TPP. An increase in enzyme activity greater than 25% is evidence of thiamine depletion.

4. **Treatment**

   A minimum thiamine intake of 1 mg daily is recommended for adults (12). The treatment of symptomatic thiamine deficiency is 50–100 mg by intravenous or intramuscular injection daily for 7–14 days, followed by an oral dose of 10 mg daily until the condition resolves (12).

B. Vitamin D Deficiency (?)

1. Vitamin D deficiency is found in as many as 50% of the general adult population (15), and it is so common in ICU patients that one study found normal blood levels of vitamin D in only 5% of the patients tested (16). The problem here may not be vitamin D deficiency, but the diagnostic criteria.

2. The diagnosis of vitamin D deficiency is based solely on a plasma level of 25-hydroxyvitamin D (a metabolite of vitamin D) that is below 50 nmol/L (20 ng/mL) (17). Evidence of adverse consequences are not required, and virtually all patients are asymptomatic. Therefore, *vita-*

min D deficiency in ICU patients is a laboratory value that is outside the expected range for healthy adults. The clinical significance of this condition is unclear.

3. There is some evidence that vitamin D deficiency is associated with an increased risk of infection in ICU patients (18), but the risk ratios (1.4–1.5) are not convincing.

4. Routine monitoring of 25(OH) vitamin D levels is not recommended (the assay is costly), and since vitamin D deficiency is asymptomatic in ICU patients, there are no real indications for pursuing the diagnosis of vitamin D deficiency.

5. Nevertheless, if confronted with a low plasma level of 25(OH) vitamin D, a single intramuscular injection of 150,000 IU of cholecalciferol can correct the blood levels in 80% of patients (19).

6. The recommended daily intake of vitamin D in adults is 600 IU up to age 70, and 800 IU after age 70.

IV. ESSENTIAL TRACE ELEMENTS

A trace element is a substance that is present in the body in amounts less than 50 mg per gram of body tissue (20). Seven trace elements are considered essential in humans (i.e., are associated with deficiency syndromes), and these are listed in Table 36.5, along with the daily requirement for each in healthy adults. As mentioned for vitamins, the daily requirement for trace elements in critically ill patients is not defined, and is probably not definable. The following trace elements deserve mention because of their relevance to oxidant cell injury.

A. Iron

The normal adult has approximately 4.5 grams of iron, yet

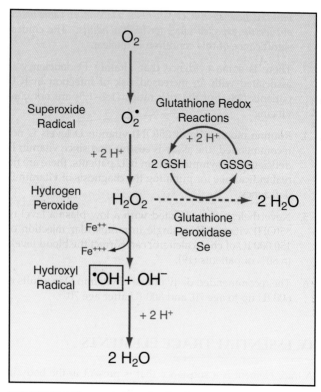

FIGURE 36.1 The metabolism of molecular oxygen to water, and the actions of the glutathione redox reactions. Symbols with a dot are free radicals. See text for explanation. Fe^{++} = reduced iron, Fe^{+++} = oxidized iron, Se = selenium, GSH = reduced glutathione, GSSG = oxidized glutathione (a dipeptide connected by a disulfide bridge).

there is virtually no free iron in plasma (28). Most of the iron is bound to hemoglobin, and the remainder is bound to ferritin in tissues and transferrin in plasma. The absence of free iron can be viewed as a defense mechanism that protects the tissues from oxidant injury (21,22), as described next.

Table 36.5	Daily Allowances for Essential Trace Elements	
Trace Element	Recommended Daily Intake	Maximum Daily Intake
Chromium	30 µg	ND
Copper	900 µg	10,000 µg
Iodine	150 µg	1,100 µg
Iron	8 mg	45 mg
Manganese	2.3 mg	11 mg
Selenium	55 µg	200 µg
Zinc	11 mg	40 mg

Recommendations for adult males, ages 51–79 yrs. From the Food & Nutrition Board, Institute of Medicine. Available at the Food and Nutrition Information Center (http://fnic.nal.usda.gov). Accessed Aug., 2016. ND = not determined.

1. **Iron and Oxidant Injury**

The metabolism of oxygen to water, which is depicted in Figure 36.1, occurs in a series of single-electron reduction reactions that generates highly-reactive intermediates. These are identified in Figure 36.1 as the *superoxide radical, hydrogen peroxide*, and the *hydroxyl radical*. (A radical is an atom or molecule with an unpaired electron in its outer orbital.) These oxygen metabolites are powerful oxidizing agents, capable of damaging cell membranes and fracturing nuclear DNA. The most reactive metabolite (and the most powerful oxidant known in biochemistry) is the hydroxyl radical, and iron (in the reduced state) is essential for the formation of hydroxyl radicals, as indicated in Figure 36.1. The following statements deserve emphasis.

a. Iron represents a major risk for oxidant cell injury, especially when transferrin levels in blood are reduced (e.g., in critically ill patients).

    b. Because of this risk, *the practice of administering iron to ICU patients to correct hypoferremia, without an associated iron-deficiency anemia, should be abandoned.*

B. Selenium

Selenium is the most recent addition to essential trace elements, and has a recommended daily allowance of 55 µg in healthy adults (see Table 36.5). Selenium utilization is increased in acute illness (23), so daily requirements are likely to be higher in critically ill patients.

1. **Selenium as an Antioxidant**

   Figure 36.1 shows that hydrogen peroxide can be reduced directly to water (thus bypassing the formation of hydroxyl radicals) with the aid of reduced glutathione (GSH) and the enzyme glutathione peroxidase, which uses selenium as a cofactor. The glutathione redox reactions represent the major intracellular antioxidant system, and thus selenium has a significant role in promoting endogenous antioxidant protection.

2. **Selenium in Sepsis**

   Reduced plasma levels of selenium are common in patients with severe sepsis, and selenium supplementation is associated with a lower mortality rate (24). Therefore, monitoring plasma selenium levels in patients with severe sepsis seems justified. The normal plasma selenium concentration is 89–113 µg/L (25). Selenium can be replaced intravenously, and the maximum daily dose is 200 µg.

REFERENCES

1. Taylor BE, McClave SA, Martindale RG, et al. Guidelines for the provision and assessment of nutrition support therapy in the adult critically ill patient: Society of Critical Care Medicine (SCCM) and American Society for Parenteral and Enteral Nutrition (A.S.P.E.N.). Crit Care Med 2016; 44:390–438.

2. Bursztein S, Saphar P, Singer P, et al. A mathematical analysis of indirect calorimetry measurements in acutely ill patients. Am J Clin Nutr 1989; 50:227–230.

3. Lev S, Cohen J, Singer P. Indirect calorimetry measurements in the ventilated critically ill patient: facts and controversies—the heat is on. Crit Care Clin 2010; 26:e1–e9.

4. Paauw JD, McCamish MA, Dean RE, et al. Assessment of caloric needs in stressed patients. J Am Coll Nutr 1984; 3:51–59.

5. Krenitsky J. Adjusted body weight, pro: Evidence to support the use of adjusted body weight in calculating calorie requirements. Nutr Clin Pract 2005; 20:468–473.

6. Marik PE, Hooper MH. Normocaloric versus hypocaloric feeding: a systematic review and meta-analysis. Intensive Care Med 2016; 42:316–323.

7. Jones PJH, Kubow S. Lipids, Sterols, and Their Metabolites. In: Shils ME, et al., eds. Modern nutrition in health and disease. 10th ed. Philadelphia, PA: Lippincott Williams & Wilkins, 2006; 92–121.

8. McConachie I, Haskew A. Thiamine status after major trauma. Intensive Care Med 1988; 14:628-631.

9. Seligmann H, Halkin H, Rauchfleisch S, et al. Thiamine deficiency in patients with congestive heart failure receiving long-term furosemide therapy: a pilot study. Am J Med 1991; 91:151–155.

10. Dyckner T, Ek B, Nyhlin H, et al. Aggravation of thiamine deficiency by magnesium depletion. A case report. Acta Med Scand 1985; 218:129–131.

11. Scheiner JM, Araujo MM, DeRitter E. Thiamine destruction by sodium bisulfite in infusion solutions. Am J Hosp Pharm 1981; 38:1911–1916.

12. Butterworth RF. Thiamine. In: Shils ME, et al., eds. Modern nutrition in health and disease. 10th ed. Philadelphia, PA: Lippincott Williams & Wilkins, 2006; 426–433.

13. Wallach J. Interpretation of diagnostic tests. 8th ed. Philadelphia: Lippincott Williams & Wilkins, 2007:580.

14. Boni L, Kieckens L, Hendrikx A. An evaluation of a modified erythrocyte transketolase assay for assessing thiamine nutritional adequacy. J Nutr Sci Vitaminol (Tokyo) 1980; 26:507–514.

15. Kennel KA, Drake MT, Hurley DL. Vitamin D deficiency in adults: when to test and how to treat. Mayo Clin Proc 2010; 85:752–758.

16. Venkatram S, Chilimuri S, Adrish M, et al. Vitamin D deficiency is associated with mortality in the medical intensive care unit. Crit Care 2011; 15:R292.

17. Holick MF, Binkley NC, Bischoff-Ferrari HA, et al. Endocrine Society: Evaluation, treatment, and prevention of vitamin D deficiency: An Endocrine Society clinical practice guideline. J Clin Endocrinol Metab 2011; 96:1911–1930.

18. de Haan K, Groeneveld ABJ, de Geus HRH, et al. Vitamin D deficiency as a risk factor for infection, sepsis and mortality in the critically ill: systematic review and meta-analysis. Crit Care 2014; 18:660.

19. Nair P, Venkatesh B, Lee P, et al. A randomized study if a single dose of intramuscular cholecalciferol in critically ill adults. Crit Care Med 2015; 43:2313–2320.

20. Fleming CR. Trace element metabolism in adult patients requiring total parenteral nutrition. Am J Clin Nutr 1989; 49:573–579.

21. Halliwell B, Gutteridge JM. Role of free radicals and catalytic metal ions in human disease: an overview. Methods Enzymol 1990;186:1–85.

22. Herbert V, Shaw S, Jayatilleke E, et al. Most free-radical injury is iron-related: it is promoted by iron, hemin, holoferritin and vitamin C, and inhibited by desferoxamine and apoferritin. Stem Cells 1994; 12:289–303.

23. Hawker FH, Stewart PM, Snitch PJ. Effects of acute illness on selenium homeostasis. Crit Care Medicine 1990; 18:442–446.

24. Alhazzani W, Jacobi J, Sindi A, et al. The effect of selenium therapy on mortality in patients with sepsis syndrome. Crit Care Med 2013; 41:1555–1564.

25. Geoghegan M, McAuley D, Eaton S, et al. Selenium in critical illness. Curr Opin Crit Care 2006; 12:136–141.

Chapter 37

Enteral Tube Feeding

When oral feeding is not possible, the preferred method of nutrition support is the infusion of liquid feeding formulas into the stomach or small bowel (enteral tube feedings). This chapter presents the fundamentals of nutrition support with enteral tube feedings, and will demonstrate how to create a tube feeding regimen for individual patients.

I. GENERAL CONSIDERATIONS

A. Trophic Effects

The preference for enteral over parenteral nutrition is based on numerous studies showing that enteral nutrition is associated with fewer infections of bowel origin (1-3). This is related to the trophic effects of enteral feeding, summarized in the following statements.

1. The presence of food or tube feedings in the lumen of the bowel has a trophic effect that preserves the structural integrity of the mucosa (4), and supports the immune defenses in the bowel (such as the production of immunoglobulin A, which blocks the attachment of pathogens to the bowel mucosa) (5).

2. These trophic effects maintain the barrier function of the bowel, which protects against invasion from enteric pathogens; a phenomenon known as *translocation* (6).

3. Periods of bowel rest are associated with progressive atrophy of the bowel mucosa (4), which can lead to

translocation and the systemic spread of enteric pathogens. Parenteral nutrition does not prevent the deleterious effects of bowel rest (7).

B. Indications & Contraindications

Patients who are unable to eat and have no contraindications are candidates for enteral tube feeding.

1. Tube feedings should be started within 24–48 hours of admission to the ICU (1) to take advantage of the protective effects of tube feedings just described. There is evidence that early institution of enteral nutrition is associated with fewer septic complications and a shorter hospital stay (8).

2. *The presence of bowel sounds is not required to initiate enteral tube feedings* (1).

3. *Absolute contraindications* to enteral tube feedings include complete bowel obstruction, bowel ischemia, ileus, and circulatory shock with high-dose vasopressor requirements (1). Tube feedings can be attempted in stable patients on low doses of vasopressors (1), but any signs of intolerance should prompt immediate cessation of feedings.

C. Trophic vs. Full Feedings

1. *Trophic feedings* (10–20 kcal/hr, or up to 500 kcal/day) can be used for the first week in patients who are not malnourished, and are not seriously ill (e.g., postop patients) (1).

2. For patients who are malnourished or seriously ill, full nutritional support should be achieved within hours of starting tube feedings (1).

II. FEEDING FORMULAS

There are at least 200 enteral feeding formulas that are commercially available, and the following is a brief description of the different types of feeding formulas. Examples are provided in Tables 37.1–37.3.

Table 37.1	Standard, Protein-Enriched, and High-Calorie Feeding Formulas			
Formula	kcal/mL	Nonprotein kcal (%)	Protein (g/L)	Osmolality (mosm/kg)
Standard:				
Osmolite	1	86%	37	300
Isocal	1	87%	34	300
Protein-Enriched:				
Replete	1	75%	63	375
Promote	1	75%	63	340
High Caloric Density:				
Nutren 2.0	2	64%	80	745
Twocal HN	2	83%	84	725
Resource 2.0	2	82%	90	790

A. Caloric Density

Feeding formulas are available with caloric densities of 1 kcal/mL, 1.5 kcal/mL, and 2 kcal/mL (see Table 37.1). Standard tube feeding regimens use formulas with 1 kcal/mL. High-calorie formulas (2 kcal/mL) are intended for patients with severe physiological stress, and are often used when volume restriction is a priority (9).

1. **Nonprotein Calories**

   The caloric density of feeding formulas includes both protein and nonprotein calories, but *daily caloric require-*

ments should be provided by nonprotein calories. In standard feeding formulas, nonprotein calories account for about 85% of the total calories (see Table 37.1).

2. **Osmolality**

The osmolality of feeding formulas is determined primarily by the caloric density. Standard feeding formulas with 1 kcal/mL have an osmolality similar to plasma (280–300 mosm/kg). Hypertonic feedings can promote diarrhea, but this risk is minimized by intragastric feeding, where the large volume of gastric secretions attenuates the osmolality.

B. Protein Content

Standard feeding formulas provide 35–40 grams of protein per liter. High-protein formulas provide about 20% more protein than the standard formulas (see Table 37.1), and are typically used to promote wound healing (9).

1. **Intact vs. Hydrolyzed Protein**

   a. Most enteral formulas contain intact proteins that are broken down into amino acids in the upper GI tract. These are called *polymeric* formulas.

   b. Feeding formulas are also available that contain small peptides (*semi-elemental* formulas) and individual amino acids (*elemental* formulas) that are absorbed more readily than intact protein. These formulas promote water reabsorption from the bowel, and could benefit patients with troublesome diarrhea (unproven). Examples of semi-elemental and elemental formulas include *Optimental, Peptamen, Perative,* and *Vivonex T.E.N.*

C. Carbohydrate Content

Carbohydrates (usually polysaccharides) provide 40–70% of the total calories in most feeding formulas. Reduced carbohydrate formulas, in which carbohydrates provide 30–40% of the calories, are available for diabetics (see Table 37.2); these formulas typically contain fiber.

Table 37.2	Selected Fiber-Enriched Feeding Formulas			
Formula	**kcal/mL**	**CHO kcal (%)**	**Fiber (g/L)**	**Osmolality (mosm/kg)**
Standard Carbohydrate:				
Jevity 1 Cal	1	51%	14	300
Promote with Fiber	1	50%	14	380
Reduced Carbohydrate:				
Glucerna	1	34%	14	355
Resource Diabetic	1	36%	15	400

CHO = carbohydrate.

D. Fiber

The term *fiber* refers to polysaccharides from plants that are not digested by humans. There are two types of fiber: fermentable and nonfermentable.

1. *Fermentable fiber* is broken down by gut microbes into short-chain fatty acids, which are an important energy source for the large bowel mucosa (13); i.e., *fermentable fiber promotes the viability of the mucosa in the large bowel* (1). The uptake of these fatty acids promotes sodium and water absorption, and reduces the water content of stool, which *reduces the risk of diarrhea* (1).

2. *Nonfermentable fiber* is not broken down by gut bacteria. This type of fiber draws water into the bowel, and *increases the risk of diarrhea*.

3. Selected fiber-enriched feeding formulas are shown in Table 37.2. The fiber in most feeding formulas is a mix-

ture of fermentable and nonfermentable fiber, so it is no surprise that the effects of mixed-fiber formulas on diarrhea have been inconsistent (1).

4. The current guidelines on nutrition support recommends the following (1):

a. For patients with diarrhea, a source of fermentable fiber (e.g., fructo-oligosaccharides) should be added to the feeding regimen in a dose of 10–20 grams daily. This is preferred to the use of mixed-fiber formulas.

b. Mixed-fiber feeding formulas should NOT be used in patients with a risk of bowel ischemia, or with severe bowel dysmotility (because of reports of bowel obstruction in such patients).

E. Lipid Content

1. Standard feeding formulas contain polyunsaturated fatty acids (PUFAs) from vegetable oils, which can serve as precursors for inflammatory mediators (eicosanoids) that are capable of promoting inflammatory cell injury.

Table 37.3	Immune-Modulating Feeding Formulas			
Feeding Formula	(kcal/mL)	ω-3 FAs (g/L)	Arginine (g/L)	Antioxidants
Impact	1	1.7	13	Selenium, β-carotene
Optimental	1	2.3	6	Vitamins C & E, β-carotene
Oxepa	1.5	4.6	0	Vitamins C & E, β-carotene

ω-3 FAs = omega-3 fatty acids.

2. PUFAs from fish oils (*omega-3 fatty acids*) do not produce inflammatory mediators, and Table 37.3 includes some of the feeding formulas that are enriched with these fatty acids. The use of feeding formulas that influence the inflammatory response is known as *immunonutrition* (10).

3. Clinical studies have shown that patients with acute respiratory distress syndrome (ARDS) derive some benefit (fewer days on the ventilator) from feeding formulas enriched with omega-3 fatty acids and antioxidants (15). However, the benefits are marginal, and there is a general reluctance to adopt these feeding formulas for patients with ARDS (1).

F. Arginine

1. Arginine is a preferred metabolic substrate for injured muscle, and can be depleted in conditions like multisystem trauma (12). Arginine also promotes wound healing, and is a precursor of nitric oxide (12).

2. At least 8 enteral feeding formulas contain arginine in concentrations of 6–19 g/L. These formulas are recommended for postoperative patients (1,10), and for patients with severe trauma or traumatic brain injury (1).

3. *Caveat:* There are reports of increased mortality associated with arginine-enriched feeding formulas in patients with severe sepsis (1,13). The presumed mechanism is arginine-induced formation of nitric oxide, with subsequent vasodilation and hypotension.

G. Recommendation

Despite the multitude of available feeding formulas, the current guidelines on nutrition support (1) recommend standard (non-specialized) feeding formulas for most ICU patients.

III. CREATING A FEEDING REGIMEN

This section describes a simple method for creating a tube feeding regimen, which is summarized in Table 37.4. There are four steps in this method.

Table 37.4	Creating an Enteral Feeding Regimen

Step 1: Estimate daily calorie and protein requirements.

$$\text{Calories (kcal/day)} = 25 \times \text{wt (kg)}$$
$$\text{Protein (g/day)} = (1.2\text{--}2.0) \times \text{wt (kg)}$$

Step 2: Select feeding formula.

Step 3: Calculate desired infusion rate.

$$\text{Feeding volume (mL)} = \frac{\text{kcal/day required}}{\text{kcal/mL in feeding formula}}$$

$$\text{Infusion rate (mL/hr)} = \frac{\text{Feeding volume (mL)}}{\text{Feeding time (hrs)}}$$

Step 4: Adjust protein intake, if necessary.

a. Calculate the projected protein intake (g/day) as:

Feeding volume (L/day) x Protein (g/L) in feedings

b. If the projected intake is less than desired intake, add protein powder to the feeding regimen to correct the discrepancy.

Step 1. Estimate daily energy and protein requirements

1. The daily requirement for calories and protein is first estimated with the simple formulas in Table 37.4 (1). Actual body weight is used.

2. For obese patients (body mass index of 30 kg/m^2 or higher), use the calorie-restricted, high-protein estimates in Table 36.2.

Step 2. Select a feeding formula

As mentioned earlier, standard feeding formulas with a caloric density of 1 kcal/mL should be sufficient for most patients (1).

Step 3. Calculate the desired infusion rate

To determine the desired infusion rate for feeding:

1. First calculate the volume of the feeding formula that must be infused to meet the daily requirement for calories, as indicated in Table 37.4.

2. Then divide the feeding volume by the number of hours each day that the feeding formula will be infused.

3. If propofol is being infused, subtract the calories provided by propofol (1 kcal/mL) from the daily calorie requirement.

4. Although nonprotein calories are recommended for providing the daily energy needs, tube feeding regimens often use the total caloric yield of the feeding formula to determine the desired volume and infusion rate. (Nonprotein calories account for about 85% of the total calories in standard feeding formulas.)

Step 4. Adjust the protein intake, if necessary

The final step in the process to determine if the feeding regimen will provide enough protein to satisfy the daily protein requirement (from Step 1). The projected protein intake is simply the daily feeding volume multiplied by the protein concentration in the feeding formula. If the projected protein

intake is less than the desired protein intake, powdered protein is added to the tube feedings to correct the discrepancy.

IV. INITIATING TUBE FEEDINGS

A. Feeding Tube Placement

1. Feeding tubes are inserted through the nares and advanced
   blindly into the stomach or duodenum. The distance required to reach the stomach can be estimated by measuring
   the distance from the tip of the nose to the earlobe and then
   to the xiphoid process (typically 50 to 60 cm) (16).

2. Advancing the tip of the feeding tube into the duodenum is not necessary in most patients (1), because *there
   is no difference in the risk of aspiration with gastric versus
   duodenal feedings* (17).

3. *A portable chest x-ray is required to verify proper tube position* before the feeding formula is infused. The common
   practice of *evaluating tube placement by pushing air
   through the tube and listening for bowel sounds is not reliable,* because sounds emanating from a misplaced tube
   in the distal airways or pleural space can be transmitted
   into the upper abdomen (18,19).

4. Feeding tubes end up in the trachea during 1% of insertions (20). Intubated patients often do not cough when
   feeding tubes enter the trachea (unlike healthy subjects);
   as a result, feeding tubes can be advanced deep into the
   lungs without any warning signs, and can puncture the
   visceral pleura and create a pneumothorax (18,19). The
   portable chest x-ray in Figure 37.1 shows a feeding tube
   that has been advanced almost to the edge of the right
   lung in a patient who displayed no signs of distress during insertion of the feeding tube.

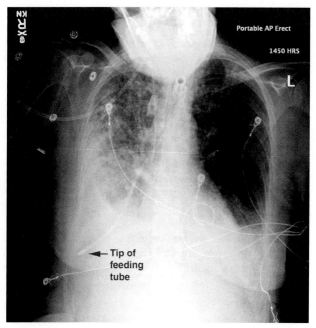

FIGURE 37.1 Routine chest x-ray following the insertion of a feeding tube. See text for explanation.

B. Starter Regimens

1. The traditional practice is to begin tube feedings at a low infusion rate (10–20 ml/hr), and then gradually advance to the target infusion rate over the next 6–8 hours. However, gastric feedings can begin at the desired (target) rate in most patients without the risk of vomiting or aspiration (21).

2. Starter regimens are more appropriate for small bowel feedings (particularly in the jejunum) because of the limited reservoir capacity of the small bowel.

V. COMPLICATIONS

The complications associated with enteral tube feedings include occlusion of the feeding tube, regurgitation of the feeding formula into the mouth and airways, and diarrhea.

A. Occlusion of Feeding Tubes

Narrow-bore feeding tubes can become occluded by protein precipitates that form when acidic gastric secretions reflux into the feeding tubes (22). Standard preventive measures include flushing the feeding tubes with 30 mL of water every 4 hours, and a 10-mL water flush after medications are instilled.

1. **Restoring Patency**

   If flow through the feeding tube is sluggish, flushing the tube with warm water can restore flow in 30% of cases (22). If this is ineffective, *pancreatic enzyme* (Viokase) can be used as follows (23):

   a. REGIMEN: Dissolve 1 tablet of Viokase and 1 tablet of sodium carbonate (324 mg) in 5 mL of water. Inject this mixture into the feeding tube and clamp for 5 minutes. Follow with a warm water flush. This should relieve the obstruction in about 75% of cases (23).

   b. If the tube is completely occluded, advance a flexible wire or a drum cartridge catheter through the feeding tube in an attempt to clear the obstruction. If this is unsuccessful, replace the feeding tube without delay.

B. Regurgitation / Aspiration

The most feared complication of enteral tube feeding is regurgitation of feeding formula and subsequent pulmonary aspiration.

1. The following measures are recommended for reducing

the risk of regurgitation and pulmonary aspiration (1):

a. Elevation of the head of the bed to 30–45° above the horizontal plane.

b. Oral care with chlorhexidine.

c. Reducing the level of sedation, when possible.

d. Jejunal feedings and prokinetic agents should be considered in patients who have an increased risk of aspiration (e.g., those who are comatose or have abnormal swallowing function).

2. *Monitoring gastric residual volumes is not recommended* (1), because residual volumes do not correlate with the incidence of pneumonia (24), regurgitation, or aspiration (25).

3. **Prokinetic Therapy**

   The prokinetic agents and recommended dosing regimens are shown in Table 37.5. Prokinetic therapy is associated with short-term improvement in gastric motility, but the clinical significance of this effect has been difficult to demonstrate (26).

   a. ERYTHROMYCIN: Erythromycin, promotes gastric emptying by stimulating motilin receptors in the GI tract (27). At a dose of 200 mg IV every 12 hours, gastric residual volumes decrease by 60% after 24 hours, but this effect diminishes rapidly over a few days (28). Erythromycin is more effective in combination with metoclopramide (29).

   b. METOCLOPRAMIDE: Metoclopramide promotes gastric emptying by antagonizing the actions of dopamine in the GI tract. At a dose of 10 mg IV every 6 hours, gastric residual volumes decrease by 30% after 24 hours, but the effect wanes rapidly (28). Metoclopramide is more effective in combination with erythromycin (29).

Table 37.5	Prokinetic Agents	
Agent	**Dosing Regimens and Comments**	
Metoclopramide	Dosing:	10 mg IV every 6 hours
	Comment:	Effect diminishes over a few days. More effective in combination with erythromycin.
Erythromycin	Dosing:	200 mg IV every 12 hours
	Comment:	Effect diminishes over a few days. More effective in combination with metoclopramide.

From References 28 and 29.

C. Diarrhea

Diarrhea is common in tube-fed patients, and is often attributed to the hyperosmolality of many feeding formulas. However, other factors may have an important role; i.e., antibiotic-associated diarrhea, *Clostridium difficile* infection (described in Chapter 32, Section II), and liquid drug preparations (which may be the culprit in a majority of cases) (30).

1. **Liquid Drug Preparations**

   Liquid drug preparations (which are favored for drug delivery through feeding tubes) have two features that create a risk for diarrhea (31): (a) they can be extremely hyperosmolar ($\geq 3,000$ mosm/kg), and (b) they can contain sorbitol, a well-known laxative that draws water into the bowel lumen.

   a. Table 37.6 includes a list of diarrhea-prone liquid preparations that are used in tube-fed ICU patients. These preparations should be discontinued in any patient who develops diarrhea of uncertain etiology during tube feedings.

Table 37.6	Liquid Drug Preparations That Promote Diarrhea	
≥3,000 mosm/kg	**Contain Sorbitol**	
Acetaminophen elixir	Acetaminophen liquid	
Dexamethasone solution	Cimetidine solution	
Ferrous sulfate liquid		
Hydroxazine syrup	Isoniazid syrup	
Metoclopramide syrup	Lithium syrup	
Multivitamin liquid		
Potassium chloride liquid	Metoclopramide syrup	
Promethazine syrup	Theophylline solution	
Sodium phosphate liquid	Tetracycline suspension	

From Reference 31.

REFERENCES

1. Taylor BE, McClave SA, Martindale RG, et al. Guidelines for the provision and assessment of nutrition support therapy in the adult critically ill patient: Society of Critical Care Medicine (SCCM) and American Society for Parenteral and Enteral Nutrition (A.S.P.E.N.). Crit Care Med 2016; 44:390–438.

2. Simpson F, Doig GS. Parenteral vs enteral nutrition in the critically ill patient: a meta-analysis of trials using the intention to treat principle. Intensive Care Med 2005; 31:12–23.

3. Moore FA, Feliciano DV, Andrassay RJ, et al. Early enteral feeding, compared with parenteral, reduces postoperative septic complications: the results of a meta-analysis. Ann Surg 1992; 216:172–183.

4. Alpers DH. Enteral feeding and gut atrophy. Curr Opin Clin Nutr Metab Care 2002; 5:679–683.

5. Ohta K, Omura K, Hirano K, et al. The effect of an additive small amount of a low residue diet against total parenteral nutrition-induced gut mucosal barrier. Am J Surg 2003; 185:79–85.

6. Wiest R, Rath HC. Gastrointestinal disorders of the critically ill. Bacterial translocation in the gut. Best Pract Res Clin Gastroenterol 2003; 17:397–425.

7. Alverdy JC, Moss GS. Total parenteral nutrition promotes bacterial translocation from the gut. Surgery 1988; 104:185–190.

8. Marik PE, Zaloga GP. Early enteral nutrition in acutely ill patients: a systematic review. Crit Care Med 2001; 29:2264–2270.

9. Lefton J, Esper DH, Kochevar M. Enteral formulations. In: The A.S.P.E.N. Nutrition Support Core Curriculum. Silver Spring, MD: American Society for Parenteral and Enteral Nutrition, 2007:209–232.

10. Heyland DK, Novak F, Drover JW, et al. Should immunonutrition become routine in critically ill patients? JAMA 2007; 286:944–953.

11. Singer P, Theilla M, Fisher H, et al. Benefit of an enteral diet enriched with eicosapentanoic acid and gamma-linolenic acid in ventilated patients with acute lung injury. Crit Care Med 2006; 34:1033–1038.

12. Kirk SJ, Barbul A. Role of arginine in trauma, sepsis, and immunity. J Parenter Ent Nutr 1990; 14(Suppl):226S–228S.

13. Bertolini G, Iapichino G, Radrizzani D, et al. Early enteral immunonutrition in patients with severe sepsis: results of an interim analysis of a randomized multicentre clinical trial. Intensive Care Med 2003; 29:834–840.

14. Rebouche CJ. Carnitine. In: Shils ME, et al., eds. Modern nutrition in health and disease. 10th ed. Philadelphia, PA: Lippincott Williams & Wilkins, 2006; 537–544.

15. Karlic H, Lohninger A. Supplementation of L-carnitine in athletes: does it make sense? Nutrition (Burbank, CA) 2004; 20:709–715.

16. Stroud M, Duncan H, Nightingale J. Guidelines for enteral feeding in adult hospital patients. Gut 2003; 52 Suppl 7:vii1–vii12.

17. Marik PE, Zaloga GP. Gastric versus post-pyloric feeding: a systematic review. Crit Care 2003; 7:R46–R51.

18. Kolbitsch C, Pomaroli A, Lorenz I, et al. Pneumothorax following

nasogastric feeding tube insertion in a tracheostomized patient after bilateral lung transplantation. Intensive Care Med 1997; 23:440–442.

19. Fisman DN, Ward ME. Intrapleural placement of a nasogastric tube: an unusual complication of nasotracheal intubation. Can J Anaesth 1996; 43:1252–1256.

20. Baskin WN. Acute complications associated with bedside placement of feeding tubes. Nutr Clin Pract 2006; 21:40–55.

21. Mizock BA. Avoiding common errors in nutritional management. J Crit Illness 1993; 10:1116–1127.

22. Marcuard SP, Perkins AM. Clogging of feeding tubes. J Parenter Enteral Nutr 1988; 12:403–405.

23. Marcuard SP, Stegall KS. Unclogging feeding tubes with pancreatic enzyme. J Parenter Enteral Nutr 1990; 14:198–200.

24. Reignier K, Mercier E, Le Gouge A, et al. Effect of not monitoring residual gastric volume on risk of ventilator-associated pneumonia in adults receiving mechanical ventilation and early enteral feeding. JAMA 2013; 309:249–256.

25. McClave SA, DeMeo MT, DeLegge MH, et al. North American Summit on Aspiration in the Critically Ill Patient: a consensus statement. JPEN: J Parenter Enteral Nutr 2002; 26:S80–S85.

26. Booth CM, Heyland DK, Paterson WG. Gastrointestinal promotility drugs in the critical care setting: a systematic review of the evidence. Crit Care Med 2002; 30:1429–1435.

27. Hawkyard CV, Koerner RJ. The use of erythromycin as a gastrointestinal prokinetic agent in adult critical care: benefits and risks. J Antimicrob Chemother 2007; 59:347–358.

28. Nguyen NO, Chapman MJ, Fraser RJ, et al. Erythromycin is more effective than metoclopramide in the treatment of feed intolerance in critical illness. Crit Care Med 2007; 35:483–489.

29. Nguyen NO, Chapman M, Fraser RJ, et al. Prokinetic therapy for feed intolerance in critical illness: one drug or two? Crit Care Med 2007; 35:2561–2567.

30. Edes TE, Walk BE, Austin JL. Diarrhea in tube-fed patients: feeding formula not necessarily the cause. Am J Med 1990; 88:91–93.

31. Williams NT. Medication administration through enteral feeding tubes. Am J Heath-Sys Pharm 2008; 65:2347–2357.

Chapter 38

Parenteral Nutrition

When full nutritional support is not possible in the alimentary canal, the intravenous route is available for nutrient delivery (1,2). This chapter describes the basic features of intravenous nutritional support, and demonstrates how to create a parenteral nutrition regimen to meet the needs of individual patients.

I. SUBSTRATE SOLUTIONS

A. Dextrose Solutions

1. Carbohydrates are the main source of nonprotein calories in parenteral nutrition (PN), and dextrose (glucose) is the carbohydrate source in PN. The available dextrose solutions are shown in Table 38.1.

Table 38.1	Intravenous Dextrose Solutions		
Strength	Concentration (g/L)	Energy Yield* (kcal/L)	Osmolarity (mosm/L)
5%	50	170	253
10%	100	340	505
20%	200	680	1,080
50%	500	1,700	2,525
70%	700	2,380	3,530

*Based on an oxidative energy yield of 3.4 kcal/g for dextrose.

2. Because the energy yield from dextrose is relatively low (3.4 kcal/g), the dextrose solutions must be concentrated to provide enough calories to satisfy daily requirements. (The standard solution is 50% dextrose, or D_{50}.) The solutions used in PN are hyperosmolar, and must be infused through large central veins.

B. Amino Acid Solutions

Protein is provided as amino acid solutions that contain varying mixtures of essential (N = 9), semiessential (N = 4), and nonessential (N = 10) amino acids. These solutions are mixed with dextrose solutions in a 1:1 volume ratio. Examples of standard and specialized amino acid solutions are shown in Table 38.2.

Table 38.2	Standard & Specialty Amino Acid Solutions		
	Aminosyn	**Aminosyn-HBC**	**Aminosyn RF**
Strengths	3.5%, 5%, 7%, 8.5%, 10%	7%	5.2%
Indications	Standard TPN	Hypercatabolism	Renal Failure
% EAA	50%	63%	89%
% BCAA	25%	46%	33%

EAA = essential amino acids; BCAA = branched chain amino acids.

1. **Standard Solutions**

    Standard amino acid solutions (e.g., Aminosyn in Table 38.2) are balanced mixtures of 50% essential amino acids and 50% nonessential and semiessential amino acids. Available concentrations range from 3.5% up to 10%, but 7% solutions (70 g/L) are used most often.

2. **Specialty Solutions**

Specially-designed amino acid solutions are available for patients with severe metabolic stress (e.g., multisystem trauma or burns), and for patients with renal or liver failure.

a. Solutions designed for metabolic stress (e.g., Aminosyn-HBC in Table 38.2) are enriched with branched chain amino acids (isoleucine, leucine, and valine), which are preferred fuels in skeletal muscle when metabolic demands are high.

b. Renal failure solutions (e.g., Aminosyn RF in Table 38.2) are rich in essential amino acids, because the nitrogen in essential amino acids is partially recycled to produce nonessential amino acids, which results in smaller increments in blood urea nitrogen (BUN) than seen with breakdown of nonessential amino acids.

c. Solutions designed for hepatic failure (e.g., HepaticAid) are enriched with branched chain amino acids, because these amino acids block the transport of aromatic amino acids across the blood-brain barrier (which are implicated in hepatic encephalopathy).

d. It is important to emphasize that *none of these specialized formulas have improved outcomes in the disorders for which they are designed* (3).

3. **Glutamine**

Glutamine is the principal metabolic fuel for rapidly-dividing cells like intestinal epithelial cells and vascular endothelial cells (4). However, based on a meta-analysis of 5 multicenter trials that showed increased mortality in patients receiving intravenous glutamine (1), the recent guidelines on nutrition support do NOT recommend IV glutamine for PN regimens (1).

C. Lipid Emulsions

1. Lipids are provided as emulsions composed of cholesterol, phospholipids, and triglycerides (5). The triglycerides are derived from vegetable oils (safflower or soybean oils) and are rich in linoleic acid, an essential fatty acid (6).

2. Lipids are used to provide 30% of daily calorie requirements, and 4% of the daily calories should be provided as linoleic acid to prevent essential fatty acid deficiency (7).

Table 38.3	Intravenous Lipid Emulsions for Clinical Use			
Feature	**Intralipid**		**Liposyn II**	
	10%	**20%**	**10%**	**20%**
Calories (kcal/mL)	1.1	2	1.1	2
% calories as EFA (Linoleic acid)	50%	50%	66%	66%
Cholesterol (mg/dL)	250–300	250–300	13–22	13–22
Osmolarity (mosm/L)	260	260	276	258
Unit Volumes (mL)	50 100 250 500	50 100 250 500	100 200 500	200 500

EFA = essential fatty acid.

3. As shown in Table 38.3, lipid emulsions are available in 10% and 20% strengths (grams of triglyceride per 100 mL of solution). The 10% emulsions provide about 1 kcal/mL, and the 20% emulsions provide 2 kcal/mL. Unlike the hypertonic dextrose solutions, lipid emul-

sions are roughly isotonic to plasma and *can be infused through peripheral veins*.

4. Lipid emulsions are available in unit volumes of 50 to 500 mL, and can be infused separately (at a maximum rate of 50 mL/hr) or added to the dextrose–amino acid mixtures. The infused triglycerides are not cleared for 8–10 hours, and lipid infusions often produce a transient lipemic appearance in plasma.

II. ADDITIVES

Commercially available mixtures of electrolytes, vitamins, and trace elements are added directly to the dextrose–amino acid mixtures.

A. Electrolytes

There are more than 15 electrolyte mixtures available. Most have a volume of 20 mL, and contain sodium, chloride, potassium, and magnesium. You must check the mixture used at your hospital to determine if additional electrolytes must be added. Additional requirements for potassium or other electrolytes can be specified in the TPN orders.

B. Vitamins

Aqueous multivitamin preparations are added to the dextrose–amino acid mixtures. One vial of a standard multivitamin preparation will provide the normal daily requirements for most vitamins in healthy adults (see Table 36.4). The daily vitamin requirement in ICU patients is not known (and probably varies with each patient), but vitamin deficiencies can be common in ICU patients despite the provision of normal daily requirements. (See Chapter 36, Section III-B, on Vitamin D deficiency.)

C. Trace Elements

1. A variety of trace element additives are available, and one of these is shown in Table 38.4, along with the recommended daily requirement for trace elements. Note the poor correlation between the daily requirements and the trace element content.

2. Trace element mixtures don't contain iron and iodine, and some don't contain selenium. Although iron can be risky because of its pro-oxidant effects (see Chapter 36, Section IV-A), selenium has an important role as an antioxidant (see Chapter 36, Section IV-B), and should be given daily to critically ill patients.

Table 38.4	Intravenous Lipid Emulsions for Clinical Use	
Trace Element	Daily Requirement[†]	Multitrace-5 Concentrated[§]
Chromium	30 µg	10 µg
Copper	900 µg	1 mg
Iodine	150 µg	—
Iron	8 mg	—
Manganese	2.3 mg	0.5 mg
Selenium	55 µg	60 µg
Zinc	11 mg	5 mg

[†]From the Food and Nutrition Information Center (http://fnic.nal.usda.gov). Accessed August, 2016. [§]Product description, America Reagent, Inc.

III. CREATING A PN REGIMEN

A. When to Start PN

PN does not offer the same benefits described for enteral tube feedings (see Chapter 37, Section I), and can be withheld for 7 days in patients who are well nourished (1). In malnourished patients (who are unable to receive tube feedings), it should be started within 24 hours of ICU admission.

B. Creating a PN Regimen

The following is a stepwise approach to creating a standard PN regimen. Each step is accompanied by an example, using the same patient, to illustrate how the method is used.

1. STEP 1: The initial task is to determine the daily requirement for calories and protein. The following simple approximations can be used:

$$\text{Daily Calories} = 25 \times \text{weight (kg)} \qquad (38.1)$$

$$\text{Daily Protein} = 1.2\text{--}2 \text{ g/kg/day} \qquad (38.2)$$

Actual or dry body weight is used in these estimates. (For obese patients, see the recommended nutritional requirements in Table 36.2.)

a. EXAMPLE: For an adult with a dry body weight of 70 kg, the daily requirement for calories is $25 \times 70 = 1{,}750$ kcal/day. Using a protein requirement of 1.4 g/kg/day, the daily protein requirement is $1.4 \times 70 = 98$ grams/day.

b. *Note:* If propofol is being used for sedation, the daily caloric requirement should be adjusted because propofol is infused in a lipid emulsion with a caloric density of about 1 kcal/mL.

2. STEP 2: Using a standard mixture of 10% amino acids (500 mL) and 50% dextrose (500 mL), the next step is to determine the volume and infusion rate of the $A_{10}D_{50}$ mixture that will deliver the estimated daily protein requirement. The volume required is equivalent to the daily protein requirement divided by the protein concentration in the $A_{10}D_{50}$ mixture (which is 50 g/L).

$$\text{Liters of } A_{10}D_{50} = \text{Protein Required (g/day)}/50 \text{ (g/L)} \quad (38.3)$$

The infusion rate is then:

$$\text{Infusion Rate} = \text{Liters of } A_{10}D_{50}/24 \text{ hours} \quad (38.4)$$

a. EXAMPLE: For the estimated protein requirement of 98 grams daily (see example in Step 1), the volume of $A_{10}D_{50}$ needed is 98/50 = 1.9 liters, and the desired infusion rate is 1,900 mL/24 hr = 81 mL/hr.

3. STEP 3: The final step is to determine how much lipid to infuse daily. This is dependent on the calories provided by dextrose in the volume of $A_{10}D_{50}$ infused. The carbohydrate (CHO) calories are determined as follows:

$$\text{CHO calories} = 250 \text{ (g/L)} \times \text{Liters of } A_{10}D_{50} \times 3.4 \text{ (kcal/g)} \quad (38.5)$$

where 250 g/L is the dextrose concentration in the $A_{10}D_{50}$ mixture, and 3.4 kcal/g is the caloric yield from dextrose. Lipids are then used to provide the remainder of the daily caloric requirement.

$$\text{Lipid calories} = \text{Daily calories} - \text{CHO calories} \quad (38.6)$$

If 10% Intralipid (1 kcal/mL) is used to provide the lipid calories, then the volume in mL is equivalent to the kcal of lipid needed.

a. EXAMPLE: For our example where 1.9 liters of $A_{10}D_{50}$ is needed to deliver 98 grams of protein daily, the carbohydrate calories are $250 \times 1.9 \times 3.4 = 1,615$ kcal, and the daily caloric need is 1,750 kcal, so the calories needed from lipid are $1,750 - 1,615 = 135$ kcal. Lipid emulsions are available in unit volumes of 50 mL, so 150 mL of 10% Intralipid (150 kcal) would be used to provide the lipid calories (to avoid wastage). The maximum infusion rate is 50 mL/hr.

b. PN ORDERS: The PN orders for the example used here would be written as follows:

1) $A_{10}D_{50}$ to run at 81 mL/hour.

2) 10% Intralipid, 150 mL, to infuse over 3 hours.

3) Add standard electrolytes, multivitamins, and trace elements.

PN orders are rewritten each day.

IV. COMPLICATIONS

A. Catheter-Related Complications

As mentioned earlier, the hyperosmolarity of the dextrose and amino acid solutions requires infusion through large veins, so central venous cannulation, or a peripherally inserted central catheter (PICC), is required. Complications related to insertion of these catheters are described in Chapter 1, Section IV; noninfectious complications of indwelling catheters are described in Chapter 2, Section II; and catheter-related infections are described in Chapter 2, Section III.

1. **Misdirected Catheter**

Insertion of subclavian vein catheters and peripherally inserted central catheters (PICCs) can occasionally

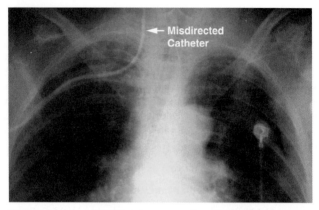

FIGURE 38.1 Portable X-ray showing a catheter that has been unintentionally advanced into the internal jugular vein. Image digitally enhanced.

result in advancement of a catheter into the internal jugular vein, like the one shown in Figure 38.1. In one survey (8), 10% of subclavian vein cannulations (mostly on the right) resulted in misplacement of the catheter in the internal jugular vein. The standard recommendation is to reposition such catheters because of the assumed risk of thrombosis (8), but there is no evidence to support this claim.

B. Carbohydrate Complications

1. **Hyperglycemia**

   Hyperglycemia is common during PN, but tight glycemic control is not recommended in critically ill patients because of the risk of hypoglycemia, which is more deleterious than hyperglycemia (9,10).

   a. The current recommendation of the nutrition support guidelines is *a target range of 140–180 mg/dL for plasma glucose in the general ICU population* (1).

b. Tighter glycemic control is recommended for patients with acute brain injury from cardiac arrest, ischemic stroke, or intracranial hemorrhage (10), because hyperglycemia can aggravate the brain injury in these patients.

2. **Insulin**

a. If insulin therapy is required, a continuous infusion of regular insulin (1 unit/mL) is preferred for patients who are unstable or have type 1 diabetes (10). This can be accomplished by adding insulin to the TPN solutions.

b. Because insulin can adsorb to the plastic tubing in IV infusion sets, insulin infusions should be primed with 20 mL of a saline solution containing 1 unit/mL of regular insulin (10). This priming procedure must be repeated each time the IV infusion set is changed (10).

c. Patients can be transitioned to a protocol-driven subcutaneous (subQ) insulin regimen when they are clinically stable, off vasopressors, and there are no planned interruptions in the nutrition regimen for procedures, etc (10). The transition to subQ insulin should begin before the insulin infusion is discontinued (10).

d. The final subQ insulin regimen will vary for each patient, but the combination of an intermediate or long-acting insulin with a rapid-acting insulin, when needed, is popular for hospitalized patients. The variety of insulin preparations is shown in Table 38.5 (11).

3. **Hypophosphatemia**

The movement of glucose into cells is associated with a similar movement of phosphate into cells, and plasma phosphate levels typically show a steady decline after PN is initiated (see Figure 30.1).

4. Hypokalemia

Glucose movement into cells is also accompanied by an intracellular shift of potassium, and continuous infusions of glucose during PN can lead to persistent hypokalemia.

Table 38.5		Insulin Preparations		
Type	**Name**	**Onset**	**Peak**	**Duration**
Rapid-Acting	Aspart	10–20 min	1–3 hr	3–5 hr
Rapid-Acting	Glulisine	25 min	45–50 min	4–5 hr
Rapid-Acting	Lispro	15–30 min	0.5–2.5 hr	3–6 hr
Short-Acting	Regular	30–60 min	1–5 hr	6–10 hr
Intermediate	NPH	1–2 hr	6–14 hr	16–24 hr
Long-Acting	Glargine	1 hr	2–20 hr	24 hr

From Reference 11.

C. Lipid Complications

1. Overfeeding with lipids may contribute to hepatic steatosis (see later).

2. A frequently overlooked feature of lipid infusions is the potential to *promote inflammation*. The lipid emulsions used in PN regimens are rich in oxidizable lipids (12), and the oxidation of infused lipids will trigger an inflammatory response. In fact, infusions of oleic acid, one of the lipids in PN, is a standard method for producing the acute respiratory distress syndrome (ARDS) in animals (13), and this might explain why *lipid infusions are associated with impaired oxygenation and prolonged respiratory failure* (14,15). The possible role of lipid infusions in promoting oxidant-induced injury deserves more attention.

D. Hepatobiliary Complications

1. **Hepatic Steatosis**

   Fat accumulation in the liver (hepatic steatosis) is common in patients receiving long-term PN, and is believed to be the result of chronic overfeeding with carbohydrates and lipids. This condition is associated with elevated liver enzymes (16), but it may not be a pathological entity.

2. **Cholestasis**

   The absence of lipids in the proximal small bowel prevents cholecystokinin-mediated contraction of the gallbladder. This results in bile stasis and the accumulation of sludge in the gallbladder, which can lead to *acalculous cholecystitis* when PN is prolonged for more than 4 weeks (see Chapter 32, Section I-A).

E. Bowel Sepsis

The bowel rest associated with PN leads to atrophy of the bowel mucosa, and impairs bowel-associated immunity, and these changes can lead to the systemic spread of enteric pathogens (see Chapter 37, Section I-A).

V. PERIPHERAL PARENTERAL NUTRITION

Peripheral parenteral nutrition (PPN) is a truncated form of PN that can be used to provide nonprotein calories in amounts that will spare the breakdown of proteins to provide energy (i.e., *protein-sparing* nutrition support) (17,18).

1. PPN can be used as a protein-sparing strategy during brief periods of inadequate nutrition (e.g., in postoperative patients), but is not intended for hypercatabolic or malnourished patients, who need full nutritional support.

2. The osmolarity of peripheral vein infusates should be kept below 900 mosm/L, to limit the risk of osmotic damage in the catheterized veins (17,18).

A. Regimen

1. A popular solution for PPN is a mixture of 3% amino acids and 20% dextrose (final concentration of 1.5% amino acids and 10% dextrose), which has an osmolarity of 500 mosm/L. The dextrose will provide 340 kcal/L, so 2.5 L of the mixture will provide 850 kcal.

2. If 250 mL of 20% Intralipid is added to the regimen (adding 500 kcal), the total nonprotein calories will increase to 1,350 kcal/day, which is close to the nonprotein calorie requirement of an average-sized, unstressed adult (20 kcal/kg/day).

REFERENCES

1. Taylor BE, McClave SA, Martindale RG, et al. Guidelines for the provision and assessment of nutrition support therapy in the adult critically ill patient: Society of Critical Care Medicine (SCCM) and American Society for Parenteral and Enteral Nutrition (A.S.P.E.N.). Crit Care Med 2016; 44:390–438.

2. Singer P, Berger MM, Van den Berghe G, et al. ESPN guidelines on parenteral nutrition: Intensive care. Clin Nutr 2009; 387–400.

3. Andris DA, Krzywda EA. Nutrition support in specific diseases: back to basics. Nutr Clin Pract 1994; 9:28–32.

4. Souba WW, Klimberg VS, Plumley DA, et al. The role of glutamine in maintaining a healthy gut and supporting the metabolic response to injury and infection. J Surg Res 1990; 48:383–391.

5. Driscoll DF. Compounding TPN admixtures: then and now. J Parenter Enteral Nutr 2003; 27:433–438.

6. Warshawsky KY. Intravenous fat emulsions in clinical practice. Nutr Clin Pract 1992; 7:187–196.

7. Barr LH, Dunn GD, Brennan MF. Essential fatty acid deficiency during total parenteral nutrition. Ann Surg 1981; 193:304–311.

8. Padberg FT, Jr., Ruggiero J, Blackburn GL, et al. Central venous catheterization for parenteral nutrition. Ann Surg 1981; 193:264–270.

9. Marik PE, Preiser J-C. Toward understanding tight glycemic control in the ICU. Chest 2010; 137:544–551.

10. Jacobi J, Bircher N, Krinsley J, et al. Guidelines for the use of an insulin infusion for the management of hyperglycemia in critically ill patients. Crit Care Med 2012; 40:3251–3276.

11. Insulins. In McEvoy GK, ed. AHFS Drug Information, 2014. Bethesda, MD: American Society of Heath System Pharmacists, 2014:3228.

12. Carpentier YA, Dupont IE. Advances in intravenous lipid emulsions. World J Surg 2000; 24:1493–1497.

13. Schuster DP. ARDS: clinical lessons from the oleic acid model of acute lung injury. Am J Respir Crit Care Med 1994; 149:245–260.

14. Suchner U, Katz DP, Furst P, et al. Effects of intravenous fat emulsions on lung function in patients with acute respiratory distress syndrome or sepsis. Crit Care Med 2001; 29:1569–1574.

15. Battistella FD, Widergren JT, Anderson JT, et al. A prospective, randomized trial of intravenous fat emulsion administration in trauma victims requiring total parenteral nutrition. J Trauma 1997; 43:52–58.

16. Freund HR. Abnormalities of liver function and hepatic damage associated with total parenteral nutrition. Nutrition 1991; 7:1–5.

17. Culebras JM, Martin-Pena G, Garcia-de-Lorenzo A, et al. Practical aspects of peripheral parenteral nutrition. Curr Opin Clin Nutr Metab Care 2004; 7:303–307.

18. Anderson AD, Palmer D, MacFie J. Peripheral parenteral nutrition. Br J Surg 2003; 90:1048–1054.

Chapter 39

Adrenal and Thyroid Dysfunction

This chapter describes the spectrum of adrenal and thyroid disorders that occur in critically ill patients, and how to identify and manage each of these disorders.

I. ADRENAL INSUFFICIENCY

A. Adrenal Suppression in Critical Illness

1. Adrenal insufficiency is common in critically ill patients. The overall prevalence is 10–20% (1), but rates as high as 60% have been reported in patients with severe sepsis and septic shock (2).

2. The adrenal suppression in critically ill patients is *often reversible*, and is called *critical illness-related corticosteroid insufficiency* (CIRCI) (3).

3. The mechanisms involved in CIRCI are complex, and not fully elucidated; Figure 39.1 shows some of the known mechanisms (1-4). As indicated, the systemic inflammatory response plays a major role in CIRCI.

4. Systemic sepsis and septic shock are the leading causes of adrenal suppression in critically ill patients, and most cases involve suppression at the hypothalamic-pituitary level (2).

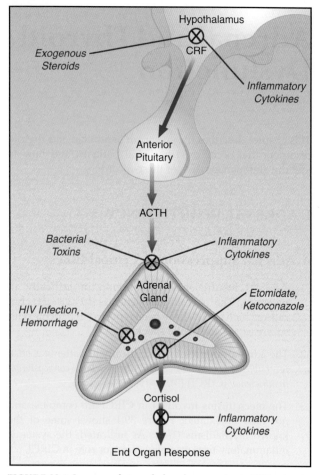

FIGURE 39.1 Sources and sites of adrenal suppression in ICU patients. CRF = corticotrophin-releasing factor, ACTH = adrenocorticotrophic hormone.

B. Clinical Manifestations

1. The principal manifestation of CIRCI is *hypotension that is refractory to volume resuscitation* (1-3).

2. The typical electrolyte abnormalities in adrenal insufficiency (i.e., hyponatremia and hyperkalemia) are uncommon in CIRCI.

C. Diagnosis

1. Adrenal suppression should be suspected in any ICU patient with unexplained or refractory hypotension.

2. A random plasma cortisol level that is 35 µg/dL or higher is evidence of normal adrenal function in critically ill (stressed) patients, while a random plasma cortisol level below 10 µg/dL is evidence of adrenal insufficiency (1,3).

3. If the random plasma cortisol level is indeterminate (10–34 µg/dL), a *rapid ACTH stimulation test* can be performed. A blood sample is obtained for a baseline plasma cortisol level, and the patient is given an IV injection of synthetic ACTH (250 µg), followed 60 minutes later by a repeat plasma cortisol level.

   a. An increment in plasma cortisol of less than 9 µg/dL is evidence of primary adrenal insufficiency (1,3).

   b. However, a larger increment in plasma cortisol (≥9 µg/dL) does not eliminate the possibility of secondary adrenal insufficiency from hypothalamic-pituitary dysfunction (which is common in septic shock, as mentioned earlier).

4. In patients with septic shock, plasma cortisol levels are not considered necessary for identifying patients who might benefit from corticosteroid therapy; in these patients, corti-

costeroid therapy is sanctioned when hypotension is refractory to volume resuscitation, and requires a vasopressor drug (5). (See Chapter 9, Section II-D, for more information on steroid therapy in septic shock.)

D. Treatment

1. The treatment of CIRCI is *intravenous hydrocortisone, 200-300 mg daily*, in 3 divided doses (1), or by continuous infusion in septic shock (5).

2. The addition of a mineralocorticoid (i.e., *fludrocortisone, 50 μg orally once daily*) is considered optional (1), because hydrocortisone has excellent mineralocorticoid activity.

3. Hydrocortisone can be discontinued after satisfactory resolution of the predisposing condition. If the period of hydrocortisone therapy exceeds 7–10 days, a gradual taper of the dosage is recommended (1).

II. EVALUATION OF THYROID FUNCTION

Laboratory tests of thyroid function can be abnormal in up to 90% of critically ill patients (6). In most cases, the abnormality is a consequence of non-thyroidal illness (i.e., *euthyroid sick syndrome*), and is not a sign of thyroid disease (6,7). This section describes the laboratory evaluation of thyroid function, and how to distinguish non-thyroidal illness from thyroid disease.

A. Thyroxine and Triiodothyronine

1. Thyroxine (T_4) is the principal hormone secreted by the thyroid gland, but the active form is triiodothyronine (T_3), which is formed by deiodination of thyroxine in extrathyroidal tissues.

2. T_3 and T_4 are extensively bound to plasma proteins, and less than 1% of either hormone is present in the free, or biologically active form (8).

3. Because of the potential for alterations in plasma proteins and protein binding in acute illness, *free T_4 levels are used to evaluate thyroid function in acutely ill patients.* (Free T_3 levels are not routinely available.)

B. Thyroid-Stimulating Hormone

1. The plasma level of thyroid-stimulating hormone (TSH) is considered *the most reliable test of thyroid function*; it is useful for identifying nonthyroidal illness, and for distinguishing between primary and secondary thyroid disorders.

   a. Plasma TSH levels are normal in a majority of patients with euthyroid sick syndrome (6). However, TSH secretion can be depressed by sepsis, corticosteroids, and dopamine infusions (9).

   b. In patients with hypothyroidism, an elevated plasma TSH level is evidence of primary hypothyroidism, while a reduced TSH level is evidence of secondary hypothyroidism (from hypothalamic–pituitary dysfunction).

2. Plasma TSH levels have a diurnal variation (with the lowest values in late afternoon and the highest values around the hour of sleep), and TSH levels can vary by as much as 40% over a 24-hour period (10). This diurnal variation must be considered when interpreting plasma TSH levels.

C. Abnormal Thyroid Function Tests

Table 39.1 shows the expected changes in plasma free T_4 and TSH levels in specific conditions.

Table 39.1	Patterns of Abnormal Thyroid Function Tests	
Condition	**Free T$_4$**	**TSH**
Euthyroid Sick Syndrome	NL or ↓	NL
Primary Hypothyroidism	↓	↑
Secondary Hypothyroidism	↓	↓
Primary Hyperthyroidism	↑	↓

1. Acute, non-thyroidal illness is associated with low plasma levels of free T$_3$, which is the result of impaired conversion of T$_4$ to T$_3$ in non-thyroidal tissue (6). With increasing severity of illness, both free T$_3$ and free T$_4$ levels are depressed, which is the pattern reported in 30–50% of ICU patients (6,7). As mentioned earlier, plasma TSH levels are normal in a majority of patients with euthyroid sick syndrome.

2. Primary hypothyroidism is characterized by reciprocal changes in free T$_4$ and TSH levels, while in secondary hypothyroidism (from hypothalamic-pituitary dysfunction), both free T$_4$ and TSH levels are depressed.

III. THYROTOXICOSIS

Thyrotoxicosis is almost always the result of primary hyperthyroidism. Notable causes include autoimmune thyroiditis, and chronic therapy with amiodarone (11).

A. Clinical Manifestations

1. The principal manifestations of thyrotoxicosis are agitation,

tachycardias (including atrial fibrillation), and fine tremors.

2. *Elderly patients with hyperthyroidism can be lethargic* rather than agitated; this condition is called *apathetic thyrotoxicosis.* The combination of lethargy and atrial fibrillation is a frequently cited presentation for apathetic thyrotoxicosis in the elderly.

3. Thyroid storm is an uncommon but severe form of hyperthyroidism that can be precipitated by acute illness or surgery.

   a. This condition is characterized by hyperpyrexia (temp. can exceed 104°F), severe agitation or delirium, and tachycardia with high-output heart failure. Advanced cases are associated with obtundation or coma, generalized seizures, and hemodynamic instability.

   b. If untreated, the outcome is uniformly fatal (11).

B. Diagnosis

1. The plasma TSH level is the most sensitive and specific diagnostic test for hyperthyroidism (11).

2. TSH levels are <0.01 mU/dL in mild cases of hyperthyroidism, and TSH levels are undetectable in most cases of overt thyrotoxicosis (11).

3. A normal TSH level excludes the diagnosis of hyperthyroidism (11).

C. Management

The acute pharmacologic management of thyrotoxicosis and thyroid storm is summarized in Table 39.2.

1. **β-Receptor Antagonists**

   Treatment with β-receptor antagonists relieves the tachycardia, agitation, and fine tremors in thyrotoxicosis.

a. *Propranolol* has been the most widely used β-receptor antagonist in hyperthyroidism, but it is a non-selective β-receptor antagonist, which makes it less than ideal for patients with asthma or systolic heart failure.

b. Selective β-receptor antagonists like *metoprolol* (25–50 mg PO every 4 hours) can be used for thyrotoxicosis, but propranolol remains the drug of choice for thyroid storm (11).

c. The ultra-rapid-acting agent *esmolol* is an appealing choice for acute rate control in atrial fibrillation associated with hyperthyroidism. (See Table 13.1 for dosing recommendations.)

2. **Antithyroid Drugs**

   Two drugs are used to suppress thyroxine production: *methimazole* and *propylthiouracil* (PTU). Both are given orally.

   a. Methimazole is preferred for the treatment of thyrotoxicosis, while PTU is favored for the treatment of thyroid storm (11).

   b. Uncommon but serious side effects include cholestatic jaundice for methimazole, and fulminant hepatic necrosis or agranulocytosis for PTU (11).

3. **Inorganic Iodine**

   In severe cases of hyperthyroidism, iodine (which blocks the synthesis and release of T_4) can be added to antithyroid drug therapy. The iodine is given orally as a saturated potassium iodide solution (Lugol's solution). In patients with an iodine allergy, lithium (300 mg orally every 8 hours) can be used as a substitute (12).

4. **Special Concerns in Thyroid Storm**

   a. Aggressive volume resuscitation is often required in thyroid storm because of vomiting, diarrhea, and heightened insensible fluid loss.

Table 39.2	Drug Therapy for Thyrotoxicosis and Thyroid Storm	
Drug	**Dosing Regimens and Comments**	
Propanolol	Dosing:	10–40 mg PO TID or QID for thyrotoxicosis, and 60–80 mg IV or PO every 4 hrs for thyroid storm.
	Comment:	Blocks conversion of T_4 to T_3 in high doses. Use cautiously in patients with systolic heart failure. Use selective β-blocker in asthmatics.
Methimazole	Dosing:	10–20 mg PO once daily for thyrotoxicosis, and 60–80 mg PO once daily for thyroid storm.
	Comment:	Blocks synthesis of T_4. Preferred to PTU for thyrotoxicosis, but not for thyroid storm.
Propylthiouracil	Dosing:	50–150 mg PO TID for thyrotoxicosis, and 500–1,000 mg PO loading dose, then 250 mg PO every 4 hrs for thyroid storm.
	Comment:	Blocks both T_4 synthesis and the conversion of T_4 to T_3. Preferred to methimazole for thyroid storm.
Iodine	Dosing:	50 drops of saturated potassium iodide (Lugol's) solution (250 mg iodine) PO every 6 hrs, for severe thyrotoxicosis or thyroid storm.
	Comment:	Blocks synthesis and secretion of T_4. Used in combination with antithyroid drugs.
Hydrocortisone	Dosing:	300 mg IV as a loading dose, then 100 mg every 8 hrs, for thyroid storm only.
	Comment:	Prophylaxis for the relative adrenal insufficiency in thyroid storm.

Dosing regimens from Reference 11.

b. Thyroid storm can accelerate glucocorticoid metabolism and create a relative adrenal insufficiency; as a result prophylactic hydrocortisone (300 mg IV as a loading dose, followed by 100 mg IV every 8 hours) is recommended (11).

IV. HYPOTHYROIDISM

Symptomatic hypothyroidism is uncommon, with a prevalence of only 0.3% in the general population (13). Most cases are the result of chronic autoimmune thyroiditis (Hashimoto's thyroiditis), while less common causes include radioiodine or surgical treatment of hyperthyroidism, hypothalamic-pituitary dysfunction from tumors and hemorrhagic necrosis (Sheehan's syndrome), and drugs (lithium, amiodarone).

A. Clinical Manifestations

1. The clinical manifestations of hypothyroidism are often subtle, and include dry skin, fatigue, muscle cramps, and constipation. Advanced cases can be accompanied by hyponatremia and a skeletal muscle myopathy, with elevated muscle enzymes (creatine kinase and aldolase), and an increase in the serum creatinine (from creatine released by skeletal muscle) in the absence of renal dysfunction (14).

2. Contrary to popular perception, *obesity is not a consequence of hypothyroidism* (13).

3. Hypothyroidism can be associated with *pleural and pericardial effusions*. The mechanism is an increase in capillary permeability, and the effusions are exudative in quality.

   a. Pericardial effusions are the most common cause of an enlarged cardiac silhouette in patients with hypothyroidism (15). These effusions usually accumulate slowly and do not cause cardiac tamponade.

4. Advanced cases of hypothyroidism are accompanied by an edematous appearance known as *myxedema*. This condition is mistaken for edema, but is caused by the intradermal accumulation of proteins (16). Myxedema is also associated with hypothermia and depressed consciousness; the latter condition is called *myxedema coma*, although total unresponsiveness is uncommon (16).

B. Diagnosis

The changes in free T_4 and TSH levels in hypothyroidism are shown in Table 39.1.

1. Serum T_3 levels can be normal in hypothyroidism, but free T_4 levels are always reduced (13).

2. Serum TSH levels are increased (often above 10 mU/dL) in primary hypothyroidism, and are depressed in hypothyroidism from hypothalamic-pituitary dysfunction.

C. Thyroid Replacement Therapy

1. For mild-to-moderate hypothyroidism, *levothyroxine* (T_4) is given orally in a single daily dose of 50 to 200 µg (17). The initial dose is usually 50 µg/day, and this is increased in 50 µg/day increments every 3 to 4 weeks. The optimal replacement dose (in primary hypothyroidism) is identified by normalization of the plasma TSH level.

2. For severe hypothyroidism, intravenous levothyroxine is favored initially, because of the risk of impaired GI motility in severe hypothyroidism. One recommendation is an initial IV dose of 250 µg, followed on the next day by an IV dose of 100 µg, and followed thereafter by

a daily IV dose of 50 µg (17). The effective IV dose of thyroxine is about half of the effective oral dose.

2. Because the conversion of T_4 to T_3 (the active form of thyroid hormone) can be depressed in critically ill patients (16), oral therapy with T_3 (25 µg every 12 hours) can be used to supplement thyroxine (T_4) replacement in seriously ill patients (18). (T_3 can be given via nasogastric tube, if necessary.) Studies evaluating the benefits of T_3 supplementation have shown mixed results (13).

REFERENCES

1. Marik PE, Pastores SM, Annane D, et al. Recommendations for the diagnosis and management of corticosteroid insufficiency in critically ill adult patients: consensus statement from an international task force by the American College of Critical Care Medicine. Crit Care Med 2008; 36:1937–1949.

2. Annane D, Maxime V, Ibrahim F, et al. Diagnosis of adrenal insufficiency in severe sepsis and septic shock. Am J Respir Crit Care Med 2006; 174:1319–1326.

3. Marik PE. Critical illness-related corticosteroid insufficiency. Chest 2009; 135:181–193.

4. Bornstein SR. Predisposing factors for adrenal insufficiency. N Engl J Med 2009; 360:2328–2339.

5. Dellinger RP, Levy MM, Rhodes A, et al. Surviving Sepsis Campaign: International guidelines for management of severe sepsis and septic shock, 2012. Intensive Care Med 2013; 39:165–228.

6. Umpierrez GE. Euthyroid sick syndrome. South Med J 2002; 95:506–513.

7. Peeters RP, Debaveye Y, Fliers E, et al. Changes within the thyroid axis during critical illness. Crit Care Clin 2006; 22:41–55.

8. Dayan CM. Interpretation of thyroid function tests. Lancet 2001; 357:619–624.

9. Burman KD, Wartofsky L. Thyroid function in the intensive care unit setting. Crit Care Clin 2001;17:43–57.

10. Karmisholt J, Andersen S, Laurberg P. Variation in thyroid function tests in patients with stable untreated subclinical hypothyroidism. Thyroid 2008; 18:303–308.

11. Bahn RS, Burch HB, Cooper DS, et al. Hyperthyroidism and other causes of thyrotoxicosis: Management guidelines of the American Thyroid Association and the American Association of Clinical Endocrinologists. Thyroid 2011; 21:593–646.

12. Migneco A, Ojetti V, Testa A, et al. Management of thyrotoxic crisis. Eur Rev Med Pharmacol Sci 2005; 9:69–74.

13. Garber JR, Cobin RH, Gharib H, et al. Clinical practice guidelines for hypothyroidism in adults. Endocr Pract 2012; 18:988–1028.

14. Lafayette RA, Costa ME, King AJ. Increased serum creatinine in the absence of renal failure in profound hypothyroidism. Am J Med 1994; 96:298–299.

15. Ladenson PW. Recognition and management of cardiovascular disease related to thyroid dysfunction. Am J Med 1990; 88:638–641.

16. Myers L, Hays J. Myxedema coma. Crit Care Clin 1991; 7:43–56.

17. Toft AD. Thyroxine therapy. New Engl J Med 1994; 331:174–180.

18. McCulloch W, Price P, Hinds CJ, et al. Effects of low dose oral triiodothyronine in myxoedema coma. Intensive Care Med 1985; 11:259–262.

Chapter 40

Disorders of Consciousness

The ability to recognize and interact with the surroundings (i.e., consciousness) is the *sina qua non* of the life experience, and loss of this ability is one of the dominant signs of a life-threatening illness. This chapter describes the principal disorders of consciousness, with emphasis on delirium, coma, and brain death.

I. ALTERED CONSCIOUSNESS

A. Consciousness

Consciousness has two components: *arousal* and *awareness*.

1. Arousal is the ability to experience your surroundings.

2. Awareness is the ability to understand your relationship to your surroundings.

3. These two components are used to identify the altered states of consciousness described next.

B. Altered States of Consciousness

1. *Anxiety* and *lethargy* are conditions where arousal and awareness are intact, but there is a change in *attentiveness* (i.e., the degree of awareness).

2. A *locked-in state* is a condition where arousal and awareness are intact, but there is almost total absence of motor responsiveness. This condition is caused by bilateral injury to the motor pathways in the ventral pons, which disrupts all voluntary movements except up-down ocular movements and eyelid blinking (1).

3. *Delirium* and *dementia* are conditions where arousal is intact, but awareness is altered. The change in awareness can be fluctuating (as in delirium) or slowly progressive (as in dementia).

4. A *vegetative state* is a condition where there is some degree of arousal (eyes can open), but there is no awareness. Spontaneous movements and motor responses to deep pain can occur, but the movements are purposeless. After one month, this condition is called a *persistent vegetative state* (2).

5. *Coma* is characterized by the total absence of arousal and awareness. Spontaneous movements and motor responses to deep pain can occur, but the movements are purposeless.

6. *Brain death* is similar to coma in that there is a total absence of arousal and awareness, but it differs from coma in two ways: (a) it involves loss of all brainstem function, including cranial nerve activity and spontaneous respirations, and (b) it is always irreversible.

C. Sources of Altered Consciousness

The identifiable causes of altered consciousness are indicated in Figure 40.1. In a prospective survey of neurologic complications in a medical ICU (3), ischemic stroke was the most frequent cause of altered consciousness on admission to the ICU, and septic encephalopathy was the most common cause of altered consciousness acquired in the ICU.

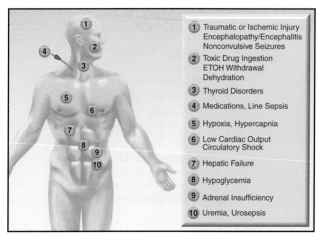

1	Traumatic or Ischemic Injury Encephalopathy/Encephalitis Nonconvulsive Seizures
2	Toxic Drug Ingestion ETOH Withdrawal Dehydration
3	Thyroid Disorders
4	Medications, Line Sepsis
5	Hypoxia, Hypercapnia
6	Low Cardiac Output Circulatory Shock
7	Hepatic Failure
8	Hypoglycemia
9	Adrenal Insufficiency
10	Uremia, Urosepsis

FIGURE 40.1 Common causes of altered consciousness.

II. ICU-RELATED DELIRIUM

Delirium is reported in 16–89% of ICU patients (4), and has an adverse effect on outcomes (5).

A. Clinical Features

The clinical features of delirium are summarized in Figure 40.2 (4,6).

1. Delirium is an acute confusional state with attention deficits, disordered thinking, and a fluctuating course (the fluctuations in behavior occur over a 24-hour period).

2. Over 40% of hospitalized patients with delirium have psychotic symptoms (e.g., visual hallucinations) (7); as a result, delirium is often inappropriately termed "ICU psychosis" (8).

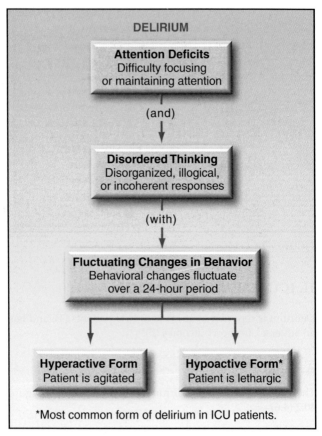

FIGURE 40.2 The clinical features of delirium.

3. **Subtypes**

The following subtypes of delirium are recognized:

a. *Hyperactive delirium* is characterized by restless agitation. This form of delirium is common in alcohol withdrawal, but it is *uncommon in hospital-acquired delirium*, accounting for 2% or fewer of cases (4).

b. *Hypoactive delirium* is characterized by lethargy and somnolence. This is *the most common form of hospital-acquired delirium*, and is responsible for 45–64% of cases (4). This type of delirium is often overlooked, and may explain why the diagnosis of delirium is often missed.

c. *Mixed delirium* involves episodes that alternate between hyperactive and hypoactive delirium. This type of delirium is reported in 6–55% of patients with hospital-acquired delirium (4).

4. **Delirium vs. Dementia**

Delirium and dementia are distinct mental disorders that are often confused because they have overlapping clinical features (i.e., attention deficits and disordered thinking). *The principal features of delirium that distinguish it from dementia are the abrupt onset and fluctuating course.*

B. Predisposing Conditions

Several conditions promote delirium in hospitalized patients, including: (a) advanced age, (b) sleep deprivation, (c) unrelieved pain, (d) prolonged bed rest, (e) major surgery, (f) encephalopathy, and (g) drugs (see next) (4,9,10).

1. **Deleriogenic Drugs**

Drugs that promote delirium include: (a) anticholinergic drugs, (b) dopaminergic drugs, (c) seritonergic drugs, and (d) benzodiazepines (10,11). *The principal drugs that promote delirium in the ICU are the benzodiazepines* (11).

C. Preventive Measures

Recommended measures for reducing the risk of delirium include: (a) adequate treatment of pain, (b) maintaining regular sleep-wake cycles, (c) promoting out-of-bed time, (d) encouraging family visitation, and (e) limiting the use of deliriogenic drugs, if possible (4,11).

1. **Dexmedetomidine**

   Sedation with dexmedetomidine is associated with fewer episodes of delirium than benzodiazepines (12,13). This drug provides an alternative to benzodiazepines for sedation in ICU patients who are at risk for delirium. For more information on dexmedetomidine, see Chapter 43, Section II-D.

D. Diagnosis

The current guidelines on the management of agitation and delirium (11) recommend periodic testing for delirium using validated screening tools like the *Confusion Assessment Method for the ICU* (CAM-ICU) (6), which is available at www.icudelirium.org.

E. Management

There is no universally-sanctioned drug therapy for hospital-acquired delirium.

1. Current guidelines on sedation in ICU patients (11) recommend *dexmedetomidine* over benzodiazepines for the treatment of delirium that is unrelated to alcohol or benzodiazepine withdrawal. However, there is no evidence to support this recommendation (11).

2. *Haloperidol* has been a popular drug for the treatment of delirium, although there is no evidence for or against its use (11). (For information on the use of haloperidol, see Chapter 43, Section II-E.)

3. There is some evidence of success in treating delirium with "atypical antipsychotics" (e.g., *quietiapine, olanzapine, risperidone*) (14), which do not have the risk of

extrapyramidal side effects associated with haloperidol. However, there is not enough evidence to warrant recommendation of these drugs (11).

III. ALCOHOL WITHDRAWAL DELIRIUM

Alcohol withdrawal delirium is characterized by increased motor activity and increased activity on the electroencephalogram (EEG), whereas hospital-acquired delirium is characterized by decreased motor activity and slowing of activity on the EEG (4).

A. Clinical Features

The clinical features of alcohol withdrawal are summarized in Table 44.1.

1. **Delirium Tremens**

    About 5% of patients who experience alcohol withdrawal will develop *delirium tremens* (DTs), which is characterized by agitated delirium, hallucinations, fever, tachycardia, hypertension, dehydration, and can also include seizures and multiple electrolyte abnormalities (especially hypokalemia and hypomagnesemia) (15). Onset is typically delayed (2 days after the last drink), and the syndrome can last for 5 days or longer. The reported mortality is 5–15% (15).

2. **Wernicke's Encephalopathy**

    Alcoholic patients who are admitted with borderline thiamine stores and receive an intravenous glucose infusion can develop acute Wernicke's encephalopathy from thiamine deficiency (18). The acute changes in mental status can occur a few days after admission, and can be confused with alcohol withdrawal delirium. The presence of *nystagmus or lateral gaze paralysis* will help to identify Wernicke's encephalopathy. (For more on thiamine deficiency, see Chapter 36, Section III-A.)

Table 40.1	Clinical Features of Alcohol Withdrawal	
Features	**Onset after last drink**	**Duration**
Early Withdrawal Anxiety Tremulousness Nausea	6–8 hours	1–2 days
Generalized Seizures	6–48 hours	2–3 days
Hallucinations Visual Auditory Tactile	12–48 hours	1–2 days
Delirium Tremens[†]	48–96 hours	1–5 days

[†]Agitated delirium, hallucinations, fever, tachycardia, hypertension, seizures, dehydration, and multiple electrolyte disorders. Adapted from Reference 15.

B. Treatment

1. The central nervous system depressant effects of ethanol are the result, in part, of stimulation of gamma-aminobutyric acid (GABA) receptors, which are a major inhibitory pathway in the brain. This is also the mechanism of action for benzodiazepines, and this is the basis for the use of *benzodiazepines* as the *drugs of choice for alcohol withdrawal agitation and delirium* (17). An added benefit of benzodiazepines is protection against generalized seizures.

2. REGIMEN: For patients who require care in the ICU, *intravenous lorazepam* is an appropriate choice for the management of DTs (17). For initial control, give 2–4 mg IV every 5–10 minutes until the patient is calm. Thereafter, administer IV lorazepam every 1–2 hours (or by continuous

infusion) in a dose that maintains calm. (Intubation and mechanical ventilation may be necessary.)

   a. It is important to taper benzodiazepines as soon as possible because they accumulate and can produce prolonged sedation and a prolonged ICU stay.

   b. An additional concern with prolonged infusion of IV lorazepam is *propylene glycol toxicity* (see Chapter 24, Section I-A-5).

3. For more information on benzodiazepines, see Chapter 43, Section II-B.

4. Because of the risk of thiamine deficiency mentioned previously, thiamine is given routinely to patients with DTs. The popular dose is 50–100 mg daily, which can be given intravenously without harm.

IV. COMA

Persistent coma is one of the most challenging conditions in critical care practice, and requires attention not only to the patient, but to the patient's family and other intimates as well.

A. Etiologies

Coma can be the result of any of the following conditions:

1. Diffuse, ischemic brain injury.

2. Toxic or metabolic encephalopathy (including drug overdose).

3. Brainstem compression from a supratentorial mass lesion with transtentorial herniation, or from a mass lesion in the posterior fossa.

4. Nonconvulsive status epilepticus.

5. Apparent coma (i.e., locked-in state, hysterical reaction).

6. *Note:* ischemic stroke does not result in coma unless there is a unilateral mass effect with midline shift and compression of the contralateral cerebral hemisphere, or brainstem involvement.

B. Bedside Evaluation

The bedside evaluation of coma should include an evaluation of cranial nerve reflexes, spontaneous eye and body movements, and motor reflexes (18,19). The following elements of the evaluation deserve mention:

1. **Motor Responses**

   a. Spontaneous myoclonus (irregular, jerking movements) can be a nonspecific sign of diffuse cerebral dysfunction, or can represent seizure activity (myoclonic seizures), while flaccid extremities can indicate diffuse brain injury or injury to the brainstem.

   b. Clonic movements elicited by flexion of the hands or feet (*asterixis*) is a sign of a diffuse metabolic encephalopathy (20).

   c. With injury to the thalamus, painful stimuli provoke flexion of the upper extremity, which is called *decorticate posturing*.

   d. With injury to the midbrain and upper pons, the arms and legs extend and pronate in response to pain; this is called *decerebrate posturing*.

   e. Finally, with injury involving the lower brainstem, the extremities remain flaccid during painful stimulation.

2. **Examination of Pupils**

   The conditions that affect pupillary size and light reactivity are shown in Table 40.2 (18,19,21). Pupillary findings can be summarized as follows:

Table 40.2	Conditions That Alter Pupillary Size and Reactivity
Pupil Size & Reactivity	**Associated Conditions**
⬤ ⬤ (+) (+)	Atropine, anticholinergic toxicity, adrenergic agonists (e.g., dopamine), stimulant drugs (e.g., amphetamines), or nonconvulsive seizures
⬤ ⬤ (−) (−)	Diffuse brain injury, hypothermia (<28° C), intracranial hypertension, or brainstem compression from an expanding intracranial mass
⬤ ◉ (−) (−)	Expanding intracranial mass (e.g., uncal herniation), ocular trauma or surgery, or focal seizure
◉ ◉ (+) (+)	Toxic/metabolic encephalopathy, sedative overdose, or neuromuscular blockade
◉ ◉ (−) (−)	Acute liver failure, postanoxic encephalopathy, or brain death
◉ ◉ (+) (+)	Horner's Syndrome
● ● (+) (+)	Opiate overdose, toxic/metabolic encephalopathy
● ● (−) (−)	Brainstem (pontine) injury

(+) and (−) indicate a reactive and nonreactive pupil, respectively. From References 18, 19, and 21.

    a. Dilated, reactive pupils can be the result of drugs (e.g., anticholinergics) or nonconvulsive seizures, while dilated, nonreactive pupils are a sign of diffuse brain injury, intracranial hypertension, or brainstem compression from an expanding intracranial mass.

b. A unilateral, dilated and fixed pupil can be the result of ocular trauma, recent ocular surgery, or third cranial nerve dysfunction from an expanding intracranial mass.

c. Midposition, reactive pupils can be the result of a metabolic encephalopathy, a sedative overdose, or neuromuscular blocking drugs, while midposition, nonreactive pupils can be seen with acute liver failure, postanoxic encephalopathy, or brain death.

d. Small, reactive pupils can be the result of a metabolic encephalopathy, while pinpoint pupils can be the result of opiate overdose (pupils reactive) or damage in the pons (pupils nonreactive).

3. **Ocular Motility**

Spontaneous eye movements are a nonspecific sign in comatose patients, but a fixed gaze preference is highly suggestive of a mass lesion or seizure activity.

4. **Ocular Reflexes**

The ocular reflexes are used to evaluate the functional integrity of the lower brainstem (19). These reflexes are illustrated in Figure 40.3.

a. OCULOCEPHALIC REFLEX: The oculocephalic reflex is assessed by briskly rotating the head from side-to-side. When the cerebral hemispheres are impaired but the lower brainstem is intact, the eyes will deviate away from the direction of rotation and maintain a forward field of view. When the lower brainstem is damaged, the eyes will follow the direction of head rotation.

b. OCULOVESTIBULAR REFLEX: The oculovestibular reflex is performed by injecting 50 ml of cold saline in

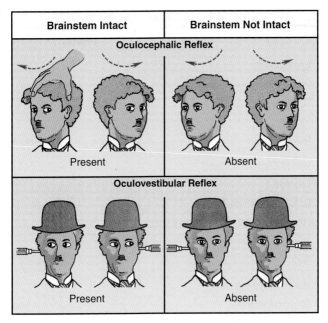

Brainstem Intact	**Brainstem Not Intact**
Oculocephalic Reflex	
Present	Absent
Oculovestibular Reflex	
Present	Absent

FIGURE 40.3 The ocular reflexes in the evaluation of coma.

the external auditory canal of each ear. When brainstem function is intact, both eyes will deviate slowly towards the irrigated ear. This conjugate eye movement is lost when the lower brainstem is damaged.

C. The Glasgow Coma Score

1. The Glasgow Coma Scale in Table 40.3 was introduced to evaluate the severity of traumatic brain injuries (22), but it has been adopted for use in nontraumatic brain injuries as well.

Table 40.3	The Glasgow Coma Scale and Score	
	Points	
Eye Opening:		
Spontaneous	4	
To speech	3	
To pain	2	
None	1	☐ Points
Verbal Communication:		
Oriented	5	
Confused conversation	4	
Inappropriate but recognizable words	3	
Incomprehensible sounds	2	
None	1	☐ Points
Motor Response:		
Obeys commands	6	
Localizes to pain	5	
Withdraws to pain	4	
Abnormal flexion (decorticate response)	3	
Abnormal extension (decerebrate response)	2	
No movement	1	☐ Points
Glasgow Coma Score (Total of 3 scales)*		☐ Points

*Worst score is 3 points, and best score is 15 points. With endotracheal intubation, the highest score is 11.

2. The Scale consists of three components: 1) eye opening, 2) verbal communication, and 3) motor response to verbal or noxious stimulation. The *Glasgow Coma Score* (GCS) is the sum of the three components; a minimum score of 3 indicates total absence of awareness and responsiveness, and a maximum score of 15 is normal.

3. Coma is identified as a GCS ≤8.

4. One of the major shortcomings of the Glasgow Coma Scale is the inability to evaluate verbal responses in intubated patients. These patients are assigned a verbal "pseudoscore" of 1 (for a maximum GCS of 11). The GCS is also unreliable in patients who are paralyzed, heavily sedated, or hypotensive.

D. Electroencephalography

1. Nonconvulsive status epilepticus can be an occult cause of coma; e.g., in one study, it accounted for 8% of the cases of coma (23).

2. Electroencephalography is advised for unexplained or persistent coma.

V. BRAIN DEATH

The Uniform Determination of Death Act states that "An individual who has sustained either 1) irreversible cessation of circulatory and respiratory functions, or 2) irreversible cessation of all functions of the entire brain, including the brainstem, is dead." (24). The second condition is the purpose of the brain death determination described here.

A. The Determination

A checklist for the diagnosis of brain death in adults is shown in Table 40.4 (25). There is a lack of consensus about minor aspects of the brain death determination, but the essential components are as follows:

1. Irreversible coma

2. The absence of brainstem reflexes

3. The absence of spontaneous respirations during a CO_2 challenge

Table 40.4	Checklist for Brain Death Determination in Adults

Instructions:

The patient can be declared legally dead if Steps 1–4 are confirmed.

Check (✔) Item if Confirmed

Step 1: Prerequisite to Exam:

All of the following conditions should be satisfied before beginning the brain death evaluation. ☐

- Systolic blood pressure ≥100 mm Hg
- Body temperature >36°C or (96.8°F)
- Normal thyroid and adrenal function
- Normoglycemia
- No CNS depressant drugs
- No neuromuscular paralysis

Step 2: Establish the Cause of Coma:

The cause of coma is known, and is sufficient to account for irreversible brain death. ☐

Step 3: Absence of Cortical and Brainstem Function:

A. The patient is comatose. ☐

B. There is no facial grimacing in response to a noxious stimulus. ☐

C. The following brainstem reflexes are absent: ☐

- Absent pupillary response to bright light
- Absent corneal reflex
- Absent gag and cough reflexes
- Absent oculocephalic reflex
- Absent oculovestibular reflex

Step 4: Absence of Spontaneous Breathing Efforts:

There are no spontaneous breathing efforts when the arterial PCO_2 is 20 mm Hg above the patient's baseline level. ☐

From the Clinical Practice Guidelines in Reference 25.

4. The brain death determination must be conducted under the following conditions:

   a. Systolic blood pressure ≥ 100 mm Hg, and body temperature $>36°C$

   b. No sedating or neuromuscular blocking drugs

   c. Euglycemia, and normal thyroid function

5. One neurologic examination is sufficient for the diagnosis of brain death in most U.S. states, but some states require 2 examinations.

B. The Apnea Test

Brain death is confirmed by the absence of spontaneous respiratory efforts in the face of an acute increase in arterial PCO_2 ($PaCO_2$). This is evaluated with the *apnea test*, which involves removing the patient from the ventilator and observing for spontaneous breathing efforts as the $PaCO_2$ rises. The following steps are involved in the apnea test (25):

1. Prior to the test, the patient is placed on 100% O_2 for at least 10 minutes. The respiratory rate on the ventilator is reduced to 10 breaths/min, and the PEEP level is reduced to 5 cm H_2O. If the O_2 saturation by pulse oximetry (SpO_2) is >95%, an arterial blood gas is obtained to establish the baseline $PaCO_2$.

2. The patient is then separated from the ventilator, and 100% O_2 is insufflated into the airways through a catheter that is advanced through the endotracheal tube (apneic oxygenation).

3. The goal of the apnea test is to allow the $PaCO_2$ to rise 20 mm Hg above baseline. The $PaCO_2$ rises about 3 mm Hg per minute during apnea at normal body temperatures (26), so a test period of 6–7 minutes should be sufficient for achieving the target $PaCO_2$. A repeat arterial blood gas is obtained at the end of the test period, and the patient is placed back on the ventilator.

4. If apnea persists despite a rise in $PaCO_2 \geq 20$ mm Hg, the diagnosis of brain death is confirmed.

5. The apnea test should be aborted when either of the following occurs (25):

   a. Systolic blood pressure falls below 90 mm Hg

   b. SpO_2 falls below 85% for longer than 30 seconds

C. Ancillary Tests

1. The ancillary tests for the diagnosis of brain death include magnetic resonance imaging and angiography (MRI and MRA), computed tomographic angiography (CTA), and somatosensory evoked potentials.

2. These tests are typically used when the neurologic examination is equivocal, or apnea testing cannot be performed safely.

3. However, *there is insufficient evidence to determine if ancillary testing can reliably identify brain death* (25), and the current guidelines on brain death determination caution physicians about the use of these tests (25).

D. Lazarus' Sign

1. Brain-dead patients can exhibit brief, spontaneous movements of the head, torso, or upper extremities (*Lazarus' Sign*), especially after they are removed from the ventilator (27).

2. These movements are the result of neuronal discharges in the cervical spinal cord, possibly in response to hypoxemia.

E. The Potential Organ Donor

Organ donation is an integral part of the brain death determination process. This topic is beyond the scope of this text, but recently published guidelines for organ procurement in the ICU (28) are included in the bibliography at the end of the chapter.

REFERENCES

1. Leon-Carrion J, van Eeckhout P, Dominguez-Morales Mdel R. The locked-in syndrome: a syndrome looking for a therapy. Brain Inj 2002; 16:555–569.

2. The Multi-Society Task Force on PVS. Medical aspects of the persistent vegetative state (Part 1). N Engl J Med 1994; 330:1499–1508.

3. Bleck TP, Smith MC, Pierre-Louis SJ, et al. Neurologic complications of critical medical illnesses. Crit Care Med 1993; 21:98–103.

4. Zaal IJ, Slooter AJC. Delirium in critically ill patients: epidemiology, pathophysiology, diagnosis and management. Drugs 2012; 72:1457–1471.

5. Ely EW, Shintani A, Truman B, et al. Delirium as a predictor of mortality in mechanically ventilated patients in the intensive care unit. JAMA 2004; 291:1753–1762.

6. Ely EW, Margolin R, Francis J, et al. Evaluation of delirium in critically ill patients: validation of the Confusion Assessment Method for the Intensive Care Unit (CAM-ICU). Crit Care Med 2001; 29:1370–1379.

7. Webster R, Holroyd S. Prevalence of psychotic symptoms in delirium. Psychosomatics 2000; 41:519–522.

8. McGuire BE, Basten CJ, Ryan CJ, et al. Intensive care unit syndrome: a dangerous misnomer. Arch Intern Med 2000; 160:906–909.

9. Inouye SK. Delirium in older persons. N Engl J Med 2006; 354:1157–1165.

10. Reade MC, Finfer S. Sedation and delirium in the intensive care unit. N Engl J Med 2014; 370:444–454.

11. Barr J, Fraser GL, Puntillo K, et al. Clinical practice guidelines for the management of pain, agitation, and delirium in adult patients in the intensive care unit. Crit Care Med 2013; 41:263–306.

12. Pandharipande PP, Pun BT, Herr DL, et al. Effect of sedation with dexmedetomidine vs lorazepam on acute brain dysfunction on mechanically ventilated patients: the MENDS randomized controlled trial. JAMA 2007; 298:2644–2653.

13. Riker RR, Shehabi Y, Bokesch PM, et al. Dexmedetomidine vs midazolam for sedation of critically ill patients: a randomized trial. JAMA 2009; 301:489–499.

14. Gilchrist NA, Asoh I, Greenberg B. Atypical antipsychotics for the treatment of ICU delirium. J Intensive Care Med 2012; 27:354–361.

15. Tetrault JM, O'Connor PG. Substance abuse and withdrawal in the critical care setting. Crit Care Clin 2008; 24:767–788.

16. Attard O, Dietermann JL, Diemunsch P, et al. Wernicke encephalopathy: a complication of parenteral nutrition diagnosed by magnetic resonance imaging. Anesthesiology 2006; 105:847–848.

17. Mayo-Smith MF, Beecher LH, Fischer TL, et al. Management of alcohol withdrawal delirium: an evidence-based practice guideline. Arch Intern Med 2004; 164:1405–1412.

18. Stevens RD, Bhardwaj A. Approach to the comatose patient. Crit Care Med 2006; 34:31–41.

19. Bateman DE. Neurological assessment of coma. J Neurol Neurosurg Psychiatry 2001; 71:i13–17.

20. Kunze K. Metabolic encephalopathies. J Neurol 2002; 249:1150–1159.

21. Wijdicks EFM. Neurologic manifestations of pharmacologic agents commonly used in the intensive care unit. In: Neurology of critical illness. Philadelphia: F.A. Davis, Co., 1995:3–17.

22. Teasdale G, Jennett B. Assessment of coma and impaired consciousness. A practical scale. Lancet 1974; 2:81–84.

23. Towne AR, Waterhouse EJ, Boggs JG, et al. Prevalence of nonconvulsive status epilepticus in comatose patients. Neurology 2000; 54:340–345.

24. National Conference of Commissioners on Uniform State Laws. Uniform Determination of Death Act. Approved July, 1980.

25. Wijdicks EFM, Varelas PNV, Gronseth GS, Greer DM. Evidence-based guideline update: determining brain-death in adults. Report of the Quality Standards Subcommittee of the American Academy of Neurology. Neurology 2010; 74:1911–1918.

26. Dominguez-Roldan JM, Barrera-Chacon JM, Murillo-Cabezas F, et al. Clinical factors influencing the increment of blood carbon dioxide during the apnea test for the diagnosis of brain death. Transplant Proc 1999; 31:2599–2600.

27. Ropper AH. Unusual spontaneous movements in brain-dead patients. Neurology 1984; 34:1089–1092.

28. Kotloff RM, Blosser S, Fulda GJ, et al. Management of the potential organ donor in the ICU: Society of Critical Care Medicine/American College of Chest Physicians/Association of Organ Procurement Organizations Consensus Statement. Crit Care Med 2015; 43:1291–1325.

Chapter 41

Disorders of Movement

This chapter describes three types of movement disorder: (a) involuntary movements (i.e., seizures), (b) weak or ineffective movements (i.e., neuromuscular weakness), and (c) no movements (i.e., drug-induced paralysis).

I. SEIZURES

A. Types of Seizures

Seizures are classified by the extent of brain involvement (generalized vs. focal seizures), the presence or absence of abnormal movements (convulsive vs. nonconvulsive seizures), and the type of movement abnormality (e.g., tonic, clonic, etc.).

1. **Abnormal Movements**

   The movements caused by seizures can be *tonic* (sustained muscle contraction), *clonic* (rhythmic movements with a regular amplitude and frequency), or *myoclonic* (irregular, twitchy movements) (1). Some movements are familiar (e.g., chewing) and repetitive; these are called *automatisms*.

2. **Generalized Seizures**

   Generalized seizures arise from synchronous, rhythmic electrical discharges that involve most of the cerebral cortex, and they are always associated with loss of consciousness. These seizures typically produce tonic-clonic movements of the extremities, but they can also occur without abnormal movements (generalized nonconvulsive seizures) (2).

3. **Partial Seizures**

   Partial seizures can arise from diffuse or localized rhythmic discharges, and the clinical manifestations can vary widely, as demonstrated by the following two examples.

   a. *Partial complex seizures* are nonconvulsive seizures that produce behavioral changes, and can be accompanied by repetitive chewing motions or lip smacking (automatisms). These seizures are a common cause of nonconvulsive status epilepticus, but they do not appear *de novo* in critically ill patients (2).

   b. *Epilepsia partialis continua* is a convulsive seizure that is characterized by persistent tonic-clonic movements of the facial and limb muscles on one side of the body.

4. **Myoclonus**

   Myoclonus (irregular, jerking movements of the extremities) can occur spontaneously, or in response to painful stimuli or loud noises (*startle myoclonus*). These movements can be seen in any type of encephalopathy (metabolic, ischemic). Myoclonus is not universally regarded as a seizure because it is not associated with rhythmic discharges on the EEG (3).

B. Status Epilepticus

Status epilepticus can be defined as *5 minutes of continuous seizure activity, or two seizures without an intervening period of consciousness* (4). This can involve any type of seizure, and can be "convulsive" (i.e., associated with abnormal movements) or "nonconvulsive" (i.e., not associated with abnormal movements).

1. **Nonconvulsive Status Epilepticus**

   Most cases of nonconvulsive status epilepticus (NSE) involve partial complex seizures (which are not common in ICU patients), but as many as 25% of generalized seizures can be nonconvulsive (5).

   a. Generalized NSE is accompanied by loss of consciousness, and can be an occult source of coma in ICU patients (see Chapter 40, Section IV-D).

C. Predisposing Conditions

A variety of conditions can promote new-onset seizures in critically ill patients. In one survey, the most common predisposing conditions were drug intoxication, drug withdrawal, and hypoglycemia (6). Other predisposing conditions include metabolic encephalopathies (e.g., liver failure, uremia), ischemic and traumatic brain injuries, intracranial mass lesions, and meningoencephalitis.

D. Acute Management

The following recommendations (unless otherwise cited) are from the most recent guidelines on convulsive status epilepticus (CSE) from the American Epilepsy Society (7).

1. **Fingerstick Blood Glucose**

   The initial encounter should include a fingerstick blood glucose level. If the blood glucose is <60 mg/dL, administer IV boluses of D_{50} (50 mL) and thiamine (100 mg).

2. **Stage 1 Drugs**

   The most effective drugs for rapid termination of CSE are the benzodiazepines, which are effective in 60–80% of cases.

   a. LORAZEPAM: Intravenous lorazepam (4 mg IV over 2 minutes) is the drug of choice for terminating CSE.

The onset of action is <2 minutes, and the full dose can be repeated after 5–10 minutes, if necessary.

b. MIDAZOLAM: The benefit of midazolam is rapid uptake when given by intramuscular (IM) injection. When IV access is not available, midazolam can be given IM in a dose of 10 mg. The efficacy in terminating CSE is equivalent to IV lorazepam, and the onset of action is only slightly longer than with IV lorazepam (e.g., one study showed a median onset of 3.3 minutes with IM midazolam vs. 1.6 minutes with IV lorazepam) (8).

3. **Stage 2 Drugs**

Stage 2 drugs are used for seizures that are refractory to benzodiazepines, or are likely to recur within 24 hours. These drugs include phenytoin, fosphenytoin, valproic acid, and levetiracetam.

a. PHENYTOIN: The IV dose of phenytoin is 20 mg/kg, or a maximum dose of 1,500 mg. Phenytoin cannot be infused faster than 50 mg/min because of the risk of cardiac depression and hypotension.

b. FOSPHENYTOIN: Fosphenytoin is a water-soluble phenytoin analogue that produces less cardiac depression, and can be infused three times faster than phenytoin (150 mg/min) (12). It is as effective as phenytoin, and is preferred because of the reduced risk of hypotension (7).

c. VALPROIC ACID: The IV dose of valproic acid is 40 mg/kg, or a maximum IV dose of 3,000 mg. Although considered equivalent to phenytoin in efficacy (7), a recent meta-analysis showed that valproic acid is superior to phenytoin for terminating benzodiazepine-resistant CSE (9).

Table 41.1	Drug Regimens for Status Epilepticus	
Drug	**Dosing Regimens and Comments**	

Stage 1 Drugs

Lorazepam	Dosing:	4 mg IV over 2 min. Repeat in 5–10 min, if necessary.
	Comment:	Initial treatment of choice. Onset of action typically <2 min.
Midazolam	Dosing:	10 mg by intramuscular (IM) injection.
	Comment:	As effective as IV lorazepam, and preferred when IV access is not available.

Stage 2 Drugs

Phenytoin	Dosing:	20 mg/kg IV or maximum single IV dose of 1,500 mg.
	Comment:	Promotes cardiac depression and hypotension.
Fosphenytoin	Dosing:	Same dose as phenytoin.
	Comment:	Equal in efficacy to phenytoin, but has a more favorable safety profile.
Valproic Acid	Dosing:	40 mg/kg IV, or maximum single IV dose of 3,000 mg.
	Comment:	Considered equivalent to phenytoin in efficacy.
Levetiracetam	Dosing:	60 mg/kg IV, or maximum single IV dose of 4,500 mg.
	Comment:	Considered equivalent to phenytoin in efficacy.

From Reference 7.

    d. LEVETIRACETAM: The newest anticonvulsant for CSE is levetiracetam which is given in a single dose of 60 mg/kg IV, or a maximum IV dose of 4,500 mg. This drug is also considered equivalent to phenytoin in efficacy (7), but a recent meta-analysis shows that it is superior to phenytoin for terminating benzodiazepine-resistant CSE (9).

4. **Refractory Status Epilepticus**

Ten percent of patients with CSE are refractory to stage 1 and 2 drugs (5). The recommended treatment at this point is anesthetic doses of one of the drugs in Table 41.2. Guidance from a neurologist (along with continuous electroencephalographic monitoring) is the best option at this stage.

Table 41.2	Drug Regimens for Refractory Status Epilepticus
Drug	**Dosing Regimens**
Pentobarbital	Load with 5–15 mg/kg IV over one hr, then infuse at 0.5–1 mg/kg/hr. If necessary, increase infusion rate up to 3 mg/kg/hr (maximum rate).
Thiopental	Start with an IV bolus of 3–5 mg/kg, and follow with 1–2 mg/kg every 2–3 min until seizures subside. Then infuse 3–7 mg/kg/hr for the next 24 hrs.
Midazolam	Load with 0.2 mg/kg IV, then infuse at 4–10 mg/kg/hr.
Propofol	Start with IV bolus of 2–3 mg/kg, and use further boluses of 1–2 mg/kg, if needed, until seizure activity subsides. Then infuse at 4–10 mg/kg/hr for 24 hrs.

Dosing regimens from Reference 3.

II. NEUROMUSCULAR WEAKNESS SYNDROMES

The neuromuscular weakness syndromes that deserve attention include myasthenia gravis, Guillain-Barré syndrome, and critical illness neuromyopathy.

A. Myasthenia Gravis

Myasthenia gravis (MG) is an autoimmune disease produced by antibody-mediated destruction of acetylcholine receptors on the postsynaptic side of neuromuscular junctions (10).

1. **Predisposing Conditions**

   MG can be triggered by major surgery or a concurrent illness. Thymic tumors are responsible for up to 20% of cases (10). Several drugs can precipitate or aggravate MG (11); the principal offenders are antibiotics (e.g., aminoglycosides, ciprofloxacin) and cardiac drugs (e.g., beta-adrenergic blockers, lidocaine, procainamide, quinidine).

2. **Clinical Feature**

   The muscle weakness in MG has the following features:

   a. The weakness worsens with activity and improves with rest.

   b Weakness is first apparent in the eyelids and extraocular muscles, and limb weakness follows in 85% of cases (12).

   c. Progressive weakness often involves the chest wall and diaphragm, and rapid progression to respiratory failure, called *myasthenic crisis*, occurs in 15–20% of patients.

   d. The deficit is purely motor, and deep tendon reflexes are preserved (see Table 41.3).

3. **Diagnosis**

   The diagnosis of MG is suggested by weakness in the eyelids or extraocular muscles that worsens with repeated use. The diagnosis is confirmed by:

   a. Increased muscle strength after the administration of *edrophonium* (Tensilon), an acetylcholinesterase inhibitor.

   b. A positive assay for acetylcholine receptor antibodies in the blood, which are present in 85% of patients of MG (10).

4. **Treatment**

   a. The first line of therapy is an acetylcholinesterase inhibitor like *pyridostigmine* (Mestinon), which is started at an oral dose of 60 mg every 6 hours, and can be increased to 120 mg every 6 hours if necessary (13,14). Pyridostigmine can be given intravenously to treat myasthenic crisis: the IV dose is 1/30th of the oral dose (12,13).

   b. Immunotherapy is added, if needed, using either *prednisone* (1–1.5 mg/kg/day), *azathioprine* (1–3 mg/kg/day), or *cyclosporine* (2.5 mg/kg twice daily) (14). To reduce the need for long-term immunosuppressive therapy, surgical thymectomy is often advised in patients under 60 years of age (14).

5. **Advanced Cases**

   In advanced cases requiring mechanical ventilation, there are two treatment options:

   a. Plasmapheresis to clear pathological antibodies from the bloodstream.

   b. IV immunoglobulin G (0.4 to 2 gm/kg/day for 2 to 5 days) to neutralize the pathologic antibodies.

   c. Both approaches are equally effective (14), but plasmapheresis produces a more rapid response.

Table 41.3	Comparative Features of Myasthenia Gravis and Guillain-Barré Syndrome	
Features	**Myasthenia Gravis**	**Guillain-Barré Syndrome**
Ocular weakness	Yes	No
Fluctuating weakness	Yes	No
Bulbar weakness	Yes	No
Deep tendon reflexes	Intact	Depressed
Autonomic instability	No	Yes
Nerve conduction	Normal	Slowed

B. Guillain-Barré Syndrome

The Guillain-Barré syndrome (GBS) is a *subacute inflammatory demyelinating polyneuropathy* that often follows an acute infectious illness (by 1 to 3 weeks) (15,16). An immune etiology is suspected.

1. **Clinical Features**

   a. GBS presents with distal paresthesias and symmetric limb weakness that evolves over a period of a few days to a few weeks.

   b. Progression to respiratory failure occurs in 25% of cases (15), and autonomic instability can be a feature in advanced cases (17).

   c. The condition resolves spontaneously in about 80% of cases, but residual neurological deficits are common (15).

2. **Diagnosis**

   The diagnosis of GBS is based on the clinical presentation (paresthesias and symmetric limb weakness), nerve conduction studies (slowed conduction) and cerebrospinal fluid analysis (elevated protein in 80% of cases) (15). The features that distinguish GBS from myasthenia gravis are shown in Table 41.3.

3. **Treatment**

   Treatment is mostly supportive, but in advanced cases with respiratory failure, *plasmapheresis or IV immunoglobulin G* (0.4 g/kg/day for 5 days) are equally effective in producing short-term improvement (16). Immunoglobulin is often preferred because it is easier to implement.

C. Critical Illness Neuromyopathy

Two neuromuscular disorders are recognized in patients with progressive systemic inflammation (18); i.e., *critical illness polyneuropathy* and *critical illness myopathy*. Both disorders often co-exist in the same patient, and become apparent when patients fail to wean from mechanical ventilation.

1. **Polyneuropathy**

   Critical illness polyneuropathy (CIP) is a diffuse sensory and motor axonal neuropathy that is found in at least 50% of patients with severe sepsis and septic shock (18-20). The onset is variable, occurring from 2 days to a few weeks after the onset of the septic episode.

2. **Myopathy**

   Critical illness myopathy (CIM) is a diffuse inflammatory myopathy that involves both limb and truncal muscles (21). In addition to severe sepsis and septic shock, CIM is associated with prolonged periods of drug-induced neuromuscular paralysis, particularly when combined with high-dose corticosteroid therapy (18,19,21), and

with status asthmaticus treated with high-dose corticosteroids (21).

3. **Clinical Features**

As mentioned, CIP and CIM often go undetected until
there is an unexplained failure to discontinue mechanical ventilation. Physical examination then reveals a flaccid quadriparesis with hyporeflexia or areflexia.

4. **Diagnosis**

a. The diagnosis of CIP is confirmed by nerve conduction studies, which show slowed conduction in sensory and motor fibers (20).

b. The diagnosis of CIM is confirmed by electromyo-
graphy (which shows myopathic changes) and by
muscle biopsy (which shows atrophy, loss of myosin
filaments, and inflammatory infiltration) (21).

5. **Outcome**

There is no specific treatment for CIP or CIM. Complete
recovery is expected in about half the patients (20), but
it can take months to recover.

III. NEUROMUSCULAR BLOCKADE

1. Drug-induced neuromuscular blockade is used to facilitate endotracheal intubation, to prevent shivering during induced hypothermia, and to facilitate mechanical
ventilation in patients who are severely agitated and
difficult to ventilate (22).

2. Neuromuscular blocking agents act by binding to
acetylcholine receptors on the postsynaptic membranes.
There are two different modes of action:

a. *Depolarizing agents* act like acetylcholine and produce
a sustained depolarization of the post-synaptic mem-

brane. *Succinylcholine* is the only depolarizing agent available for clinical use.

b. *Non-depolarizing agents* act by inhibiting depolarization at the post-synaptic membrane. These agents include *pancuronium, vecuronium, rocuronium, atracurium,* and *cisatracurium.*

A. Selected Neuromuscular Blockers

The comparative features of three commonly used neuromuscular blocking agents are shown in Table 41.4 (23).

Table 41.4	Features of Commonly Used Neuromuscular Blocking Agents		
	Succinylcholine	**Rocuronium**	**Cisatracurium**
IV Bolus Dose	1 mg/kg	0.6 mg/kg	0.15 mg/kg
Onset Time	1–1.5 min	1.5–3 min	5–7 min
Recovery Time	10–12 min	30–40 min	40–50 min
Infusion Rate	—	5–10 mg/kg/min	1–3 mg/kg/min
Cardiovascular Effects	Bradycardia	None	None
Contraindications	Multiple†	None	None

†Hyperkalemia, malignant hyperthermia, rhabdomyolysis, burns, muscular dystrophy, spinal cord injuries. Adapted from Reference 23.

1. Succinylcholine

Succinylcholine is a depolarizing agent with a rapid onset

of action (60–90 seconds) and a rapid recovery time (10–12 minutes). Because of these features, succinylcholine is used to facilitate endotracheal intubation.

a. SIDE EFFECTS: Succinylcholine-induced depolarization of skeletal muscle promotes the efflux of K^+ from muscle cells, which can be problematic in the following conditions: hyperkalemia, malignant hyperthermia, rhabdomyolysis, burns, muscular dystrophy, and spinal cord injuries. Succinylcholine also promotes bradycardia.

2. **Rocuronium**

Rocuronium is a non-depolarizing agent with a rapid onset of action (1.5–3 minutes) and an "intermediate" recovery time (30–40 min). Because of its rapid onset of action, rocuronium is suitable for endotracheal intubation (e.g., when succinylcholine is not advised). The drug is well tolerated, and has no cardiovascular side effects.

3. **Cisatracurium**

Cisatracurium is a non-depolarizing agent with a prolonged onset of action (5–7 min) and an "intermediate" recovery time. It is an isomer of atracurium, and does not have the risk of histamine release associated with atracurium. Like rocuronium, cisatracurium is well tolerated, and has no cardiovascular side effects.

B. Monitoring

The standard method of monitoring drug-induced paralysis is to apply a series of four low-frequency (2 Hz) electrical pulses to the ulnar nerve at the forearm, and observe for adduction of the thumb. Total absence of thumb adduction is evidence of excessive block. The desired goal is 1 or 2 perceptible twitches, and the drug infusion is adjusted to achieve that end-point (23).

C. Complications

Monitoring the adequacy of sedation during neuromuscular paralysis is not possible, and being awake while paralyzed is both horrifying and painful (24). Additional complications of prolonged neuromuscular paralysis include the following:

1. Critical illness myopathy (described earlier)

2. "Hypostatic" pneumonia (from pooling of respiratory secretions in dependent lung regions)

3. Venous thromboembolism

4. Pressure ulcers of the skin

REFERENCES

1. Chabolla DR. Characteristics of the epilepsies. Mayo Clin Proc 2002; 77:981–990.

2. Holtkamp M, Meierkord H. Nonconvulsive status epilepticus: a diagnostic and therapeutic challenge in the intensive care setting. Ther Adv Neurol Disorders 2011; 4:169–181.

3. Meierkord H, Boon P, Engelsen B, et al. EFNS guideline on the management of status epilepticus in adults. Eur J Neurol 2010; 17:348–355.

4. Brophy GM, Bell R, Claassen J, et al. Guidelines for the evaluation and management of status epilepticus. Neurocrit Care 2012; 17:3–23.

5. Marik PE, Varon J. The management of status epilepticus. Chest 2004; 126:582–591.

6. Wijdicks EF, Sharbrough FW. New-onset seizures in critically ill patients. Neurology 1993; 43:1042–1044.

7. Glauser T, Shinnar S, Gloss D. Evidence-based guideline: Treatment of convulsive status epilepticus in children and adults: Report of the Guideline Committee of the American Epilepsy Society. Epilepsy Currents 2016; 16:48–61.

8. Silbergleit R, Durkalski V, Lowenstein D, et al. for the NETT Investigators. Intramuscular vs intravenous therapy for prehospital status epilepticus. N Engl J Med 2012; 366:591–600.

9. Yasiry Z, Shorvon SD. The relative effectiveness of five antiepileptic drugs in the treatment of benzodiazepine-resistant convulsive status epilepticus: a meta-analysis of published studies. Seizure 2014; 23:167–174.

10. Vincent A, Palace J, Hilton-Jones D. Myasthenia gravis. Lancet 2001; 357:2122–2128.

11. Wittbrodt ET. Drugs and myasthenia gravis. An update. Arch Intern Med 1997; 157:399–408.

12. Drachman DB. Myasthenia gravis. N Engl J Med 1994; 330:1797–1810.

13. Berrouschot J, Baumann I, Kalischewski P, et al. Therapy of myasthenic crisis. Crit Care Med 1997; 25:1228–1235.

14. Saperstein DS, Barohn RJ. Management of myasthenia gravis. Semin Neurol 2004; 24:41–48.

15. Hughes RA, Cornblath DR. Guillain-Barré syndrome. Lancet 2005; 366:1653–1666.

16. Hund EF, Borel CO, Cornblath DR, et al. Intensive management and treatment of severe Guillain-Barré syndrome. Crit Care Med 1993; 21:433–446.

17. Pfeiffer G, Schiller B, Kruse J, et al. Indicators of dysautonomia in severe Guillain-Barré syndrome. J Neurol 1999; 246:1015–1022.

18. Hund E. Neurological complications of sepsis: critical illness polyneuropathy and myopathy. J Neurol 2001; 248:929–934.

19. Bolton CF. Neuromuscular manifestations of critical illness. Muscle & Nerve 2005; 32:140–163.

20. van Mook WN, Hulsewe-Evers RP. Critical illness polyneuropathy. Curr Opin Crit Care 2002; 8:302–310.

21. Lacomis D. Critical illness myopathy. Curr Rheumatol Rep 2002; 4:403–408.

22. Murray MJ, Cowen J, DeBlock H, et al. Clinical practice guidelines for sustained neuromuscular blockade in the adult critically ill patient. Crit Care Med 2002; 30:142–156.

23. Brull SJ, Claudius C. Neuromuscular blocking agents. In: Barash PG, Cullen BF, Stoelting RK, et al, eds. Clinical Anesthesia Fundamentals. Philadelphia: Wolters Kluwer Health, 2015:185–207.

24. Parker MM, Schubert W, Shelhamer JH, et al. Perceptions of a critically ill patient experiencing therapeutic paralysis in an ICU. Crit Care Med 1984; 12:69–71.

Chapter 42

Acute Stroke

This chapter describes the initial evaluation and management of acute stroke, with an emphasis on the use of thrombolytic therapy, and the recommendations in the current clinical practice guidelines on acute stroke (1).

I. DEFINITIONS

1. Stroke is defined as "an acute brain disorder of vascular origin accompanied by neurological dysfunction that persists for longer than 24 hours" (2).

2. Stroke is classified according to the underlying mechanism:

   a. *Ischemic stroke* accounts for 87% of all strokes (3): 80% of ischemic strokes are *thrombotic strokes*, and 20% are *embolic strokes*. Most emboli originate from thrombi in the left side of the heart, but some originate from venous thrombi in the legs that reach the brain through a patent foramen ovale (4).

   b. Hemorrhagic stroke accounts for 13% of all strokes: 97% of hemorrhagic strokes involve intracerebral hemorrhage, and 3% are the result of subarachnoid hemorrhage (3). Epidural and subdural hematomas are not considered to be strokes (2).

3. *A transient ischemic attack* (TIA) is an acute episode of ischemia with focal loss of brain function that lasts less than 24 hours (2). The feature that distinguishes TIA from stroke is the *reversibility of clinical symptoms.* This

does not apply to reversibility of cerebral injury, because *one-third of TIAs are associated with cerebral infarction* (5,6).

II. INITIAL EVALUATION

The evaluation of a patient with suspected acute stroke must proceed quickly; i.e., each minute of cerebral infarction results in the destruction of 1.9 million neurons and *7.5 miles of myelinated nerves* (7).

A. Bedside Evaluation

The clinical presentation of acute stroke is determined by the area of brain that is injured, as demonstrated in Figure 42.1.

1. **Mental Status**

    a. Most cerebral infarctions are unilateral, and do not result in loss of consciousness (8).

    b. When focal neurological deficits are accompanied by coma, the most likely conditions are intracerebral hemorrhage, brainstem infarction, or nonconvulsive seizures.

2. **Aphasia**

    Injury in the left cerebral hemisphere (the dominant hemisphere for speech in 90% of the population) produces *aphasia*, which is a disturbance in the comprehension and/or formulation of language. There can be difficulty with verbal comprehension (*receptive aphasia*), difficulty with verbal expression (*expressive aphasia*), or both (*global aphasia*).

3. **Sensorimotor Loss**

    Injury involving one cerebral hemisphere results in weakness on the opposite or contralateral side of the body (i.e.,

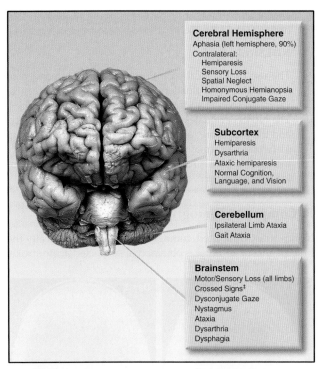

Cerebral Hemisphere
Aphasia (left hemisphere, 90%)
Contralateral:
    Hemiparesis
    Sensory Loss
    Spatial Neglect
    Homonymous Hemianopsia
    Impaired Conjugate Gaze

Subcortex
Hemiparesis
Dysarthria
Ataxic hemiparesis
Normal Cognition,
Language, and Vision

Cerebellum
Ipsilateral Limb Ataxia
Gait Ataxia

Brainstem
Motor/Sensory Loss (all limbs)
Crossed Signs‡
Dysconjugate Gaze
Nystagmus
Ataxia
Dysarthria
Dysphagia

FIGURE 42.1 Areas of brain injury and corresponding neurological abnormalities. ‡Indicates deficits involving the same side of the face and the opposite side of the body.

hemiparesis). Hemiparesis has also been reported in patients with hepatic and septic encephalopathy (9,10).

4. **Stroke Mimics**

As many as 30% of patients with suspected stroke based on clinical findings will have another condition that mimics an acute stroke (11). The most common *stroke mimics* are nonconvulsive seizures, sepsis, metabolic encephalopathies, and space-occupying lesions (in that order) (11).

5. **NIH Stroke Scale**

The use of a clinical scoring system is recommended to standardize the evaluation of acute stroke (1), and the most validated scoring system is the NIH Stroke Scale (NIHSS). The NIHSS evaluates 11 different aspects of performance, and the total score ranges from zero (best performance) to 41 (worst performance); a score of 22 or higher generally indicates a poor prognosis. (The NIHSS can be downloaded from http://stroke.nih.gov/documents.)

B. Computed Tomography

Noncontrast computed tomography (NCCT) is typically the first diagnostic test that is obtained in suspected acute stroke.

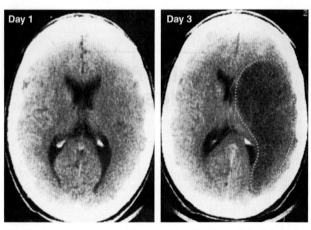

FIGURE 42.2 Noncontrast CT images from the first and third day following an ischemic stroke. The image on day 1 is unrevealing, but the image on day 3 shows a large hypodense area (outlined by the dotted line) with mass effect, representing extensive tissue destruction with intracerebral edema. Images from Reference 13.

1. NCCT has a sensitivity close to 100% for detecting intracranial hemorrhage (5), and the results of NCCT are essential for decisions regarding thrombolytic therapy.

2. NCCT is *not* reliable for visualizing ischemic changes. One-half of ischemic strokes are not apparent on NCCT (12), and the diagnostic yield is even lower in the first 24 hours after an acute stroke (13). The nonvalue of CT imaging in the early post-infarct period is shown in Figure 42.2 (13). The CT image on day 3 shows a large area of infarction with mass effect, which is not apparent in the CT image on day 1 (the day of the stroke).

C. Magnetic Resonance Imaging

1. MRI with diffusion-weighted imaging is the most sensitive and specific technique for the detection of ischemic stroke (1). This technique (which is based on water movement through tissues) can detect ischemic changes within 5–10 minutes after onset (14), and it has a sensitivity of 90% for the detection of ischemic stroke in the early period after stroke onset (5).

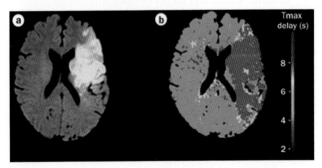

FIGURE 42.3 Diffusion-weighted MRI showing an area of ischemic change (image on the left). The colored image on the right shows areas of hypoperfusion (in red and yellow). Digital subtraction of the ischemic area (on the left) from the area of hypoperfusion (on the right) will reveal areas of threatened infarction. Images from Reference 15.

2. The appearance of diffusion-weighted MRI in ischemic stroke is shown in Figure 42.3 (15). The image on the left shows a large, hyperdense area representing ischemic change. (This differs from CT scans, which show ischemic changes as hypodense areas.) The image on the right is a time-delay technique that detects regions of hypoperfusion using the adjacent color palette.

3. If the ischemic area (on the left) is digitally subtracted from the hypoperfused area (on the right), the remaining colored area represent a region of threatened infarction. This allows an assessment of continued risk in patients with acute ischemic stroke.

D. Echocardiography

Echocardiography has two diagnostic roles in acute stroke:

1. To identify a source of cerebral emboli when ischemic stroke is associated with atrial fibrillation, acute MI, or left-sided endocarditis.

2. To identify a patent foramen ovale in patients with ischemic stroke and recent or prior thromboembolism.

III. THROMBOLYTIC THERAPY

When the initial evaluation identifies a patient with suspected acute stroke, the next step is to determine if the patient is a candidate for thrombolytic therapy.

A. Selection Criteria

The selection criteria for thrombolytic therapy in ischemic stroke are presented as a checklist in Table 42.1. The following points deserve emphasis:

1. Thrombolytic therapy can be used only if it is started within 4.5 hours of symptom onset (1).

Table 42.1	Checklist for Thrombolytic Therapy in Ischemic Stroke

Step 1: Inclusion Criteria

☑ Time of symptom onset can be identified accurately.

☑ Thrombolytic therapy can be started within 4.5 hrs of symptom onset.

If both boxes are checked, proceed to Step 2.

Step 2: Exclusion Criteria

☐ Evidence of active bleeding

☐ Systolic pressure ≥185 mm Hg or diastolic pressure ≥110 mm Hg

☐ History of previous intracranial hemorrhage

☐ Intracranial neoplasm, aneurysm, or AV malformation

☐ Intracranial/intraspinal surgery, serious head trauma, or stroke in past 3 mos.

☐ Thrombin inhibitor or factor Xa inhibitor in past 2 days

☐ Laboratory evidence of a coagulopathy (e.g., platelets <100,000/μL)

☐ Blood glucose <50 mg/dL (2.7 mmol/L)

☐ CT scan shows multilobar infarction (hypodense area >1/3 cerebral hemispheres)

If no boxes are checked, proceed to Step 3.

Step 3: Relative Exclusion Criteria

☐ Major surgery or serious trauma in past 14 days

☐ GI or urinary tract bleeding within past 21 days

☐ Acute MI within past 3 months

☐ Seizure since onset with continued postictal state

Additional criteria for thrombolytic therapy at 3–4.5 hrs after symptom onset:

☐ Age >80 years   ☐ Oral anticoagulant therapy, regardless of INR

☐ Severe stroke   ☐ Diabetes plus a previous stroke (NIHSS >25)

Proceed to Step 4 when no boxes are checked, or when 1 or more boxes are checked, but a risk-benefit analysis favors thrombolytic therapy.

Step 4: Thrombolytic Therapy (begin immediately)

From Reference 1.

2. The time restriction for thrombolytic therapy makes it essential to pinpoint the time of symptom onset, which can be difficult.

3. One of the exclusion criteria for thrombolytic therapy is a systolic pressure ≥185 mm Hg, or a diastolic pressure ≥110 mm Hg. If the patient is otherwise a candidate for thrombolytic therapy, the blood pressure can be lowered to qualify for thrombolytic therapy using the drug regimens in Table 42.2 (1). Following thrombolytic therapy, the blood pressure should be maintained below 180/105 for the next few days to limit the risk of intracranial hemorrhage.

Table 42.2	Blood Pressure Control in Acute Stroke
Trigger	**Drugs & Dosing Regimens**
†SBP >185 mm Hg or DBP >110 mm Hg	Labetalol: 10–20 mg IV over 1–2 min. Can repeat once after 10 min.
	Nicardipine: Infuse at 5 mg/hr, and increase by 2.5 mg/hr every 5–15 min, if necessary, up to 15 mg/hr.
SBP >220 mm Hg or DBP >120 mm Hg	Labetalol: 10 mg IV bolus, then infuse at 2–8 mg/min.
	Nicardipine: Infuse at 5 mg/hr, and increase by 2.5 mg/hr every 5–15 min, if necessary, up to 15 mg/hr.
DBP >140 mm Hg	Nitroprusside: Infuse at 0.2 µg/kg/min and titrate to effect.

†Blood pressure reduction to allow thrombolytic therapy. Adapted from Reference 1.

B. Thrombolytic Regimen

1. Thrombolytic therapy should be initiated as soon as possible, because earlier initiation is associated with better outcomes (1).

2. Recombinant tissue plasminogen activator (tPA) is the only thrombolytic agent approved for use in acute stroke.

3. *Dosing Regimen:* The dose of tPA is 0.9 mg/kg, up to a maximum dose of 90 mg. Ten percent of the dose is given IV over 1–2 minutes, and the remainder is infused over 60 minutes (1).

4. The infusion should be stopped for any signs of possible intracerebral hemorrhage, such as a deteriorating neurological status, a sudden rise in blood pressure, or a complaint of headache.

5. The administration of anticoagulant or antiplatelet agents is contraindicated for the first 24 hours after thrombolytic therapy.

C. Antithrombotic Therapy

1. Several studies have failed to show a beneficial effect of heparin anticoagulation in ischemic stroke (1). Therefore heparin anticoagulation is not recommended in ischemic stroke (1). Low-dose heparin is, however, recommended for thromboprophylaxis (see Chapter 4, Section II).

2. Despite an apparent lack of benefit with aspirin therapy in ischemic stroke, aspirin therapy is recommended as a routine measure in ischemic stroke (1). The initial dose is 325 mg (oral), which is given 24–48 hours after stroke onset (or after thrombolytic therapy), and the daily maintenance dose is 75–150 mg (1).

D. Mechanical Thrombectomy

1. Several (N=8) clinical trials have shown that endovascular thrombectomy is superior to thrombolytic therapy in acute ischemic strokes caused by proximal occlusion of the middle cerebral and internal carotid arteries (16).

2. The thrombectomy was performed within 8 hours of symptom onset in most of the clinical trials.

3. Proceeding to endovascular thrombectomy (if available) does not preclude the early use of thrombolytic therapy.

IV. PROTECTIVE MEASURES

The measures described in this section are designed to limit the extent of ischemic brain injury in acute stroke.

A. Oxygen

1. Oxygen inhalation has been a routine practice in patients with ischemic stroke, even when arterial oxygenation is adequate. This practice has no proven benefit (17), and it neglects the potential for reactive oxygen metabolites (see Figure 36.1) to cause reperfusion injury in the brain. In addition, *oxygen promotes cerebral vasoconstriction* (18), which is counterproductive in ischemic stroke.

2. The current guidelines on stroke management acknowledge the potential for harm from the unrestricted use of oxygen, and recommend supplemental oxygen only when the arterial O_2 saturation falls below 94% (1).

B. Antipyretic Therapy

1. Fever develops within 48 hours in 30% of patients with acute stroke (1), and the presence of fever has adverse effects on the extent of ischemic injury, and the clinical outcome in patients with acute stroke (19). Therefore, aggressive measures to control fever are advised in patients with acute stroke.

2. Antipyretic therapy is described in Chapter 35, Section V.

3. Although post-stroke fever is typically attributed to tissue injury, some studies have found infections in a majority of patients with stroke-related fever (20), so antipyretic therapy should be combined with a search for infection.

C. Glycemic Control

1. Hyperglycemia is common following acute stroke (21), and there is evidence that hyperglycemia aggravates ischemic brain injury and adversely affects outcomes (22). Although there is no evidence that preventing hyperglycemia has clinical benefits (21), attention to glycemic control in poststroke patients seems warranted.

2. Current guidelines recommend a target range of 140–180 mg/dL for plasma glucose in ICU patients (see Reference 1 in Chapter 38). Stricter glycemic control can be hazardous because of the risk of hypoglycemia, which can also aggravate brain injury.

D. Hypertension

1. Hypertension is reported in over half of patients with acute stroke (23), and blood pressures typically return to baseline levels in 2–3 days.

2. There is a reluctance to recommend blood pressure reduction in the early period following acute stroke because of the risk of compromising flow in peri-infarct areas, which could extend the ischemic brain injury.

3. The current guidelines on stroke management (1) recommend blood pressure reduction in the first 24 poststroke hours only when the systolic pressure exceeds 220 mm Hg, or the diastolic blood pressure exceeds 120 mm Hg (unless thrombolytic therapy is used, as described earlier) as long as there are no apparent complications of hypertension (e.g., heart failure).

4. If acute blood pressure reduction is required, the drug regimen in Table 42.2 are recommended (1).

REFERENCES

1. Jauch EC, Saver JL, Adams HP, et al. Guidelines for the early management of patients with acute ischemic stroke. A guideline for healthcare professionals from The American Heart Association/American Stroke Association. Stroke 2013; 44:1–78.

2. Special report from the National Institute of Neurological Disorders and Stroke. Classification of cerebrovascular diseases III. Stroke 1990; 21:637–676.

3. Go AS, Mozaffarian D, Roger VL, et al. Heart disease and stroke statistics—2013 update: A report from the American Heart Association. Circulation 2013; 127:e6–e245.

4. Kizer JR, Devereux RB. Clinical practice. Patent foramen ovale in young adults with unexplained stroke. N Engl J Med 2005; 353:2361–2372.

5. Culebras A, Kase CS, Masdeu JC, et al. Practice guidelines for the use of imaging in transient ischemic attacks and acute stroke. A report of the Stroke Council, American Heart Association. Stroke 1997; 28:1480–1497.

6. Ovbiagele B, Kidwell CS, Saver JL. Epidemiological impact in the United States of a tissue-based definition of transient ischemic attack. Stroke 2003; 34:919–924.

7. Saver JL. Time is brain—quantified. Stroke 2006; 37:263–266.

8. Bamford J. Clinical examination in diagnosis and subclassification of stroke. Lancet 1992; 339:400–402.

9. Atchison JW, Pellegrino M, Herbers P, et al. Hepatic encephalopathy mimicking stroke. A case report. Am J Phys Med Rehabil 1992; 71:114–118.

10. Maher J, Young GB. Septic encephalopathy. Intensive Care Med 1993; 8:177–187.

11. Hand PJ, Kwan J, Lindley RI, et al. Distinguishing between stroke and mimic at the bedside: the brain attack study. Stroke 2006; 37:769–775.

12. Warlow C, Sudlow C, Dennis M, et al. Stroke. Lancet 2003; 362:1211–1224.

13. Graves VB, Partington VB. Imaging evaluation of acute neurologic disease. In: Goodman LR Putman CE, eds. Critical care imaging. 3rd ed. Philadelphia: W.B. Saunders, Co., 1993; 391–409.

14. Moseley ME, Cohen Y, Mintorovich J, et al. Early detection of regional cerebral ischemia in cats: comparison of diffusion- and T_2-weighted MRI and spectroscopy. Magn Reson Med 1990; 14:330–346.

15. Asdaghi N, Coutts SB. Neuroimaging in acute stroke—where does MRI fit in? Nature Rev Neurol 2011; 7:6–7.

16. Chen CJ, Starke RM, Mehndiratta P, et al. Endovascular vs medical management of acute ischemic stroke. Neurology 2015; 85:1980–1990.

17. Ronning OM, Guldvog B. Should stroke victims routinely receive supplemental oxygen: A quasi-randomized controlled trial. Stroke 1999; 30:2033–2037.

18. Kety SS, Schmidt CF. The effects of altered tensions of carbon dioxide and oxygen on cerebral blood flow and cerebral oxygen consumption of normal young men. J Clin Invest 1984; 27:484–492.

19. Reith J, Jorgensen HS, Pedersen PM, et al. Body temperature in acute stroke: relation to stroke severity, infarct size, mortality, and outcome. Lancet 1996; 347:422–425.

20. Grau AJ, Buggle F, Schnitzler P, et al. Fever and infection early after ischemic stroke. J Neurol Sci 1999; 171:115–120.

21. Radermecker RP, Scheen AJ. Management of blood glucose in patients with stroke. Diabetes Metab 2010; 36(Suppl 3):S94–S99.

22. Baird TA, Parsons MW, Phanh T, et al. Persistent poststroke hyperglycemia is independently associated with infarct expansion and worse clinical outcome. Stroke 2003; 34:2208–2214.

23. Qureshi AI, Ezzeddine MA, Nasar A, et al. Prevalence of elevated blood pressure in 563,704 adult patients with stroke presenting to the ED in the United States. Am J Emerg Med 2007; 25:32–38.

Chapter 43

Analgesia & Sedation

Our principal role in caring for the sick is not to save lives (since this is impossible on a consistent basis), but to *relieve pain and suffering*. The analgesic and sedative drug regimens described in this chapter will allow you to serve in this role.

I. ANALGESIA

A. Monitoring Pain

1. Treating pain in critically ill patients requires a reliable pain assessment tool to determine the adequacy of pain relief (1).

   a. A horizontal numeric rating scale can be used for intubated patients who are able to self-report (1). This scale has 10 equally-spaced divider markings, numbered 1 (no pain) to 10 (maximal pain). The patient points to one of the numbered markings to indicate the severity of pain. A score of 3 or less indicates adequate pain control.

   b. When patients are unable to self-report, the Behavioral Pain Scale (BPS) shown in Table 43-1 is a reliable tool for use at the bedside (2).

   c. *Vital signs* (e.g., heart rate) *correlate poorly with* patients' reports of *pain intensity*, and are not recommended to assess pain (1,3).

Table 43.1	The Behavioral Pain Scale	
Item	**Description**	**Score**
Facial Expression	Relaxed	1
	Partially tightened	2
	Fully tightened	3
	Grimacing	4
Upper Limbs	No movement	1
	Partially bent	2
	Fully bent, fingers flexed	3
	Permanently retracted	4
Compliance with Ventilation	Tolerating ventilator	1
	Coughing, but tolerating ventilator	2
	Fighting ventilator	3
	Unable to control ventilator	4
	Total Score	

Score	Interpretation
1	No pain
1–5	Acceptable pain control
12	Maximal pain

From Reference 2.

B. Opioid Analgesia

Pain relief in ICU patients is achieved almost exclusively with *opioids*, which are natural derivatives of opium (opiates) that produce their effects by stimulating discrete opioid receptors in the central nervous system. Stimulation of opioid receptors can produce a variety of beneficial effects, which include analgesia, sedation, and euphoria, but no amnesia (4–6). The most frequently used intravenous opioids are morphine, hydromorphone, and fentanyl. A comparison of these agents is shown in Table 43-2.

Table 43.2	Commonly Used Intravenous Opioids		
	Morphine	**Hydromorphone**	**Fentanyl**
Onset	5–10 min	5–10 min	1–2 min
Bolus Dosing	2–4 mg q 1–2 hr	0.3–0.6 mg q 1–2 hr	0.35–0.5 µg/kg q 0.5–1 hr
Infusion rate	2–30 mg/hr	0.5–3 mg/hr	0.5–2 µg/hr
PCA Demand (bolus)	0.5–3 mg	0.1–0.5 mg	15–75 µg
Lockout interval	10–20 min	5–15 min	3–10 min
Lipid Solubility	x	0.2x	600x
Active Metabolites	Yes	No	No
Histamine Release	Yes	No	No
Dose Adjustment for Renal Failure	↓50%	None	None
Analgesic Potency	x	7x	100x

Dosing recommendations from Reference 1.

1. **Fentanyl**

   a. Fentanyl is the most popular opioid analgesic used in ICUs (7).

   b. The advantages of fentanyl over morphine include a more rapid onset of action (because fentanyl is 600 times more lipid soluble), less risk of hypotension (because fentanyl does not release histamine), and the absence of active metabolites.

   c. The major disadvantage with fentanyl is the tendency of the drug to accumulate in the brain during prolonged infusions (due to the high lipid solubility of the drug).

2. **Hydromorphone**

   a. Hydromorphone is a morphine derivative that may produce more effective analgesia compared to morphine (8,9).

   b. Additional benefits of hydromorphone include lack of active metabolites and no requirement for dose modification in renal failure.

3. **Morphine**

   a. Morphine has several active metabolites that can accumulate in renal failure. One metabolite (morphine 3-glucuronide) can produce central nervous system excitation with myoclonus and seizures (10), while another metabolite (morphine-6-glucuronide) has more potent analgesic effects than the parent drug (5).

   b. To avoid accumulation of these metabolites, *the maintenance dose of morphine should be reduced by 50% in patients with renal failure* (11).

   c. Morphine also promotes the release of histamine, and this can produce systemic vasodilation and a decrease in blood pressure (5).

4. **Remifentanil**

   a. Remifentanil is an ultra-short acting opioid that is given by continuous IV infusion, using the dosing regimen shown below (19).

   DOSING REGIMEN: 1.5 µg/kg as a loading dose, followed by a continuous infusion at 0.5–15 µg/kg/hr (1).

   b. Analgesic effects are lost 8–10 min after stopping the

drug infusion, owing to the breakdown of remifentanil by plasma esterases.

c. Dose adjustments are not required in hepatic or renal failure.

d. Remifentanil's short duration of action is advantageous in conditions that require frequent evaluation of cerebral function (e.g., traumatic brain injury). The abrupt cessation of opioid activity can precipitate acute withdrawal, which can be prevented by combining remifentanil with a longer-acting opioid.

C. Adverse Effects of Opioids

1. **Respiratory Depression**

   a. Opioids produce a centrally-mediated, dose-dependent decrease in respiratory rate and tidal volume, but *respiratory depression and hypoxemia are uncommon when opioids are given in the usual doses* (12,13). Opioid doses that impair arousal also impair ventilation and produce hypercapnia (12).

   b. Patients with sleep apnea syndrome or chronic hypercapnia are particularly prone to respiratory depression from opioids.

2. **Cardiovascular Effects**

   a. Opioid analgesia is often accompanied by decreases in blood pressure and heart rate, which are the result of decreased sympathetic activity and increased parasympathetic activity. These effects are usually mild and well tolerated, at least in the supine position (14).

   b. Decreases in blood pressure can be pronounced in patients with hypovolemia or heart failure (where there is an increased baseline sympathetic tone), or when opioids are given in combination with benzodiazepines (27). Opioid-induced hypotension is rarely a threat to tissue perfusion, and the blood pressure responds to intravenous fluids or small bolus doses of vasopressors.

3. **Intestinal Motility**

   a. Opioids depress bowel motility via activation of opioid receptors in the GI tract. Impaired GI motility can promote reflux of enteral tube feedings into the oropharynx, creating a risk for aspiration pneumonitis.

   b. Opioid-induced bowel hypomotility can be partially reversed with enteral *naloxone* (8 mg every 6 hours) or *naltrexone* (50 mg once a day by mouth) without affecting opioid analgesia (15).

4. **Nausea and Vomiting**

   a. Opioids can promote vomiting via stimulation of the chemoreceptor trigger zone in the lower brainstem (12). All opioids are equivalent in their ability to promote vomiting, but vomiting induced by one opioid occasionally resolves when another opioid is used.

D. Patient-Controlled Analgesia (PCA)

1. For patients who are awake and capable of drug self-administration, *patient-controlled analgesia* (PCA) can be an effective method of pain control, and may be superior to intermittent opioid dosing.

2. The PCA method uses an electronic infusion pump that can be activated by the patient. When pain is sensed, the patient presses a button connected to the pump to receive a small intravenous bolus of drug. After each bolus, the pump is disabled for a mandatory time period called the *lockout interval*, to prevent overdosing.

3. The opioid dosing regimens for PCA are shown in Table 43.2. The minimum lockout interval is a function of the time to achieve peak drug effect (22).

E. Non-Opioid Analgesia

A variety of non-opioid analgesics are available, but only a few of these drugs can be given intravenously. Most of these drugs are used for analgesia in the early postoperative period. They can be used alone for mild pain, but are commonly used in combination with an opioid analgesic for moderate to severe pain. Dosing regimens for non-opioid analgesics are presented in Table 43.3.

1. **Ketorolac**

   a. Ketorolac is a nonsteroidal anti-inflammatory drug (NSAID) that is 350 times more potent than aspirin as an analgesic (16). It does not cause respiratory depression, but other toxic effects limit its use. It is usually given as an adjunct to opioid analgesia, and has an *opioid-sparing effect*.

   b. IM injection of ketorolac can produce hematomas (16), so IV bolus injection is preferred.

   c. The beneficial actions of ketorolac and other NSAIDs are attributed to inhibition of prostaglandin production, but this also creates a risk for adverse effects, particularly gastric mucosal injury, upper GI hemorrhage, and impairment of renal function (16). These side effects are uncommon when use of the drug is limited to 5 days (16).

   d. Ketorolac inhibits platelet aggregation, and should not be used in patients with a high risk of bleeding.

2. **Ibuprofen**

   a. Ibuprofen is very similar to ketorolac because it is an NSAID that can be given intravenously, has an opioid-sparing effect, and is safe when used for short-term pain control (17).

   b. Unlike ketorolac, the treatment period for ibuprofen

has no recommended time limit. Clinical trials of IV ibuprofen typically employ a treatment period of 24–48 hours, and serious complications are uncommon over that time period.

Table 43.3	Intravenous Non-Opioid Analgesia	
Agent	**Dosing Regimens and Comments**	
Ketorolac	Dosing:	30 mg IV or IM every 6 hrs, for up to 5 days. Reduce dose by 50% for age ≥65 yrs or body weight <50 kg.
	Comment:	Ketorolac is an NSAID, and has anti-inflammatory and antipyretic effects. Serious complications are uncommon when treatment is limited to 5 days.
Ibuprofen	Dosing:	400–800 mg IV every 6 hrs.
	Comment:	Ibuprofen is an NSAID, like ketorolac, but has no limit on duration of use.
Acetaminophen	Dosing:	1 g IV every 6 hrs. Daily dose should not exceed 4 g.
	Comment:	No anti-inflammatory effects (which is a major disadvantage in critically ill patients).
Ketamine	Dosing:	0.1–0.5 mg/kg IV loading dose followed by 0.05–0.4 mg/kg/hr.
	Comment:	Attenuates the development of acute tolerance to opioids. May cause hallucinations, psychological disturbances, and hypersalivation.

Dosing recommendations from Reference 1.

3. Acetaminophen

   a. Acetaminophen was approved for intravenous use in 2010, and is intended for the short-term treatment of pain and fever in postoperative patients who are unable to receive acetaminophen via the oral or rectal routes (18).

b. Acetaminophen has an opioid-sparing effect in postoperative patients.

c. Acetaminophen has no anti-inflammatory activity, which is a major disadvantage in critically ill patients, who often have pain as a result of systemic or localized inflammation. Furthermore, *although the daily dose limitation of 4 grams is intended to avoid hepatotoxicity, the toxic dose has not been evaluated in critically ill patients.*

4. **Oral agents for neuropathic pain**

   a. Non-opioid analgesia is usually required for neuropathic pain (e.g., from diabetic neuropathy), and the recommended drugs for this type of pain are *gabapentin, pregabalin* and *carbamazepine* (1).

   b. Effective drug doses vary in individual patients, but typical doses are 600 mg every 8 hours for gabapentin, 50–100 mg every 8 hours for pregabalin, and 100 mg every 6 hours for carbamazepine (oral suspension) (1).

5. **Ketamine**

   a. Ketamine induces a dissociative state of anesthesia but also has potent analgesic effects (19).

   b. At low doses, ketamine has been shown to prevent secondary hyperalgesia and chronic pain after surgery (19).

   c. Ketamine is most commonly used as an analgesic adjunct in cases where patients fail to respond to escalating doses of opioids (e.g., in chronic opioid users).

   d. The lack of adverse hemodynamic and respiratory effects makes ketamine potentially desirable as both an analgesic adjunct and sedative.

   e. The effective dose remains unclear, and the long-term safety effects of ketamine are unknown. A suggested dosing regimen is listed in Table 43.3.

II. SEDATION

Anxiety and related disorders (agitation and delirium) are observed in as many as 85% of patients in the ICU (20). The common denominator in these disorders is the *absence of a sense of well-being*. These disorders can be defined as follows:

1. Anxiety is characterized by exaggerated feelings of fear or apprehension that are sustained by internal mechanisms more than external events.

2. Agitation is a state of anxiety that is accompanied by increased motor activity.

3. Delirium is an acute confusional state that may, or may not, have agitation as a component. Although delirium is often equated with agitation, there is a hypoactive form of delirium that is characterized by lethargy (delirium is described in more detail in Chapter 40).

A. Assessment of Sedation

1. The routine use of sedation scales is instrumental in achieving effective sedation in the ICU (1). The sedation scales that are most reliable in ICU patients are the Sedation-Agitation Scale (SAS) and the Richmond Agitation-Sedation Scale (RASS) (1). The latter scale is shown in Table 43.4 (20).

   a. The added advantage of RASS is the ability to monitor serial changes in a patient's mental state (21). This feature allows the RASS score to be used as the end-point of sedative drug therapy (sedative drug infusions can be titrated to achieve a RASS score of -1 to -2, which represents light sedation).

Table 43.4	Richmond Agitation-Sedation Scale (RASS)	

Score	Term	Description
+4	Combative	Overly combative or violent; immediate danger to staff
+3	Very agitated	Pulls on or removes tube(s)/catheter(s), or aggressive behavior
+2	Agitated	Frequent non-purposeful movement or patient-ventilator asynchrony
+1	Restless	Anxious or apprehensive but movements not aggressive or vigorous
0	Alert & calm	
−1	Drowsy	Not fully alert, but awakens for >10 sec, with eye contact, to voice
−2	Light sedation	Briefly awakens (<10 sec), with eye contact, to voice
−3	Moderate sedation	Any movement (but no eye contact) to voice
−4	Deep sedation	No response to voice, but movement to physical stimulation
−5	Unarousable	No response to voice or physical stimulation

To determine the RASS proceed as follows:

Step 1 Observation: Observe the patient without interaction. If patient is alert, assign the appropriate score (0 to +4). If patient is not alert, go to Step 2.

Step 2 Verbal Stimulation: Address patient by name in a loud voice and ask the patient to look at you. Can repeat once if necessary. If patient responds to voice, assign the appropriate score (−1 to −3). If there is no response, go to Step 3.

Step 3 Physical Stimulation: Shake the patient's shoulder. If there is no response, rub the sternum vigorously. Assign the appropriate score (−4 to −5).

From Reference 21, adapted from *Am J Respir Crit Care Med.* 2002; 166: 1338-1344.

Table 43.5	Sedation with Intravenous Benzodiazepines	
Feature	**Midazolam**	**Lorazepam**
Loading Dose	0.01–0.05 mg/kg	0.02–0.04 mg/kg (max = 2 mg)
Onset of Action	2–5 min	5–20 min
Duration of Effect	1–2 hrs	2–6 hr
Continuous Infusion	0.02–0.1 mg/kg/hr	0.01–0.1 mg/kg/hr (max =10 mg/hr)
Intermittent Bolus Dosing	—	0.02–0.06 mg/kg q 2–6 hrs, prn
Lipophilicity	+++	++
Specific Concerns	Active Metabolite[†]	Propylene Glycol Toxicity[§]

[†]The active metabolite prolongs sedation, especially in renal failure.

[§]Lorazepam (2mg/mL) contains propylene glycol (830 mg/mL) as a solvent.

Dosing recommendations from Reference 1.

B. Benzodiazepines

Once the most popular sedative drugs in the ICU (1), benzodiazepines are gradually falling out of favor because of the *propensity for drug accumulation and prolonged sedation*. Two benzodiazepines are used for sedation in ICUs: midazolam and lorazepam (diazepam is no longer used because of excessive sedation with prolonged use). Both drugs are given intravenously; a brief profile of each drug is presented in Table 43.5.

1. **Midazolam**

   a. Midazolam (Versed) is a rapid-acting drug (by virtue

of its high lipid solubility); sedative effects are apparent within 1–2 minutes after an intravenous bolus dose of the drug.

b. Avid uptake of midazolam into tissues results in rapid clearance from the bloodstream, resulting in a short duration of action (22).

c. Because of the short-lived effect (1–2 hrs), midazolam is given as a continuous IV infusion for more prolonged sedation. However, because the brief drug effect is due to avid drug uptake into tissues (rather than drug elimination from the body), a continuous infusion of midazolam will result in progressive drug accumulation in tissues. To avoid excessive sedation from drug accumulation, *midazolam infusions should be limited to ≤48 hours* (22).

d. Midazolam is metabolized by the cytochrome P450 enzyme system, and drugs that interfere with this enzyme system (e.g., diltiazem, erythromycin) can inhibit midazolam metabolism and potentiate its effects.

e. Midazolam has one active metabolite that is cleared by the kidneys, so alterations in renal function can influence midazolam dosing.

2. **Lorazepam**

a. Lorazepam (Ativan) is a longer-acting drug than midazolam, with effects lasting up to 6 hours after a single IV dose of the drug (1).

b. Lorazepam can given by intermittent IV injections, or by continuous IV infusion.

c. The IV preparation of lorazepam contains propylene glycol, a solvent used to increase drug solubility in plasma. This solvent has adverse effects (see later), which is why lorazepam dosing has a maximum allowable dose (2 mg for bolus doses, and 10 mg/hr for continuous infusions).

    d. Lorazepam has no active metabolites.

3. **Advantages of Benzodiazepines**

    a. Benzodiazepines have a dose-dependent amnestic effect that is distinct from the sedative effect. This effect extends beyond the sedation period (antegrade amnesia).

    b. Benzodiazepines have anticonvulsant effects (see Chapter 41).

    c. Benzodiazepines are the sedatives of choice for drug withdrawal syndromes, including alcohol, opiate, and (surprise) benzodiazepine withdrawal.

4. **Disadvantages of Benzodiazepines**

    a. PROLONGED SEDATION: Both midazolam and lorazepam accumulate in tissues with prolonged use, and this produces deeper levels of sedation, and prolongs the time for awakening when the drugs are discontinued. Prolonged sedation is more of a problem with midazolam, because of its greater lipid solubility, and the accumulation of its active metabolite.

        1) Daily interruption of benzodiazepine infusions (until the patient awakens) curtails drug accumulation, and has been shown to hasten weaning from mechanical ventilation (23).

        2) Titration of benzodiazepine infusions to maintain light levels of sedation, using routine monitoring with a sedation scale (SAS or RASS), has been proposed in the most recent guidelines on sedation in ICUs (3).

    b. DELIRIUM: Benzodiazepines produce their effects by binding to receptors for gamma aminobutyric acid (GABA), the principal inhibitory neurotransmitter in the brain, and GABA-mediated neurotransmission is also involved in the development of delirium (24).

Sedation with drugs that do not involve GABA receptors is associated with fewer cases of delirium in ICU patients (1).

c. PROPYLENE GLYCOL TOXICITY: Intravenous preparations of lorazepam contain propylene glycol (830 mg/mL per lorazepam vial of 2 mg/mL) to enhance drug solubility in plasma. Propylene glycol is converted to lactic acid in the liver, and excessive intake of propylene glycol can produce a toxidrome characterized by a metabolic (lactic) acidosis, delirium (with hallucination), hypotension, and (in severe cases) multiorgan failure.

1) An unexplained metabolic acidosis during prolonged (>24 hours) infusions of lorazepam should prompt a measurement of the serum lactate levels, and an elevated lactate should raise suspicion of propylene glycol toxicity.

2) Plasma levels of propylene glycol can be measured, but the results may not be immediately available. If this is the case, an *elevated osmolal gap* (see Chapter 27, Section I-D for a description) can be a marker of propylene glycol accumulation.

d. WITHDRAWAL SYNDROME: Abrupt termination of prolonged benzodiazepine infusions can produce a withdrawal syndrome, characterized by agitation, disorientation, hallucinations, and seizures (25). However, this does not appear to be a common occurrence with benzodiazepine use in the ICU.

C. Propofol

Propofol is a rapidly-acting general anesthetic that acts through an interaction with the inhibitory neurotransmitter γ-aminobutyric acid (GABA) (26).

1. **Actions and Uses**

   a. Propofol has sedative and amnestic effects, but no analgesic effects (26).

   b. Because of its short duration of action, propofol is given as a continuous infusion. When the infusion is stopped, awakening occurs within 10–15 minutes, even with prolonged infusions (26).

   c. Propofol can be useful in head injuries and neurosurgical patients because it reduces intracranial pressure (26), and the rapid arousal allows for frequent evaluations of mental status.

2. **Preparation and Dosage**

   a. Propofol is suspended in a 10% lipid emulsion to enhance solubility in plasma. This lipid emulsion is almost identical to 10% Intralipid used in parenteral nutrition formulas, and has a caloric density of 1 kcal/mL (which should be included as part of the daily caloric intake).

   b. Dosing recommendations for propofol are shown in Table 43.6. *Dosing is based on ideal rather than actual body weight,* and no dose adjustment is required for renal failure or hepatic insufficiency (26). Loading doses are not advised in patients who are hemodynamically unstable (because of the risk of hypotension) (1).

   c. Green urine is occasionally noted during propofol infusions, and is caused by harmless phenolic metabolites (26).

3. **Adverse Effects**

   a. Propofol is a respiratory depressant, and should only be used during mechanical ventilation.

   b. Propofol-induced hypotension is attributed to systemic vasodilation (22), and can be profound in conditions like hypovolemia and heart failure (where blood pressure is maintained by systemic vasoconstriction).

c. Anaphylactoid reactions to propofol are uncommon but can be severe (26).

d. The lipid emulsion in propofol preparations can promote hypertriglyceridemia. However, hypertriglyceridemia is common in ICU patients, and is not associated with adverse outcomes (27).

e. *Propofol infusion syndrome* is a rare and poorly understood condition that is characterized by the abrupt onset of bradycardic heart failure, lactic acidosis, rhabdomyolysis, and acute renal failure (28).

   1) This syndrome almost always occurs during prolonged, high-dose propofol infusions (>4–6 mg/kg/hr for longer than 24–48 hrs) (28).

   2) The mortality rate is 30% (28).

   3) Avoiding propofol infusion rates above 5 mg/kg/hr for longer than 48 hrs is recommended to reduce the risk of this condition (28).

D. Dexmedetomidine

1. **Actions and Uses**

   a. Dexmedetomidine is a selective alpha-2 adrenergic agonist that has sedative, amnestic, and mild analgesic effects, yet does not depress ventilation. A brief profile of the drug is presented in Table 43.6.

   b. The sedation produced by dexmedetomidine is unique because *arousal is maintained, despite deep levels of sedation*. Patients can be aroused from sedation without discontinuing the drug infusion, and when awake, patients are able to communicate and follow commands. When arousal is no longer required, the patient is allowed to return to the prior state of sedation. This property makes dexmedetomidine an appealing sedative for weaning patients from mechanical ventilation.

c. Clinical studies have shown a lower prevalence of delirium in patients who are sedated with dexmedetomidine instead of midazolam, and based on these studies, *dexmedetomidine is recommended over benzodiazepines for the sedation of patients with ICU-acquired delirium* (1).

Table 43.6	Sedation with Rapid-Arousal Drugs	
Feature	**Propofol**	**Dexmedetomidine**
Loading Dose	25 μg/kg over 5 min†	1 μg/kg over 10 min†
Onset of Action	<1 min	1–3 min
Maintenance Infusion	5–50 μg/kg/min	0.2–0.7 μg/kg/hr§
Time to Arousal	10–15 min	6–10 min
Respiratory Depression	Yes	No
Adverse Effects	Hypotension Hyperlipidemia Propofol Infusion Syndrome	Hypotension Bradycardia Sympathetic Rebound

†Use loading dose only in hemodynamically stable patients.

§Infusion rate may be increased to 1.5 mg/kg/hr as tolerated.

Dosing recommendations from Reference 1.

2. Dosage

a. Dosing recommendations are summarized in Table 43.6. Prolonged (>24 hrs) drug infusions do not adversely affect arousal, even at higher than recommended doses (up to 1.5 μg/kg/hr) (1).

3. **Adverse Effects**

   a. The most common side effects of dexmedetomidine are hypotension and bradycardia (sympatholytic effects) (1,29). Hypotension is most prominent in patients with hypovolemia or heart failure.

   b. Hypertension and hypotension have been observed following loading doses. Hypertension is attributed to activation of peripheral α-2b receptors (which promote vasoconstriction) and hypotension is a consequence of central α-2a receptor activation (which promote vasodilation) (30).

E. Haloperidol

1. **Actions and Uses**

   a. Haloperidol (Haldol) is a first-generation antipsychotic agent that has a long history of treating agitation and delirium (31).

   b. Haloperidol produces its effects by blocking dopamine receptors in the central nervous system.

   c. Following an IV bolus dose of haloperidol, sedation is evident in 10–20 minutes, and the effect lasts 3–4 hours. *Because haloperidol has a delayed onset of action, this agent is not appropriate when rapid sedation is required.*

   d. The lack of respiratory depression makes haloperidol well suited for sedation during weaning from mechanical ventilation (31). Hypotension is unusual in the absence of hypovolemia.

2. **Dosing**

   a. The dosing recommendation for intravenous haloperidol are shown in Table 43.7.

Table 43.7	Intravenous Haloperidol for the Agitated Patient

Severity of Anxiety	Dose
Mild	0.5–2 mg
Moderate	5–10 mg
Severe	10–20 mg

1. Administer dose by IV push.
2. Allow 10–20 min for response:
3. If no response, double the drug dose, or add lorazepam (1 mg).
4. If still no response, switch to another sedative.
5. Give ¼ of the loading dose every 6 hr for maintenance of sedation.

Adapted from References 1 and 31.

b. Individual patients show a wide variation in serum drug levels after a given dose of haloperidol (1,31). Therefore, if there is no evidence of a sedative response after 10–20 min, the dose should be doubled. If there is a partial response, a second dose can be given along with 1 mg lorazepam (preferred to midazolam because of the longer duration of action) (31).

c. Lack of response to a second dose of haloperidol should prompt a switch to another agent.

3. **Adverse Effects**

a. *Extrapyramidal reactions* (e.g., rigidity, spasmodic movements) are dose-related side effects of oral haloperidol, but *are uncommon when haloperidol is given intravenously* (for unclear reasons) (31).

b. The *neuroleptic malignant syndrome* (described in Chapter 35) is an idiosyncratic reaction to neuroleptic agents like haloperidol, and presents with hyperpyrexia, severe muscle rigidity, and rhabdomyolysis. This condition has been reported with IV haloperidol (31), and should be considered in all cases of unexplained fever in patients receiving haloperidol.

c. *Prolongation of the QT interval* can trigger *polymorphic ventricular tachycardia*, which has been reported in up to 3.5% of patients receiving IV haloperidol (31).

REFERENCES

1. Barr J, Fraser GL, Puntillo K, et al. Clinical practice guidelines for the management of pain, agitation, and delirium in adult patients in the intensive care unit. Crit Care Med 2013; 41(1):263–306.

2. Chanques G, Sebbane M, Barbotte E, et al. A prospective study of pain at rest: incidence and characteristics of an unrecognized symptom in surgical and trauma versus medical intensive care unit patients. Anesthesiology 2007; 107:858–860.

3. Jacobi J, Fraser GL, Coursin DB, et al. Clinical practice guidelines for the sustained use of sedatives and analgesics in the critically ill adult. Crit Care Med 2002; 30:119–141.

4. Murray MJ, Plevak DJ. Analgesia in the critically ill patient. New Horizons 1994; 2:56–63.

5. Pasternak GW. Pharmacological mechanisms of opioid analgesics. Clin Neuropharmacol 1993; 16:1–18.

6. Veselis RA, Reinsel RA, Feshchenko VA, et al. The comparative amnestic effects of midazolam, propofol, thiopental, and fentanyl at equisedative concentrations. Anesthesiology 1997; 87:749–764.

7. Payen J-F, Chanques G, Mantz J, et al, for the DOLOREA Investigators. Current practices in sedation and analgesia for mechanically ventilated critically ill patients. Anesthesiology 2007; 106:687–695.

8. Quigley C. A systematic review of hydromorphone in acute and chronic pain. J Pain Symptom Manag 2003; 25:169–178.

9. Felden L, Walter C, Harder S, et al. Comparative clinical effects of hydromorphone and morphine: a meta-analysis. Br J Anesth 2011; 107:319–328.

10. Smith MT. Neuroexcitatory effects of morphine and hydromorphone: evidence implicating the 3-glucuronide metabolites. Clin Exp Pharmacol Physiol 2000; 27:524–528.

11. Aronoff GR, Berns JS, Brier ME, et al. Drug Prescribing in Renal Failure: Dosing Guidelines for Adults. 4th ed. Philadelphia: American College of Physicians, 1999.

12. Bowdle TA. Adverse effects of opioid agonists and agonist-antagonists in anaesthesia. Drug Safety 1998; 19:173–189.

13. Bailey PL. The use of opioids in anesthesia is not especially associated with nor predictive of postoperative hypoxemia. Anesthesiology 1992; 77:1235.

14. Schug SA, Zech D, Grond S. Adverse effects of systemic opioid analgesics. Drug Safety 1992; 7:200–213.

15. Meissner W, Dohrn B, Reinhart K. Enteral naloxone reduces gastric tube reflux and frequency of pneumonia in critical care patients during opioid analgesia. Crit Care Med 2003; 31:776–780.

16. Ketorolac Tromethamine. In: McEvoy GK, ed. AHFS Drug Information, 2012. Bethesda: American Society of Health System Pharmacists, 2012:2139–2148.

17. Scott LJ. Intravenous ibuprofen. Drugs 2012; 72:1099–1109.

18. Yeh YC, Reddy P. Clinical and economic evidence for intravenous acetaminophen. Pharmacother 2012; 32:559–579.

19. Parashchanka A, Schelfout S, Coppens M. Role of novel drugs in sedation outside the operating room: dexmedetomidine, ketamine, and remifentanil. Curr Opin Anesthesiol 2014; 27(4):442–447.

20. Ely EW, Inouye SK, Bernard GR, et al. Delirium in mechanically ventilated patients: validity and reliability of the confusion assessment method for the intensive care unit (CAM-ICU). JAMA 2001; 286:2703–2710.

21. Ely EW, Truman B, Shintani A, et al. Monitoring sedation status over time in ICU patients: reliability and validity of the Richmond Agitation-Sedation Scale (RASS). JAMA 2003; 289:2983–2991.

22. Devlin JW, Roberts RJ. Pharmacology of commonly used analgesics and sedatives in the ICU: benzodiazepines, propofol, and opioids. Crit Care Clin 2009; 25:431–449.

23. Kress JP, Pohlman AS, O'Connor MF, et al. Daily interruption of sedative infusions in critically ill patients undergoing mechanical ventilation. N Engl J Med 2000; 342:1471–1477.

24. Zaal IJ, Slooter AJC. Delirium in critically ill patients: epidemiology, pathophysiology diagnosis and management. Drugs, 2012; 72:1457–1471.

25. Shafer A. Complications of sedation with midazolam in the intensive care unit and a comparison with other sedative regimens. Crit Care Med 1998; 26:947–956.

26. McKeage K, Perry CM. Propofol: a review of its use in intensive care sedation of adults. CNS drugs 2003; 17:235–272.

27. Devaud JC, Berger MM, Pannatier A. Hypertriglyceridemia: a potential side effect of propofol sedation in critical illness. Intensive Care Med 2012; 38:1990–1998.

28. Fodale V, LaMonaca E. Propofol infusion syndrome: an overview of a perplexing disease. Drug Saf 2008; 31:293–303.

29. Parashchanka A, Schelfout S, Coppens M. Role of novel drugs in sedation outside the operating room: dexmedetomidine, ketamine, and remifentanil. Curr Opin Anesthesiol 2014; 27(4):442–447.

30. Carollo DS, Nossaman BD, Ramadhyani U. Dexmedetomidine: a review of clinical applications. Curr Opin Anaesthesiol 2008; 21:457–461.

31. Haloperidol. In: McEvoy GK, ed. AHFS Drug Information, 2012. Bethesda: American Society of Health System Pharmacists, 2012:2542–2547.

Chapter 44

Antimicrobial Therapy

This chapter describes the intravenous antibiotics you are most likely to use in the ICU. Each is presented in the order shown below.

1. Aminoglycosides (gentamicin, tobramycin, amikacin)

2. Antifungal agents (amphotericin B, fluconazole, echinocandins)

3. Carbapenems (imipenem, meropenem)

4. Cephalosporins (ceftriaxone, ceftazidime, cefepime)

5. Fluoroquinolones (ciprofloxacin, levofloxacin, moxifloxacin)

6. Penicillins (piperacillin-tazobactam)

7. Vancomycin and alternatives (linezolid, tigecycline, daptomycin)

I. AMINOGLYCOSIDES

The aminoglycosides (gentamicin, tobramycin, and amikacin) were once the darlings of critical care antibiotics, but their popularity has waned because of nephrotoxicity.

A. Activity & Clinical Uses

1. Aminoglycosides are active against staphylococci and gram-negative aerobic bacilli, including *Pseudomonas aeruginosa* (1). Amikacin has the greatest antibacterial activity of the aminoglycosides, and (as indicated in

Table 44.1) it is currently the most active antibiotic against *Pseudomonas aeruginosa* (2).

2. Aminoglycosides can be used to treat any serious infection caused by gram-negative bacilli. However, because of the risk of nephrotoxicity, they are generally reserved for life-threatening infections involving *P. aeruginosa*.

3. In cases of gram-negative bacteremia associated with neutropenia or septic shock, there is evidence that empiric antibiotic therapy is more effective if an aminoglycoside is added to another drug with activity against gram-negative bacilli (3).

Table 44.1	Antibiotic Susceptibilities for the Most Frequently Isolated Gram-Negative Organisms in ICU Patients in the U.S.		
Antibiotic	E. coli	Klebsiella spp	P. aeruginosa
Amikacin	100%	95%	97%
Tobramycin	86%	89%	89%
Imipenem	100%	96%	72%
Meropenem	100%	95%	73%
Cefepime	91%	88%	76%
Ceftazidime	91%	88%	76%
Ciprofloxacin	65%	87%	71%
Levofloxacin	65%	89%	67%
Piperacillin/ Tazobactam	91%	86%	71%

From Reference 2, which includes data from 65 hospitals collected over a 2-year period (2009–2011). The 3 organisms in the table accounted for 57% of total (3,946) gram-negative isolates.

B. Dosage

Aminoglycoside dosing is based on body weight and renal function.

1. Aminoglycoside dosing is based on *ideal body weight* (see Appendix 2 for tables on ideal body weight).

2. For obese patients (body weight >20% above ideal body weight), dosing is based on an adjusted body weight, which is the ideal body weight plus 45% of the difference between the actual body weight (ABW) and the ideal body weight (IBW) (1); i.e.,

$$\text{Adjusted Weight} = \text{IBW} + 0.45\,(\text{ABW} - \text{IBW}) \quad (44.1)$$

3. Recommended dosing regimens for the aminoglycosides are shown in Table 44.2 (1).

   a. Standard doses of aminoglycosides often produce subtherapeutic drug levels in critically ill patients (4), so higher doses are recommended (at least initially) for ICU patients.

   b. Once-daily dosing is favored for aminoglycosides because outcomes are not adversely affected, and the onset of nephrotoxicity is delayed (1).

   c. Dose reduction is necessary when renal function is impaired (1). This is achieved by extending the dosing interval and/or reducing the amount of drug that is administered.

C. Drug Levels

Monitoring serum drug levels is essential for optimal dosing of aminoglycosides, especially in patients with renal insufficiency.

1. Peak drug levels (drawn one hour after initiating a dose) are used as an indication of therapeutic effect. The

target peak levels for once-daily dosing are 56–64 µg/mL for amikacin, and 16–24 µg/mL for gentamicin and tobramycin (5).

2. When a pathogen is isolated and a minimum inhibitory concentration (MIC) is available, the ratio of peak drug concentration (C_{max}) to MIC is a more reliable measure of therapeutic effect. Aminoglycosides are most effective when C_{max}/MIC ratio is 8–10 (4).

Table 44.2	Aminoglycoside Dose Recommendations		
Creatinine Clearance (mL/min)	Gentamicin Tobramycin (mg/kg)	Amikacin (mg/kg)	Dosing Interval
≥80	7	20	24 hr
60–79	5	15	24 hr
40–59	4	12	24 hr
20–39	4	12	48 hr
10–19	3	10	48 hr
<10	2.5	7.5	48 hr

From Reference 1.

D. Adverse Effects

1. **Nephrotoxicity**

   a. Aminoglycosides are known as *obligate nephrotoxins* because renal impairment will eventually develop in all patients. Increases in serum creatinine usually appear after one week of therapy (9).

   b. The mechanism is accumulation of aminoglycosides in renal tubular cells, which culminates in lethal cell injury and acute tubular necrosis (1).

c. Nephrotoxic effects are enhanced by hypovolemia, renal disease, hypokalemia, loop diuretics, and vancomycin (1,6).

2. **Less Frequent Toxicities**

a. Aminoglycosides can produce irreversible hearing loss and vestibular damage (1). The incidence of ototoxicity is unclear, but low-frequency hearing loss has been reported in 13% of patients who received gentamicin (7). There is no clear relationship between aminoglycoside dose and the risk of ototoxicity.

b. Aminoglycosides can inhibit acetylcholine release from presynaptic nerve terminals (8), but clinically apparent muscle weakness has only been reported on rare occasions in patients with myasthenia gravis (9).

II. ANTIFUNGAL AGENTS

The pathogenic fungi of concern in critically ill patients are *Candida* species (primarily *Candida albicans),* so the description of antifungal agents is limited to their role in treating *Candida* infections.

A. Amphotericin B

1. **Activity & Clinical Uses**

Amphotericin B (AmB) is active against all *Candida* species except *C. lusitaniae* (a rare pathogen) (10), but it is not favored for treating *Candida* infections because of the risk of adverse effects. Instead, AmB is reserved for cases of intolerance or resistance to other antifungal drugs (11).

2. **Dosage**

a. Central venous cannulation is preferred for AmB infusions to reduce the risk of infusion-related phlebitis (10).

b. AmB is given once daily in an intravenous dose of 0.5–1 mg/kg (10,12). The dose is usually delivered over 4 hours, but it can be delivered in one hour, if tolerated.

c. The total AmB dose is 0.5–4 grams, and is determined by the type and severity of the fungal infection.

3. **Adverse Effects**

a. SYSTEMIC INFLAMMATORY RESPONSE: Infusions of AmB are accompanied by fever, chills, and rigors in about 70% of instances (12). This reaction is most pronounced with the initial infusion, and diminishes in intensity with repeated infusions. The following measures help to reduce the severity of this reaction (12):

1) Thirty minutes before the infusion, give acetaminophen (10 to 15 mg/kg orally) and diphenhydramine (25 mg orally or IV).

2) If rigors are a problem, give meperidine (25 mg IV).

3) If the above measures do not provide adequate relief, add hydrocortisone to the AmB infusate (0.1 mg/mL).

b. NEPHROTOXICITY: AmB can damage the renal tubules and produce a *renal tubular acidosis* (distal type), with increased urinary excretion of potassium and magnesium (13). Hypokalemia and hypomagnesemia are common consequences.

1) The serum creatinine rises above 2.5 mg/dL in 30% of patients after 2–3 weeks of AmB infusions, and 15% of these patients may eventually require dialysis (14). Therefore, a rise in serum creatinine to 2.5 mg/dL during AmB therapy should prompt cessation of the drug for a few days, or a switch to a lipid AmB preparation (see next).

4. **Lipid Preparations**

Specialized lipid preparations of AmB have been developed to reduce the binding of AmB to mammalian cells (thereby reducing the risk of renal injury). Two lipid preparations are available: *liposomal AmB*, and *AmB lipid complex*. The dose for both preparations is 3–5 mg/kg daily (10). A comparison study showed a lower incidence of renal injury with the liposomal AmB preparation (13).

B. Fluconazole

Fluconazole is an azole antifungal agent (like itraconazole and voraconazole) that was introduced in 1990 as the first oral antifungal agent.

1. **Activity & Clinical Uses**

   a. Fluconazole is active against *Candida albicans, C. tropicalis*, and *C. parapsilosis*, but is not active against *C. krusei* and *C. glabrata* (10).

   b. According to the 2016 guidelines on treating candidiasis (11), fluconazole is a second-line drug for invasive candidiasis involving susceptible organisms, and is suitable only for patients who are not seriously ill (i.e., non-ICU patients) and have no prior exposure to azole drugs.

   c. Fluconazole is the preferred agent for symptomatic urinary tract infections involving susceptible organisms, and for infections involving *C. parapsilosis* (11).

2. **Dosage**

   a. Fluconazole can be given orally or IV using the same dose.

   b. The dose for invasive candidiasis is 800 mg IV initially, then 400 mg IV daily (11).

   c. A 50% dose reduction is recommended for a creatinine clearance <50 mL/min (10).

3. **Adverse Effects**

   a. Fluconazole is a potent inhibitor of cytochrome P450 isoenzymes, and drugs that are metabolized by the same P450 isoenzymes will accumulate during therapy with fluconazole. Drugs in this category include drugs that prolong the QT interval (cisapride, erythromycin, quinidine), CNS drugs (carbamazepine, phenytoin, haloperidol, benzodiazepines, opiates) coumadin, and theophylline. Concurrent therapy with fluconazole and cisapride is contraindicated (10), while combined therapy with other interacting drugs can be continued, using serum drug levels to determine the need for dose reduction.

   b. Fluconazole has been implicated in cases of severe and even fatal hepatic injury in HIV patients (16).

C. Echinocandins

The echinocandins are antifungal agents with a broader spectrum of activity than fluconazole. There are 3 drugs in this class: *caspofungin, micafungin,* and *anidulafungin.* Most of the early clinical experience has been with caspofungin.

1. **Activity & Clinical Uses**

   a. The echinocandins are active against all *Candida* species, but have reduced activity against *C. parapsilosis* (17).

   b. The echinocandins are *the preferred antifungal agents for the treatment of invasive candidiasis* (except cases involving *C. parapsilosis*), including patients with septic shock or neutropenia (11). This preference is based on convincing evidence of a survival benefit when invasive candidiasis is treated with echinocandins instead of the other antifungal agents (11,18).

2. **Dosage**

Echinocandins are given intravenously in once-daily doses. The doses for invasive candidiasis are shown below. No dose modification is necessary for renal impairment.

   a. Caspofungin: 70 mg IV initially, then 50 mg IV daily.

   b. Micafungin: 100 mg IV daily.

   c. Anidulafungin: 200 mg IV initially, then 100 mg IV daily.

3. **Adverse Effects**

The echinocandins are relatively free of troublesome side effects. Transient elevations in liver enzymes can occur (17), and a reversible thrombocytopenia has been reported (5).

III. CARBAPENEMS

The carbapenems have the *broadest spectrum of activity of all the available antibiotics.* There are 4 carbapenems (*imipenem, meropenem, doripenem,* and *ertapenem*), but the clinical experience with these drugs has mostly involved imipenem and meropenem.

A. Activity

1. Imipenem and meropenem are active against the following organisms (5):

   a. All aerobic gram-negative bacilli, including *Pseudomonas aeruginosa.*

   b. Most aerobic gram-positive cocci, including *Strep pneumoniae*, methicillin-sensitive *Staph aureus* (MSSA), and *Staph epidermidis.*

c. All gram-positive and gram-negative anaerobic organisms, including *Enterococcus faecalis* and *Bacteroides fragilis*.

2. Carbapenems are NOT active against methicillin-resistant *Staph aureus* (MRSA) and vancomycin-resistant enterococci (VRE) (5). Activity against *P. aeruginosa* has also been declining in recent years, as demonstrated in Table 44.1.

B. Clinical Uses

1. Because of their broad antibacterial spectrum, carbapenems are popular for empiric antibiotic coverage in critically ill or neutropenic patients who develop a fever (24).

2. The carbapenems have been effective when used alone for empiric antibiotic coverage (24), but a second antibiotic is necessary in ICUs where MRSA or multidrug resistance is prevalent.

3. Meropenem readily crosses the blood-brain barrier, and can be used for gram-negative meningitis.

C. Dosage

The dosing recommendations for imipenem and meropenem are summarized in Table 43.3. Dose reduction is necessary in patients with impaired renal function.

D. Adverse Effects

1. There is an increased risk of seizures in patients treated with carbapenems, but the risk is small (2 seizures per 1000 patients treated) (22). Failure to reduce the carbapenem dose in renal failure may be a contributory factor. Despite early claims that meropenem is less epileptogenic than imipenem, the pooled data from 21 clinical trials shows no difference in the risk of seizures with imipenem and meropenem (22).

Table 44.3	Dose Recommendations for the Carbapenems

Imipenem:

1. Usual dose is 500 mg IV every 6 hr, or 1g IV every 6 hr for *Psuedomonas* infections.

2. Dose reduction is required for creatinine clearance <70 mL/min.

Cr CL (mL/min): 51–70: 500–750 mg every 8 hr
21–50: 250–500 mg every 6 hr
6–20: 250–500 mg every 12 hr
<6: 250–500 mg every 12 hr
plus dialysis every 48 hr

Meropenem:

1. Usual dose is 1 g IV every 8 hr, or 2 g IV every 8 hr for meningitis.

2. Dose reduction is required for creatinine clearance <50 mL/min.

Cr CL (mL/min): 26–50: usual dose every 12 hr
10–25: ½ usual dose every 12 hr
<10: ½ usual dose every 24 hr

From References 5 and 19.

2. Meropenem can reduce serum levels of valproic acid, and this could indirectly precipitate seizures (23).

3. Patients with hypersensitivity reactions to penicillin can occasionally have a hypersensitivity reaction to carbapenems. These reactions usually include a rash or urticaria, and are rarely life-threatening (24).

IV. CEPHALOSPORINS

There are more than 25 cephalosporins available for clinical use, but only 3 (ceftriaxone, ceftazidime, and cefepime) are used more than infrequently in ICU patients.

Table 44.4	Dose Recommendations for the Cephalosporins

Ceftriaxone:

1. Usual dose is 1 g IV daily, or 2 g IV every 12 hr for meningitis.

2. Dose modification is not necessary for renal impairment.

Ceftazidime:

1. Usual dose is 2 g IV every 8 hr for life-threatening infections, and for empiric R_x of neutropenic patients with fever.

2. Dose reduction is required for creatinine clearance ≤ 80 mL/min. In this case, an initial dose of 2 g is given, followed by:

   Cr CL (mL/min): 30–80: 2 g IV every 12–24 hr
   10–29: 2 g IV every 24–36 hr
   <10: 2 g IV every 36–48 hr

Cefepime:

1. Usual dose is 1–2 g IV every 12 hr for life-threatening infections, and 2 g IV every 8 hr for empiric R_x of neutropenic patients with fever.

2. Dose reduction is required for creatinine clearance ≤ 60 mL/min.

   a. For renal dosing, the initial dose is equivalent to the usual dose (1–2 g), followed by:

      Cr CL (mL/min): 30–60: usual dose every 24 hr
      11–29: ½ usual dose every 24 hr
      <11: ¼ usual dose every 24 hr

   b. For empiric R_x of neutropenic patients with fever, the initial dose is 2 g, followed by:

      Cr CL (mL/min): 30–60: 2 g every 12 hr
      11–29: 2 g every 24 hr
      <11: 1 g every 24 hr

From Reference 26.

A. Ceftriaxone

1. Ceftriaxone (Rocephin) is active against gram-negative bacilli (except *Pseudomonas* spp), gram-positive cocci (except MRSA and *Staph epidermidis*), and *Hemophilus influenza*.

2. The principal use of ceftriaxone is for community-acquired pneumonias that require hospital (or ICU) admission (25). Combination therapy with a macrolide (azithromycin) is recommended (25). The rationale for ceftriaxone is its activity against penicillin-resistant pneumococci, which are associated with a poor outcome.

3. Ceftriaxone is also a preferred agent for pneumococcal meningitis, and is a suitable alternative to penicillin G for meningococcal meningitis (26).

4. Dosing recommendations for ceftriaxone are shown in Table 44.4 (26).

B. Ceftazidime

1. Ceftazidime (Ceftaz) is active against gram-negative bacilli, including *P. aeruginosa*, but has limited activity against gram-positive organisms.

2. Ceftazidime was the first non-toxic alternative to the aminoglycosides for *Pseudomonas* infections. However, its popularity has waned as a result of increasing resistance in *Pseudomonas* isolates (see Table 44.1), as well as the introduction of other antipseudomonal agents with a broader spectrum of activity (like cefepime, described next).

3. Dosing recommendations for ceftazidime are shown in Table 44.4 (26).

C. Cefepime

1. Cefepime (Maxipime) is active against gram-negative

bacilli, including *P. aeruginosa*, but has additional activity against gram-positive cocci other than MRSA.

2. Cefepime has become a popular drug for empiric therapy of ICU patients with suspected sepsis, and it is one of the preferred drugs for neutropenic patients with fever (24).

3. Dosing recommendations for cefepime are included in Table 44.4 (26).

D. Adverse Effects

1. Adverse reactions to cephalosporins are uncommon and nonspecific (e.g., rash, diarrhea).

2. There is a 5–15% incidence of cross-antigenicity with penicillin (26), and cephalosporins should be avoided in patients with a history of *serious* (anaphylactic) reactions to penicillin.

V. FLUOROQUINOLONES

The fluoroquinolone antibiotics include ciprofloxacin, levofloxacin and moxifloxacin.

A. Activity & Clinical Uses

1. Fluoroquinolones are active against aerobic gram-negative bacilli, including *Pseudomonas aeruginosa*. However, their current activity against common ICU pathogens is relatively poor (see Table 44.1). As a result, fluoroquinolones are not preferred for serious gram-negative infections in ICU patients.

2. The newer fluoroquinolones (i.e., levofloxacin and moxifloxacin) provide added coverage for respiratory pathogens; i.e., *Strep pneumoniae* (including penicillin-resistant strains), *Mycoplasma pneumoniae*, *Hemophilus influenza*, and *Legionella* species (27).

3. In the ICU, the newer fluoroquinolones are used primarily for community-acquired pneumonias (25) and exacerbations of chronic obstructive lung disease.

B. Dosage

Table 44.5 shows the dosing recommendations for the quinolones (27). These agents can be given orally or IV in the same doses, but IV delivery is advised, at least initially, in ICU patients. The newer agents have longer half-lives than ciprofloxacin, and only require once-daily dosing.

Table 44.5	Dose Recommendations for the Quinolones

Ciprofloxacin:

1. Usual dose is 400 mg IV every 12 hr for serious infections.
2. Dose reduction to 200–400 mg IV every 18–24 hr is required for creatinine clearance <30 mL/min.

Levofloxacin:

1. Usual dose is 750 mg PO or IV every 24 hr for community-acquired pneumonia.
2. Dose reduction is required for creatinine clearance <50 mL/min.

   Cr CL (mL/min): 20–49: 750 mg IV every 48 hr
   10–19: 750 mg initially, then
   500 mg IV every 48 hr

Moxifloxacin:

1. Usual dose is 400 mg PO or IV every 24 hr.
2. Dose modification is not necessary for renal impairment.

From Reference 27.

C. Adverse Effects

1. Ciprofloxacin interferes with the hepatic metabolism of theophylline and warfarin and can potentiate the actions of both drugs (27). The newer fluoroquinolones do not share these drug interactions.

2. Neurotoxic reactions (confusion, hallucinations, seizures) have been reported in 1–2% of patients receiving quinolones (28).

3. Prolongation of the QT interval and polymorphic ventricular tachycardia (*torsades de pointes*) have been reported in association with all quinolones except moxifloxacin. However, this is a rare occurrence (29).

4. Quinolones can aggravate the muscle weakness in patients with myasthenia gravis (27).

5. All quinolones can produce a false-positive urine drug screen for opiates (5).

VI. THE PENICILLINS

Penicillin use in the ICU is restricted largely to the *antipseudomonal* penicillins, which include the carboxypenicillins (carbenicillin, ticarcillin), and the ureidopenicillins (azlocillin, mezlocillin, and piperacillin) (30). Of these, piperacillin is the overwhelming favorite in critically ill patients.

A. Piperacillin-Tazobactam

1. Piperacillin has a broad spectrum of activity, which includes streptococci, enterococci, methicillin-sensitive staphylococci (but not MRSA), *Staph epidermidis*, and aerobic gram-negative bacilli, including *P. aeruginosa*. This spectrum contains most nosocomial bacterial pathogens (except MRSA), although the activity against *P. aeruginosa* is waning (see Table 44.1).

2. The intravenous piperacillin preparation contains tazobactam, a β-lactamase inhibitor that has synergistic activity with piperacillin (39).

3. Because of its broad spectrum of activity, piperacillin-tazobactam (Pip-Tazo) is a preferred agent for empiric antibiotic coverage in critically ill and neutropenic patients (24). However, it should not be used alone when MRSA is a potential pathogen.

4. The usual dose of Pip-Tazo in critically ill patients is 3.375 grams (3 g piperacillin, 0.375 mg tazobactam) IV every 6 hrs (31).

5. Dose reduction is required for a creatinine clearance (Cr CL) ≤40 mL/min (31). For Cr CL = 20–40 mL/min, the dose is 2.25 g every 6 hrs, and for Cr CL <20 ml/min, the dose is 2.25 g every 8 hrs (31).

VII. VANCOMYCIN

Vancomycin is the most frequently used antibiotic in the ICU, but concerns about emerging resistance have prompted a general mandate to limit its use.

A. Activity & Clinical Uses

1. Vancomycin is active against all gram-positive cocci, including all strains of *Staphylococcus aureus* (coagulase-positive, coagulase-negative, methicillin-sensitive, methicillin-resistant) as well as aerobic and anaerobic streptococci (including pneumococci and enterococci) (32).

2. Vancomycin is the drug of choice for infections caused by methicillin-resistant *Staph aureus* (MRSA), *Staph epidermidis*, *Enterococcus faecalis*, and penicillin-resistant pneumococci.

3. About ²/₃ of the vancomycin use in ICUs is attributed to

empiric antibiotic therapy, rather than treatment of pathogen-specific infections (33).

B. Dosage

1. Weight-based dosing is recommended for vancomycin (34). Actual body weight can be used unless the patient is obese (weight >20% above ideal body weight), in which case an adjusted body weight is calculated using Equation 44.1.

2. The standard loading dose is 15–20 mg/kg , but a larger *loading dose of 25–30 mg/kg is recommended for critically ill patients* (34).

3. Maintenance dosing is determined by body weight, renal function, and a target vancomycin level (trough) in blood. A vancomycin dosing nomogram based on these variables is shown in Table 44.6. Note that the target vancomycin level (trough) is 10–20 mg/L for this nomogram.

4. Monitoring vancomycin blood levels is recommended when the drug is used to treat serious infections. Steady-state levels are usually reached after the fourth dose (42). Trough blood levels should be >10 mg/L to prevent the development of resistance. *For serious infections, trough blood levels of 15–20 mg/L are recommended* (34).

C. Adverse Effects

1. **Red Man Syndrome**

   Rapid infusions of vancomycin can be accompanied by vasodilation, flushing, and hypotension (*red man syndrome*) as a result of histamine release from mast cells (32). An infusion rate below 10 mg/min usually prevents this problem.

Table 44.6	Vancomycin Dosing Nomogram*			
Creatinine Clearance (mL/min)	Weight (kg)			
	60–69	70–79	80–89	90–99
>80	1,000 mg q 12 hr	1,250 mg q 12 hr	1,250 mg q 12 hr	1,500 mg q 12 hr
70–79	1,000 mg q 12 hr	1,250 mg q 12 hr	1,250 mg q 12 hr	1,250 mg q 12 hr
60–69	750 mg q 12 hr	1,000 mg q 12 hr	1,000 mg q 12 hr	1,250 mg q 12 hr
50–59	1,000 mg q 18 hr	1,000 mg q 18 hr	1,250 mg q 18 hr	1,250 mg q 18 hr
40–49	750 mg q 18 hr	1,000 mg q 18 hr	1,250 mg q 18 hr	1,250 mg q 18 hr
30–39	750 mg q 24 hr	1,000 mg q 24 hr	1,250 mg q 24 hr	1,250 mg q 24 hr
20–29	750 mg q 24 hr	1,000 mg q 36 hr	1,250 mg q 36 hr	1,250 mg q 36 hr
10–19	1,000 mg q 48 hr	1,000 mg q 48 hr	1,250 mg q 48 hr	1,250 mg q 48 hr
<10	Repeat dose when spot serum vancomycin <20 mg/L			

From UpToDate (www.uptodate.com). Accessed 1/2016.
*Based on a target vancomycin level (trough) of 10–20 mg/L.

2. Ototoxicity

Vancomycin can cause reversible hearing loss for high-frequency sounds when serum drug levels exceed 40 mg/L (35), and permanent deafness has been reported when serum levels exceed 80 mg/L.

3. **Nephrotoxicity**

    Renal insufficiency has been reported in patients receiving vancomycin (36), although some studies have not observed nephrotoxicity when vancomycin is used alone (32).

4. **Hematologic Effects**

    An immune-mediated thrombocytopenia has been reported in 20% of patients receiving vancomycin (37), and neutropenia has been reported in 2–12% of patients who receive the drug for more than 7 days (38).

D. Alternatives to Vancomycin

Vancomycin continues to be a solid performer as a critical care antibiotic, but alternative antibiotics are needed for vancomycin-resistant enterococci (VRE), and for patients with MRSA infections who do not tolerate vancomycin. The following are some proposed alternatives for vancomycin.

1. **Linezolid**

    a. Linezolid (Zyvox) is a synthetic antibiotic that has the same spectrum of activity as vancomycin (including MRSA), but is also active against VRE (32).

    b. The dose is 600 mg IV every 12 hrs.

    c. Linezolid has much better penetration into lung secretions than vancomycin, but original studies suggesting improved outcomes with linezolid in MRSA pneumonia have not been confirmed (39).

    d. Adverse effects attributed to linezolid include thrombocytopenia (with prolonged use) (32), a partially-reversible optic neuropathy (rare) (40), and serotonin syndrome.

2. **Daptomycin**

   a. Daptomycin (Cubicin) is a naturally occurring antibiotic that is active against gram-positive cocci, including MRSA and VRE (32,41).

   b. The recommended dose is 4–6 mg/kg IV once daily. Dose reductions are advised for creatinine clearance <30 mL/min (41).

   c. Daptomycin can be used to treat soft tissue infections or bacteremias involving MRSA and VRE (32). However, it *cannot be used to treat pneumonias* (41) because the drug is inactivated by surfactants in the lung.

   d. The major adverse effect is a skeletal muscle myopathy, and serum CPK levels should be monitored during therapy with daptomycin (41).

3. **Tigecycline**

   a. Tigecycline (Tygacil) is a tetracycline derivative with activity against difficult-to-treat pathogens such as MRSA, VRE, *Acinetobacter baumannii,* and gram-negative bacilli that produce extended-spectrum β-lactamases (42).

   b. The usual dose is 50 mg IV every 12 hrs, and dose modification is not required for renal insufficiency.

   c. A major concern with tigecycline is a meta-analysis of 13 clinical trials showing *increased mortality* associated with the drug (43). The reason for this mortality effect is not clear, but the FDA issued a black box warning about tigecycline (FDA MedWatch, Sept 27, 2013), and the current recommendation is that the drug should be reserved only for cases where alternative therapies are not suitable.

REFERENCES

1. Craig WA. Optimizing aminoglycoside use. Crit Care Clin 2011; 27:107–111.

2. Sader HS, Farrell DJ, Flamm RK, Jones RN. Antimicrobial susceptibility of Gram-negative organisms isolated from patients hospitalized in intensive care units in United States and European hospitals (2009-2111). Diagn Microbiol Infect Dis 2014; 78:443–448.

3. Martinez JA, Cobos-Triqueros N, Soriano A, et al. Influence of empiric therapy with a beta-lactam alone or combined with an aminoglycoside on prognosis of bacteremia due to gram-negative organisms. Antimicrob Agents Chemother 2010; 54:3590–3596.

4. Matthaiou DK, Waele JD, Dimopoulos G. What is new in the use of amino-glycosides in critically ill patients? Intensive Care Med 2014; 40:1553–1555.

5. Gilber DN, Chambers HF, Eliopoulos GM, et al. (eds). The Sanford Guide to Antimicrobial Therapy, 45th ed. Sperryville, VA: Antimicrobial Therapy, Inc, 2015:96–111.

6. Wilson SE. Aminoglycosides: assessing the potential for nephrotoxicity. Surg Gynecol Obstet 1986; 171(Suppl):24–30.

7. Sha S-H, Qiu J-H, Schacht J. Aspirin to prevent gentamicin-induced hearing loss. N Engl J Med 2006; 354:1856–1857.

8. Lippmann M, Yang E, Au E, Lee C. Neuromuscular blocking effects of tobramycin, gentamicin, and cefazolin. Anesth Analg 1982; 61:767–770.

9. Drachman DB. Myasthenia gravis. N Engl J Med 1994; 330:179–1810.

10. Groll AH, Gea-Banacloche JC, Glasmacher A, et al. Clinical pharmacology of antifungal compounds. Infect Dis Clin N Am 2003; 17:159–191.

11. Pappas PG, Kauffman CA, Andes DR, et al. Clinical practice guideline for the management of candidiasis: 2016 update by the Infectious Disease Society of America. Clin Infect Dis 2016; 62:e1–50.

12. Bult J, Franklin CM. Using amphotericin B in the critically ill: a new look at an old drug. J Crit Illness 1996; 11:577–585.

13. Carlson MA, Condon RE. Nephrotoxicity of amphotericin B. J Am Coll Surg 1994; 179:361–381.

14. Wingard JR, Kublis P, Lee L, et al. Clinical significance of nephrotoxicity in patients treated with amphotericin B for suspected or proven aspergillosis. Clin Infect Dis 1999; 29:1402–1407.

15. Wade WL, Chaudhari P, Naroli JL, et al. Nephrotoxicity and other adverse events among inpatients receiving liposomal amphotericin B and amphotericin B lipid complex. Diag Microbiol Infect Dis 2013; 76:361–367.

16. Gearhart MO. Worsening of liver function with fluconazole and a review of azole antifungal hepatotoxicity. Ann Pharmacother 1994; 28:1177–1181.

17. Echinocandins. In: McEvoy GK, ed. AHFS Drug Information, 2014. Bethesda: American Society of Health-System Pharmacists, 2014:511–521.

18. Andes DR, Safdar N, Baddley JW, et al. Impact of treatment strategy on outcomes in patients with candidemia or other forms of invasive candidiasis: A patient-level quantitative review of randomized trials. Clin Infect Dis 2012; 54:1110–1122.

19. Carbapenems. In: McEvoy GK, ed. AHFS Drug Information, 2014. Bethesda: American Society of Health-System Pharmacists, 2014:143–160.

20. Freifeld AG, Bow EJ, Sepkowitz KA, et al. Clinical practice guideline for the use of antimicrobial agents in neutropenic patients with cancer: 2010 update by the Infectious Disease Society of America. Clin Infect Dis 2011; 52:e56–e93.

21. Golightly LK, Teitelbaum I, Kiser TH, et al. (eds). Renal pharmacotherapy: Dosage adjustment of medications eliminated by the kidneys. New York: Springer, 2013.

22. Cannon JP, Lee TA, Clatk NM, et al. The risk of seizures among the carbapenems: a meta-analysis. J Antimicrob Chemother 2014; 69:2043–2055.

23. Baughman RP. The use of carbapenems in the treatment of serious infections. J Intensive Care Med 2009; 24:230–241.

24. Asbel LE, Levison ME. Cephalosporins, carbapenems, and monobactams. Infect Dis Clin N Am 2000; 14:1–10.

25. Mandell LA, Wunderink RG, Anzueto A, et al. Infectious Diseases Society/American Thoracic Society consensus guide-

lines on the management of community-acquired pneumonia in adults. Clin Infect Dis 2007; 44:S27–S72.

26. Third and fourth generation cephalosporins. In: McEvoy GK, ed. AHFS Drug Information, 2014. Bethesda: American Society of Health-System Pharmacists, 2014:82–140.

27. Quinolones. In: McEvoy GK, ed. AHFS Drug Information, 2014. Bethesda: American Society of Health-System Pharmacists, 2014:329–390.

28. Finch C, Self T. Quinolones: recognizing the potential for neuro-toxicity. J Crit Illness 2000; 15:656–657.

29. Frothingham R. Rates of torsade de pointes associated with ciprofloxacin, ofloxacin, levofloxacin, gatifloxacin, and moxi-floxacin. Pharmacother 2001; 21:1468–1472.

30. Wright AJ. The penicillins. Mayo Clin Proc 1999; 74:290–307.

31. Piperacillin and Tazobactam. In: McEvoy GK, ed. AHFS drug information, 2014. Bethesda: American Society of Hospital Pharmacists, 2014:319–324.

32. Nailor MD, Sobel JD. Antibiotics for gram-positive bacterial infections: vancomycin, teicoplanin, quinupristin/dalfopristin, oxazolidinones, daptomycin, dalbavancin, and telavancin. Infect Dis Clin N Am 2009; 23:965–982.

33. Ena J, Dick RW, Jones RN. The epidemiology of intravenous van-comycin usage in a university hospital. JAMA 1993; 269:598–605.

34. Rybak M, Lomaestro B, Rotschafer JC, et al. Therapeutic monitor-ing of vancomycin in adult patients: A consensus review of the American Society of Health System Pharmacists, the Infectious Disease Society of America, and the Society of Infectious Diseases Pharmacists. Am J Heath-Syst Pharm 2009; 66:82–98.

35. Saunders NJ. Why monitor peak vancomycin concentrations? Lancet 1994; 344: 1748–1750.

36. Hanrahan TP, Harlow G, Hutchinson J, et al. Vancomycin-associ-ated nephrotoxicity in the critically ill: A retrospective multivari-ate regression analysis. Crit Care Med 2014; 42: 2527–2536.

37. Von Drygalski A, Curtis B, Bougie DW, et al. Vancomycin-induced immune thrombocytopenia. N Engl J Med 2007; 356:904–910.

38. Black E, Lau TT, Ensom MHH. Vancomycin-induced neutropenia. Is it dose- or duration-related? Ann Pharmacother 2011; 45:629–638.

39. Kali AC, Murthy MH, Hermsen ED, et al. Linezolid versus vancomycin or teicoplanin for nosocomial pneumonia: A systematic review and meta-analysis. Crit Care Med 2010; 38:1802–1808.

40. Rucker JC, Hamilton SR, Bardenstein D, et al. Linezolid-associated toxic optic neuropathy. Neurology 2006; 66:595–598.

41. Daptomycin. In: McEvoy GK, ed. AHFS drug information, 2012. Bethesda: American Society of Hospital Pharmacists, 2012:454–457.

42. Stein GE, Babinchak T. Tigecycline: an update. Diagn Microbiol Infect Dis 2013; 75(4):331–6.

43. Prasad P, Sun J, Danner RL, Natanson C. Excess deaths associated with tigecycline after approval based on noninferiority trials. Clin Infect Dis 2012; 54:1699–1709.

Chapter 45

Hemodynamic Drugs

This chapter focuses on drugs that are given by intravenous infusion to modulate blood pressure and blood flow. The following drugs are described: dobutamine, dopamine, epinephrine, nicardipine, nitroglycerin, nitroprusside, norepinephrine, and phenylephrine. Each is presented in alphabetical order.

I. DOBUTAMINE

Dobutamine is a synthetic catecholamine with both positive inotropic and vasodilator effects (i.e., an *inodilator*).

A. Actions

1. Dobutamine is a β-adrenergic receptor agonist, and binds to β_1- and β_2-receptors in a 3:1 ratio (see Table 45.1) (1,2). Activation of β_1-receptors (in cardiac muscle) produces positive inotropic and chronotropic effects, while activation of β_2-receptors (in vascular smooth muscle) promotes vasodilation.

2. The principal effects of dobutamine include (1,2):

   a. A dose-dependent increase in cardiac output (due to augmentation of stroke volume more than heart rate).

   b. A decrease in ventricular filling pressures.

   c. A decrease in systemic vascular resistance.

   d. Blood pressure can be decreased, unchanged, or increased, depending on the balance between changes in stroke volume and systemic vascular resistance.

Table 45.1	Dosing and Receptor Binding Affinities for Catecholamine Drugs			
Drug	**Usual Dose Range**	**Adrenergic Receptors**		
		α_1	β_1	β_2
Dobutamine	3–20 µg/kg/min	—	+++++	++
Dopamine	3–10 µg/kg/min	—	++++	++
	11–20 µg/kg/min	+++	++++	++
Epinephrine	1–15 µg/min	+++++	++++	+++
Norepinephrine	2–20 µg/min	+++++	+++	++
Phenylephrine	0.1–0.2 mg/min	+++++	—	—

B. Clinical Uses

1. According to the American Heart Association guidelines on the management of heart failure (3), dobutamine should be reserved for cases of severe systolic dysfunction that have progressed to cardiogenic shock or impending shock. Because dobutamine does not reliably raise the blood pressure, hypotension should be corrected with a vasoconstrictor agent before dobutamine is used.

2. The Surviving Sepsis Campaign guidelines on severe sepsis and septic shock (4) recommends dobutamine when fluids and vasoconstrictor drugs do not normalize the central venous O_2 saturation (see Chapter 9).

3. Dobutamine is NOT appropriate for the management of heart failure caused by impaired ventricular filling (i.e., "diastolic" heart failure).

C. Drug Administration

1. Dobutamine is given by continuous intravenous infusion without an initial loading dose.

2. The initial dose rate is 3–5 µg/kg/min, which can be increased in increments of 3–5 µg/kg/min, if necessary. At dose rates above 20 µg/kg/min, the risk of adverse events usually outweighs the benefit (3,4).

D. Adverse Effects

The adverse effects of dobutamine are related to cardiac stimulation:

1. Dobutamine infusions are usually accompanied by a mild increase in heart rate (10–15 beats/min), but greater increments in heart rate (≥30 beats/min) can occur in individual patients (2). Malignant tachyarrhythmias are uncommon during dobutamine infusions.

2. Dobutamine increases myocardial O_2 consumption, and this can hasten depletion of energy stores in the failing myocardium. This concern is one of the reasons that dobutamine is recommended only as a short-term (≤72 hrs) intervention (3).

II. DOPAMINE

Dopamine is an endogenous catecholamine that serves as both a neurotransmitter and a precursor for norepinephrine synthesis. About 25% of a dose of dopamine is taken up into adrenergic nerve terminals and metabolized to norepinephrine (5).

A. Actions

1. **Low Dose Rates**

   At low dose rates (<3 µg/kg/min), dopamine selectively activates dopamine-specific receptors in the renal and splanchnic circulations, which promotes vasodilation and enhanced blood flow in these regions (5). The renal effects of low-dose dopamine are minimal or absent in patients with acute renal failure (6).

2. **Intermediate Dose Rates**

   At intermediate dose rates (3–10 µg/kg/min), dopamine stimulates β-receptors in the heart and systemic circulation, and produces cardiovascular changes very similar to those described for dobutamine.

3. **High Dose Rates**

   At high dose rates (>10 µg/kg/min), dopamine produces a dose-dependent activation of α-receptors, resulting in widespread vasoconstriction and a progressive increase in blood pressure.

B. Clinical Uses

The popularity of dopamine as a hemodynamic support drug has waned considerably in recent years because of troublesome tachyarrhythmias and reports of increased mortality associated with the drug (7). Relevant issues regarding dopamine use are summarized below.

1. Low-dose dopamine was once used in an attempt to increase glomerular filtration rate in patients with acute renal failure, but this practice does not hasten renal recovery (6) and is no longer recommended.

2. Dopamine is no longer a preferred vasopressor in septic shock, and is recommended only for patients with relative or absolute bradycardia and a minimal risk of tachyarrhythmias (4).

3. Dopamine is a consideration in cardiogenic shock because the combined α- and β-agonist actions can raise the blood pressure while also providing positive inotropic support.

C. Drug Administration

1. Like all vasoconstrictors, dopamine can cause extensive tissue necrosis if extravasation occurs, so the drug should be delivered into a large, central vein.

2. Dopamine is given by continuous intravenous infusion, without an initial loading dose.

   a. The initial dose rate is 3–5 µg/kg/min, and this can be titrated upwards every few minutes, if necessary, to achieve the desired effect.

   b. Dose rates of 3–10 µg/kg/min are optimal for augmenting cardiac output.

   c. Dose rates >10 µg/kg/min are usually needed to raise the blood pressure.

   d. The maximum dose rate is usually 20 µg/kg/min; higher dose rates are often accompanied by undesirable levels of tachycardia without additional vasopressor effects.

D. Adverse Effects

1. Tachyarrhythmias are the most common adverse effect; sinus tachycardia and atrial fibrillation are reported in 25% of patients receiving dopamine infusions (7).

2. Other adverse effects of dopamine include gangrene of the digits (5), splanchnic hypoperfusion (5), increased intraocular pressure (9), and delayed gastric emptying (10).

III. EPINEPHRINE

Epinephrine is an endogenous catecholamine that is released by the adrenal medulla in response to physiological stress. It is the most potent naturally-occurring β-agonist.

A. Actions

1. Epinephrine is a non-selective α- and β-receptor agonist, and produces dose-dependent increases in heart rate, stroke volume, and blood pressure (11,12).

2. α-receptor stimulation produces a non-uniform peripheral vasoconstriction, with the most prominent effects in the subcutaneous, renal, and splanchnic circulations. The risk of splanchnic ischemia is one of the major concerns with epinephrine administration (12).

3. Epinephrine has the following metabolic effects (11,12):

   a. β-receptor activation promotes lipolysis and glycolysis, and increases lactate production; the latter effect is often accompanied by hyperlactatemia. (These effects are not prominent with the other, less potent, β-agonists.)

   b. α-receptor stimulation inhibits insulin secretion and promotes hyperglycemia.

B. Clinical Uses

1. Epinephrine is a first-line drug in the resuscitation of cardiac arrest and anaphylactic shock (see Chapters 9 and 15).

2. Epinephrine is also a popular hemodynamic support drug in the early postoperative period following cardiopulmonary bypass surgery.

3. Concerns about the risk for adverse effects have limited the popularity of epinephrine as a vasopressor drug in septic shock, and it is usually reserved for cases that are refractory to conventional vasopressor agents (e.g., norepinephrine) (12).

C. Drug Administration

1. Because of its vasoconstrictor actions, epinephrine should be delivered into a large, central vein.

2. The epinephrine dosing regimens for circulatory support are as follows (11):

   a. CARDIAC ARREST: 1 mg as IV bolus every 3–5 minutes until return of spontaneous circulation.

   b. ANAPHYLACTIC SHOCK: Start infusion at 5 µg/min, and increase dose rate by 2–5 µg/min, if necessary, to achieve the target blood pressure. Usual dose range is 5–15 µg/min.

   c. SEPTIC SHOCK OR POST-BYPASS CIRCULATORY SUPPORT: Start infusion at 1–2 µg/min, and increase dose rate by 1–2 µg/min, if necessary, to achieve the desired blood pressure. Usual dose range is 1–10 µg/min.

D. Adverse Effects

1. Adverse effects of epinephrine include tachyarrhythmias (risk greater than with other catecholamine drugs), hyperglycemia, hypermetabolism with increased whole-body O_2 demands, and splanchnic ischemia (11,12).

2. The hyperlactatemia associated with epinephrine is not considered an adverse effect because it reflects an increased rate of glycolysis, not tissue hypoxia, and the lactate can be used for hepatic gluconeogenesis (the Cori Cycle).

IV. NICARDIPINE

Nicardipine is a calcium channel blocker that acts as an antihypertensive agent.

A. Actions

1. Nicardipine promotes vasodilation by inhibiting calcium influx into vascular smooth muscle cells (13).

2. Vasodilator effects are not uniform, and are greatest in the cerebral circulation (13,14).

3. Nicardipine has negative inotropic effects, but does not affect the function of the sinus or AV nodes (14).

Table 45.2	Continuous Infusion Vasodilator Therapy	
Vasodilator	**Drug Administration**	
Nicardipine	Dosing:	Start infusion at 5 mg/hr, and increase by 2.5 mg/hr every 5–15 min, if needed, to a maximum dose of 15 mg/hr.
	Comment:	Popular drug for hypertensive emergencies.
Nitroglycerin	Dosing:	Start infusion at 5–10 µg/min, and increase by 5–10 µg/min every 5 min to achieve desired effect. Effective dose usually ≤100 µg/min.
	Comment:	Risk of propylene glycol toxicity and nitrate tolerance with prolonged infusions at high dose rates.
Nitroprusside	Dosing:	Start infusion at 0.2–0.3 µg/kg/min, and gradually increase dose every few minutes, if needed to a maximum dose of 3 µg/kg/min (or 1 µg/kg/min in patients with renal failure).
	Comment:	Add thiosulfate to the infusate to limit the risk of cyanide accumulation.

B. Clinical Uses

1. Nicardipine is used for acute control of troublesome hypertension, including postoperative hypertension (15), and hypertensive emergencies (16). It is also a first-line agent in cases of acute ischemic stroke that require

urgent blood pressure reduction to allow thrombolytic therapy (17).

C. Drug Administration

1. Nicardipine is available as an oral medication, but is given by continuous IV infusion for rapid blood pressure control. The drug can be given safely via a peripheral vein.

2. The initial infusion rate is 5 mg/h, and this can be increased in increments of 2.5 mg/h every 5–10 minutes, if needed, to a maximum dose of 15 mg/h (18).

3. Although nicardipine is metabolized in the liver and excreted in the urine, no dose adjustments are required for hepatic or renal insufficiency (18).

D. Adverse Effects

1. Frequently reported adverse effects include headache, facial flushing, hypotension, and (reflex) tachycardia (16,18).

2. Nicardipine can produce profound hypotension in patients with advanced aortic stenosis, and the drug is contraindicated in this condition (18).

V. NITROGLYCERIN

Nitroglycerin (NTG) is an organic nitrate (glyceryl trinitrate) with vasodilator, antiplatelet, and antianginal effects.

A. Actions

1. **Vasodilator Effects**

   a. NTG acts as a vasodilator by virtue of its conversion to nitric oxide, which promotes the relaxation of vascular smooth muscle (19).

    b. The vasodilator effects of NTG are dose-dependent, and involve both arteries and veins; venodilator effects are prominent at low dose rates (<50 µg/min), while arterial vasodilator effects predominate at higher dose rates (20,21).

    c. At low dose rates, NTG produces a decrease in cardiac filling pressures with little or no change in cardiac output (20). As the dose rate is increased, the cardiac output begins to rise as a result of the arterial vasodilator effects. Blood pressure may be unchanged initially, but progressive increases in dose rate will eventually produce a drop in blood pressure.

2. **Antiplatelet Effects**

The conversion of NTG to nitric oxide leads to inhibition of platelet aggregation, and this effect may be responsible for the antianginal effects of NTG (22).

B. Clinical Uses

1. NTG has 3 principal uses in critically ill patients:

    a. Augmenting cardiac output in patients with acute, decompensated heart failure.

    b. Relieving chest pain in patients with unstable angina.

    c. Treating hypertensive emergencies.

C. Drug Administration

1. **Adsorption to Plastic**

    a. As much as 80% of the NTG in infusates can be lost by adsorption to polyvinylchloride (PVC) in standard intravenous infusion systems (21).

    b. NTG does not bind to glass or hard plastics like polyethylene (PET), so drug loss via adsorption can be eliminated by using glass bottles and PET tubing.

2. **Dosing**

a. NTG should be started at a dose rate of $5–10$ μg/min. The rate is then increased in $5–10$ μg/min increments every 5 minutes until the desired effect is achieved.

b. The effective dose is usually ≤ 100 μg/min.

D. Adverse Effects

1. **Adverse Hemodynamic Effects**

a. NTG-induced venodilation can promote hypotension in patients with hypovolemia or right heart failure. In either of these conditions, volume loading is required prior to infusion of NTG.

b. NTG can also produce a precipitous fall in blood pressure in patients who have taken a phosphodiesterase inhibitor for erectile dysfunction within the past 24 hours (20).

c. NTG-induced increases in cerebral blood flow can lead to increased intracranial pressure (23).

d. In patients with ARDS, the pulmonary vasodilator effects of NTG can result in an increase in intrapulmonary shunt fraction and a subsequent decrease in arterial oxygenation (24).

2. **Methemoglobinemia**

The metabolism of NTG produces inorganic nitrites, which can oxidize the iron moiety in hemoglobin to produce methemoglobin. However, overt methemoglobinemia is not a common complication of NTG infusions, and occurs only with prolonged infusions at high dose rates (23).

3. **Solvent Toxicity**

NTG does not readily dissolve in aqueous solutions, and nonpolar solvents such as ethanol and propylene glycol are required to keep the drug in solution. These solvents can accumulate during prolonged infusions.

a. Both ethanol intoxication (25) and propylene glycol toxicity (26) have been reported as a result of NTG infusions.

b. Propylene glycol toxicity is a particular concern because this solvent makes up 30–50% of some NTG preparations (23). (Propylene glycol toxicity is described in Chapter 24, Section I-A-5.)

E. Nitrate Tolerance

1. Tolerance to the vasodilator and antiplatelet actions of NTG can appear after only 24 hours of continuous drug administration (23,27). The underlying mechanism may involve oxidation-induced endothelial dysfunction (27).

2. The most effective measure for preventing or reversing nitrate tolerance is a daily drug-free interval of at least 6 hours (23).

VI. NITROPRUSSIDE

Nitroprusside (NTP) is a rapidly-acting vasodilator with a dangerous tendency to promote cyanide accumulation.

A. Actions

1. The vasodilator actions of NTP, like those of nitroglycerin, are mediated by nitric oxide (19). NTP dilates both arteries and veins, but it is less potent than nitroglycerin as a venodilator, and more potent as an arterial vasodilator.

2. NTP has variable effects on cardiac output in patients with normal cardiac function (28), but it increases cardiac output in patients with decompensated heart failure (29).

B. The Cyanide Burden

1. The NTP molecule is a ferricyanide complex that contains 5 cyanide (CN) atoms bound to an oxidized iron core, and these cyanide moieties are released into the bloodstream when NTP exerts is vasodilator effects.

2. The mechanisms for promoting cyanide clearance are described in Chapter 47 (see Equations 47.1 and 47.2).

   a. The principal mechanism for clearing CN involves the transfer of sulfate ions from thiosulfate (S_2O_3) to CN to produce thiocyanate (SCN), which is then cleared by the kidneys. Healthy adults have enough endogenous thiosulfate to detoxify about 68 mg of NTP (23); at an NTP infusion rate of 2 µg/kg/min (upper therapeutic range) in an 80-kg adult, the ability to detoxify 68 mg of NTP will be lost after only 500 min (8.3 hrs).

   b. A secondary (minor) clearance mechanism for CN involves the binding of CN by methemoglobin to form cyanomethemoglobin.

C. Clinical Uses

1. NTP is used primarily in conditions where rapid reduction of blood pressure is desirable (e.g., hypertensive emergencies, acute aortic dissection).

2. NTP has also been used in the short-term management of acute, decompensated heart failure (29).

3. Despite the proven efficacy of NTP as a vasodilator, the potential for cyanide toxicity has severely curtailed the popularity of this drug (30).

D. Drug Administration

1. Thiosulfate must be added to the NTP infusate to limit CN accumulation. About 500 mg of thiosulfate should be added for every 50 mg of NTP (31).

2. NTP infusions are started at 0.2–0.3 μg/kg/min, and then titrated upward every few minutes to achieve the desired result. The dose rate should not exceed 3 μg/kg/min (31), to limit cyanide accumulation.

3. In renal failure, the dose rate of NTP should not exceed 1 μg/kg/min (31), to limit the risk of thiocyanate toxicity (see later).

E. Cyanide Toxicity

1. The clinical presentation and management of CN intoxication is described in Chapter 47 (see Section II and Table 47.1).

2. One of the early signs of CN intoxication during NTP infusions is a progressive increase in the dose requirement for NTP (*tachyphylaxis*) (23). Signs of impaired oxygen utilization (e.g., lactic acidosis) do not appear until the late stages of CN intoxication (31).

F. Thiocyanate Toxicity

1. When renal function is impaired, thiocyanate can accumulate and produce a neurotoxic syndrome characterized by agitation, hallucinations, generalized seizures, tinnitus and pupillary constriction (32). This clinical picture can be difficult to distinguish from CN intoxication; however, thiocyanate toxicity is not accompanied by a metabolic acidosis (which is characteristic of CN intoxication).

2. The diagnosis is established by the serum thiocyanate

level. Normal levels are below 10 mg/L, and levels above 100 mg/L are associated with clinical toxicity (32).

3. Thiocyanate toxicity can be treated by hemodialysis.

VII. NOREPINEPHRINE

Norepinephrine is a an endogenous catecholamine that serves as an excitatory neurotransmitter. As a clinical drug, norepinephrine is used for its ability to promote widespread vasoconstriction .

A. Actions

1. Norepinephrine is a prominent α-receptor agonist and a mild β_1-receptor agonist. The overall effect is systemic vasoconstriction with variable effects on cardiac output (33).

2. The vasoconstrictor response to norepinephrine is normally accompanied by a decrease in renal blood flow (33). This is not the case in septic shock, where renal blood flow is preserved (or slightly augmented) during norepinephrine infusions (34,35).

B. Clinical Uses

Norepinephrine is currently preferred to dopamine for vasopressor therapy in septic shock (36). This preference is based on studies showing fewer adverse effects (7) and a lower mortality rate (4,36) when norepinephrine is used instead of dopamine in septic shock.

C. Drug Administration

1. Like all vasoconstrictors, norepinephrine should be administered through a large, central vein.

2. Norepinephrine is given by continuous infusion without a loading dose. The initial dose is 2–3 µg/min, and this can be increased in increments of 2–3 µg/min every few minutes, if needed, to achieve the desired response.

3. The effective dose can can vary widely in individual patients. The usual dose range is 2–20 µg/min, and dose rates above 40 µg/min are not advised (33).

D. Adverse Effects

The adverse effects of norepinephrine are primarily related to exaggerated vasoconstriction, which can produce hypoperfusion in vital organs (especially the bowel and kidneys) and can also produce a reflex bradycardia. These adverse effects are magnified by hypovolemia.

VIII. PHENYLEPHRINE

Phenylephrine is a potent vasoconstrictor that has few advantages, and several disadvantages, when compared to other vasopressor drugs.

A. Actions

Phenylephrine is a pure α-receptor agonist that produces intense and widespread vasoconstriction. This effect is usually accompanied by a reflex bradycardia and a decrease in cardiac output (37).

B. Clinical Uses

1. The principal use of phenylephrine is the reversal of hypotension resulting from spinal anesthesia. However, pure α-receptor agonists are not universally favored in this situation because they can aggravate the decrease in cardiac output associated with spinal anesthesia (37).

2. Phenylephrine is NOT recommended for vasopressor support in septic shock because of its deleterious effects on cardiac output and renal perfusion (4).

C. Drug Administration

1. Phenylephrine can be given as a slow IV injection; the initial dose is 0.2 mg (200 µg), and this can be repeated every 5–10 min, using increments of 0.1 mg to a maximum dose of 0.5 mg (37).

2. Phenylephrine can also be infused at a dose rate of 0.1–0.2 mg/min, which is titrated *downward* as soon as feasible (37).

D. Adverse Effects

The adverse effects of phenylephrine are related to exaggerated vasoconstriction, and include reflex bradycardia, low cardiac output, and generalized hypoperfusion of vital organs. These effects are magnified by hypovolemia.

REFERENCES

1. Overgaard CB, Dzavik V. Inotropes and vasopressors: review of physiology and clinical use in cardiovascular disease. Circulation 2008; 118:1047–1056.

2. Dobutamine hydrochloride. In McEvoy GK, ed. AHFS Drug Information, 2014. Bethesda: American Society of Health-System Pharmacists, 2014:1350–1352.

3. Yancy CW, Jessup M, Bozkurt B, et al. 2013 ACCF/AHA guideline for the management of heart failure: a report of the American College of Cardiology Foundation/American Heart Association Task Force on Practice Guidelines. J Am Coll Cardiol 2013; 62:e147–e239.

4. Dellinger RP, Levy MM, Rhodes A, et al. Surviving Sepsis Campaign: International guidelines for management of severe sepsis and septic shock. Crit Care Med 2013; 41:580–637.

5. Dopamine Hydrochloride. In McEvoy GK, ed. AHFS Drug Information, 2014. Bethesda: American Society of Health-System Pharmacists, 2014:1352–1356.

6. Kellum JA, Decker JM. Use of dopamine in acute renal failure: A meta-analysis. Crit Care Med 2001; 29:1526–1531.

7. De Backer D, Biston P, Devriendt J, et al. Comparison of dopamine and norepinephrine in the treatment of shock. N Engl J Med 2010; 362:779–789.

8. Ellender TJ, Skinner JC. The use of vasopressors and inotropes in the emergency medical treatment of shock. Emerg Med Clin N Am 2008; 26:759–786.

9. Brath PC, MacGregor DA, Ford JG, Prielipp RC. Dopamine and intraocular pressure in critically ill patients. Anesthesiology 2000; 93:1398–1400.

10. Johnson AG. Source of infection in nosocomial pneumonia. Lancet 1993; 341:1368 (Letter).

11. Epinephrine. In McEvoy GK, ed. AHFS Drug Information, 2014. Bethesda: American Society of Health-System Pharmacists, 2014:1402–1408.

12. Levy B. Bench-to-bedside review: Is there a place for epinephrine in septic shock? Crit Care 2005; 9:561–565.

13. Amenta F, Tomassoni D, Traini E, et al. Nicardipine: a hypotensive dihydropyridine-type calcium antagonist with a peculiar cerebrovascular profile. Clinical and Experimental Hypertension 2008; 30:808–826.

14. Struyker-Boudier HAJ, Smits JFM, De Mey JGR. The pharmacology of calcium antagonists: a review. J Cardiovasc Pharmacol 1990; 15 (Suppl. 4):S1–S10.

15. Kaplan JA. Clinical considerations for the use of intravenous nicardipine in the treatment of postoperative hypertension. Am Heart J 1990; 119:443–6.

16. Peacock WF, Hilleman DE, Levy PD, et al. A systematic review of nicardipine vs. labetalol for the management of hypertensive crises. Am J Emerg Med 2012; 30:981–993.

17. Ayagari V, Gorelick PB. Management of blood pressure for acute and recurrent stroke. Stroke 2009; 40:2251–2256.

18. Nicardipine hydrochloride [package insert]. Bedminster, NJ: EKR Therapeutics, Inc., 2010.

19. Anderson TJ, Meredith IT, Ganz P, et al. Nitric oxide and nitrovasodilators: similarities, differences and potential interactions. J Am Coll Cardiol 1994; 24:555–566.

20. Nitroglycerin. In: McEvoy GK, ed. AHFS Drug Information, 2014. Bethesda: American Society of Health System Pharmacists, 2014:1860–1863.

21. Elkayam U. Nitrates in heart failure. Cardiol Clin 1994; 12:73–85.

22. Stamler JS, Loscalzo J. The antiplatelet effects of organic nitrates and related nitroso compounds in vitro and in vivo and their relevance to cardiovascular disorders. J Am Coll Cardiol 1991; 18:1529–1536.

23. Curry SC, Arnold-Cappell P. Nitroprusside, nitroglycerin, and angiotensin-converting enzyme inhibitors. In: Blumer JL, Bond GR, eds. Toxic effects of drugs used in the ICU. Crit Care Clin 1991; 7:555–582.

24. Radermacher P, Santak B, Becker H, Falke KJ. Prostaglandin F_1 and nitroglycerin reduce pulmonary capillary pressure but worsen ventilation–perfusion distribution in patients with adult respiratory distress syndrome. Anesthesiology 1989; 70:601–606.

25. Korn SH, Comer JB. Intravenous nitroglycerin and ethanol intoxication. Ann Intern Med 1985; 102:274.

26. Demey HE, Daelemans RA, Verpooten GA, et al. Propylene glycol-induced side effects during intravenous nitroglycerin therapy. Intensive Care Med 1988; 14:221–226.

27. Münzel T, Gori T. Nitrate therapy and nitrate tolerance in patients with coronary artery disease. Curr Opin Pharmacol 2013; 13:251–259.

28. Sodium Nitroprusside. In: McEvoy GK, ed. AHFS Drug Information, 2014. Bethesda: American Society of Health System Pharmacists, 2014:1848–1851.

29. Guiha NH, Cohn JN, Mikulic E, et al. Treatment of refractory heart failure with infusion of nitroprusside. New Engl J Med 1974; 291:587–592.

30. Robin ED, McCauley R. Nitroprusside-related cyanide poisoning. Time (long past due) for urgent, effective interventions. Chest 1992; 102:1842–1845.

31. Hall VA, Guest JM. Sodium nitroprusside-induced cyanide intoxication and prevention with sodium thiosulfate prophylaxis. Am J Crit Care 1992; 2:19–27.

32. Apple FS, Lowe MC, Googins MK, Kloss J. Serum thiocyanate concentrations in patients with normal or impaired renal function receiving nitroprusside. Clin Chem 1996; 42:1878–1879.

33. Norepinephrine Bitartrate. In: McEvoy GK, ed. AHFS Drug Information, 2014. Bethesda: American Society of Health System Pharmacists, 2014:1410–1413.

34. Bellomo R, Wan L, May C. Vasoactive drugs and acute kidney injury. Crit Care Med 2008; 36(Suppl):S179–S186.

35. Desairs P, Pinaud M, Bugnon D, Tasseau F. Norepinephrine therapy has no deleterious renal effects in human septic shock. Crit Care Med 1989; 17:426–429.

36. Fawzy A, Evans SR, Walkey AJ. Practice patterns and outcomes associated with choice of initial vasopressor therapy for septic shock. Crit Care Med 2015; 43:2141–2146.

37. Phenylephrine Hydrochloride. In: McEvoy GK, ed. AHFS Drug Information, 2014. Bethesda: American Society of Health System Pharmacists, 2014:1342–1347.

Chapter 46

Pharmaceutical Drug Overdoses

This chapter describes the manifestations and management of overdoses with the following pharmaceutical agents: acetaminophen, benzodiazepines, β-receptor antagonists, opioids, and salicylates. Each is presented in alphabetical order.

I. ACETAMINOPHEN

Acetaminophen is a ubiquitous analgesic-antipyretic agent that is included in over 600 commercial drug preparations. It is also a hepatotoxin, and is the *most common cause of acute liver failure in the United States* (1). Acetaminophen overdoses are responsible for half of all cases of acute liver failure in the United States, and *half of the overdoses are unintentional* (2).

A. Pathophysiology

The toxicity of acetaminophen is related to its metabolism in the liver (1).

1. A small fraction (5–15%) of acetaminophen is metabolized to form a toxic metabolite that can promote oxidant injury in hepatocytes. This metabolite is normally inactivated by conjugation with glutathione, an intracellular antioxidant.

2. The metabolic burden created by acetaminophen overdose can deplete hepatic glutathione reserves. When this occurs, the toxic metabolite accumulates and promotes hepatocellular injury.

3. **Toxic Dose**

   a. The maximum recommended daily dose of acetaminophen is 3–4 grams (1).

   b. The toxic dose can vary widely in individual patients, but is typically between 7.5 and 15 grams for most adults (3,4).

   c. Malnutrition, ethanol abuse, and chronic illness can increase the susceptibility to acetaminophen toxicity. In these conditions, an acute ingestion of 4 grams of the drug can result in liver damage (1).

B. Clinical Features

1. Symptoms are either absent or nonspecific (e.g., nausea, vomiting) in the first 24 hours after a toxic ingestion.

2. Liver enzymes are not elevated until 24–36 hours postingestion (3).

   a. Elevated aspartate aminotransferase (AST) is the most sensitive marker of acetaminophen toxicity. The rise in AST precedes hepatic dysfunction, and often peaks by 72–96 hours.

3. Evidence of hepatic injury manifests 24–48 hours after ingestion, with steadily rising liver enzymes, jaundice, and coagulopathy.

4. Peak hepatic injury occurs at 3–5 days after the toxic ingestion. Hepatic encephalopathy, acute oliguric renal failure, and lactic acidosis appear during this time period.

C. Predictive Nomogram

The initial patient contact often occurs within 24 hours after drug ingestion, prior to the onset of overt hepatic injury. In this situation, a nomogram is available (see Figure 46.1) that

predicts the risk of hepatic injury based on the plasma acetaminophen level obtained between 4 and 24 hours after drug
ingestion (4).

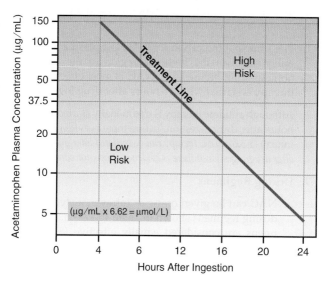

FIGURE 46.1 Nomogram for predicting the risk of acetaminophen
hepatotoxicity. From Reference 4.

1. This nomogram is useful only when the time of drug
   ingestion can be identified, and when the plasma drug
   level can be measured between 4 and 24 hours post-
   ingestion (4).

2. If the plasma level is in the high-risk region of the nomogram, the risk of developing hepatotoxicity is 60% or higher, and antidote therapy is indicated (see next section).

3. If the plasma level is in the low-risk region of the nomogram, the risk of hepatotoxicity is only 1–3%, and antidote therapy is not required.

D. N–Acetylcysteine (Antidote)

The antidote for acetaminophen hepatotoxicity is N-acetyl-cysteine (NAC), a glutathione analogue that crosses cell membranes (which glutathione does not) and inactivates the toxic acetaminophen metabolite (5).

1. The principal indication for NAC is a plasma acetaminophen level in the high-risk region of the predictive nomogram in Figure 46.1. NAC is most effective when therapy is started within 8 hours after drug ingestion (1).

2. Although antidote therapy is traditionally started within 24 hours after drug ingestion (before there is evidence of liver injury) (1,3,6), *NAC therapy can be initiated later than 24 hours after drug ingestion if there is evidence of hepatotoxicity* (1).

3. **Dosing Regimens**

   a. NAC can be given orally or intravenously using the dosing regimens shown in Table 46.1 (7-9). Both regimens are considered equally effective (8), but the intravenous route is preferred because drug delivery is more reliable and there are fewer adverse reactions.

   b. The standard duration of treatment is 21 hours for the intravenous regimen and 72 hours for the oral regimen. If NAC is started after the onset of overt liver injury, antidote therapy can be continued beyond the normal course of therapy, until liver enzyme levels begin to decline and the INR is <1.3 (1).

4. **Adverse Effects**

   a. Intravenous NAC can cause anaphylactoid reactions, and fatal reactions have been reported in asthmatics (10).

   b. Oral NAC has a very disagreeable taste (because of the sulfur content), and often causes nausea and vomiting. The oral NAC regimen produces diarrhea in about 50% of patients, but this usually resolves with continued therapy (11).

Table 46.1	Treatment of Acetaminophen Overdose with N-Acetylcysteine (NAC)

Use 20% NAC (200 mg/mL) for each of the doses below and infuse in sequence.

    1. 150 mg/kg in 200 mL D_5W over 60 min

    2. 50 mg/kg in 500 mL D_5W over 4 hrs

    3. 100 mg/kg in 1,000 mL D_5W over 16 hrs

Total dose: 300 mg/kg over 21 hrs

Oral Regimen:

Use 10% NAC (100 mg/mL) and dilute 2:1 in water or juice to make a 5% solution (50 mg/mL).

    Initial dose: 140 mg/kg

    Maintenance dosage: 70 mg/kg every 4 hrs for 17 doses

Total dose: 1,330 mg/kg over 72 hrs

From Reference 9.

E. Activated Charcoal

1. Acetaminophen is rapidly absorbed from the GI tract, and activated charcoal (1 g/kg) is recommended if given within 4 hours after drug ingestion (12).

2. In cases of massive drug ingestion, charcoal may provide a benefit when given as late as 16 hours post-ingestion (1).

3. Activated charcoal does not interfere with the efficacy of oral NAC (1).

F. Liver Transplantation

Liver transplantation may be required in severe or refractory cases of acetaminophen hepatotoxicity (13).

II. BENZODIAZEPINES

Benzodiazepines are second only to opiates as the drugs most frequently involved in medication-related deaths (14). However, benzodiazepines are rarely fatal when ingested alone (15), and other respiratory depressant drugs (e.g., opiates) are almost always involved in benzodiazepine-related fatalities (14).

A. Clinical Features

Since benzodiazepine overdoses frequently involve other drugs, the clinical presentation may vary, depending on the other agent(s) that have been ingested.

1. Pure benzodiazepine overdoses produce deep sedation but rarely result in coma (15).

2. Benzodiazepine overdoses can also precipitate an agitated state of delirium with hallucinations, which can be mistaken for alcohol withdrawal (15).

3. Uncommon side effects of pure benzodiazepine overdose include respiratory depression (2–12% of cases), bradycardia (1–2% of cases) and hypotension (5–7% of cases) (15).

4. Qualitative tests for benzodiazepines in urine are unreliable because of a limited spectrum of detection (16). The diagnosis of benzodiazepine intoxication is based primarily on the clinical history.

B. Flumazenil (Antidote)

The antidote for benzodiazepine overdoses is flumazenil, a pure antagonist that binds to benzodiazepine receptors but does not exert any agonist actions (17). Flumazenil is effective in reversing benzodiazepine-induced sedation, but is inconsistent in reversing benzodiazepine-induced respiratory depression (18).

1. **Drug Administration**

   a. Flumazenil is given as an intravenous bolus of 0.2 mg, which can be repeated at 1 to 6-minute intervals if necessary, to a total dose of 1 mg (17).

   b. The response is rapid (onset in 1–2 min), and peak effect occurs at 6–10 min (19). The effect lasts about one hour.

   c. Since flumazenil has a shorter duration of action than benzodiazepines, recurrence of sedation is common. To avoid this risk, the bolus dose(s) of flumazenil can be followed by a continuous infusion at 0.3–0.4 mg/hr (20).

2. **Adverse Effects**

   a. Flumazenil can precipitate withdrawal symptoms in patients with a longstanding history of benzodiazepine use, but this is uncommon (21).

   b. Flumazenil can precipitate seizures in patients receiving benzodiazepines for seizure control, and in patients with concomitant overdose with tricyclic antidepressants (22).

III. β-RECEPTOR ANTAGONISTS

Intentional β-blocker overdoses are uncommon, but can be life-threatening. Unintentional β-blocker toxicity is a more common concern in the ICU, where β-blockers are used to manage a number of conditions, including hypertension, tachyarrhythmias, and acute coronary syndromes.

A. Clinical Toxicity

1. The most common manifestations of β-blocker overdose are bradycardia and hypotension (23).

a. The bradycardia is usually sinus in origin, and is often asymptomatic.

b. The hypotension can be due to peripheral vasodilatation (renin blockade), or a decrease in cardiac output (β_1 receptor blockade). Sudden or refractory hypotension is usually a reflection of a decrease in cardiac output, and is an ominous sign.

2. β-blockers can also prolong atrioventricular (AV) conduction via a membrane stabilizing effect that is independent of β-receptor blockade. This can result in complete heart block (24).

3. β-blocker overdoses are often accompanied by neurologic manifestations such as lethargy, depressed consciousness, and generalized seizures (25). These are not the result of β-receptor blockade, and are likely related to membrane stabilizing activity (25).

B. Glucagon (Antidote)

Glucagon can antagonize the cardiovascular effects of β-blockade by virtue of glucagon receptors on cardiac muscle that have the same mechanism of action as β-receptors. This allows glucagon to produce β-like effects that are independent of β-receptor blockade.

1. Indications

a. Glucagon is indicated for the treatment of hypotension and *symptomatic* bradycardia associated with toxic exposure to β-blockers.

b. Glucagon is *not* indicated for reversing the prolonged AV conduction or neurologic manifestations of β-blocker overdose because these effects are not mediated by β-receptor blockade.

Table 46.2	Glucagon as an Antidote
Indications	**Dosing Regimen**
When the actions of β-receptor antagonists or calcium channel blockers result in: 1. Hypotension, or 2. Symptomatic bradycardia	1. Start with 50 µg/kg (or 3 mg) as IV bolus. 2. If response is not satisfactory, give a second IV bolus of 70 µg/kg (or 5 mg). 3. Follow a satisfactory response with a continuous infusion at 70 µg/kg/hr (or 5 mg/hr).

From References 26 and 27.

2. **Dosing Considerations**

   a. The dosing regimen for glucagon is described in Table 46-2 (26,27). A favorable response to the IV bolus dose can be short-lived (5 min), and should be followed by a continuous infusion (5 mg/hr).

   b. When used in the appropriate doses, glucagon will elicit a favorable response within 3 minutes in 90% of patients (26). The chronotropic response to glucagon is optimal when the plasma ionized calcium is normal (28).

3. **Adverse Effects**

   a. Nausea and vomiting are common at glucagon doses above 5 mg/hr.

   b. Mild hyperglycemia is common, and is the result of glucagon-induced glycogenolysis. The insulin response to hyperglycemia can drive K^+ into cells and promote hypokalemia.

   c. Glucagon also stimulates catecholamine release from the adrenal medulla, and this can aggravate an underlying hypertension.

4. **Calcium Antagonist Overdose**

   Glucagon can also antagonize the effects of calcium channel blockers (27), but it is less effective in reversing the cardiac depression produced by calcium antagonist overdoses.

C. Adjunctive Therapy

Phosphodiesterase inhibitors (e.g., milrinone) can increase cardiac output in the setting of β-blockade (29), and this could add to the antagonist effects of glucagon. However, these drugs are vasodilators, and can produce undesired decreases in blood pressure. As a result, these drugs are reserved for cases of β-blocker toxicity that are refractory to glucagon.

IV. OPIOIDS

Opioids are implicated in 75% of fatal drug overdoses in the United States, and given the widespread prevalence of opioid abuse (30), opioid overdoses are likely to remain one of the most common overdoses requiring ICU support.

A. Clinical Features

1. The classic description of opioid intoxication is a patient with stupor, pinpoint pupils, and slow breathing (bradypnea), but these findings are nonspecific and may be absent. As a result, it is often not possible to identify an opiate overdose based on the clinical presentation (30). (See Chapter 43, Section I-C for more information on the adverse effects of opioids.)

2. The response to the opioid antagonist, naloxone, is probably the most reliable method of identifying an opioid overdose.

B. Naloxone (Antidote)

The antidote for opioid intoxication is naloxone, a pure opioid antagonist that binds to endogenous opioid receptors but does not elicit agonist responses. It is most effective in blocking the opioid receptors responsible for analgesia, euphoria, and respiratory depression (30,31).

1. **Routes of Administration**

   Naloxone is usually given as an IV bolus, and the response is apparent within 3 minutes. Alternate routes of delivery include intramuscular injection (onset in 15 min), intraosseous or intralingual injection, and endotracheal instillation (32).

2. **Dosing Considerations**

   Dosing recommendations for naloxone are shown in Table 46.3. Reversing the sedative effects of opioids usually requires smaller doses of naloxone than reversing the respiratory depression.

Table 46.3	Naloxone Dosing Regimens
Depressed Sensorium	**Respiratory Depression**
1. Start with 0.4 mg IV bolus.	1. Start with 2 mg IV bolus.
2. If no response in 2–3 min, give another 0.4 mg IV bolus.	2. If no response in 2–3 min, give 4 mg IV bolus.
3. If no response in 2–3 min, give 2 mg IV bolus.	3. If no response in 2–3 min, give 10 mg IV bolus.
4. If no response in 2–3 min, STOP and reassess.	4. If no response in 2–3 min, give 15 mg IV bolus.
	5. If no response in 2–3 min, STOP and reassess.

From References 21 and 30.

a. For patients with a depressed sensorium but no respiratory depression, the initial dose of naloxone should be 0.4 mg IV push. This can be repeated in 2 minutes, if necessary. *A total dose of 0.8 mg should be effective in reversing the mental status changes induced by opioids* (21).

b. For patients with respiratory depression (e.g., hypercapnia), the initial dose of naloxone should be 2 mg IV push. If there is no response in 2–3 minutes, the initial dose should be doubled. Incremental doses can be given, if necessary, until the dose reaches 15 mg (30). *Opioids are an unlikely cause of respiratory depression if there is no response to 15 mg of naloxone.*

c. The effects of naloxone last about 60 to 90 minutes, which is less than the duration of action of most opioids. Therefore, a favorable response to naloxone should be followed by repeat doses at one-hour intervals, or by a continuous infusion.

d. For a continuous naloxone infusion, the hourly dose of naloxone should be two-thirds of the effective bolus dose (diluted in 250–500 ml of isotonic saline and infused over 6 hours) (33). To achieve steady-state drug levels in the early infusion period, a second bolus of naloxone (at one-half the original bolus dose) is given 30 minutes after the infusion is started. The duration of treatment varies (according to the drug and the dose ingested), but averages 10 hours (21).

3. **Adverse Effects**

Naloxone has few undesirable effects. The most common adverse effect is the opioid withdrawal syndrome (anxiety, abdominal cramps, vomiting, and piloerection). There are case reports of acute pulmonary edema (most in the early postoperative period) and generalized seizures following naloxone administration (21), but these are rare occurrences.

4. **Empiric Therapy**

Empiric therapy with naloxone (0.2–8 mg IV bolus) has been used in patients who present with altered mentation to identify occult cases of opioid overdose. However, this practice identifies opioid overdose in fewer than 5% of cases (34). An alternative approach has been proposed where *empiric naloxone is indicated only for patients with pinpoint pupils and circumstantial evidence of opioid abuse* (e.g., needle tracks) (21,34). When naloxone is used in this manner, a favorable response is expected in about 90% of patients (34).

V. SALICYLATES

Despite a steady decline in prevalence, salicylate intoxication remains the 14th leading cause of drug-induced deaths in the United States (35).

A. Pathophysiology

Ingestion of 10–30 grams of aspirin (150 mg/kg) can have fatal consequences. Once ingested, acetylsalicylic acid (aspirin) is promptly converted to salicylic acid, which is the active form of the drug. Salicylic acid is readily absorbed from the upper GI tract, and is metabolized in the liver. Most of the drug is cleared in the first 2 hours after ingestion.

1. **Respiratory Alkalosis**

Within hours after a toxic ingestion of aspirin, there is an increase in respiratory rate and tidal volume. This is the result of direct stimulation of brainstem respiratory neurons by salicylic acid, and the subsequent increase in minute ventilation results in a decrease in arterial PCO_2 (i.e., acute respiratory alkalosis).

2. **Metabolic Acidosis**

   Salicylic acid is a weak acid that does not readily dissociate, and thus does not produce a metabolic acidosis. However, salicylic acid activates proteins in the mitochondria that uncouple oxidative phosphorylation, and this results in a marked increase in the anaerobic production of lactate, which is the principal source of the metabolic acidosis in salicylate intoxication.

B. Clinical Features

1. The early stages of salicylate toxicity are characterized by nausea, vomiting, tinnitus, tachypnea, and agitation.

2. Progression of the toxidrome is associated with neurologic changes (delirium, seizures, and progression to coma), fever (from the uncoupled oxidative phosphorylation), and acute respiratory distress syndrome (ARDS).

3. The hallmark of salicylate intoxication is the *combination of a respiratory alkalosis and a metabolic (lactic) acidosis.* This results in a low arterial PCO_2 and a low serum bicarbonate level. The arterial pH initially remains in the normal range, but the pH will decrease if the lactic acidosis progresses. A low arterial pH (acidemia) is a poor prognostic sign (36).

C. Diagnosis

1. The plasma salicylate level (which is usually elevated by 4–6 hrs after a toxic ingestion) is used to confirm or exclude the diagnosis of salicylate intoxication.

2. The therapeutic range for plasma salicylates is 10–30 mg/L (0.7–2.2 mmol/L), and plasma levels >40 mg/L (2.9 mmol/L) are considered toxic (36).

D. Management

1. Multiple-dose activated charcoal (25 grams every 2 hrs for 3 doses) is recommended if it can be started within 2–3 hrs of salicylate ingestion.

2. **Urine Alkalinization**

   a. Alkalinization of the urine is the cornerstone of management for salicylate intoxication. An alkaline pH promotes the dissociation of salicylic acid, and this essentially "traps" the salicylic acid in the renal tubules, where it can be excreted in the urine.

   b. A bicarbonate infusion regimen for raising the urine pH is shown in Table 46.4.

Table 46.4	Protocol for Alkalinization of the Urine

1. Start with a bicarbonate loading dose of 1–2 mEq/kg.
2. Create a bicarbonate solution by adding 3 amps $NaHCO_3$ to 1 L D_5W, and infuse this solution at 2–3 mL/kg/hr.
3. Maintain a urine output of 1–2 mL/kg/hr, and a urine pH ≥7.5.

From Reference 34.

   c. Bicarbonate infusions promote hypokalemia (by driving K^+ into cells), and this hampers the ability to alkalinize the urine (because hypokalemia promotes the secretion of H^+, instead of K^+, by the distal tubules). Therefore, K^+ should be added to the bicarbonate solution (40 mEq/L) to reduce the risk of hypokalemia.

3. **Hemodialysis**

   Hemodialysis is the most effective method of clearing salicylates from the body (37).

a. Indications for dialysis include a serum salicylate level >100 mg/L, the presence of renal failure or ARDS, and progressive illness despite alkali therapy (35).

REFERENCES

1. Hodgman M, Garrard AR. A review of acetaminophen poisoning. Crit Care Clin 2012; 28(4):499–516.

2. Larson AM, Polson J, Fontana RJ, et al. Acetaminophen-induced acute liver failure: results of a United States multicenter, prospective study. Hepatology 2005; 42:1364–1372.

3. Hendrickson RG, Bizovi KE. Acetaminophen. In: Flomenbaum NE, et al., eds. Goldfrank's Toxicologic Emergencies. 8th ed. New York: McGraw-Hill, 2006; 523–543.

4. Rumack BH. Acetaminophen hepatotoxicity: the first 35 years. J Toxicol Clin Toxicol 2002; 40:3–20.

5. Holdiness MR. Clinical pharmacokinetics of N-acetylcysteine. Clin Pharmacokinet 1991; 20:123–134.

6. Rumack BH, Peterson RC, Koch GG, et al. Acetaminophen overdose. 662 cases with evaluation of oral acetylcysteine treatment. Arch Int Med 1981; 141:380–385.

7. Howland MA. Flumazenil. In: Flomenbaum NE, et al., eds. Goldfrank's Toxicologic Emergencies. 8th ed. New York: McGraw-Hill, 2006; 1112–1117.

8. Buckley NA, Whyte IM, O'Connell DL, et al. Oral or intravenous N-acetylcysteine: which is the treatment of choice for acetaminophen (paracetamol) poisoning? J Toxicol Clin Toxicol 1999; 37:759–767.

9. Temple AR, Bagish JS. Guideline for the Management of Acetaminophen Overdose. Camp Hill, PA: McNeil Consumer & Specialty Pharmaceuticals, 2005.

10. Appelboam AV, Dargan PI, Knighton J. Fatal anaphylactoid reaction to N-acetylcysteine: caution in patients with asthma. Emerg Med J 2002; 19:594–595.

11. Miller LF, Rumack BH. Clinical safety of high oral doses of acetylcysteine. Semin Oncol 1983; 10:76–85.

12. Spiller HA, Krenzelok EP, Grande GA, et al. A prospective evaluation of the effect of activated charcoal before oral N-acetylcysteine in acetaminophen overdose. Ann Emerg Med 1994; 23:519–523.

13. Lopez AM, Hendrickson RG. Toxin-induced hepatic injury. Emerg Med Clin North Am 2014; 32(1):103–25.

14. Centers for Disease Control and Prevention. National Vital Statistics System. 2010 Multiple Cause of Death File. Hyattsville, MD: US Department of Health and Human Services, Centers for Disease Control and Prevention; 2012.

15. Gaudreault P, Guay J, Thivierge RL, Verdy I. Benzodiazepine poisoning. Drug Saf 1991; 6:247–265.

16. Wu AH, McCay C, Broussard LA, et al. National Academy of Clinical Biochemistry laboratory medicine practice guidelines: Recommendations for the use of laboratory tests to support poisoned patients who present to the emergency department. Clin Chem 2003; 49:357–379.

17. Howland MA. Flumazenil. In: Flomenbaum NE, et al., eds. Goldfrank's Toxicologic Emergencies. 8th ed. New York: McGraw-Hill, 2006; 1112–1117.

18. Shalansky SJ, Naumann TL, Englander FA. Effect of flumazenil on benzodiazepine-induced respiratory depression. Clin Pharm 1993; 12:483–487.

19. Roche Laboratories. Romazicon (flumazenil) package insert. 2004.

20. Bodenham A, Park GR. Reversal of prolonged sedation using flumazenil in critically ill patients. Anaesthesia 1989; 44:603–605.

21. Doyon S, Roberts JR. Reappraisal of the "coma cocktail". Dextrose, flumazenil, naloxone, and thiamine. Emerg Med Clin North Am 1994; 12:301–316.

22. Haverkos GP, DiSalvo RP, Imhoff TE. Fatal seizures after flumazenil administration in a patient with mixed overdose. Ann Pharmacother 1994; 28:1347–1349.

23. Newton CR, Delgado JH, Gomez HF. Calcium and beta receptor antagonist overdose: a review and update of pharmacological principles and management. Semin Respir Crit Care Med 2002; 23:19–25.

24. Henry JA, Cassidy SL. Membrane stabilising activity: a major cause of fatal poisoning. Lancet 1986; 1:1414–1417.

25. Weinstein RS. Recognition and management of poisoning with beta-adrenergic blocking agents. Ann Emerg Med 1984; 13:1123–1131.

26. Kerns W, 2nd, Kline J, Ford MD. Beta-blocker and calcium channel blocker toxicity. Emerg Med Clin North Am 1994; 12:365–390.

27. Howland MA. Glucagon. In: Flomenbaum NE, et al., eds. Goldfrank's Toxicologic Emergencies. 8th ed. New York: McGraw-Hill, 2006:942–945.

28. Chernow B, Zaloga GP, Malcolm D, et al. Glucagon's chronotropic action is calcium dependent. J Pharmacol Exp Ther 1987; 241:833–837.

29. Travill CM, Pugh S, Noblr MI. The inotropic and hemodynamic effects of intravenous milrinone when reflex adrenergic stimulation is suppressed by beta adrenergic blockade. Clin Ther 1994; 16:783–792.

30. Boyer EW. Management of opioid analgesic overdose. N Engl J Med 2012; 367:146–155.

31. Handal KA, Schauben JL, Salamone FR. Naloxone. Ann Emerg Med 1983; 12:438–445.

32. Naloxone hydrochloride. In: McEvoy GK, ed. AHFS Drug Information, 2012. Bethesda: American Society of Hospital Systems Pharmacists, 2012:2236–2239.

33. Goldfrank L, Weisman RS, Errick JK, et al. A dosing nomogram for continuous infusion intravenous naloxone. Ann Emerg Med 1986; 15:566–570.

34. Hoffman JR, Schriger DL, Luo JS. The empiric use of naloxone in patients with altered mental status: a reappraisal. Ann Emerg Med 1991; 20:246–252.

35. Bronstein AC, Spyker DA, Cantilena LR, et al. 2011 Annual Report of the American Association of Poison Control Centers' National Poison Data System (NPDS): 29th Annual Report. Clin Toxicol 2012; 50:911–1164.

36. O'Malley GF. Emergency department management of the salicylate-poisoned patient. Emerg Med Clin N Am 2007; 25:333–346.

37. Fertel BS, Nelson LS, Goldfarb DS. The underutilization of hemodialysis in patients with salicylate poisoning. Kidney Int 2009; 75:1349–1353.

Chapter 47

Nonpharmaceutical Toxidromes

This chapter describes toxic syndromes that are not the result of medications, and includes poisonings caused by carbon monoxide, cyanide, the toxic alcohols (methanol and ethylene glycol), and organophosphates.

I. CARBON MONOXIDE

Carbon monoxide (CO) is a gaseous end-product of incomplete oxidation of organic matter. The principal cause of CO intoxication is smoke inhalation during structural fires. Less frequent sources include faulty furnaces, inadequate ventilation of flame-based heating sources, and the exhaust from hydrocarbon-powered engines (1).

A. Pathophysiology

1. CO binds to the heme moieties in hemoglobin (at the same site that binds O_2) to produce carboxyhemoglobin (COHb). The affinity of CO for binding to Hb is 200–300 times greater than the affinity of O_2 (1,2).

2. Progressive increases in COHb are accompanied by proportional decreases in arterial O_2 content: if severe enough, this can result in inadequate tissue oxygenation and impaired aerobic energy production (1-3).

3. In addition to the deleterious effects of COHb on tissue oxygenation, CO poisoning can promote cell injury via: (a) inhibition of cytochrome oxidase (which further impairs the oxidative production of ATP), (b) genera-

tion of peroxynitrite (a potent oxidant capable of widespread cell injury), and (*c*) enhanced lipid peroxidation by neutrophils (which damages cell and mitochondrial membranes) (1,2,4).

B. Clinical Features

The diagnosis of CO poisoning is based on a history of recent CO exposure, the presence of symptoms, and an elevated COHb level (4).

1. There is no combination of symptoms that confirms or excludes a diagnosis of CO poisoning; COHb levels *do not* correlate with clinical manifestations of CO poisoning (1,4).

2. Headache (usually frontal) and dizziness are the earliest and most common complaints in CO poisoning (reported in 85% and 90% of patients, respectively) (1).

3. Progressive exposure to CO can produce ataxia, confusion, delirium, generalized seizures, and coma (1).

4. Cardiac effects of CO poisoning include elevated biomarkers with normal coronary angiography, and transient LV systolic dysfunction (5).

5. Advanced cases of CO poisoning can be accompanied by rhabdomyolysis, lactic acidosis, and acute respiratory distress syndrome (ARDS) (1).

6. The "cherry red" skin color in classic descriptions of CO poisoning (because COHb is a brighter shade of red than hemoglobin) is a *rare* finding (4).

7. Delayed neurological sequelae are possible (within about one year), usually consisting of cognitive deficits (ranging from mild confusion to severe dementia) and parkinsonism (1,4,6). These occur most frequently following prolonged (24 hrs) exposure to CO, and in patients with loss of consciousness or COHb levels above 25% (4).

C. Diagnosis

The measurement of Hb in its different forms (oxygenated and deoxygenated Hb, COHb, and methemoglobin) is based on light absorption; i.e., each form of hemoglobin reflects light of specific wavelengths. This technique of spectrophotometry is called *oximetry* when it applies to hemoglobin. The following statements summarize the use of oximetry to measure COHb levels in blood:

1. Pulse oximetry is *NOT* reliable for the detection of COHb. Pulse oximeters use two wavelengths of light to measure oxygenated and deoxygenated Hb in blood. Light absorbance at one of the wavelengths (660 nm) is very similar for oxygenated Hb and COHb, *so COHb is measured as oxygenated Hb by pulse oximeters,* and this results in spuriously high readings for O_2 saturation (4).

2. The measurement of COHb requires an 8-wavelength co-oximeter, which measures the relative abundance of all 4 forms of Hb in blood.

3. COHb levels are negligible (<1%) in healthy nonsmokers, but smokers have COHb levels of 3–5% or even higher (4). The threshold for elevated COHb levels is 3–4% for nonsmokers, and 10% for smokers (4).

D. Treatment

1. The principal treatment for CO poisoning is inhalation of 100% oxygen. The elimination half-life of COHb is 320 minutes while breathing room air, and 74 minutes while breathing 100% oxygen (1,4), so only a few hours of breathing 100% oxygen is needed to return COHb levels to normal (<3%).

2. In patients with severe neurologic manifestations, hyperbaric oxygen has been used (with variable results) to reduce the risk and severity of delayed neurologic sequelae (1,7).

II. CYANIDE

The principal source of cyanide (CN) poisoning is inhalation of hydrogen cyanide gas during domestic fires (8,9). Infusion of the vasodilator, sodium nitroprusside, is an additional source of CN toxicity in ICU patients (see Chapter 45).

A. Pathophysiology

1. Cyanide ions have a high affinity for metalloproteins, most notably the oxidized iron (Fe^{3+}) in cytochrome oxidase, the last enzyme system in the electron-transport chain within mitochondria (where the electrons collected during ATP production are used to reduce O_2 to H_2O).

2. CN-induced inhibition of cytochrome oxidase halts the process of oxidative metabolism in mitochondria, which halts the uptake of pyruvate into mitochondria and results in excess production of lactic acid. The accumulation of lactate in plasma produces *a progressive metabolic (lactic) acidosis,* which *is one of the hallmarks of CN poisoning.*

3. Cyanide Clearance

   There are two mechanisms for clearing CN from the body.

   a. The principal clearance mechanism is a transsulfuration reaction, where sulfur is transferred from thiosulfate (S_2O_3) to CN to form thiocyanate (SCN).

   $$S_2O_3 + CN \rightarrow SCN + SO_3 \qquad (47.1)$$

   Thiocyanate is cleared by the kidneys, and can accumulate in patients with renal failure, precipitating an acute psychosis (10).

   b. The second (minor) mechanism for CN clearance is

the reaction of CN with methemoglobin ($Hb\text{-}Fe^{3+}$) to form cyanomethemoglobin.

$$Hb\text{-}Fe^{3+} + CN \rightarrow Hb\text{-}Fe^{2+}\text{-}CN \qquad (47.2)$$

c. These two clearance mechanisms are easily overwhelmed, especially in the setting of thiosulfate deficiency (i.e., in smokers).

B. Clinical Features

1. Early signs of CN poisoning include agitation, tachycardia, and tachypnea. Progressive CN accumulation eventually results in loss of consciousness, bradycardia, hypotension, and cardiac arrest.

2. Plasma lactate levels are typically elevated (>10 mmol/L), and venous blood may appear "arterialized" because of the marked decrease in tissue O_2 utilization.

3. Cyanide poisoning should be strongly suspected if a smoke inhalation victim exhibits a severe metabolic acidosis (pH <7.2) or a markedly elevated lactate level. The time to onset of symptoms after smoke inhalation is rapid, and progression to cardiac arrest can occur in less than 5 minutes (8).

C. Diagnosis

1. Cyanide poisoning is a clinical diagnosis. Whole blood cyanide levels, while useful for purposes of documentation, are typically not readily available. Cyanide antidotes must be administered rapidly and empirically if poisoning is suspected. Diagnosis can be challenging because many of the clinical features of cyanide poisoning are indistinguishable from CO poisoning.

2. As a general rule of thumb, severe metabolic (lactic) aci-

dosis and hemodynamic instability are the clinical features that distinguish CN from CO poisoning in victims of smoke inhalation (8,9).

D. Treatment

Antidote therapy should begin immediately after CN poisoning is suspected. Antidotes for CN poisoning are presented in Table 47.1.

1. **Hydroxocobalamin**

   a. The antidote of choice for CN poisoning is hydroxocobalamin, a cobalt-containing precursor of vitamin B_{12} that combines with CN to form cyanocobalamin, which is then excreted in the urine. The recommended dose is 5 grams, as an IV bolus. A second dose of 5 grams is recommended for patients with cardiac arrest (8).

   b. Hydroxocobalamin is relatively safe to use; urine and other body fluids can have a reddish color for a few days.

2. **Sodium Thiosulfate**

   a. Sodium thiosulfate converts CN to thiocyanate (see Equation 47.1), and is used in combination with hydroxocobalamin. The recommended dose is 12.5 grams as an IV bolus.

   b. Since thiocyanate can accumulate in renal failure and cause an acute psychosis (10), thiosulfate should not be used in patients with renal failure. If thiosulfate is given before evidence of renal failure is available, watch for signs of thiocyanate toxicity (which requires hemodialysis).

3. **Nitrates**

   a. Nitrates promote CN clearance by promoting the formation of methemoglobin (see Equation 47.2).

   b. Nitrates are *contraindicated in smoke inhalation* be-

cause they cause a leftward shift in the oxyhemoglobin dissociation curve, which aggravates the similar
effect of carbon monoxide.

c. The only role for nitrates in CN poisoning is the use
of inhaled amyl nitrate as a temporary measure
when IV access is not available (see Table 47.1 for
dosing regimen).

Table 47.1	Antidotes for Cyanide Poisoning	
Agent	**Dosing Regimens & Comments**	
Hydroxocobalamin	Dosing:	5 grams as IV bolus (10 grams for cardiac arrest).
	Comment:	The antidote of choice for cyanide poisoning. May cause reddish color in urine.
Sodium Thiosulfate (25%)	Dosing:	50 mL (12.5 g) as IV bolus.
	Comment:	Used in combination with hydroxo-cobalamin. Avoid, if possible, in patients with renal failure.
Amyl Nitrate Inhalant	Dosing:	Inhale for 30 sec. each min, for up to 5 min.
	Comment:	Used only for temporary relief when IV access is not available. Contraindicated in smoke inhalation.

From References 8 and 9.

4. **Cyanide Antidote Kits**

a. There are specialized antidote kits for cyanide poisoning (e.g., Akorn Cyanide Antidote Kit) that contain amyl nitrate for inhalation, sodium nitrite
(300 mg in 10 mL) for IV injection, and sodium thiosulfate (12.5 g in 50 mL) for IV injection.

b. These kits can be used as a source of thiosulfate, but they *do not contain hydroxocobalamin* (at least at the present time), and *should not be used alone to treat CN poisoning*.

III. TOXIC ALCOHOLS

Ethylene glycol and methanol are common components of household, automotive, and industrial products, and ingestion of these alcohols produces toxidromes that share many features (see Table 47.2).

A. Ethylene Glycol

Ethylene glycol is the main ingredient in many automotive antifreeze products. It has a sweet, agreeable taste, which makes it a popular method of attempted suicide.

1. Pathophysiology

   a. Ethylene glycol is readily absorbed from the GI tract, and 80% of the ingested dose is metabolized in the liver.

   b. The metabolism of ethylene glycol involves the formation of a series of acids, with the participation of alcohol dehydrogenase and lactate dehydrogenase enzymes, ending with the formation of oxalic acid (Figure 47.1) (12). Each of the intermediate reactions involves the conversion of NAD to NADH, which promotes the conversion of pyruvate to lactate. As a result, serum lactate levels are elevated in ethylene glycol poisoning (12).

   c. Each of the acid intermediates in ethylene glycol metabolism is a strong acid that readily dissociates, and can contribute to a metabolic acidosis with a high anion gap.

Table 47.2	Comparative Features of Poisoning with Toxic Alcohols	
Feature	**Ethylene Glycol**	**Methanol**
Acid-Base	Metabolic Acidosis	Metabolic Acidosis
Anion-Gap	Elevated	Elevated
Osmolar Gap	Elevated	Normal[†]/Elevated
Other Findings	Crystalluria	Visual Impairment
Primary Rx	Fomepizole Hemodialysis	Fomepizole Hemodialysis
Adjunctive Rx	Thiamine Pyridoxine	Folinic Acid

[†]Osmolar gap can be normal in the later stages of illness.

2. **Clinical Features**

a. Early signs of ethylene glycol intoxication include nausea, vomiting, and apparent inebriation. Ethylene glycol is odorless, so there is no odor of alcohol on the breath.

b. Severe cases are accompanied by depressed consciousness, coma, generalized seizures, renal failure, pulmonary edema, and cardiovascular collapse (12). Renal failure can be a late finding (24 hours after ingestion).

c. The oxalic acid formed during ethylene glycol metabolism combines with calcium to form insoluble calcium oxalate crystals, which precipitate in several tissues, particularly the renal tubules. These crystals are a source of renal tubular injury, and are visible on urine microscopy. The shape of the crystals (i.e., thin, monohydrate crystals as opposed to box-shaped dihydrate crystals) is most specific for ethylene glycol poisoning (12).

3. Treatment

a. *Fomepizole*

Fomepizole inhibits alcohol dehydrogenase, the enzyme involved in the initial step of ethylene glycol metabolism (see Figure 47.1). The dosing regimen for both ethylene glycol and methanol poisoning is

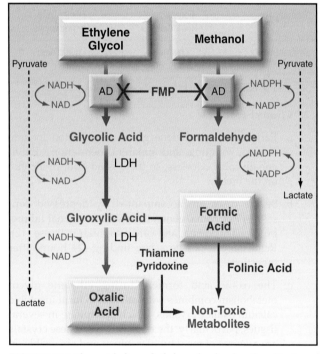

FIGURE 47.1 The metabolism of ethylene glycol and methanol in the liver. AD = alcohol dehydrogenase, LDH = lactate dehydrogenase, FMP = fomepizole.

shown in Table 47.3. Therapy should commence within 4 hours of ingestion for optimal results.

Table 47.3	Dosing Regimen for Fomepizole

1. Start with an IV loading dose of 15 mg/kg.

2. Follow with a dose of 10 mg/kg IV every 12 hrs for 4 doses.

3. Then increase the dose to 15 mg/kg IV every 12 hrs[†], and continue until the following end-points are reached:

    (a) the plasma toxin level is <20 mg/dL,

    (b) the plasma pH is normal,

    (c) the patient is asymptomatic.

4. If more than one hemodialysis session is required, change the dose to 15 mg/kg IV every 4 hrs until dialysis is no longer necessary.

[†]The increased dose is compensation for a drug-induced increase in metabolism. From Reference 12.

b. *Hemodialysis*

The clearance of ethylene glycol and all its metabolites is enhanced by hemodialysis. The indications for immediate hemodialysis include severe acidemia (pH<7.1) and evidence of significant end-organ damage (e.g., coma, seizures, and renal insufficiency) (12). Multiple courses of hemodialysis may be necessary, and fomepizole dosing should be adjusted if hemodialysis is continued (see Table 47.3).

c. *Adjuncts*

Thiamine (100 mg IV daily) and pyridoxine (100 mg IV daily) are recommended to divert glyoxylic acid to the formation of non-toxic metabolites (see Figure 47.2).

B. Methanol

Methanol (also known as *wood alcohol* because it was first distilled from wood) is a common ingredient in shellac, varnish, windshield washer fluid, and solid cooking fuel (Sterno) (12).

1. Pathophysiology

   a. Like ethylene glycol, methanol is readily absorbed from the upper GI tract, and is metabolized by alcohol dehydrogenase in the liver (see Figure 47.1).

   b. The principal metabolite is formic acid, a strong acid that readily dissociates and produces a metabolic acidosis with a high anion gap. Formic acid is also a mitochondrial toxin that inhibits cytochrome oxidase and blocks oxidative energy production. Tissues that are particularly susceptible to damage are the retina, optic nerve, and basal ganglia (12).

   c. Methanol metabolism promotes the conversion of pyruvate to lactate in the same manner described for ethylene glycol metabolism, and lactate production is increased further by the toxic effects of formic acid (see Figure 47.1).

2. Clinical Features

   a. Early manifestations include signs of apparent inebriation without the odor of alcohol on the breath.

   b. Later signs (6–24 hours after ingestion) include visual disturbances (e.g., scotoma, blurred vision, complete blindness), depressed consciousness, coma, and generalized seizures (12).

   c. Visual disturbances are characteristic of methanol poisoning, and are not a feature of ethylene glycol poisoning. Examination of the retina can reveal papilledema and generalized retinal edema.

3. **Laboratory Findings**

   a. Laboratory studies show a metabolic acidosis with a high anion gap, similar to ethylene glycol poisoning. However, there is no crystalluria in methanol poisoning.

   b. A plasma assay for methanol is available, and a level above 20 mg/dL is considered toxic. However, the results of the plasma assay are not immediately available, and are not used in the decision to initiate therapy.

4. **Treatment**

   Treatment for methanol poisoning is the same as described for ethylene glycol poisoning, except for the following:

   a. Visual impairment is an indication for dialysis.

   b. Folinic acid is used as adjunctive therapy in methanol poisoning (instead of thiamine and pyridoxine). Folinic acid (leucovorin) can convert formic acid to non-toxic metabolites. The recommended dose is 1 mg/kg IV, up to 50 mg, at 4-hour intervals (12). Folic acid should be used if folinic acid is unavailable.

IV. ORGANOPHOSPHATES

Exposure to the organic phosphorus compounds in insecticides (e.g., parathion) may cause more deaths worldwide each year than any other xenobiotic (13), and exposure to organophosphates in "nerve agents" (e.g., sarin) is an increasing threat. The mortality rate in organophosphate (OP) poisoning is 10–40% (13-15).

A. Pathophysiology

1. OPs are readily absorbed through the lungs, GI tract, and oral mucosa. Absorption through intact skin is limited, but skin absorption can be prominent in severe exposures (13).

2. The principal action of OPs is the *inhibition of acetyl-cholinesterase* and the subsequent accumulation of acetylcholine (Ach) at cholinergic receptors (muscarinic and nicotinic receptors) in nerve and muscle tissue. The resulting cholinergic activation is responsible for the clinical features of OP poisoning, which is also known as *cholinergic syndrome* (or *cholinergic crisis* in severe cases).

B. Clinical Features

1. The characteristic features of OP poisoning are summarized below (13,14):

   a. *CNS* – Agitation and confusion appear early, with rapid progression to lethargy and coma. Seizures are uncommon following exposure to insecticides, while nerve agents can precipitate status epilepticus (14).

   b. *Pupils* – Pupillary constriction (miosis) is one of the most consistent signs of cholinergic activation in OP poisoning.

   c. *Muscle* – Stimulation of nicotinic receptors can produce muscle fasciculations, and continued receptor stimulation can lead to downregulation and subsequent muscle weakness (a late finding) (14).

   d. *Exocrine Glands* – Cholinergic activation promotes hypersecretion in exocrine glands, resulting in diaphoresis, lacrimation, salivation, and bronchorrhea.

   e. *Respiratory* – Acute respiratory failure can appear at any time following exposure to OPs. Contributing factors include bronchorrhea, respiratory muscle weakness (14), and hypoventilation of brainstem origin (15).

   f. *GI* – Vomiting, and diarrhea are prominent features of OP poisoning, and the GI fluid loss, together with the exocrine gland hypersecretion, can result in profound hypovolemia.

g. *Urinary Tract* – Bladder spasticity and urinary incontinence are common consequences of cholinergic activation.

2. The principal manifestations of OP poisoning are summarized by the SLUDGEM mnemonic: Salivation, Lacrimation, Urination, Diarrhea, Gastrointestinal upset, Emesis, and Miosis.

C. Treatment

1. **Atropine**

   a. Atropine blocks muscarinic receptors, and is the first-line treatment for OP poisoning (13,14,16).

   b. The initial dose is 2 mg IV or IM. If severe symptoms develop, two additional doses can be administered, each 10 minutes apart (13). If symptoms are severe at initial presentation, the sequential 2 mg doses can be administered in rapid succession.

   c. Atropine does not block nicotinic receptors, and thus does not prevent the muscle manifestations of OP poisoning.

2. **Glycopyrrolate**

   a. Glycopyrrolate blocks muscarinic receptors (like atropine), but does not cross the blood brain barrier (unlike atropine), and thus does not block the CNS manifestations of OP poisoning (13).

   b. This agent can be used in combination with atropine when atropine causes antimuscarinic CNS toxicity (e.g., agitation) but does not completely reverse the effects of peripheral muscarinic receptor stimulation.

   c. The usual dose of glycopyrrolate is 1–2 mg IV, which can be repeated as needed until symptoms subside (10). Higher doses may be required in severe cases (10).

3. **Pralidoxime (2-PAM)**

   a. Pralidoxime (2-PAM) reactivates phosphorylated acetylcholinesterase by binding to the OP molecule (16). This agent is only effective if started early in the course of OP poisoning (because of acetylcholinesterase ageing) (14).

   b. One recommended dosing regimen for 2-PAM is 1 g (over 1 hour) every 4 hours until reversal of cholinergic signs and symptoms (14). Alternatively, 2-PAM can be given as a high-dose continuous infusion at 1g/hr (17).

   c. Treatment may be required for several days (14).

4. **Benzodiazepines**

   Benzodiazepines (midazolam, lorazepam) are preferred for the treatment of OP-induced agitation and seizures (see Table 43.5 for dosing information on benzodiazepines).

5. **GI Decontamination**

   a. Activated charcoal is recommended for patients with suspected OP poisoning, but only if it can be given within the first hour after toxic exposure to OPs (14).

   b. Gastric lavage may be considered before administration of activated charcoal, but only in patients who are intubated (14).

6. **Skin Decontamination**

   While absorption of OPs via the skin is variable, disrobing and washing exposed patients is a reasonable measure to limit exposure and prevent transmission of OPs among healthcare workers (14). This should be accomplished immediately, before admission to the ICU. Gloves, gowns, and eye protection are mandatory during decontamination.

REFERENCES

1. Guzman JA. Carbon monoxide poisoning. Crit Care Clin 2012; 28:537–548.

2. Hall JE. Medical Physiology, 12th ed. Philadelphia: Elsevier, W.B. Saunders, Co, 2011:495–504.

3. Lumb AB. Nunn's Applied Respiratory Physiology. 7th ed. Philadelphia: Elsevier, 2010:179–215.

4. Hampson NB, Piantadosi CA, Thom SR, Weaver LK. Practice recommendations in the diagnosis, management, and prevention of carbon monoxide poisoning. Am J Resp Crit Care Med 2012; 186:1095–1101.

5. Kalay N, Ozdogru I, Cetinkaya Y, et al. Cardiovascular effects of carbon monoxide poisoning. Am J Cardiol 2007; 99:322–324.

6. Choi IS. Delayed neurologic sequelae in carbon monoxide intoxication. Arch Neurol 1983; 40:433–435.

7. Buckley NA, Juurlick DN, Isbister G, et al. Hyperbaric oxygen for carbon monoxide poisoning. Cochrane Database Syst Rev 2011; 4:CD002041.

8. Anseeuw K, Delvau N, Burill-Putze G, et al. Cyanide poisoning by fire smoke inhalation: a European expert consensus. Eur J Emerg Med 2013; 20:2–9.

9. Baud FJ. Cyanide: critical issues in diagnosis and treatment. Hum Exp Toxicol 2007.

10. Weiner SW. Toxic alcohols. In: Nelson LS, Lewin NA, Howland MA, et al., eds. Goldfrank's Toxicologic Emergencies. 9th ed. New York: McGraw-Hill, 2011:1400–1410.

11. Bronstein AC, Spyker DA, Cantilena LR, Jr, et al. 2011 Annual Report of the American Association of Poison Control Centers' National Poison Data System (NPDS): 29th Annual Report. Clin Toxicol 2012; 50:911–1164.

12. Kruse PA. Methanol and ethylene glycol intoxication. Crit Care Clin 2012; 28:661–711.

13. Eddlestrom M, Clark, RF. Insecticides: Organic Phosphorus compounds and Carbamates. In: Nelson LS, Lewin NA, Howland MA, Hoffman RS, Goldfrank LR, Flomenbaum NE, eds.

Goldfrank's Toxicologic Emergencies. 9th ed. New York: McGraw-Hill, 2011:1450–1466.

14. Blain PG. Organophosphorus poisoning (acute). Clinical Evidence 2011; 05:2102.

15. Carey JL, Dunn C, Gaspari RJ. Central respiratory failure during acute organophosphate poisoning. Respiratory Physiology Neurobiology 2013; 189:403–10.

16. Weissman BA, Raveh L. Multifunctional drugs as novel antidotes for organophosphates' poisoning. Toxicology 2011; 149–155.

17. Pawar KS, Bhoite RR, Pillay CP, et al. Continuous Pralidoxime infusion versus repeated bolus injection to treat organophosphorus pesticide poisoning: a randomized controlled trial. Lancet 2006; 368:2136–2141.

Units and Conversions

Units of Measurement in the Système Internationale (SI)

Parameter	Basic SI Unit (Symbol)	Useful Conversions
Length	Meter (m)	1 meter = 3.28 feet 2.54 cm = 1 inch
Area	Square meter (m^2)	1 m^2 = 10.76 square feet
Volume	Cubic meter (m^3)	1 m^3 = 1,000 liters 1 cm^3 = 1 mL
Mass	Kilogram (kg)	1 kg = 2.2 lbs
Density	Kilogram per cubic meter (kg/m^3)	1 kg/m^3 = density of H_2O
Velocity	Meters per second (m/sec)	1 m/sec = 3.28 feet/sec = 2.23 miles/hr
Force	Newton (N) = kg x (m/sec^2)	1 dyne = 10^{-5} N
Pressure	Pascal (Pa) = N/m^2	1 kPa = 7.5 mm Hg = 10.2 cm H_2O
Heat	Joule (J) = N x m	1 kcal = 4,184 J
Viscosity	Newton x second per square meter (N • sec/m^2)	1 N • sec/m^2 = 10^{-3} Centipoise (cP)
Amount of a substance	Mole (mol) = molecular weight in grams	mol x valence = Equivalent (Eq)

Part 1	Converting Units of Solute Concentration

1. For ions that exist freely in an aqueous solution, the concentration is expressed as milliequivalents per liter (mEq/L). To convert to millimoles per liter (mmol/L):

$$\frac{mEq/L}{valence} = mmol/L$$

   a. For a univalent ion like potassium (K^+), the concentration in mmol/L is the same as the concentration in mEq/L.

   b. For a divalent ion like magnesium (Mg^{++}), the concentration in mmol/L is one-half the concentration in mEq/L.

2. For ions that are partially bound or complexed to other molecules (e.g., plasma Ca^{++}), the concentration is usually expressed as milligrams per deciliter (mg/dL). To convert to mEq/L:

$$\frac{mg/dL \times 10}{mol\ wt} \times valence = mEq/L$$

   where mol wt is molecular weight, and the factor 10 is used to convert deciliters (100 mL) to liters.

   EXAMPLE: Ca^{++} has a molecular weight of 40 and a valence of 2, so a plasma Ca^{++} concentration of 8 mg/dL is equivalent to:

$$(8 \times 10/40) \times 2 = 4\ mEq/L$$

3. The concentration of uncharged molecules (e.g., glucose) is also expressed as milligrams per deciliter (mg/dL). To convert to (mmol/L):

$$\frac{mg/dL \times 10}{mol\ wt} = mmol/L$$

   EXAMPLE:
   Glucose has a molecular weight of 180, so a plasma glucose concentration of 90 mg/dL is equivalent to: $(90 \times 10/180) = 5\ mmol/L$.

Part 2 | Converting Units of Solute Concentration

4. The concentration of solutes can also be expressed in terms of osmotic pressure, which determines the distribution of water in different fluid compartments. Osmotic activity in aqueous solutions (called osmolality) is expressed as milliosmoles per kg water (mosm/kg H_2O or mosm/kg).

The following formulas can be used to express the osmolality of solute concentrations (n is the number of nondissociable particles per molecule).

$$\text{mmol/L} \times n = \text{mosm/kg}$$

$$\frac{\text{mEq/L}}{\text{valence}} \times n = \text{mosm/kg}$$

$$\frac{\text{mg/dL} \times 10}{\text{mol wt}} \times n = \text{mosm/kg}$$

EXAMPLE:
a. A plasma Na^+ concentration of 140 mEq/L has the following osmolality:

$$\frac{140}{1} \times 1 = 140 \text{ mosm/kg}$$

b. A plasma glucose concentration of 90 mg/dL has the following osmolality:

$$\frac{90 \times 10}{180} \times 1 = 5 \text{ mosm/kg}$$

The sodium in plasma has a much greater osmotic activity than the glucose in plasma because osmotic activity is determined by the number of particles in solution, and is independent of the size of the particles (i.e., one sodium ion has the same osmotic activity as one glucose molecule).

Temperature Conversions			
°C	°F	°C	°F
41	105.8	35	95
40	104	34	93.2
39	102.2	33	91.4
38	100.4	32	89.6
37	98.6	31	87.8
36	96.8	30	86
$°F = (9/5 \ °C) + 32$		$°C = 5/9 \ (°F - 32)$	

Apothecary and Household Conversions	
Apothecary	**Household**
1 grain=60 mg	1 teaspoonful=5 mL
1 ounce=30 mg	1 tablespoonful=15 mL
1 fluid ounce=30 mL	
1 pint=500 mL	1 wineglassful=60 mL
1 quart=947 mL	1 teacupful=120 mL

Pressure Conversions

mm Hg	kPa	mm Hg	kPa	mm Hg	kPa
41	5.45	61	8.11	81	10.77
42	5.59	62	8.25	82	10.91
43	5.72	63	8.38	83	11.04
44	5.85	64	8.51	84	11.17
45	5.99	65	8.65	85	11.31
46	6.12	66	8.78	86	11.44
47	6.25	67	8.91	87	11.57
48	6.38	68	9.04	88	11.70
49	6.52	69	9.18	89	11.84
50	6.65	70	9.31	90	11.97
51	6.78	71	9.44	91	12.10
52	6.92	72	9.58	92	12.24
53	7.05	73	9.71	93	12.37
54	7.18	74	9.84	94	12.50
55	7.32	75	9.98	95	12.64
56	7.45	76	10.11	96	12.77
57	7.58	77	10.24	97	12.90
58	7.71	78	10.37	98	13.03
59	7.85	79	10.51	99	13.17
60	7.98	80	10.64	100	13.90

Kilopascal (kPa) = 0.133 × mm Hg; mm Hg = 7.5 × kPa

Measures of Body Size

Measures of Body Size

Ideal Body Weight*

Males: IBW (kg) = 50 + 2.3 (Ht in inches − 60)

Females: IBW (kg) = 45.5 + 2.3 (Ht in inches − 60)

Body Mass Index[†]

$$BMI = \frac{Wt\ (in\ lbs)}{Ht\ (in\ inches)^2 \times 703}$$

Body Surface Area

Dubois Formula[‡]

$$BSA\ (m^2) = Ht\ (in\ cm) + Wt\ (in\ kg)^{0.425} \times 0.007184$$

Jacobson Formula[§]

$$BSA\ (m^2) = \frac{Ht\ (in\ cm) + Wt\ (in\ kg) - 60}{100}$$

---

[*]Devine BJ. Drug Intell Clin Pharm 1974; 8:650.

[†]Matz R. Ann Intern Med 1993; 118:232.

[‡]Dubois EF. Basal metabolism in health and disease. Philadelphia: Lea & Febiger, 1936.

[§]Jacobson B. Medicine and clinical engineering. Englewood Cliffs, NJ: Prentice-Hall, 1977.

Ideal Body Weights (in lbs.) for Adult Males*

Height		Small	Medium	Large
Feet	Inches	Frame	Frame	Frame
5	2	128–134	131–141	138–150
5	3	130–136	133–143	140–153
5	4	132–138	135–145	142–156
5	5	134–140	137–148	144–160
5	6	136–142	139–151	146–164
5	7	138–145	142–154	149–168
5	8	140–148	145–157	152–172
5	9	142–151	148–160	155–176
5	10	144–154	151–163	158–180
5	11	146–157	154–166	161–184
6	0	149–160	157–170	164–188
6	1	152–164	160–174	168–192
6	2	155–168	164–178	172–197
6	3	158–172	167–182	172–202
6	4	162–176	171–187	181–207

*Unclothed weights associated with the highest life expectancies. From the statistics bureau of Metropolitan Life Insurance Company, 1983.

Ideal Body Weights (in lbs.) for Adult Females*

Height		Small Frame	Medium Frame	Large Frame
Feet	**Inches**			
4	10	102–111	109–121	112–131
4	11	103–113	111–123	120–134
5	0	104–115	113–126	122–137
5	1	106–118	115–129	125–140
5	2	108–121	118–132	128–143
5	3	111–124	121–135	131–147
5	4	114–127	124–138	134–151
5	5	117–130	127–141	137–155
5	6	120–133	130–144	140–159
5	7	123–136	133–147	143–163
5	8	126–139	136–150	146–167
5	9	129–142	139–153	149–170
5	10	132–145	142–156	152–173
5	11	135–148	145–159	155–176
6	1	138–151	148–162	158–179

*Unclothed weights associated with the highest life expectancies. From the statistics bureau of Metropolitan Life Insurance Company, 1983.

Predicted Body Weight (PBW)/Tidal Volume Chart for Males

Height		PBW	mL/kg				
Feet	Inches		4	5	6	7	8
4'10"	58	45.4	180	230	270	320	360
4'11"	59	47.7	190	240	290	330	380
5' 0"	60	50.0	200	250	300	350	400
5' 1"	61	52.3	210	260	310	370	420
5' 2"	62	54.6	220	270	330	380	440
5' 3"	63	56.9	230	280	340	400	460
5' 4"	64	59.2	240	300	360	410	470
5' 5"	65	61.5	250	310	370	430	490
5' 6"	66	63.8	260	320	380	450	510
5' 7"	67	66.1	260	330	400	460	530
5' 8"	68	68.4	270	340	410	480	550
5' 9"	69	70.7	280	350	420	490	570
5'10"	70	73.0	290	370	440	510	580
5'11"	71	75.3	300	380	450	530	600
6' 0"	72	77.6	310	390	470	540	620
6' 1"	73	79.9	320	400	480	560	640
6' 2"	74	82.2	330	410	490	580	660
6' 3"	75	84.5	340	420	510	590	680
6' 4"	76	86.8	350	430	520	610	690
6' 5"	77	89.1	360	450	530	620	710
6' 6"	78	91.4	370	460	550	640	730

Predicted Body Weight (PBW)/Tidal Volume Chart for Females

Height		PBW	mL/kg				
Feet	Inches		4	5	6	7	8
4' 7"	55	34.0	140	170	200	240	270
4' 8"	56	36.3	150	180	220	250	290
4' 9"	57	38.6	150	190	230	270	310
4'10"	58	40.9	160	200	250	290	330
4'11"	59	43.2	170	220	260	300	350
5' 0"	60	45.5	180	230	270	320	360
5' 1"	61	47.8	190	240	290	330	380
5' 2"	62	50.1	200	250	300	350	400
5' 3"	63	52.4	210	260	310	370	420
5' 4"	64	54.7	220	270	330	380	440
5' 5"	65	57.0	230	290	340	400	460
5' 6"	66	59.3	240	300	360	420	470
5' 7"	67	61.6	250	310	370	430	490
5' 8"	68	63.9	260	320	380	450	510
5' 9"	69	66.2	260	330	400	460	530
5'10"	70	68.5	270	340	410	480	550
5'11"	71	70.6	280	350	420	500	570
6' 0"	72	73.1	290	370	440	510	580
6' 1"	73	75.4	300	380	450	530	600
6' 2"	74	77.7	310	390	470	540	620
6' 3"	75	80.0	320	400	480	560	640

Body Mass Index

Underweight | Healthy | Overweight | Obese | Extremely Obese

HEIGHT in	cm	100	105	110	115	120	125	130	135	140	146	150	155	160	165	170	175	180	185	190	195	200	205	210	215
	kg	45.5	47.7	50.0	52.3	54.5	56.8	59.1	61.4	63.6	65.9	68.2	70.5	72.7	75.0	77.3	79.5	81.8	84.1	86.4	88.6	90.9	93.2	95.5	97.7
5.'0"	– 152.4	19	20	21	22	23	24	25	26	27	28	29	30	31	32	33	34	35	36	37	38	39	40	41	42
5.'1"	– 154.9	18	19	20	21	22	23	24	25	26	27	28	29	30	31	32	33	34	35	36	36	37	38	39	40
5.'2"	– 157.4	18	19	20	21	22	22	23	24	25	26	27	28	29	30	31	32	33	33	34	35	36	37	38	39
5.'3"	– 160.0	17	18	19	20	21	22	23	24	24	25	26	27	28	29	30	31	32	32	33	34	35	36	37	38
5.'4"	– 162.5	17	18	18	19	20	21	22	23	24	24	25	26	27	28	29	30	31	31	32	33	34	35	36	37
5.'5"	– 165.1	16	17	18	19	20	20	21	22	23	24	25	25	26	27	28	29	30	30	31	32	33	34	35	35
5.'6"	– 167.6	16	17	17	18	19	20	21	21	22	23	24	25	25	26	27	28	29	29	30	31	32	33	34	34
5.'7"	– 170.1	15	16	17	18	18	19	20	21	22	22	23	24	25	25	26	27	28	29	29	30	31	32	33	33
5.'8	– 172.7	15	16	16	17	18	19	19	20	21	22	22	23	24	25	25	26	27	28	28	29	30	31	32	32
5.'9"	– 175.2	14	15	16	17	17	18	19	20	20	21	22	23	24	24	25	26	27	28	28	29	30	31	31	32
5.'10"	– 177.8	14	15	15	16	16	17	18	19	20	20	21	22	23	23	24	25	25	26	27	28	28	29	30	30
5.'11"	– 180.3	14	14	15	16	16	17	18	18	19	20	21	21	22	23	23	24	25	25	26	27	28	28	29	30
6.'0"	– 182.8	13	14	14	15	16	16	17	17	18	19	20	21	21	22	23	23	24	25	25	26	27	27	28	29
6.'1"	– 185.4	13	13	14	15	15	16	17	17	18	19	19	20	21	21	22	23	23	24	25	25	26	27	27	28
6.'2"	– 187.9	12	13	14	14	15	16	16	17	18	18	19	20	21	21	22	23	23	24	25	25	26	26	27	27
6.'3"	– 190.5	12	13	13	14	15	15	16	16	17	18	18	19	20	20	21	21	22	23	23	24	25	25	26	26
6.'4"	– 193.0	12	12	13	14	14	15	15	16	17	17	18	18	19	20	20	21	22	22	23	23	24	25	25	26

Needles and Catheters

Gauge Sizes		
Gauge Size	**Outside Diameter***	
	Inches	**mm**
26	0.018	0.45
25	0.020	0.50
24	0.022	0.56
23	0.024	0.61
22	0.028	0.71
21	0.032	0.81
20	0.036	0.91
19	0.040	1.02
18	0.048	1.22
16	0.040	1.62
14	0.080	2.03
12	0.104	2.64

*Diameters can vary with manufacturers.

French Sizes		
French Size	**Outside Diameter***	
	Inches	mm
1	0.01	0.3
4	0.05	1.3
8	0.10	2.6
10	0.13	3.3
12	0.16	4.0
14	0.18	4.6
16	0.21	5.3
18	0.23	6.0
20	0.26	6.6
22	0.28	7.3
24	0.31	8.0
26	0.34	8.6
28	0.36	9.3
30	0.39	10.0
32	0.41	10.6
34	0.44	11.3
36	0.47	12.0
38	0.50	12.6

*Diameters can vary with manufacturers. However, a useful rule of thumb is OD (mm) x 3 = French size.

Flow Rates in Peripheral Venous Catheters		
Gauge Size	Length	Flow Rate (L/hr)
16	30 mm (1.2 in)	13.2
18	30 mm (1.2 in)	6.0
	50 mm (2 in)	3.6
20	30 mm (1.2 in)	3.6

From Ann Emerg Med 1983; 12:149, and Emergency Medicine Updates (emupdates.com). Flow rates are for the gravity-driven flow of water.

Flow Rates in Triple-Lumen Central Venous Catheters				
French Size	Length	Lumens	Lumen Size	Flow Rate (L/h)
7	16 cm (6 in)	Distal	16 ga	3.4
		Medial	18 ga	1.8
		Proximal	18 ga	1.9
7	20 cm (8 in)	Distal	16 ga	3.1
		Medial	18 ga	1.5
		Proximal	18 ga	1.6
7	30 cm (12 in)	Distal	16 ga	2.3
		Medial	18 ga	1.0
		Proximal	18 ga	1.1

Flow rates are for the gravity-driven flow of saline from a height of 40 inches above the catheter. From Arrow International. ga = gauge size.

Flow Rates in Peripherally Inserted Central Catheters

French Size	Length	Lumens	Lumen Size	Flow Rate (L/hr)
5	50 cm (19.5 in)	Single	16 ga	1.75
5	70 cm (27.5 in)	Single	16 ga	1.30
5	50 cm (19.5 in)	Distal	18 ga	0.58
		Proximal	20 ga	0.16
5	70 cm (27.5 in)	Distal	18 ga	0.44
		Proximal	20 ga	0.12

Flow rates are for the gravity-driven flow of saline from a height of 40 inches above the catheter. From Arrow International. ga = gauge size.

Flow Rates in Hemodialysis Catheters

French Size	Length	Lumens	Lumen Size	Flow Rate (L/hr)
12	16 cm (6 in)	Proximal	12 ga	23.7
		Distal	12 ga	17.4
12	20 cm (8 in)	Proximal	12 ga	19.8
		Distal	12 ga	15.5

Flow rates are for the gravity-driven flow of saline from a height of 40 inches above the catheter. From Arrow International. ga = gauge size.

Miscellany

Sequential Organ Failure Assessment (SOFA)					
Parameter	Score				
	0	1	2	3	4
PaO$_2$/FiO$_2$ (mm Hg)	≥400	<400	<300	<200	<100
				with respiratory support	
Platelets (10^3/μL)	≥150	<150	<100	<50	<20
Bilirubin (mg/dL)	<1.2	1.2–1.9	2–5.9	6–11.9	>12
MAP (mm Hg)	>70	<70	dopa (<5) or dobutamine (any dose)†	dopa (5–15) or epi (≤0.1) or norepi (≤0.1)†	dopa (>15) or epi (>0.1) or norepi (>0.1)†
Glasgow Coma Score	15	13–14	10–12	6–9	<6
Creatinine (mg/dL) or Urine Output (mL/d)	<1.2	1.2–1.9	2–3.4	3.5–4.9 or <500	≥5 or <200

Adapted from Vincent et al, Intensive Care Med 1996; 22:707–710.
Abbreviations: MAP = mean arterial pressure; dopa = dopamine; epi = epinephrine; norepi = norepinephrine. †Catecholamine doses are in μg/kg/min.

The CHA$_2$DS$_2$-VASc Score and the Risk of Stroke in Patients with Nonvalvular Atrial Fibrillation

Risk Factor (Points)		Total Score	Stroke Rate (% per year)
CHF	(1)	0	0.0
Hypertension	(1)	1	1.3
Age ≥75 yrs	(2)	2	2.2
Diabetes	(1)	3	3.2
		4	4.0
Stroke/TIA/TE	(2)	5	6.7
Vascular Disease (1) (Prior MI, PAD)		6	9.8
		7	9.6
Age 65–74 yrs	(1)	8	6.7
Female Sex	(1)	9	15.20

CHA$_2$DS$_2$-VASc = Congestive heart failure, Hypertension, Age ≥75 yrs (doubled), Diabetes mellitus, prior Stroke, TIA or thromboembolism (doubled), Vascular disease, Age 65–74 yrs, Sex category (female sex).
From Circulation 2014; 130:e199.

Measures of Test Performance

	Disease is Present	Disease is Not Present
Positive Test	True Positive **a**	False Positive **c**
Negative Test	False Negative **b**	True Negative **d**

Parameter	Derivation	Definition
Sensitivity	$\dfrac{a}{a+b}$	The percentage of patients with the disease who have a positive test result.
Specificity	$\dfrac{d}{c+d}$	The percentage of patients without the disease who have a negative test result.
Positive Predictive Value	$\dfrac{a}{a+c}$	The percentage of patients with a positive test result who have the disease.
Negative Predictive Value	$\dfrac{d}{b+d}$	The percentage of patients with a negative test result who do not have the disease.

Note: Page number followed by f and t indicates figure and table respectively.